P. Santoni-Rugiu · P. J. Sykes

A History of Plastic Surgery

P. Santoni-Rugiu · P. J. Sykes

A History of Plastic Surgery

With 407 Figures

Springer

Professor Paolo Santoni-Rugiu, MD., PhD
Dept. of Plastic Surgery
S. Chiara University Hospital
Pisa
Italy

Philip J. Sykes, MA., FRCS
Consultant Plastic Surgeon
Welsh Regional Plastic Surgery Unit
Morriston Hospital
Swansea, S. Wales
UK

ISBN 978-3-662-51821-2 ISBN 978-3-540-46241-5 (eBook)
DOI 10.1007/978-3-540-46241-5
Springer Berlin Heidelberg New York

Springer is a part of Springer Science+Business Media
springer.com

Softcover reprint of the hardcover 1st edition 2007

Editor: Gabriele Schröder, Heidelberg, Germany
Desk Editor: Ellen Blasig, Heidelberg, Germany
Typesetting and Production: LE-TEX Jelonek, Schmidt & Vöckler GbR, Leipzig, Germany
Cover Design: eStudio, Calamar, Spain

Printed on acid-free paper 24|3180|YL 5 4 3 2 1 0

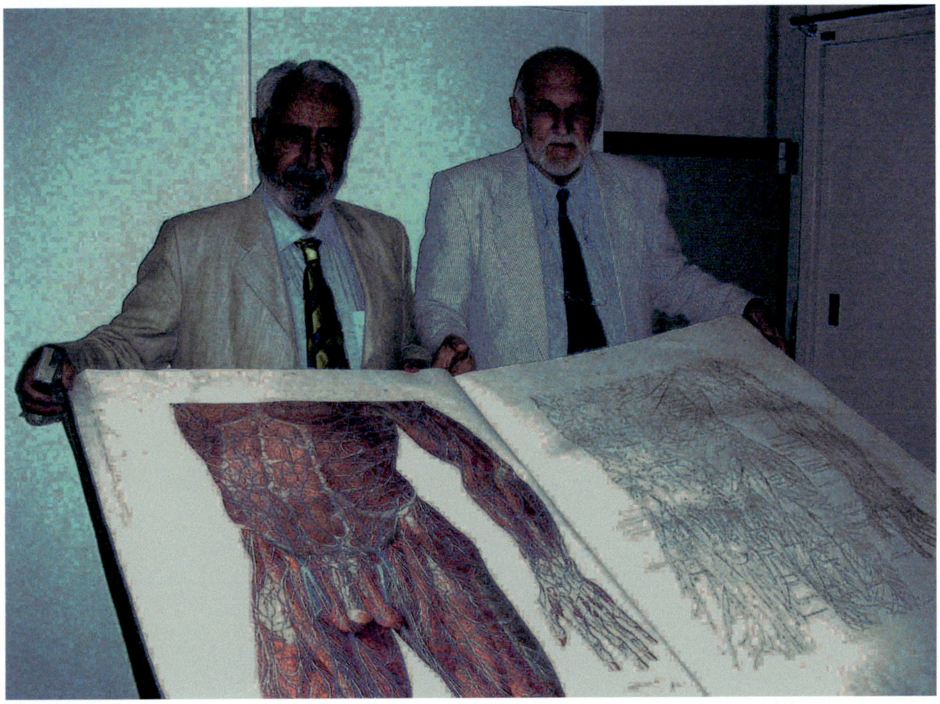

Paolo Santoni-Rugiu
formerly Professor of Plastic Surgery in Pisa and Past President of European Association of Plastic Surgeons with

Philip Sykes
once Consultant Plastic Surgeon in Wales and Past President of the British Association of Plastic Surgeons.

They are holding *Anatomiae Universae* by Mascagni published in Pisa in 1823, one of only three existing copies. *Courtesy of C. de L. Flaminio Farnesi, Pisa*

Dedication

This book is dedicated to the memory of Gustavo Sanvenero-Rosselli (1897–1974) the first Italian plastic surgeon of the modern age, pioneer of European Plastic Surgery and passionate bibliophile.

Gustavo Sanvenero-Rosselli was born in Savona in 1897. After training in ear, nose and throat surgery he went to Paris in 1927 to work with Lemaitre and Ferris Smith, who had a special interest in facial clefts. When the unit known as the "Padiglione dei Mutilati del Viso" opened in Milan he was appointed as its first director in 1929. This was the first hospital devoted solely to plastic surgery in Italy and became a National referral centre. It was visited by many foreign surgeons including Johannes Esser who, with Sanvenero, planned to open an International Centre for Injuries of the Face in Florence. The start of World War II put an end to their plan.

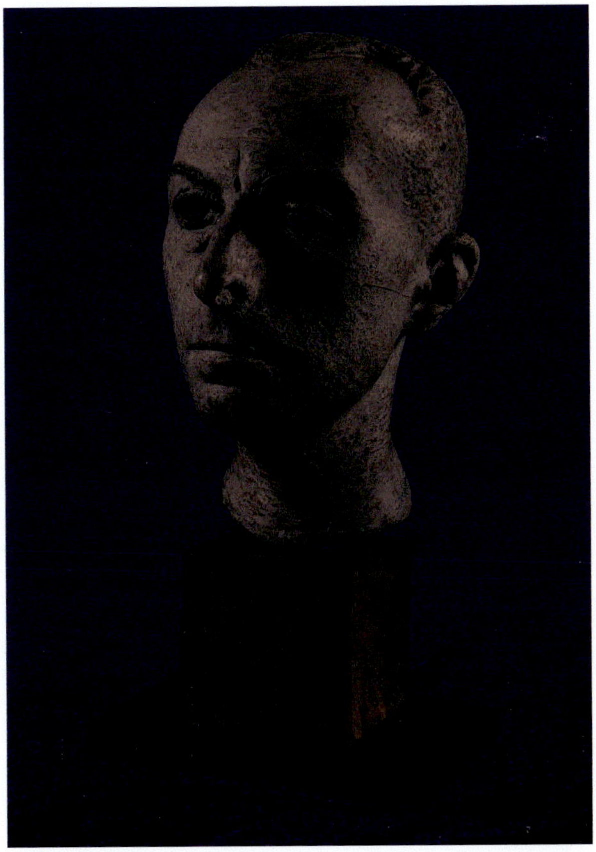

Sanvenero was a Member of the Editorial board of *La Revue de Chirurgie Plastique* in Belgium from 1931. This subsequently became *Revue de Chirurgie Structive*. In 1939 he founded the Italian *Plastica Chirurgica* which disappeared during the war. He was one of the founding members of the Italian Society of Plastic Surgery in 1934 and of the International Confederation of Plastic Reconstructive and Aesthetic Surgery (IPRAS) in Sweden in 1955. He organized a large number of congresses including the Third Congress of the European Society in 1938 in Milan. In 1966 he was the President of the Fourth International Congress of the IPRAS in Rome. His contributions to plastic surgery were many, particularly in the field of facial clefts, and he wrote many articles and two books.

He started collecting rare books in the 1930s when there were many on the market and little demand. His library competes with that of his friend Jerome P. Webster at Columbia University in New York. When he brought his first Tagliacozzi he did not dare tell his family since the price was that of an apartment in Milan!

He died in 1974 aged 77. His memory is preserved by the Foundation established by his nephew Riccardo Mazzola. It houses an extended library and organizes seminars and live surgical courses.

Foreword

Dear Readers,

You have in your hands a work that should become a milestone of our understanding of medical history. In it Professor Paolo Santoni-Rugiu and Mr Philip Sykes trace the development of plastic surgery and much of medicine in general, over three millennia. With his extensive knowledge of clinical plastic surgery, no one could be better placed than the senior author to gather this valuable material from historical documents. As well as using the great historical libraries of Italy, the authors were able to refer to the many books in the Sanvenero-Rosselli Foundation in Milan. This library contains a unique collection of ancient and rare surgical texts and original manuscripts which were acquired over many years by the late Professor Sanvenero-Rosselli. His nephew, Professor Riccardo Mazzola has added to the collection and is now its curator.

They have also gathered material from The Gillies' Archive at Queen Mary's Hospital, Sidcup, UK where Major Gillies, later to become Sir Harold, and his team treated the wounded from World War I and performed over 15,000 reconstructive operations on badly injured servicemen. The libraries of the British Association of Plastic Surgery and of the Royal College of Surgeons in London have also kindly opened their doors to the authors.

The book is cleverly organised in three groups of chapters: The Basis of Plastic Surgery (Chapters 1–6), Reconstructive Surgery of Various Organs (Chapters 7–11) and Cosmetic Surgery (Chapters 12–15). The first section deals with anatomy and the healing of wounds, discusses old and new plastic surgical procedures, and outlines the history of anaesthesia. The second covers the methods used from ancient times to reconstruct various areas of the body and is the most extensive. The last section discusses the history of cosmetic surgery and the origin of present day procedures.

The pages ring with the names of giants of the medical sciences such as Hippocrates, Leonardo da Vinci, William Harvey and Iginio Tansini, to say nothing of plastic surgeons from the nineteenth and twentieth centuries.

We plastic surgeons can be justifiably proud of our heritage. The book reveals the breadth of our speciality, covering as it does conditions of the whole body and many basic areas such as wound healing and surgical techniques as well as the ever popular topic of cosmetic surgery. New procedures are being introduced all the time, yet, incredible though it may seem, there are some that have been in use for thousands of years. This book deserves a place in every plastic surgeon's library as it teaches that all medical skill is based on the intuition, dedication and hard work of previous generations. It will enlighten and inform every reader.

Sirpa Asko-Seljavaara, MD
Former Professor of Plastic Surgery
at Helsinki University
Member of the Finnish Parliament

Preface

Why write a book about the history of plastic surgery? The publishers asked the same question and it is difficult to give a simple answer. Mountain climbers accept that the challenge is sufficient to make the effort worthwhile. There is personal satisfaction while travelling and euphoria at the end. This book has been such a journey.

There are several excellent short accounts of the history of plastic surgery in general and specific areas of the speciality in particular but the fact that a book had not appeared recently was an incentive.

In truth these were not the main reasons why the senior author embarked on this task during his early retirement. There was no one point when the decision to write a book was taken. The idea developed gradually while preparing papers on historical topics using the resources in the Sanvenero-Rosselli foundation in Milan, sometimes in cooperation with its curator Dr Riccardo Mazzola. The Italian influence on nasal reconstruction is exceptional and this is where the historical interest began.

Reading old and sometimes obscure works frequently served to confirm that very little is new and opportunities have been missed in the past. The old literature was fascinating and so the exploration continued.

A study of early anatomy followed and then moved to cleft lip and palate. One topic led to another and gradually the beginnings of a book emerged. Some knowledge of the important basic works made progress easier. This is possibly why the book is not written chronologically as one might expect. It begins with the basics, proceeds to the reconstruction surgery of different areas and ends with the origins of cosmetic surgery.

A similar approach was chosen to Antony Wallace in his excellent book published in 1984 and it seemed a good idea to follow his lead. The giants of the early days made advances in many fields so inevitably their names recur in several chapters. This does at least serve to emphasize their importance.

The book does not aim to be a work of any great scholarship but more a personal interpretation of the different events which contributed to the birth of the speciality. The numerous illustrations please the publishers, perhaps because they encourage sales. We feel that they and the footnotes will add some interest but they are not intended to make this a coffee table text.

Our speciality has become increasingly sophisticated in recent times. This answered the problem about where to stop. One could fill a whole book with the developments of the last 25 years alone and this has been resisted. For better or for worse we have drawn the line around the advent of microsurgery although unavoidably some mention is made about the beginnings of this new era. Where the origins of plastic surgery lie is a matter of opinion and we have purposely chosen a title commencing with the indefinite article together with a suitably vague historical time span!

We have not attempted to be comprehensive and have omitted some specialized clinical areas which plastic surgeons share with other disciplines. Burns, maxillofacial and cranio-facial surgery together with hand surgery have been left out even though they developed from the same basic origins.

Because of their historical importance some priority has been given to topics which are now rarities. Nasal reconstruction, for example, has been allocated a whole chapter because of its contribution to the development of plastic surgery principles. This and other ideas, largely dating from the Renaissance, receive a good deal of attention and we hope that different nationalities will not feel left out. There have been many significant contributions from the rest of Europe, Asia and the Americas. We trust we have done them justice.

As amateur historians our reference list will not bear close scrutiny by an experienced academic especially where very old books are concerned. This deficiency will be obvious to those who are familiar with the scholarly works of authors like Tom Patterson. His translations of the Zeis Index and his own work on the literature from 1864 to 1920 are masterly and have been very valuable to us. This is also true of the historical works of Frank McDowell.

We have tried to be accurate and take full responsibility for the inevitable errors which have crept in. Citing very rare old books is hazardous for all but the expert. Different editions frequently exist as do pirated copies. Some authors published different books on similar topics within a short period. We have attempted to choose the most appropriate work but where books and papers by the same author have equal merit we have attempted to include them all.

The senior author started this book in English about ten years ago and despite revisions of the text by the co-author the result did not make easy reading. The book was re-written in Italian and then translated by experts. It is interesting to note that each chapter became shorter, sometimes by as many as five pages. We hope it is also easier to digest.

The authors' friendship extends back 30 years to microsurgical training in Melbourne. It has continued professionally and socially over the years in Italy and the UK. When serious illness overtook the senior author his recovery and convalescence allowed time for both of us to enjoy each other's company and to work on the book. This was no hardship and our friends and family were very tolerant of the hours we spent working together.

Another reason helped us decide to continue with the project. In the last decade traditional plastic surgery has changed. Many operations that were exclusively performed by a plastic surgeon are now carried out by other specialists who have learnt the techniques. Plastic surgeons have also combined with other disciplines to provide a comprehensive service in specialized clinical areas. There are now *super specialists* in all the areas that once combined to form plastic surgery. Like general surgery, plastic surgery as we knew it, no longer exists. This progress is inevitable and necessary. By recalling the past we hope this book will provide present and future plastic surgeons some knowledge of the origins of our speciality.

Paolo Santoni-Rugiu and Philip Sykes
Keswick, Cumbria
October 2006

Acknowledgements

We wish to acknowledge the help and encouragement we have received from many people. Above all this book would not have been possible without access to the Library of the Sanvenero-Rosselli Foundation in Milan and we are indebted to Riccardo Mazzola for his permission and assistance in using all the facilities in that institution. His help was invaluable and the constructive criticism he offered from the onset kept us on the right path. The secretary of the foundation, Danila Beatrice, provided unstinting help during our visits to Milan and but for her assistance we would have been lost amongst the bookshelves.

Sirpa Asko-Seljavaara has written the foreword and given sound advice and encouragement. We thank her sincerely.

Brian Morgan shared his knowledge and made available material from the Antony Wallace Archive of the British Association of Aesthetic and Reconstructive Plastic Surgeons. Andrew Bamji, Curator of the Gillies Archive at Queen Mary's Hospital, Sidcup, Kent, supplied illustrations and a wealth of entertaining information about the origins of plastic surgery during the First World War.

Lisa Chang and Shona Dryburgh did an expert job translating the text from the Italian. Colette Derrick helped assemble and type the reference list.

We are also indebted to our colleagues Ron Pigott, Grazia Salimbeni, Hamish Laing, Alessandro Massei and Daniele Gandini who have all been helpful in different ways. Ravin Thatte of Mumbai helped interpret various Sanskrit texts and Raju Usgaocar of Goa searched them out for us. We thank them sincerely.

For technical support we are particularly grateful to Leopoldo Nicotra, who miraculously extracted high definition illustrations from old slides and photographs. Others who gave their help are Roberto Zuchelli, David Mart, Pablo Patanè, Rosanna Prato, Michael Connick, Maggie Climie and the photographic department at Morriston Hospital, Swansea. Gabriele Schröder and Ellen Blasig at the publishers have always been ready to give advice when problems arose.

Finally, several institutions have provided information or allowed us to use material from their collections and we are particularly grateful to the University of Padua, the Museum of Piacenza, the Royal College of Surgeons of England and the Worshipful Company of Barber Surgeons in London.

Last but not least we express our gratitude to our families. The project has taken several years, involved many trips abroad and taken hours incarcerated at the computer keyboard. They have always given uncomplaining support.

Contents

T

W

Z

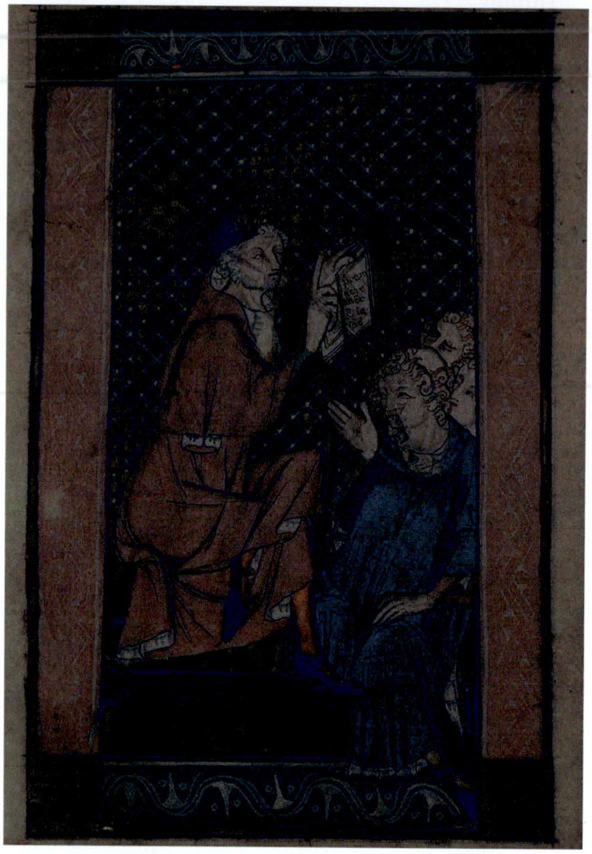

Fig. 1.1 Henry de Mondeville (1260–1320) lecturing to students. The illustration is taken from a fourteenth century illuminated manuscript of his book *Chirurgie*, probably the first on surgery published in France. *By permission of the Biblioteque Nationale de France, Paris*

The surgeon Henry de Mondeville (c.1260–1320) (Fig. 1.1) [682, 731], who had under his care the sovereigns Philippe le Bel and his son Louis X of France and whom we will encounter frequently in our survey of the origins of plastic surgery, affirmed at the beginning of his text *Chirugie*: "No craftsman should work on an object without knowing it. Being the human body the object of the whole medical art, of which surgery is one of the instruments, it is obvious that a surgeon who practises incisions on the different areas of the body and on its limbs without being aware of their anatomy will never operate well." This declaration, made more than 700 years ago underlines the close relationship that exists between anatomy and surgery and the fact that without a sufficient knowledge of anatomy the practice of surgery, and of plastic surgery in particular, could never have evolved over the centuries.

The history of anatomy may be divided into the following three periods:

- The Pre-Scientific Period, extending from the Palaeolithic Age to the middle of the fifteenth century, during which anatomical observation was intermingled with philosophical speculation. Dissections were infrequent and in general conducted on animals; human dissections were extremely rare. Findings were documented in the form of drawings.
- The Scientific Period, from the second half of the fifteenth century to the nineteenth century. During this period various factors converged to transform anatomy into a modern science, some of the most important being:
  A. The increasing accuracy of anatomical drawings, produced by artists in the form of woodcuts and engravings that were not only detailed and accurate, but of high artistic quality. Well-known artists began to take an interest in the human body and were asked to illustrate anatomical texts. Among them were Jacopo Bellini, van Calcaar, Paolo Veronese, Giambattista Piazzetta and Leonardo da Vinci. A crucial figure in this period was Andrea Vesalius, a great innovator who completely revised the methods that were used to teach anatomy.
  B. The spread of the practice of human dissections. There were obstacles from the onset. The Church was in opposition and Academics considered the use of cadavers to be a lowly occupation. Dissection gradually won acceptance, leading to a more profound knowledge of anatomy and more accurate drawings.
  C. The development of printing, which made possible the reproduction and wider dissemination of anatomical illustrations.

The Scientific Period can be further divided into the times before and after the reforms of Vesalius.

- The Modern Period, from the nineteenth century to the present day. For the last 200 years anatomical studies have focused with increasing precision on specific organs, systems and regions such as the lymph vessels, the cutaneous vascular system, and the strata and substrata of the skin. Many of these studies, as we will see, would have direct consequences for the development of plastic surgery.

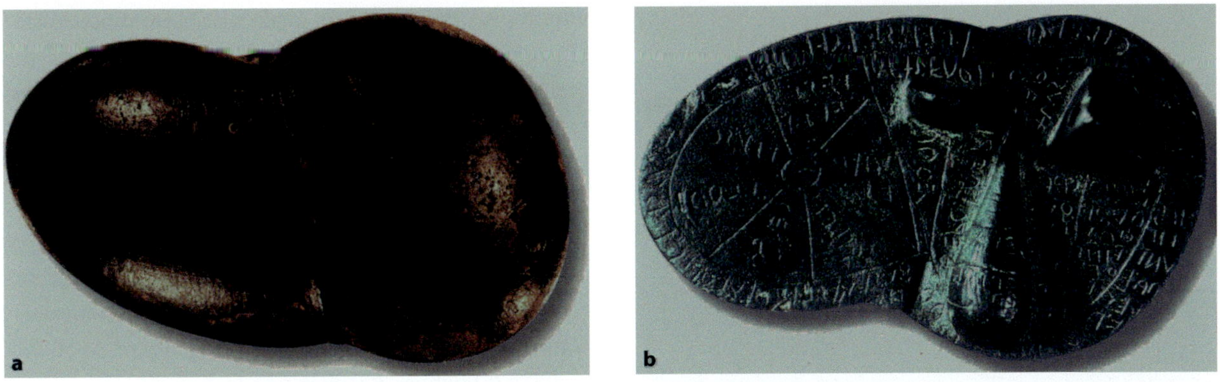

Fig. 1.2a,b A bronze Etruscan sheep's liver found near Piacenza in Italy during the nineteenth century and dated around the third century B.C. It was probably used for religious purposes. The accurate detail highlights the Etruscan's knowledge of anatomy. *Courtesy of the Musei Civici di Palazzo Farnese, Piacenza*

The Pre-Scientific Period

Man's interest in anatomy dates back to prehistoric times, although it was not originally motivated by the desire to acquire scientific knowledge that could be applied to the practice of medicine. In the Palaeolithic Age, for example, our ancestors knew perfectly well where the hearts of their victims were located, as is shown on wall paintings in the caves of Paindal in Spain and Niaux in the Ariège Mountains of France. The study of anatomy started in Classical times as highlighted by the statement of Charles Singer [932]: "In anatomy the Greeks had no predecessors."

While we have no proof that dissections were conducted in antiquity—certainly not on humans, or in the pursuit of medical knowledge—some notions of anatomy did exist. A few rather crude representations have come down to us, such as the bronze model of a liver discovered in the ruins of a Babylonian temple in Mesopotamia and dating from approximately 2000 B.C. Another is the bronze model of a sheep's liver (Fig. 1.2a, b) found at an Etruscan settlement near Piacenza in Italy. It dates from the third century B.C. and shows the gall bladder as well as the two principle lobes on the anterior surface with the caudate lobe beneath. The Etruscans were very familiar with the anatomy of the liver since another in terracotta was found in Faleri, north of Rome. Again it dates from around the fourth to third century B.C. and is kept in the Etruscan Museum at Villa Giulia in Rome. It is possible that the use of these artefacts was mainly religious but they testify of an accurate knowledge of anatomy.[1]

The ancient Egyptians began recording anatomical observations around 2900 B.C. Given their well established practice of mummification, they had ample opportunity to study the viscera of the human body and it is not surprising that some practitioners attempted to make a record of their observations. Thus, stylized representations of the heart, lungs and trachea can be found among Egyptian hieroglyphs and carved on amulets. W.M.F. Petrie [795], F.L. Griffith [396], N. de G. Davies [221]. Unfortunately, it is not possible to determine whether these represent fortuitous observations made during the mummification procedure, or if they were the result of dissections carried out for the purposes of study, although the latter hypothesis seems somewhat unlikely.

Anatomy During Classical Antiquity

The birth of anatomy as a science may be traced back to the Hellenistic period. It is no coincidence that many

1 The use of the liver by priests for auspicious predictions was not uncommon [Carini AM, Govi E (2000) *Il Fegato di Piacenza.* Pallazzo Farnese, Piacenza]. Another terracotta liver, found in Mesopotamia, now in the British Museum, was used by the Caldeans but its anatomical accuracy is not of the high standard as the Etruscan model.

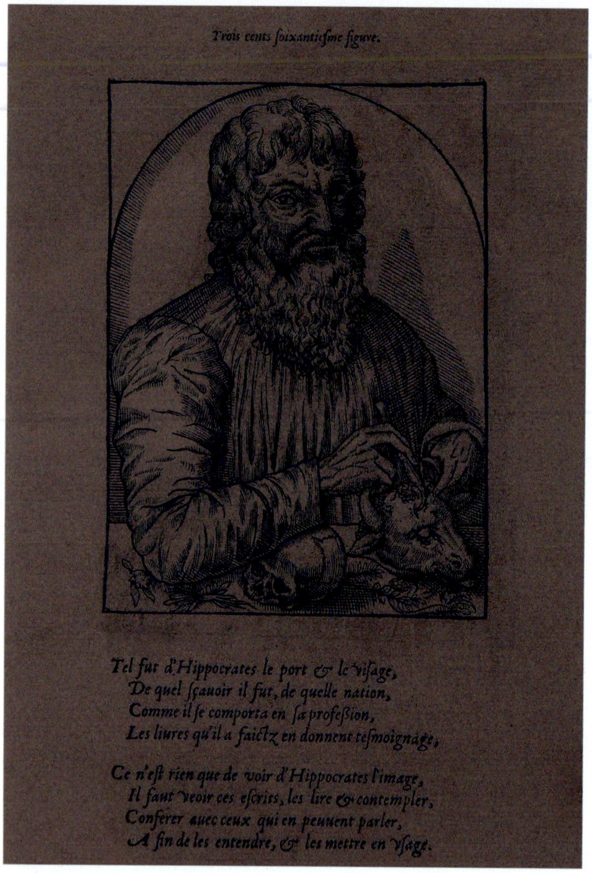
Trois cents ſoixantiſme figure.
Tel fut d'Hippocrates le port & le viſage,
De quel ſçauoir il fut, de quelle nation,
Comme il ſe comporta en ſa profeßion,
Les liures qu'il a faictz en donnent teſmoignage,
Ce n'eſt rien que de voir d'Hippocrates l'image,
Il faut veoir ces eſcrits, les lire & contempler,
Conferer auec ceux qui en peuuent parler,
A fin de les entendre, & les mettre en vſage.

Fig. 1.3 Hippocrates (ca. 460–370 B.C.). Portrait taken from *Les Oeuvres* by Ambroise Paré. *Courtesy of Riccardo Mazzola, M.D., Milan*

beautiful bronze statues cast in accurate anatomical detail were produced during this epoch and the island of Sicily, which was encompassed in the Greek sphere of influence, made significant contributions to the development of this science.

Important observations were made by Alcmaenon, who lived in Sicily around 500 B.C. It is certain that he dissected animals and it appears that the original discovery of the auditory tube, which would later be named after the sixteenth century anatomist Bartolomeo Eustachius, can be attributed to him. He also conducted the earliest studies in embryology, and has left us a description of the head of the fetus.

The most common subject of early observations was the anatomy of the vascular system. Acron, Pamanias, Empedocles of Agrasi (all c.480 B.C.) and Philiston of Locri (c.380 B.C.) were all Sicilians who left behind interesting traces of their work. We have a diagram illustrating the circulatory system by Diogenes of Apollonia (c.400 B.C.), whose *Regimen* was included in the *Corpus Hippocraticus* [932]. Anaximenes (c.580 B.C.) described the functions of the *pneuma* in the following terms: "Just as our soul, being of air, sustains us, so the pneuma and air pervade the entire world", while Empedocles held the theory that "blood is life" and the hypothesis that the heart was the most vital organ in the vascular and respiratory systems. He used the term *pneuma* to designate the soul and life, which he identified with air and the act of breathing [932]

Hippocrates of Cos (c.400–355 B.C.) (Fig. 1.3) [434–437] was without question the most important figure in anatomy and medicine in ancient Greece. We know very little about his life except that he was born on the island of Cos and his father Eraclides was a physician who established a celebrated school of medicine on the island. Not all of the fifty-nine works contained in what is referred to as the *Corpus Hippocraticus* are by his hand. There is strong evidence to suggest that at least forty of them (including some of the most famous, such as *On the Sacred Illnesses*, *Head Injuries* and *Fractures and Dislocations*) are apocryphal and were actually written by his students [932]. In any event the *Corpus* covers the entire field of medicine as it was practised during the time of Hippocrates. No less than nine of the works are dedicated exclusively to anatomy and another nine to surgery. Aldo Mieli [666].[2] Many demonstrate an astonishing knowledge of the human organs. For example, we find the first description of the brain as an organ divided into two symmetrical lobes, although curiously the Greeks were persuaded that the

2 Of pertinence to anatomy are Hippocrates' works *De Anatomia*, *De Corde* (*On the Heart*), *De Carne* (also known as *De Musculi*), *De Glandulis*, *De Natura Ossium*, *De Natura Hominis*, *De Natura Pueri* and finally *De Morbis*. Many details regarding the anatomy of human organs and systems were based on the dissections of goats. Among his other writings, *The Aphorisms*, *Treatise on Prognoses*, *Epidemic Diseases*, *Diet in Acute Diseases*, *On Injuries to the Head*, *Luxations*, *Fractures and Ulcers* and finally *On Airs, Waters and Places* deserve mention.

right lobe received blood directly from the liver while the left lobe was fed by blood from the spleen.

Beginning in the second half of the fourth century B.C., medicine was strongly influenced by the philosopher Aristotle (384–322 B.C.) [32] who wrote a number of treatises on animals [3] and during the course of his reflections on natural history elaborated a theory of "organic evolution". He is considered to be the founder of the discipline of comparative anatomy and the first scientist to record his observations in the form of anatomical drawings. The earliest work on embryology can also be attributed to Aristotle. In it he discusses the processes of reproduction in different animals and his theories concerning them. He succeeded in studying a 3-day-old chick embryo and describing its development. Aristotle does not appear to have ever conducted human dissections, but he nevertheless has left descriptions, with clear schematic diagrams, of the aorta and the male and female genito-urinary systems, with names assigned to each of the organs.

The influence of Aristotle on the science of anatomy lasted for many centuries. The philosopher was tutor and then friend to Alexander the Great, who founded the Egyptian city of Alexandria with its legendary library of 700,000 volumes. Thanks to this institution Alexandria became the centre of culture and learning in the antique world. At least two famous anatomists were active there around 250 B.C. One was Herophilus of Chalcedon who, according to Claudius Galen (131–221 A.D.) [348–354] "was the first to carry out dissections on the corpses of both man and animals". This assertion was not quite exact, since dissections—especially on animals—were being conducted long before Herophilus, but he certainly was the first to write about his studies in a scientific manner, in his work *On Anatomy* and then in his treatise *On the Eyes*.[4] The breadth of his research has justly earned Herophilus the title of "the father of anatomy". Another illustrious Alexandrian and contemporary of Herophilus, Erasistratus of Chios, is regarded as "the father of physiology" because in his studies he sought to understand not only the structure but also the functioning of the body's organs [932].

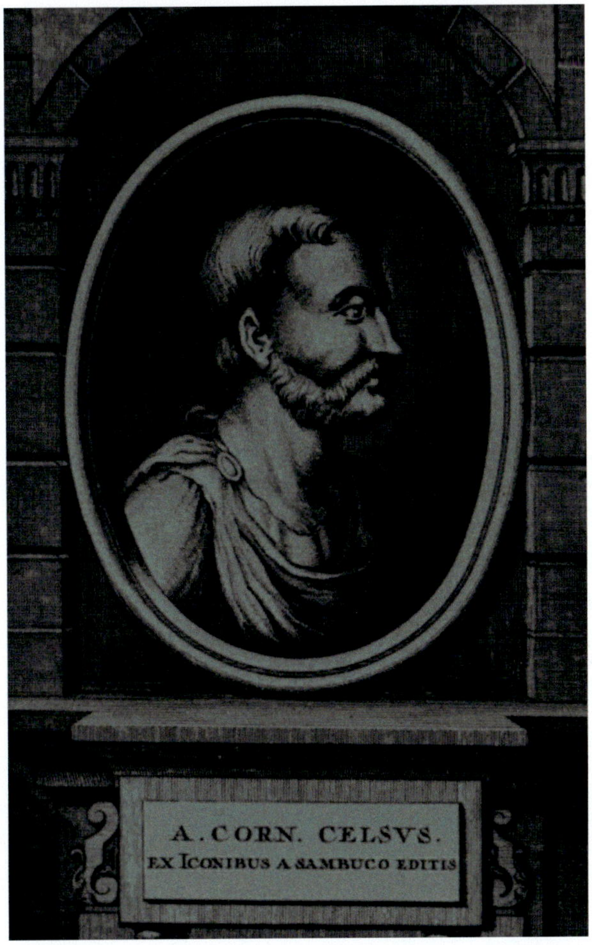

Fig. 1.4 Aulus Cornelius Celsus (second century A.D.), author of *De Medicina. Courtesy of FMR Art.spa, Bologna*

For religious reasons the ancient Romans disapproved of the dissection of both human beings and animals. Their knowledge was therefore based entirely upon the texts of their Greek predecessors. In Egypt under Roman rule the antique practice of dissection which had been perpetuated in the city of Alexandria was interrupted. Notwithstanding this Aulus Cornelius Celsus (25 B.C. to 50 A.D.) (Fig. 1.4) has left us surprisingly accurate anatomical descriptions, some of which—for example, his

3 See, for example, *The History of Animals* and *On the Parts of Animals*.

4 Herophilus is also known for having written a text on obstetrics and for identifying the brain as the seat of the intelligence, thus challenging Aristotle who retained that the soul was located in the heart. Herophilus also made the distinction between the motor and sensory nerves, describing the whole as a "miraculous network".

studies on the genitalia [5] and the skeleton[6]—are of special interest to plastic surgery [167, 168]. Apart from the works of Celsus, however, the medical literature in Latin during the first one hundred and fifty years A.D. is almost non-existent, although it must not be forgotten that all educated Romans could read and write in Greek.

A genuine revival of the study of medicine took place in Rome with the advent of Galen whose influence was destined to last for centuries. The son of a celebrated mathematician and architect, Galen was born in Pergamum, a city with a well-known medical school located in the province of Anatolia, which was then under Greek rule. At the age of twenty Galen went to Smyrna to study under Pelope and it was there that he wrote his first work *On the Movement of the Thorax and Lungs*. After spending several years in Alexandria, he returned to Pergamum at the age of twenty-eight. Four years later he moved permanently to Rome, where he eventually became personal physician to the emperor Marcus Aurelius.

According to Galen, the physician who lacked a firm grounding in anatomy was like an architect working without a blueprint, and he therefore dedicated much of his time to giving public anatomical demonstrations using animals, in particular monkeys. Garofalo and Vegetti [359]. The dissection of human cadavers was prohibited in Rome for religious reasons, although Bettman and Hench [89] claim that Galen carried out at least one dissection, on a man who had died by drowning. In any case Galen's knowledge of animal anatomy must have been encyclopaedic if it is true that he even dissected an elephant and a hippopotamus. He was quite aware of the anatomical differences between animals and man, and may in a certain sense be regarded as a comparative anatomist *ante litteram*. While in Alexandria he had carried out unprecedented studies on the skeleton (*On the Bones, for Beginners*), gathering data for the first known description of the marrow of the long bones. Other fundamental works on the motor apparatus followed, including *On the Anatomy of the Muscles*, which is considered to be his most important contribution to the study of anatomy.[7] Galen's systematic classification of the cranial nerves—a truly astonishing achievement for his time—would remain in use until the seventeenth century. Other noteworthy contributions included his accurate and detailed descriptions of the pulmonary artery (which he called the "arterial vein") and the recurrent laryngeal nerve with its intricately branching course, not to mention his fascinating comparative studies of the hands of the monkey and man (Fig. 1.5).

In the tradition of Aristotle, Galen believed that nothing was created by Mother Nature without a reason and therefore each organ must have been constructed so as to best fulfil the function for which it was designed [359, 932]. He wrote: "Indeed, the theory of finalism can be applied to the study of animal organs. Each part, being perfectly adapted to its end, could not have been constructed in any other manner than it was."

The teachings of Galen would remain a reference point for almost fifteen centuries; his authority was undisputed and all medical questions were resolved on the basis of his teachings. Unfortunately, this meant that his errors were perpetuated as well and in time became an obstacle to progress in medicine. Andrea Vesalius, in the sixteenth century, was one of the first to dare to challenge Galen's way of thinking.

The Middle Ages

After Galen interest in anatomy declined in the Western world. The cultural heritage of Athens, Rome and Alexandria instead passed into the safekeeping of the Nestorians in Mesopotamia and later the Arabs, who would go on copying and teaching from the classical texts during the centuries corresponding to the Dark Ages in Europe. For this entire period however, which lasted until the year 1000, the respect of both Arab and Oriental cultures for the bodies of the deceased was such that no human dissections could be carried out (Figs. 1.6a, b, 1.7a, b).

In western Europe after the fall of the Roman Empire the study of medicine was carried on almost exclusively in the monasteries and under the strict control of the Church. Given that Catholic doctrine included the com-

5 See *De Medicina*, Book VII, Chapters 28, 36, 37 and 45.

6 See *De Medicina*, Book VIII, Chapters 17–32.

7 While still a young man Galen wrote many other important works such as *Anatomical Procedures* (in 16 books of which only 9 have come down to us) and *The Anatomy of the Uterus*. He later also wrote a work entitled *On the Use of the Parts of the Body*.

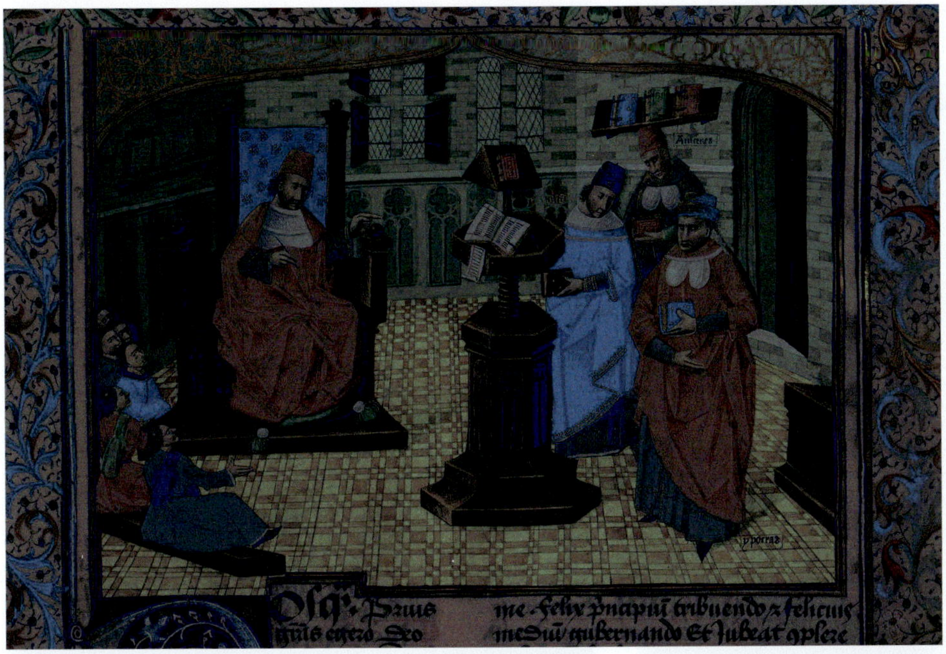

Fig. 1.5 Guy de Chauliac (1300–1368) lecturing to students with his predecessors Galen, Avicenna and Hippocrates in the background. From an illuminated manuscript in Guy's book *Chirurgie*, probably commissioned by Duke Charles d'Orleans, dated 1461. *By permission of the Biblioteque Nationale de France, Paris*

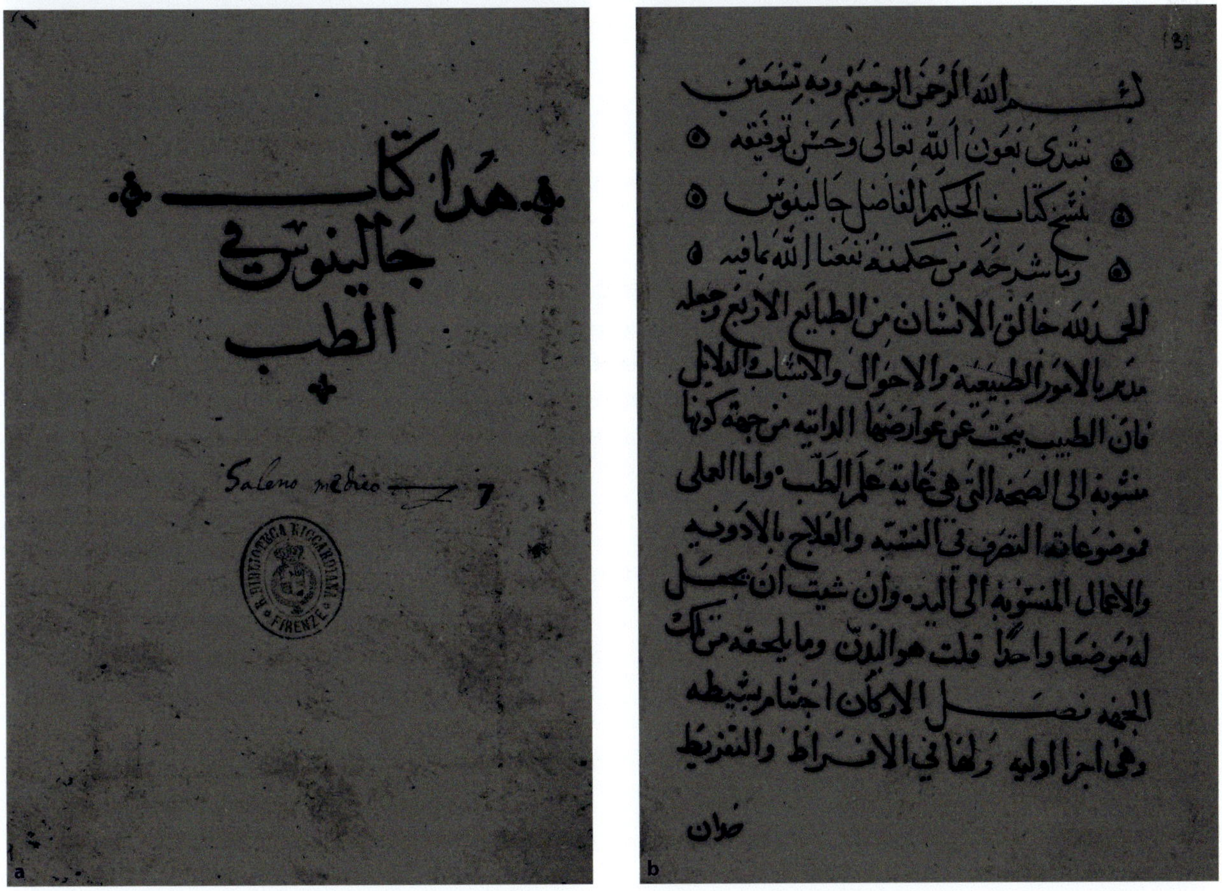

Fig. 1.6a,b Arabic translation of the works *Liber Sapientiae* by Hippocrates (Kitāb Hikmat Abuqrāt) from the Middle Ages. The translator was probably Abū Zakariya Yahyā (777–857 A.D.), doctor to Califf Hārūn ar-Rašīd who appointed him leader of a group charged with translating the Greek manuscripts acquired in Asia Minor and Egypt. *By permission of the Dipartimento per i Beni Archivistici e Librari Biblioteca Riccardiana, Florence*

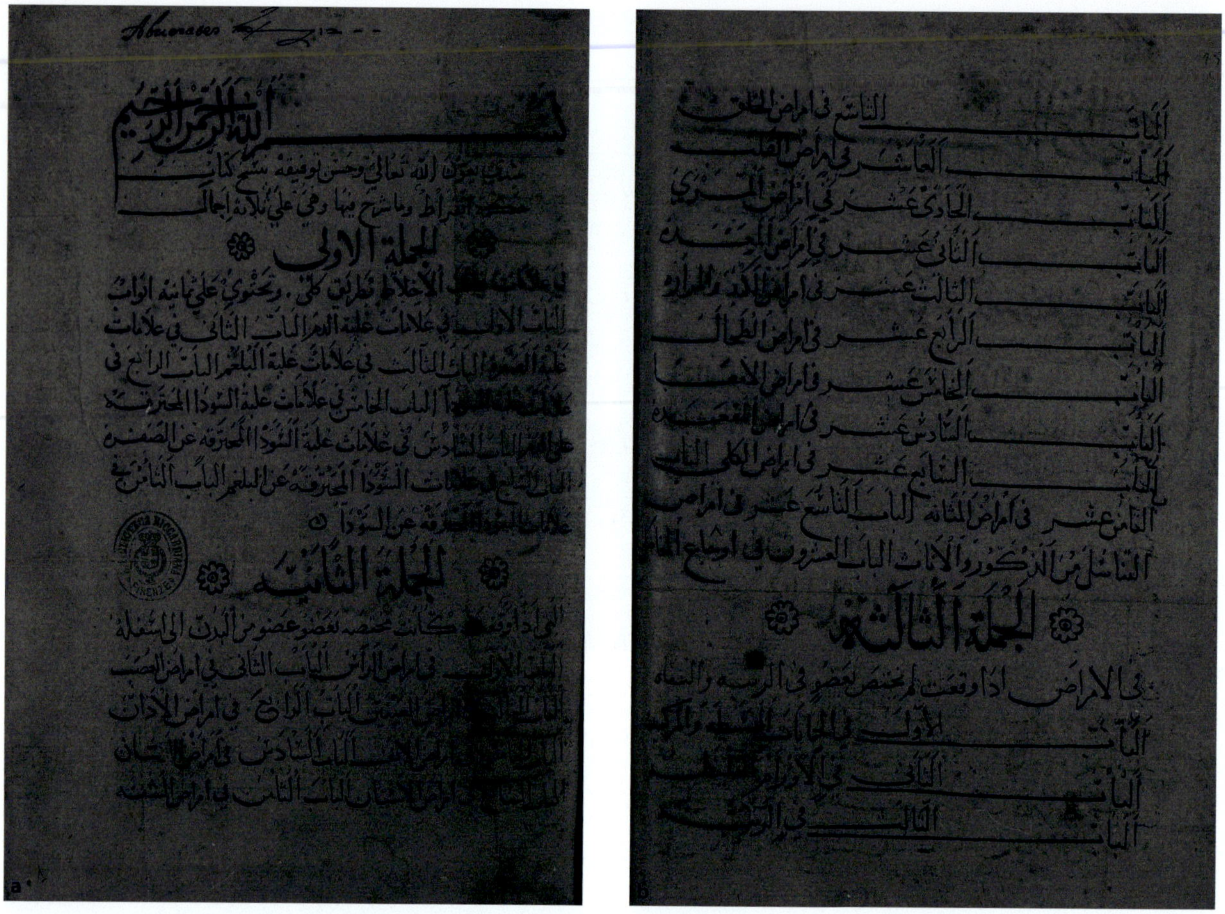

Fig. 1.7a,b Arabic translation of the works of Galen *De Arte Medica* (Kitāb Galīnūs fi't-Tibb) from the Middle Ages. Most of the original works of Galen in Greek have been lost. Those we have were preserved through the Middle Ages by the Arabic translations. The translator was probably Girğis ibn Gibrā īl, a member of the "House of the Wisdom", created in 830 A.D. in Bagdad by al-Ma'mūn, son of the mythical Califf Hārūn ar Rašīd. Many of the classic texts were translated in this House. *By permission of the Dipartimento per i Beni Archivistici e Librari Biblioteca Riccardiana, Florence*

mandment *Ecclesia abhorret a sanguine*, any procedure regarded as being unusually cruel, including dissection, was strictly prohibited. Scholasticism, the medieval system of theology and philosophy based on Aristotelian logic and the writings of the early Church Fathers, dominated medical studies as it did all the other branches of knowledge.

In Italy there was one noteworthy exception to the rule that bound the practice of medicine to the religious orders, the famous *Scuola Salernitana*. The Arab tradition had been kept alive in southern Italy and above all in Sicily, which for a long period of time remained under the influence of the Arabs. According to Bettman and Hench [89] the *Scuola Salernitana* was founded in Salerno near Naples sometime around the ninth century by four physicians of different religious faiths: one Greek Orthodox, one Jew, one Arab Muslim and one Italian Catholic. This made it possible for the school to develop unhampered by medieval superstition and above all free from the influence of the Church.[8] In this haven the

8 At the Council of Reims in 1131 the Catholic Church prohibited the practice of medicine outside the monasteries. Who knows if this was one of the reasons why Constantine, one of the founders of Western medicine (who brought many medical texts from his native Tunisia to Salerno), abandoned his profession and joined the Benedictine order in the Abbey of Montecassino.

practice of surgery flourished, and the school counted such illustrious figures as Roger of Salerno and Rolando of Parma among its teachers. The study of anatomy did not reach such impressive heights, however.[9] This seeming anomaly can be explained in part by the fact that, despite its name, the *Scuola Salernitana* was a clinic whose principle function was not teaching but the treatment of patients. In 1240 King Frederick II founded the University of Naples where dissections were permitted and this contributed to the gradual decline in importance of the *Scuola*, although it remained in existence until the Napoleonic era.

The Role of the Earliest Universities in the Teaching of Anatomy

During the thirteenth century an important development took place in the teaching of medicine which until that time, at least in the West, had been, like the arts, based on a direct relationship between teacher and student without the existence of true schools. In reality there had been schools in the past in Mesopotamia and Arabia for the teaching of medicine, but in Europe the sole example was the *Scuola Salernitana*. Eventually in the thirteenth century, European universities began to teach medicine, including anatomy (Fig. 1.8). This included the renowned university of Bologna, which had already been in existence for more than one hundred years. Unlike many of its sister institutions, the *studio* of Bologna had not been founded by ecclesiastic charter and its teachers and students were regarded with some suspicion by the Church. The faculty of law succeeded in maintaining a considerable degree of independence from the ecclesiastic authorities, becoming completely autonomous in 1306 and this contributed significantly to the development of a school of anatomy at the university. In fact, the jurists themselves requested dissections in order to gather evidence for their cases and what began as a medical-legal procedure led to increasing scientific knowledge.

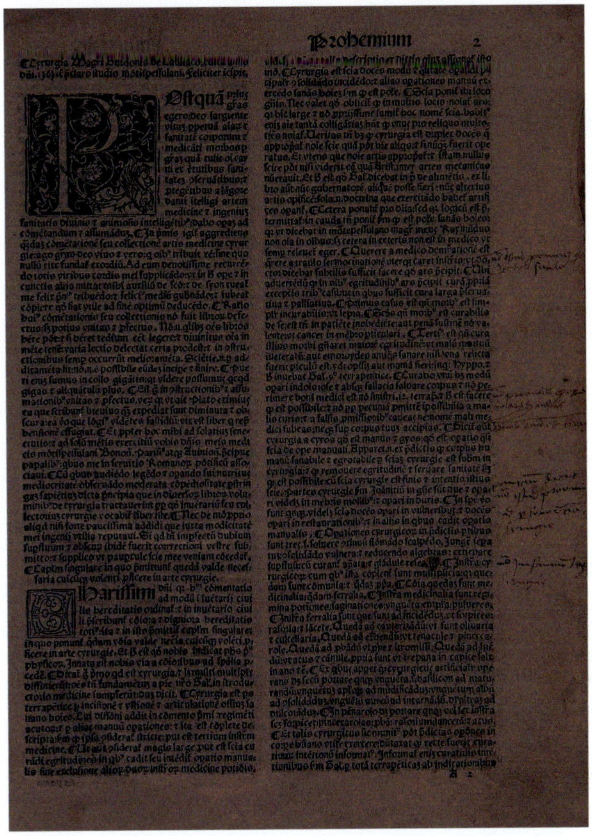

Prohemium

Fig. 1.8 The first page of Guy de Chauliac's *Chirurgia Magna* which also contains the writings of the ten most celebrated surgeons of the time, including Mondeville and Lanfranchi. *Courtesy of Riccardo Mazzola, M.D., Milan*

The founder of the school of anatomy in Bologna was Ugo Borgognoni of Lucca (1170–1240), whose work was continued by his son Theodorico of Cervia (1205–1298). Theodorico managed to have human dissections included for the first time as an integral part of the medical curriculum, even if cadavers were extremely difficult to obtain and when available, could only be used for a limited period of time due to the lack of means for their preservation [979]. In the absence of human cadavers, dissections were conducted on animals, most often pigs. The advances introduced by Theodorico were consolidated by Guglielmo da Saliceto (1215–1276), who described for the first time the motor nerves that govern the con-

9 The earliest surviving documents relating to the *Scuola Salernitana* date from 848 and concern Giuseppe da Salerno and another physician by the name of Josan. The oldest text produced by the school has been attributed to a certain Alfano (1058–1083) and is entitled *De Quatuor Humoribus Corporis Humanis* (*The Four Humours of the Human Body*).

traction of the voluntary and involuntary muscles [880, 881].[10]

Taddeo Alderotto of Florence (1223–1303) continued Theodorico's practices, while his student and successor Henry de Mondeville [682, 731] introduced the use of anatomical diagrams, carefully prepared on the basis of actual dissections, as a teaching instrument. These proved to be an invaluable aid to the students, who could in this way review what they had learned during the faculty's all too rare anatomy demonstrations.[11] Detailed and accurately drawn, these charts were considered by de Mondeville to be absolutely fundamental in the education of future surgeons.

By the end of the 1300s dissections had become an accepted and officially recognized procedure in Bologna, although cadavers remained difficult to come by. This situation favoured the introduction by Mondino de Liucci (1270–1326) innovations which generated significant impetus and helped transform anatomy into a genuine science [683–685].

Mondino was born, it seems in 1275, to a Florentine family; his father was a pharmacist. He studied medicine in Bologna where Taddeo Alderotti, a fellow Florentine, was teaching and received his degree in 1300. After further studies under Henry de Mondeville, he became a professor and taught medicine at the university of Bologna from 1306 to 1326. During this time he managed to institute the rule that lessons in anatomy should always be conducted on the basis of human dissections (Fig. 1.9) or when this was not possible, studies on animals, preferably monkeys or pigs. He realized that lectures illustrated with diagrams such as those prepared by his professor Henry de Mondeville were not sufficient. Mondino did not sully his hands personally during the anatomical demonstrations; instead he sat in an imposing chair and from there directed an assistant called an *ostensor*, who indicated the lines of dissection to a *demonstrator* who carried out the actual manual labour of cutting the cadaver (Fig. 1.10). This lofty approach to the teaching of anatomy would persist until the arrival of Vesalius, who prided himself on conducting his dissections in person.

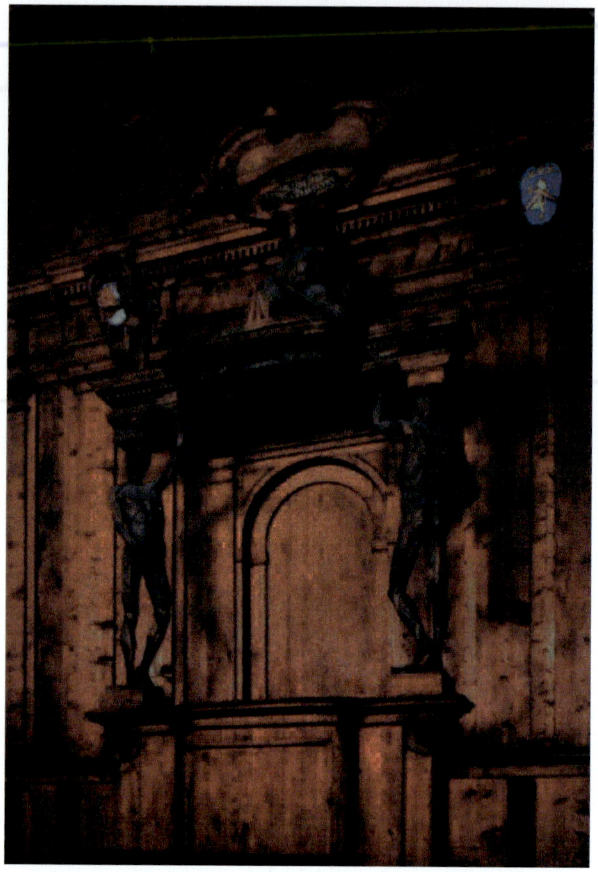

Fig. 1.9 The Anatomical Theatre of the University of Bologna dated 1637. The picture shows the "Baldacchino degli Spellati" (Canopy of the Skinned men) added in 1734. *PJS*

Nonetheless, with Mondino's reforms anatomy was taught more systematically and dissection became the fulcrum of the discipline. Thanks to this *Restauratore dell'Anatomia*, as he was regarded by his contemporaries,

10 Guglielmo da Saliceto's work *Vulgare in Chirurgia* contains many sections that are of relevance to plastic surgery. We may cite from Book II his descriptions of treatments for injuries of the nose (chapter III) and the auricle (chapter VI). Guglielmo was an advocate of the use of the scalpel for surgical procedures in a period when, due to the influence of the Arab school of medicine, cautery was the preferred practice.

11 Henri de Mondeville's famous anatomical diagrams which he prepared for his lessons as professor at Montpellier, are now conserved at the Bibliotheque Nationale de France.

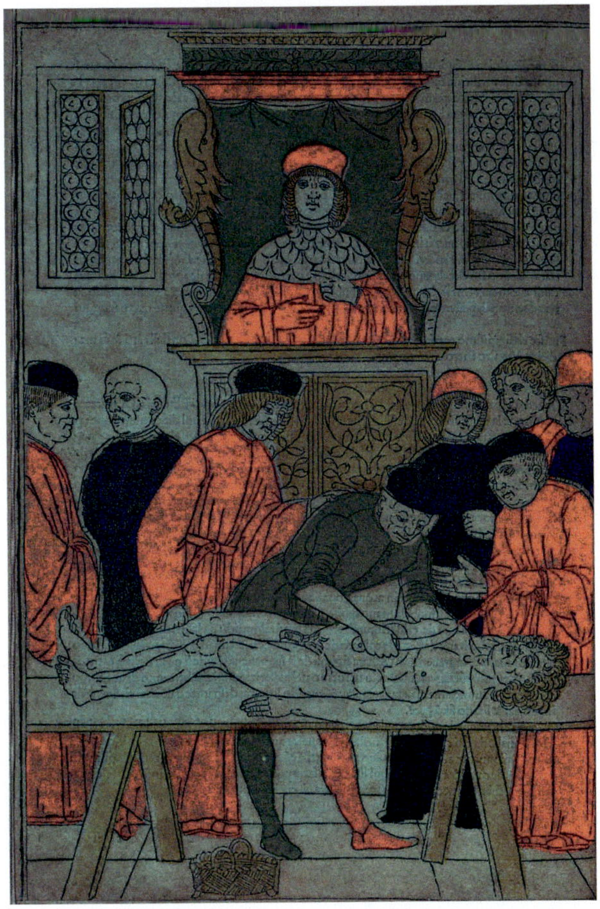

Fig. 1.10 Mondino de Liucci (1270–1326) lecturing in Bologna. He was the first anatomist to base his lectures on dissections rather then on diagrams. He did not perform the dissection himself but directed the *ostensors* and *demonstrators* from a chair. The picture, a woodcut, is taken from *Fascicula Medicinae* by John de Ketham (fifteenth century Italian School). This is probably the first illustrated book dealing only with anatomy and the first with colour illustrations. *Fondazione Giorgio Cini, Venice, Italy. Archives Charmet – Bridgeman Art Library*

Italy maintained its primacy as the most important centre for anatomical studies until the Renaissance.[12]

Traditionally the subject of anatomy had been covered in texts on surgery, but in 1316 Mondino wrote *Anathomia*,[13] perhaps the first work exclusively devoted to anatomy. Mondino's medical principles did not depart radically from those of Galen and the Arab authorities, but his teachings differed in that they were always based upon direct observation and dissections. Since there were no techniques available for the conservation of cadavers, he was obliged to conduct his demonstrations as quickly as possible. Depending upon the season, the longest delay he could afford was four days. For this reason his lessons could not be carried out systematically and organs were examined one by one as they were exposed during the course of the dissection. Nevertheless Mondino did manage to follow a logical sequence and during the dissection customarily delivered "four lectures on the body. The first concerned the nutritive organs because they were the ones that tended to putrefy the most quickly; second the 'spiritual' organs [the head and brain], third the natural organs [for example, the thoracic cavity], and finally the fourth on the extremities and the spinal column" [684, 685].

The cadavers obtained were generally those of executed criminals, a practice which would continue in Bologna until the sixteenth century. Mondino complained bitterly of the lack of corpses and experimented with various solutions to compensate for this dearth of bodies. For example, he developed a procedure for drying specimens in the sun, an approach that was particularly effective for the preservation of tendons, ligaments and bones. Skeletons were obtained by maceration, a practice that would continue for many centuries. Mondino introduced many other innovations. He was probably the first anatomist to inject coloured liquids into the blood vessels which when solidified, made it possible to study the circulatory system. In his work *De Omnibus Humanii Corporus Interioribus Membris*, printed in 1513, he

12 It was in 1300 and hence during the time of Mondino that Pope Boniface VIII issued his famous papal bull *de Sepoltura* which excommunicated anyone who conserved skeletons by boiling their bones. In reality this practice arose for a completely different reason. The remains of persons of rank who died far from home, particularly during the Crusades, were cleaned in this way so that they could be brought home for burial. The papal bull was not directed against anatomists in particular, but could not be ignored by them.

13 *Anathomia* was published in Padua in 1476 by the printer Pietro Maufer.

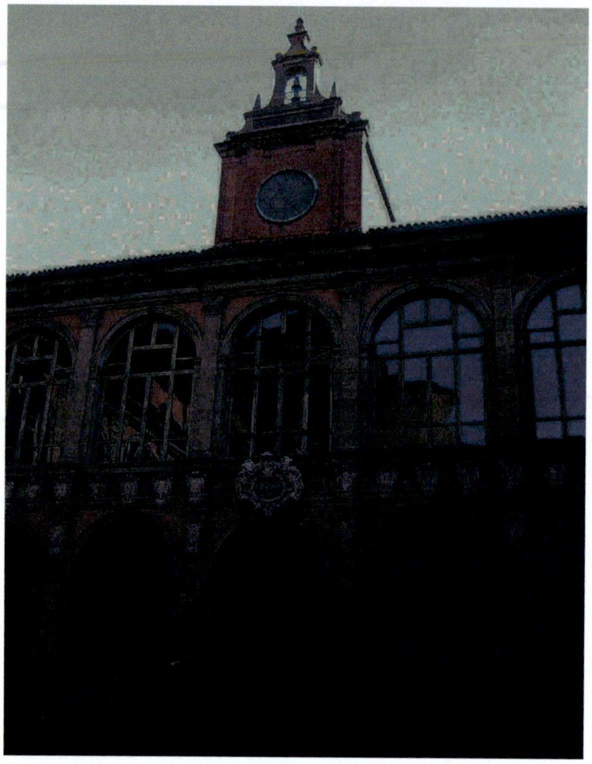

Fig. 1.11 The Archigimnasium of the University of Bologna was built in 1562. Since 1637 it has housed the Anatomical Theatre. It was bombed in World War II. *PJS*

provides a description of the palate and its role in the process of speaking.

Much of Mondino's work was inspired by his study of the Arab medical literature and many of the terms devised by him, such as *basilica*, *cephalica*, *saphena* and *retina*, reflect this. Certainly the University of Bologna (Fig. 1.11) was remarkably advanced for its time, the *Studio Generale* having boldly asserted its right to self-governance and its independence from the Church: "The students wanted to practise Medicine without having to don the cleric's habit" [89]. Medicine was taught on the basis of scientific logic, rather than by theoretical deduction as was still the practice in many other European universities. The professor of anatomy was required to perform two official dissections during the course of the year while his four assistants were responsible for the remainder. Unofficial demonstrations could be held on request at the home of the professor or one of his assistants, but for these the students had to furnish their own cadaver and pay an honorarium.

It may be said that Mondino's innovations marked the end of the Pre-Scientific Period and opened the way for the pre-Vesalian Scientific Period, at the end of which we find the masters who were destined to transform the science of anatomy.

The Scientific Period

Before Vesalius

During the fourteenth and fifteenth centuries many eminent figures such as Berengario da Carpi, Alessandro Benedetti, Leonardo da Vinci and Johannes de Ketham helped to lay the foundations for the scientific era of anatomy.

Berengario da Carpi (1460–1530), the son of a well-known Bolognese physician and surgeon, was the first of these. After completing his studies and receiving his degree on 3 August 1489, Berengario held the chair in anatomy and surgery at Bologna from 1502 to 1527. He was the author of two important works, *Isagoge Breves Perlucide in Anatomiam Humana Corpori* and *Carpi Commentarii*, in which we find the first description of organs such as the appendix, the thymus, the vas deferens and the synovia [75–77]. Of particular relevance to the area of plastic surgery, given their important role in breast reconstruction today, is his description of the abdominal muscles. Furthermore Berengario described the differences between the male and female pelvis[14] with excellent illustrations that were probably prepared by Ugo da Carpi, a talented painter in Bologna (Fig. 1.12a, b). Berengario's treatise on cranial trauma [74], written after

14 See in *Isagoge Breves Perlucide in Anatomian Humani Corpori* (published in Bologna in 1522), Chapter II entitled *Anatomia Ventris Medii*. The same work contains interesting descriptions of the reproductive organs. The illustrations, which were the work of Ugo da Carpi, are noteworthy.

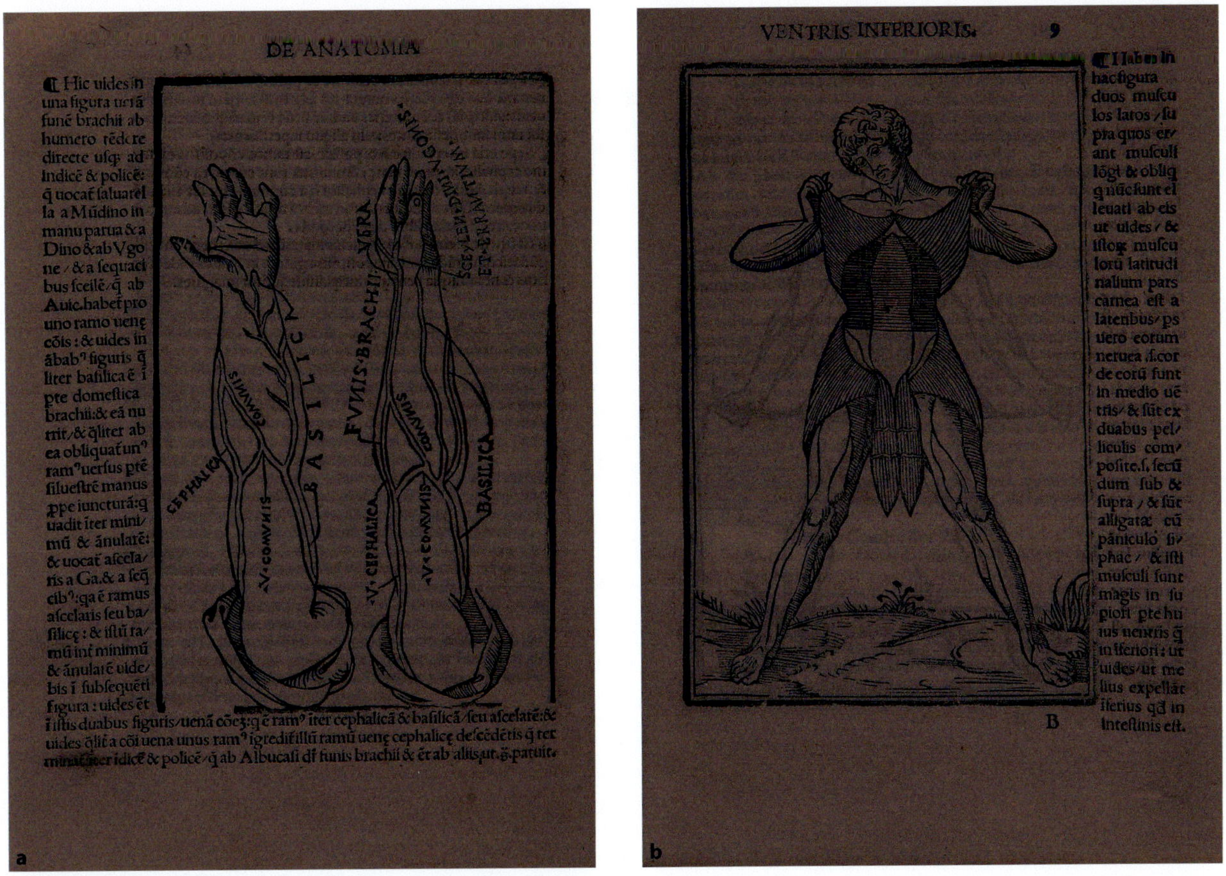

Fig. 1.12 Diagrams of **a** the venous circulation of the arm and **b** abdominal muscles, from the *Isogae* by Berengario da Carpi. *Courtesy of Riccardo Mazzola, M.D., Milan*

he had treated Lorenzo de' Medici for a head injury, is also of interest and we will consider it in more detail in our chapter on cranioplasty.[15]

Among the many distinguished anatomists who taught at the University of Bologna was Giulio Cesare Aranzid (1628–1694). He conducted pioneering studies on the human fetus and also deserves credit for having discovered and encouraged the gifted Gaspare Tagliacozzi, whom he seems to have taught the procedure of rhinoplasty. Other prestigious figures include Giovanni Alfonso Borelli (1608–1679) and Marcello Malpighi (1628–1694), but not long afterwards the study of anatomy, followed by that of surgery, experienced a decline in Italy as attention shifted to another area. Indeed, once the organs of the human body had been identified and their structure determined, it was inevitable that physicians should begin to ask themselves how they functioned; thus, the study of physiology was born.

15 See *De Fractura Calvariae sive Crani*, published in Bologna in 1516, where in Part II, Chapter IV the author provides an account of his operation on Lorenzo de' Medici for a skull fracture caused by a gunshot wound.

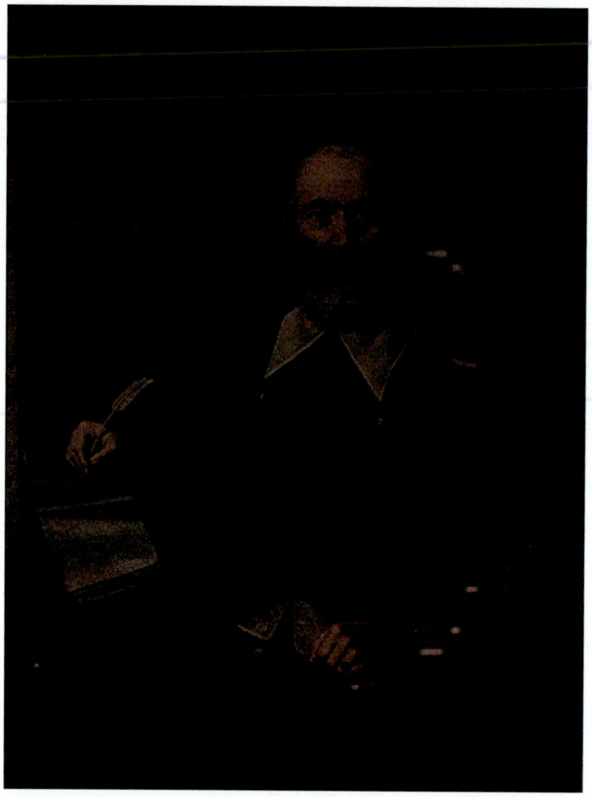

Fig. 1.13 Portrait of A. Benedetti (1460–1525). *Courtesy of the Mayor of Legnago, Verona*

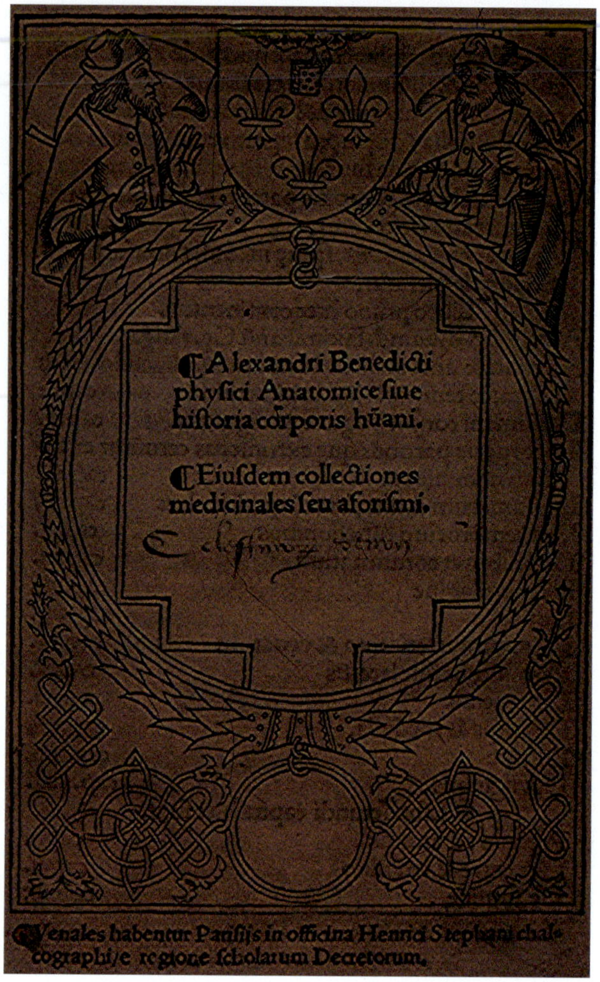

Fig. 1.14 Frontispiece of Alessandro Benedetti's *Anatomia*. He designed and started the construction of the famous Anatomical Theatre of the University of Padua. *Courtesy of Riccardo Mazzola, M.D., Milan*

The University of Padua Before Vesalius

During the second half of the fifteenth century Padua, like Bologna, experienced a significant revival in the teaching of medicine, which initially took the form of a rediscovery of the classical authors and the re-publication of their texts in Latin. Editions of the works of Hippocrates and Galen appeared in 1544 (the works of Celsus had already been printed in Florence in 1478), while many other texts were discovered *ex novo* and interpreted in the light of the most recent scientific knowledge.

This development grew out of the general movement known as *Humanism*, and one of its proponents was Alessandro Benedetti (1460–1525) (Fig. 1.13). Born in Legnago near Verona, Benedetti attended the university of Padua and completed his studies in 1475, after which he practised surgery for seventeen years in the Greek archipelago, where he also mastered the Greek language. In 1490 he was nominated professor of anatomy and surgery at the university of Padua, and was able to dedicate himself to the task of translating some of the most important medical texts from Antiquity. These authorities are amply cited in his *Anatomiae sive Historia Corporis Humanis* (Fig. 1.14), which was published in 1502 [70, 71].[16] Benedetti fully embraced the reforms of Mondino and his lessons were always based on direct observation.

The author of numerous books, he also designed and began constructing the famous anatomy theatre of Padua (Fig. 1.15) whose form was inspired by that of the Roman amphitheatre, in particular the Arena of Verona.[17] He became extremely well known and served as the personal physician to many eminent figures in the Republic of Venice, as well as the Emperor Maximilian I of Germany.

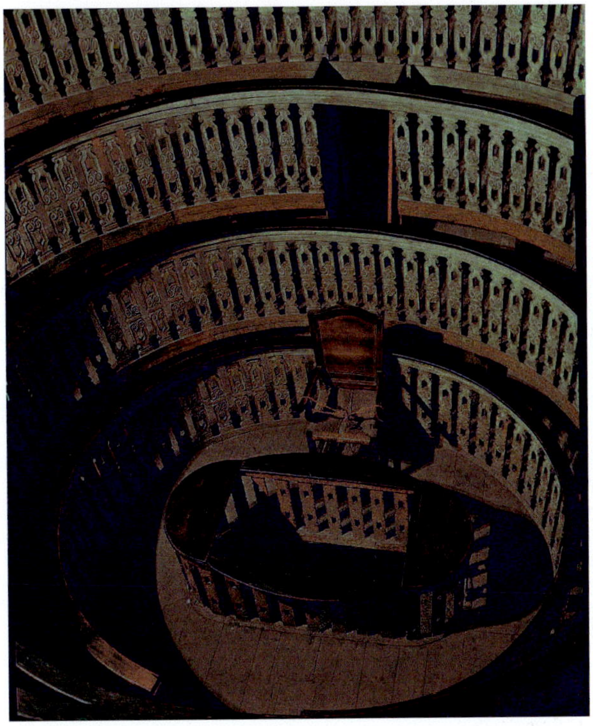

Fig. 1.15 Anatomical Theatre of Padua. The building was started by Alessandro Benedetti and completed in 1591 by Gerolamo Fabricius ab Aquapendente (1533–1619) (Fig. 1.30). This was the theatre where Vesalius gave his lectures. *University of Padua, Italy, Giraudon – Bridgeman Art Library*

The Birth of the Anatomical Illustration

During the second half of the fifteenth century the practice of human dissection became more widely accepted and spread beyond Padua and Bologna, reaching such a point that even scientists and physicians not directly involved in the teaching of medicine could perform the procedure [815]. For example, public dissections were often held in the city of Venice, which did not even have a school of medicine.

During this period a mutually beneficial collaboration between artists and anatomists arose. Artists could finally satisfy their curiosity regarding what lay beneath the surface of the living form, while anatomists had their observations recorded in drawings that were both accurate and artistic. In this way artists developed an interest in the morphology of the human body at a time when the spread of the technique of printing facilitated the diffusion of their work. It seems that for a certain period artists regularly attended dissections. In one of his accounts Vesalius describes: "… questi pittori e scultori che svolazzano attorno a me durante le dissezioni" ("these painters and sculptors who flutter around me during the dissections").

Among those who profited from the more liberal intellectual climate was Leonardo da Vinci (1452–1519), who produced anatomical drawings of astonishing accuracy and also demonstrated a lively curiosity with regard to the functioning of individual organs, in particular muscles and bones [550–552]. Born in the Tuscan village of Vinci in 1452, the illegitimate son of a local nobleman, Leonardo moved to Florence when he was still quite young. There he joined the studio of Andrea Verrocchio

16 As we will see in the chapter on nose reconstructions, in *Anatomiae sive Historia Corporsi Humanis* (Volume IV, Chapter 39, *De naso*) Benedetti describes a procedure for the reconstruction of the nose almost one hundred years before Tagliacozzi.

17 This famous anatomy theatre was completed by Fabrizio ab Aquapendente in 1591. An exact copy may be seen at the University of Uppsala in Sweden—the *Gustavianum* constructed by Olof Rudbeck in 1622. Rudbeck had studied anatomy in Padua, where he initiated his research on the lymph vessels. Other remarkable anatomy theatres are to be found in Leiden (1596) and Bologna (1637).

(1435–1488), a famous Florentine artist who understood how important it was for a painter and sculptor to have a thorough knowledge of anatomy. When he was invited to Milan by the ruling Sforza family in 1483, Leonardo took advantage of the opportunity to conduct dissections at the Ospedale Maggiore, producing five drawings of the human skull between 1487 and 1493. He continued his studies, eventually dissecting the entire human body, and produced his first anatomical work, *La Figura Umana*. When Leonardo left Milan and returned to Florence in 1506, he began collaborating with Marcantonio della Torre (1481–1512) on an anatomy treatise, but this project was interrupted by the premature death of the physician, thus depriving us of what would certainly have been a most fascinating work.

Leonardo emphasized the importance of the anatomical drawing in teaching: "How could you describe this heart in words without having to fill an entire book? In addition, the more details you write on the subject the more you risk confusing the mind of the reader." Irrefutable support for this argument can be found in his meticulous scientific drawings. For the plastic surgeon, Leonardo's two drawings of the palate showing every detail of the musculature of the soft palate (*velum palatinum*) are of enormous interest, but the quality of his other studies of the human body can never cease to amaze us (Fig. 1.16). He completed more than one hundred drawings of the heart, lungs, brain, uterus and muscles, which are all the more remarkable because we know that he conducted his dissections by candlelight. With endless inventiveness Leonardo developed various techniques to help him in his studies. For example he injected coloured wax into organs before sectioning them and this made possible his detailed studies of the cerebral ventricles. He also constructed wire cages around various joints so that he could study the movement and function of the muscles.

Leonardo was the first scientist to study the fetal membranes. He boiled eyes in albumin so that they could be sectioned for examination. The modern convention of illustrating the bones in three views, anterior, lateral and posterior, was introduced by Leonardo. Another field in which he excelled was angiology; in one drawing of the interior of the heart we can recognize such details as the septomarginal trabecula (muscle bundle) of the right ventricle, which was first described in anatomical texts many centuries later.

If Leonardo's purpose, at least initially,[18] was to establish an anatomical basis for his paintings, there is no doubt that very quickly his scientific curiosity took over. Hence his drawings are works of art, but also incomparable anatomical studies which were so useful in the teaching of anatomy that it is said even Vesalius was inspired by his work.[19]

Up until this time the highly inaccurate diagrams compiled by the anatomists themselves were copied by scribes who had no specific knowledge of anatomy and therefore added error to error. For this reason, until the fifteenth century when artists began to make their contribution, anatomical illustrations were poor. Indeed very little had changed since the time of Aristotle, who in his *Generatione Animalium* suggested the use of paradigms, schemata and diagrams to illustrate the anatomy of the body.

As Louis Choulant [178] wrote, the requirements of teaching were best met by: "an ideal human figure based on the constant use of proportions" and this model was generally followed after Mondino. Choulant divided the evolution of the anatomical illustration into six stages:

- The period before Berengario da Carpi (1521), when knowledge of anatomy was still based on schematic drawings.
- The period from Berengario to Vesalius (1521–1543), during which more accurate illustrations, made possible by the technique of woodcut engravings, were introduced.
- The period from Vesalius to Casserio (1543–1600), when the practice of dissection spread and increasing

18 Many famous artists of the period, including Andrea Mantegna (1431–1506) and Luca Signorelli (1445–1523), shared Andrea Verrocchio's conviction that a knowledge of anatomy could be useful in their work.

19 When Leonardo died his drawings were conserved by his student Francesco Melzi. The son of Melzi sold most of these to the sculptor Pompeo Leoni, who later took them with him to Spain. Two volumes remained there on the sculptor's death and were only recently rediscovered in the National Library of Madrid. A third volume was sold in 1630 to Lord Thomas Howard, Count of Arundel and adviser on matters of art to King Charles I; it is now conserved at the Royal Library of Windsor in England.

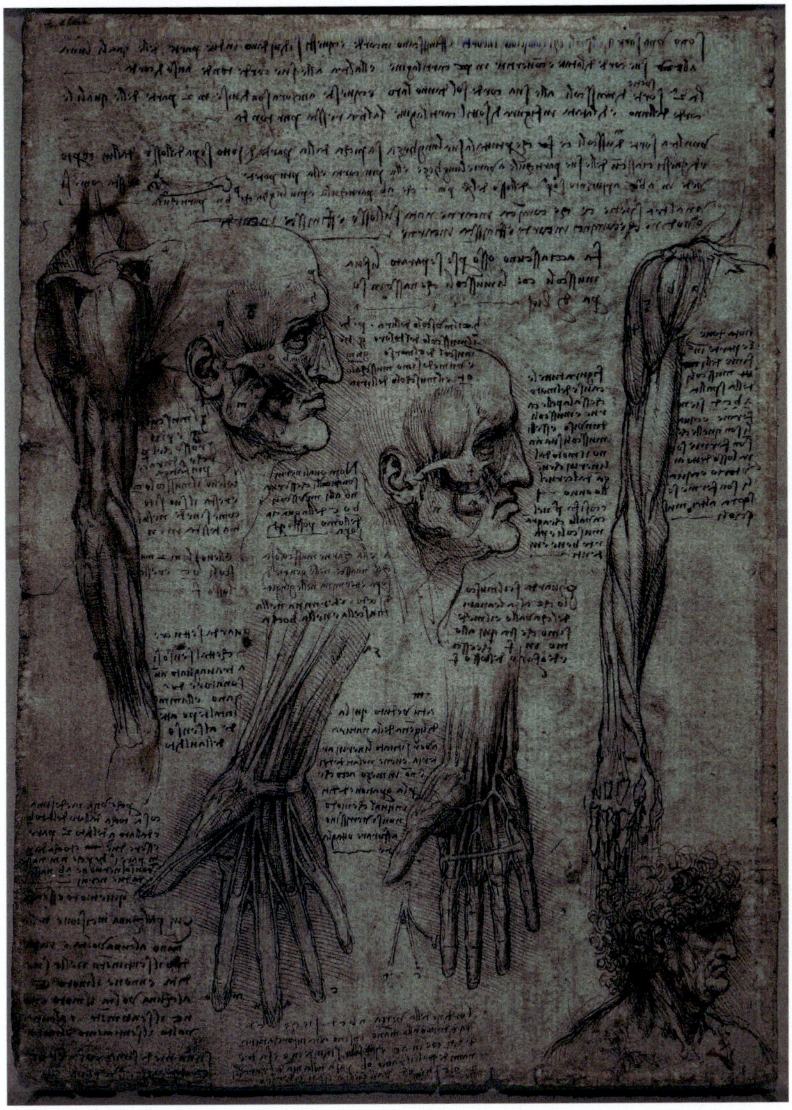

Fig. 1.16 The muscles of the arm, hand and face by Leonardo da Vinci. (RL19012v) *The Royal Collection © 2005, Her Majesty Queen Elizabeth II*

numbers of artists began to take an interest in anatomy. The quality of woodcut illustrations improved markedly.

- The period from Casserio to Albinus (1627–1737), as anatomical drawings became increasingly accurate and were reproduced in the form of highly artistic engravings.
- The period from Albinus to Sömmering (1737–1770) witnessed the zenith of the anatomical drawing, which was now exact in every detail and meticulously reproduced through the medium of the copperplate engraving.
- From Sömmering to the present day. With the introduction of the technique of lithography, anatomical illustrations became technically perfect, but their artistry was lost.

In Germany at the end of the fifteenth century, for example, modest booklets on medicine were published in the form of almanacs. *Der Tierkreiszeichenmann* or *The Zodiac Man* (Fig. 1.17) depicted "the different parts of the human body which are influenced by different planetary conjunctions, [and] indicated the appropriate times for blood-letting and purging under each sign of the Zodiac,

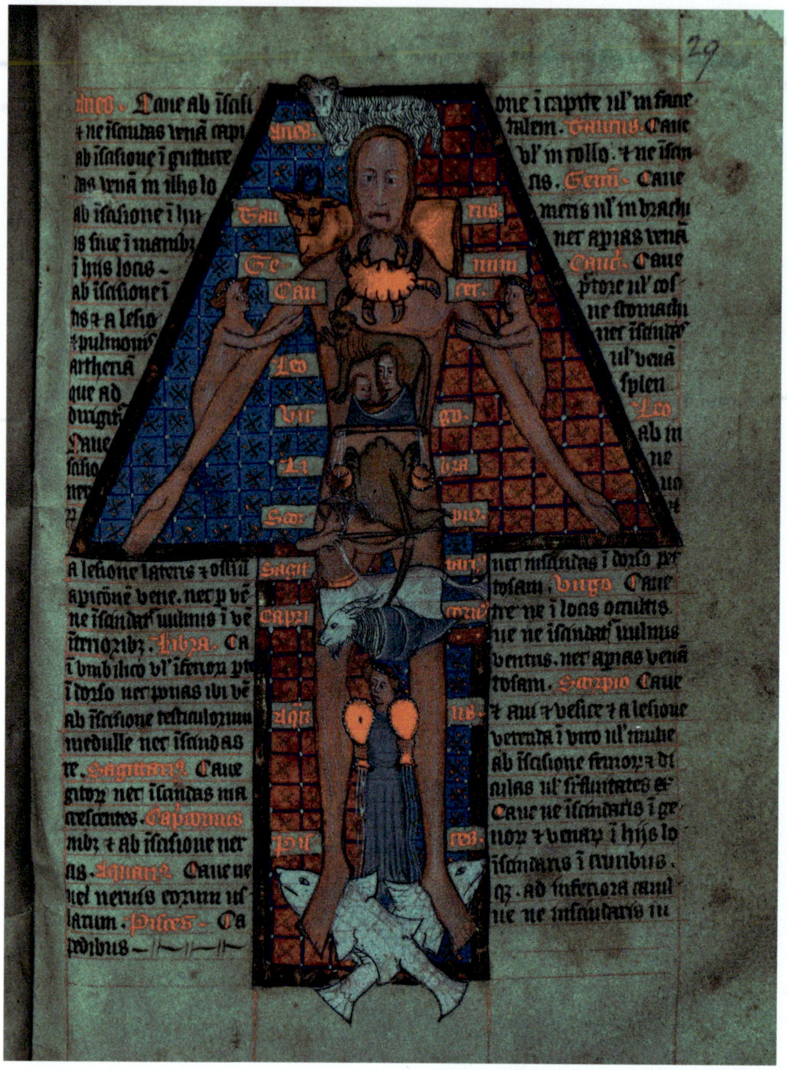

Fig. 1.17 Zodiac Man, from a calendar or astrological notes, fourteenth to fifteenth century English (on parchment). © *Corpus Christi College, Oxford, UK – Bridgeman Art Library*

with gloomy prognostications of terrible diseases" [360, 361]. The anatomical illustrations are reasonably accurate as is much of the information in the accompanying text, apart from the horoscopes.

Soon however, scientific texts with much more reliable anatomical images were being published and disseminated. Some of the first noteworthy illustrations appeared in the fifteenth century in Johannes de Ketham's *Fascicula Medicinae* [491].[20] He was a lecturer in anatomy in Vienna who diligently compiled six pre-existing anatomical texts, including that of Mondino, into a single work which was published in Latin in Venice in 1491. Heralded in Italy as the most outstanding book of the period, the first edition included five full-page

20 The identity of Johannes de Ketham has been questioned since his name does not appear in history of medicine except for this book. It has been suggested that the collector of the *Fascicula* is probably to be identified as an obscure professor of anatomy in Vienna by the name of Hans von Kircheim. The first edition was printed by the brothers Giovanni and Gregorio de Gregori in Venice in 1491. In the second edition, translated into Italian and printed in February 1494 by the same de Gregori, the name of Ketham has disappeared.

woodcuts, while the second edition contained no less than ten. One of these illustrations is quite famous. It portrays the professor of anatomy Pietro di Montagnana of Padua surrounded by the books of Pliny, Aristotle, Galen, Avicenna, and others, with three patients in the background.[21] It appears that the painter of these illustrations was the Venetian Gentile Bellini (1429–1507) or one of his students.

The illustrations in de Ketham's book were not only far more accurate than anything that came before, they also reflected the transition from a medieval to a modern concept of the science of anatomy. For example, de Ketham was the first to label the various parts of his figures with lines running to explanatory notes in the margins. Another fine woodcut (XXIII) illustrates an anatomy class. In it we can see the professor presiding over his students from a raised seat, with the *ostensor* and the *demonstrator* carrying out the dissection, and a skeleton in the background. *Fascicula Medicinae* was an immediate success because it made available to the general public for the first time a text containing accurate anatomical illustrations and it was soon translated into Italian and Spanish.[22] The originality of the illustrations is questionable [624].

Another work that deserves mention is an anatomical drawing of the abdominal muscles executed by Pietro de Abano (1250–1315) for his treatise *Conciliator*, which was published posthumously in 1497 [1].

In addition to Johannes de Ketham of Vienna, several other prominent anatomists could be found working outside Italy during the period preceding Vesalius. One of these was the surgeon Hieronimus Brunschwig of Strasbourg (1450–1534) who in 1479 published a work on wounds, fractures and other surgical problems that included excellent anatomical descriptions, particularly of the skeleton [138, 139]. It confirmed the close link between anatomy and surgery and was translated into English and other languages.

Another German working in the same period was Johannes Dryander (1500–1560) who after studying in Paris was eventually appointed professor at Marburg. In 1536 he obtained permission to conduct dissections from the prince of Hesse, to whom he dedicated his book *Anatomia Capitis Humani* (Fig. 1.18). One year later Dryander published the first part of his projected *opus magnum* on the subject, *Anatomia Hoc Est, Corporis Humani Dissectiones Pars Prior…* [252], but unfortunately the second part was never completed (Fig. 1.19). The two works that have come down to us present the results of his studies on the anatomy of the head. One series of illustrations shows the various layers of the scalp including, for the first time, the *galea capitis* and the *pericranium* (see figures in Chapter 11). Also of interest is an engraving of the soft and hard palates together with the floor of the mouth (see figure in Chapter 8), which is similar to, although less accurate than Leonardo's drawing.[23]

In 1541 Dryander published *Anatomia Mundini*, an updated version of Mondino's *Anathomia* illustrated with a fresh set of woodcuts drawn from other sources. Eighteen were copied from the *Commentaria* that Berengario wrote on Mondino's work in 1521, another twenty

21 The nine other woodcuts in the second edition illustrate: (1) Pietro and his students examining a urine sample; (2) diagrams of the four humours and twenty-three varieties of urine; (3) the bleeding of a patient; (4) the Zodiac; (5) a pregnant woman seated with her genitals exposed for examination; (6) an injured man; (7) a sick man; (8) a physician examining a patient with the plague; and (9) an anatomy session, with Mondino seated in state, overlooking the *demonstrator* and the *ostensor* who are carrying out the dissection (Fig. 1.10).

22 *Fascicula Medicinae* was generally believed to be the first illustrated text on anatomy and it is certainly the first to be printed in colour. The inexperience of the printer can be easily demonstrated by the less than accurate distribution of the colours (one of the hand of the professor in painted in red, and so is one of the hands of the *demonstrator* while the yellow of the chair is very irregular). Further research, however, suggests that some of the illustrations were copied, or at least inspired, by the illustrations on medical subjects to be found in various medieval manuscripts. Furthermore, a dissection scene by Bartolomeo Anglico (c.1200–1240) published in the encyclopaedia *De Proprietatibus Rerum* in 1491 [see 624] and other works conserved in the Bibliotheque Nationale de Paris, certainly date to an earlier period.

23 The illustrations are signed with the initials "GVB", "VB" or simply "G" which identify, at least according to Choulant, various engravers of the school of Brosamer.

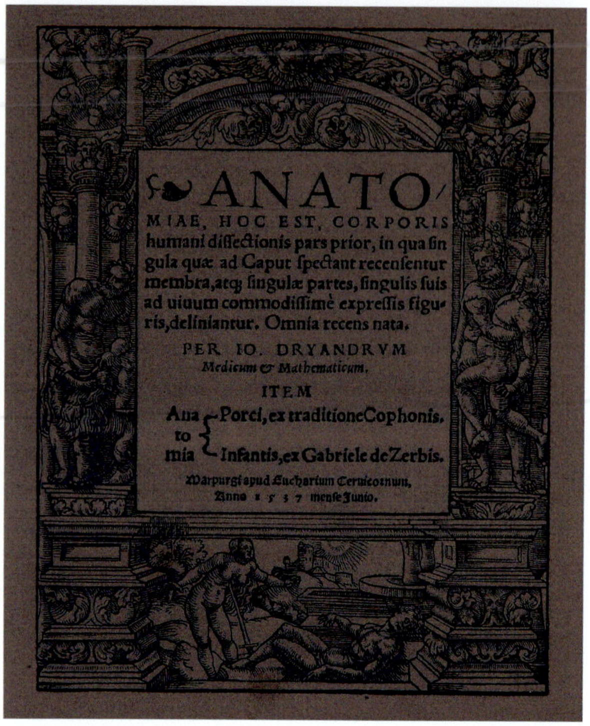

ANATOMIAE, HOC EST, CORPORIS humani dissectionis pars prior, in qua singula quæ ad Caput spectant recensentur membra, atq; singulæ partes, singulis suis ad uiuum commodissimè expressis figuris, deliniantur. Omnia recens nata.

PER IO. DRYANDRVM Medicum & Mathematicum.

ITEM

Anatomia Porci, ex traditione Cophonis. Infantis, ex Gabriele de Zerbis.

Marpurgi apud Eucharium Ceruicornum, Anno 1537 mense Junio.

Fig. 1.18 Frontispiece of *Anatomiae* by Johan Dryander (1500–1560). *Courtesy of Riccardo Mazzola, M.D., Milan*

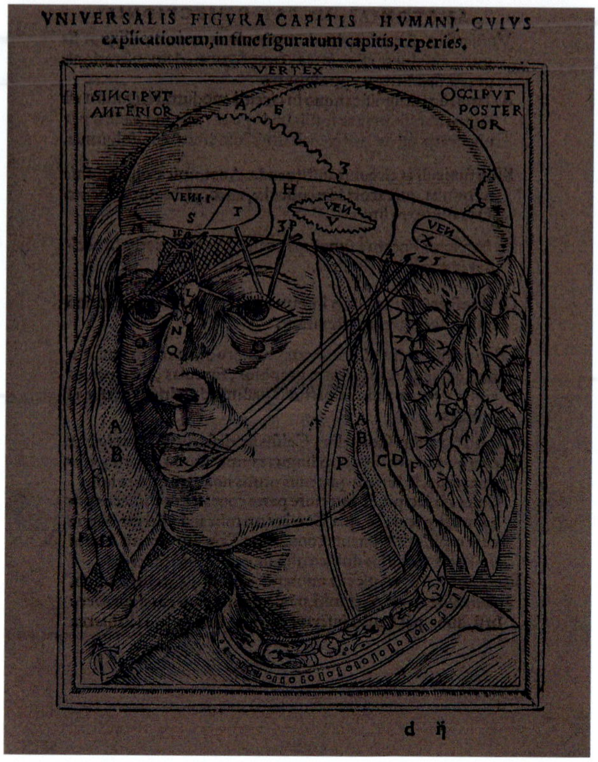
VNIVERSALIS FIGVRA CAPITIS HVMANI, CVIVS
explicationem, in fine figurarum capitis, reperies.
VERTEX
SINCIPVT ANTERIOR
OCCIPVT POSTERIOR

Fig. 1.19 One of the images of the layers of the skull by Johan Dryander (1500–1560). *Courtesy of Riccardo Mazzola, M.D., Milan*

were borrowed from Dryander's own *Anatomiae Capitis Humani*, while the remaining eight were, according to Choulant, entirely original. It has been suggested that they may have been prepared for Vesalius and stolen by Dryander, for in the preface to his *Fabrica* Vesalius complains that "a man from Marburg seems to have copied several illustrations and published them without permission."

Probably the most outstanding illustrated anatomy text to appear before Vesalius' *Fabrica* was *De Dissectione Portium Corporis Humani Libri Tres* by Charles Estienne (1503–1564) also known as Stephanus. It contains very accurate descriptions of the brain, the eye with its muscles and nerves, and other parts of the body including the male and female genital organs [283].

The publication of this work was delayed by a three-sided dispute between the author, the publisher Simon de Colines (who also happened to be his godfather) and Etienne de la Riviere, a barber-surgeon with some artistic talent who appeared to be an ideal collaborator. However in 1539 the project was interrupted by a court order (when the book was actually being printed), because de la Riviere had brought an accusation of plagiarism against Estienne. The legal battle took six years to resolve, and it was finally ordered that the name of Etienne de la Riviere should appear as one of the authors while the copyright would remain with Charles Estienne.

The publication of the book was suspended and when it finally appeared in 1545 its merits were obscured by the overwhelming success of Vesalius' *Fabrica*, which had been published just a short time before. This is a great pity because *De Dissectione Portium Corporis …* was an excellent work that included a set of highly original illustrations based on the author's own dissection studies. One, for example, describes the superficial nervous and vascular systems for the first time. Book III entitled *Prima Oculi Nudi, Tantum a Capite* is important for its detailed description of the eye with its nerves and muscles. If Estienne's work had not been preempted by Vesalius' *Fabrica*, it would have represented the first anatomical

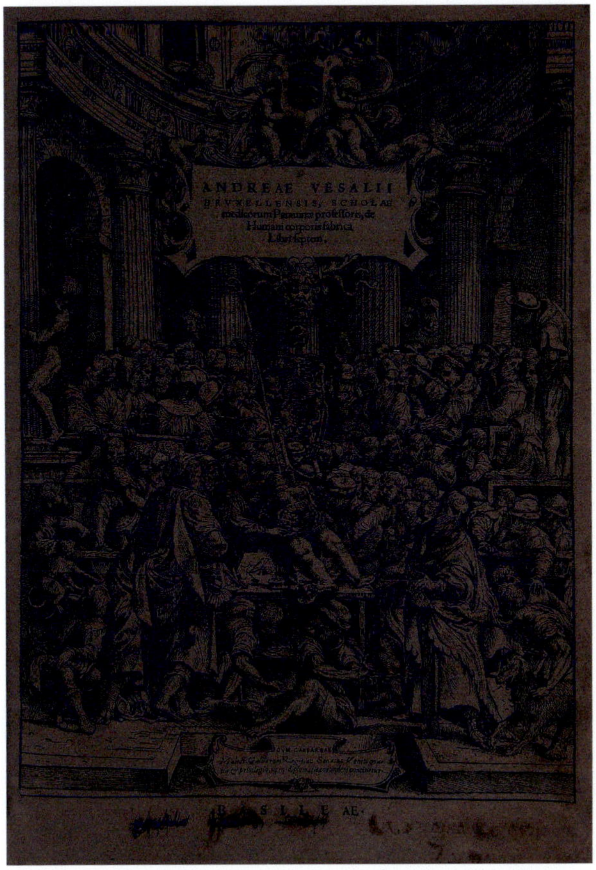

Fig. 1.20 Frontispiece of the *Humana Corporis Fabrica* by Vesalius. The first edition was published in Basel by Joannis Oporinus in 1543. *Courtesy of Riccardo Mazzola, M.D., Milan*

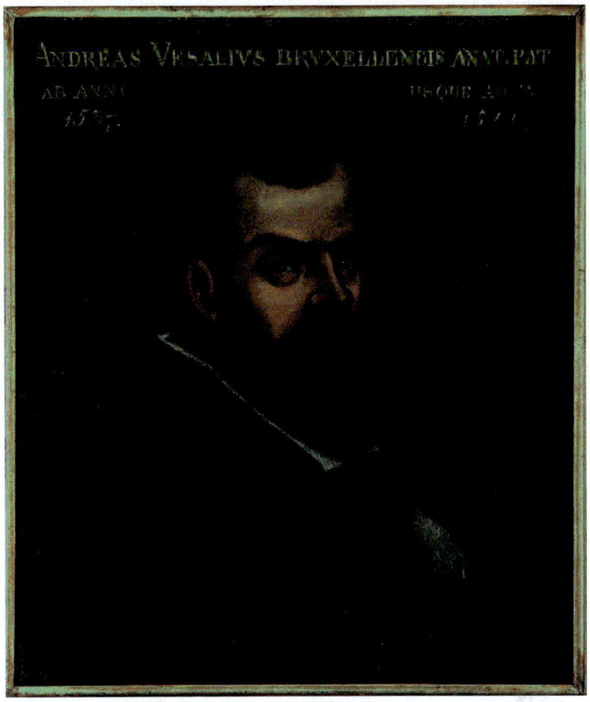

Fig. 1.21 Andrea Vesalius (1514–1564), "the Reformer of Anatomy". The picture is in the Hall of the Medical School of the University of Padua. *Courtesy of the Rector of the University of Padua*

text entirely illustrated with figures based on dissections carried out by the author himself.

The Revolutionary Reforms of Andrea Vesalius (1514–1564)

By the beginning of the sixteenth century the teaching of anatomy had changed substantially. There now were schools where the subject was taught more or less systematically following a specific programme and instruction was based on the observation of actual dissections. In addition, the preparation of accurate anatomical illustrations and the possibility of printing them made the dissemination of knowledge much easier than it had been in the past. Of this improved climate Bettman wrote: "Modern medicine was born with the publication of the first complete treatise on human anatomy." This was *Humani Corporis Fabrica* (Fig. 1.20), commonly referred to as *Fabrica*, by Andrea Vesalius (Fig. 1.21).

Born into a family of physicians and pharmacists on 31 December 1515 in the Belgian town of Wesen, from which he derived his name, Vesalius carried out meticulous dissections on small animals as a boy, demonstrating an interest in the organs and inner workings of living things that was precocious and out of the ordinary. It has been suggested that his fascination with human anatomy may have been stimulated by the conversations he overheard between his father and artists who came to the shop to purchase pigments and solvents.

After attending lectures in the liberal arts at the university in Louvain for three and a half years, Vesalius went to Paris in August 1533 to study medicine under

Jean Femel, Johan Guenther and above all Jacobus Dubois, better known as Sylvius (1478–1555). Dubois was a follower of Galen's school of medicine who conducted anatomical studies on animals and human cadavers (with the help of a barber-surgeon, who did the actual dissecting) in order to test the theories of the Greek physician [253, 254]. These sessions no doubt failed to satisfy Vesalius' thirst for knowledge through direct experience. While still a student he obtained permission to carry out public dissections in front of the Faculty of Medicine and his demonstrations were so impressive that he was officially appointed Sylvius' teaching assistant. The young Vesalius however did not appreciate his professor's conventional approach to anatomy, and differences soon arose between them: "I do not consider him to be an anatomist, and suffer when I see him inflict as many cuts as I have seen him attempt on men and on every other animal, except when … I am at table with him."

Vesalius had been received with favour at the French court, and indeed originally considered dedicating *Fabrica* to the queen, but he left Paris in 1536 when war seemed imminent between the Emperor Charles V and the French army. He returned to Louvain, where it seems that he stole the cadaver of a criminal which had been left hanging on the public gallows outside the city wall, and used it to prepare an articulated skeleton (Fig. 1.22). This impious act scandalized the conservative Catholic town and Vesalius left once again, this time settling in Padua where he received his degree on 5 December 1537. In the following year he was nominated professor of anatomy at the university.

Vesalius immediately revolutionized the teaching methods at Padua, which were still based on Mondino's system of *ostensor* and *demonstrator*, and began to conduct dissections personally (Fig. 1.23). He generally used human cadavers but made additional comparative studies on animals, often *in vivo*. His courses were a remarkable success and sometimes drew as many as five hundred observers, not only students but also practising physicians. He delivered his lessons in an anatomical theatre that had been prepared especially for him based on the design by Alessandro Benedetti. Since this was the period of the Inquisition, Vesalius' operating table was constructed in such a way that it could be turned over to disguise the room's purpose, a stratagem which seems to have been sufficient to mislead the authorities of the Church.

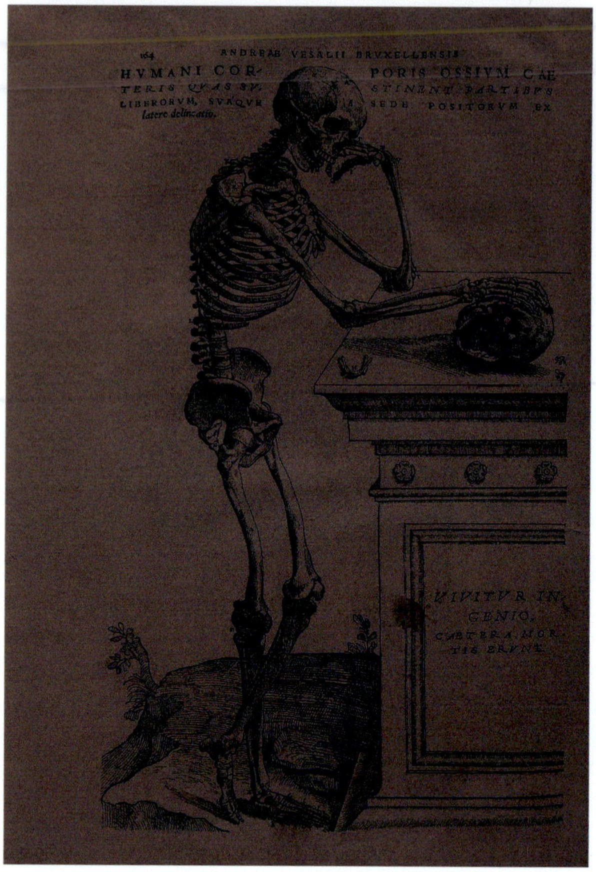

Fig. 1.22 *Tabula* of a skeleton taken from the *Fabrica* by Vesalius. The anatomical accuracy is not affected by the artistic pose. *Courtesy of Riccardo Mazzola, M.D., Milan*

Vesalius carried out his dissections with the most conscientious attention to detail. This allowed him to correct many inaccuracies and errors that had been passively transmitted since the time of Galen due to the fact that most dissections had been conducted on animals. Just one year after his appointment in 1538 Vesalius published his *Tabulae Anatomicae*, also known as *Tabulae Sex* since it contained six anatomical illustrations, magnificent works prepared from his dissections. These became extremely well known, in part because pirated copies were printed in large numbers and sold all over Europe to meet the demand for accurate anatomical drawings.

Vesalius published his most important book, *De Humani Corpori Fabrica Libri Septem* [1014–1016] at the

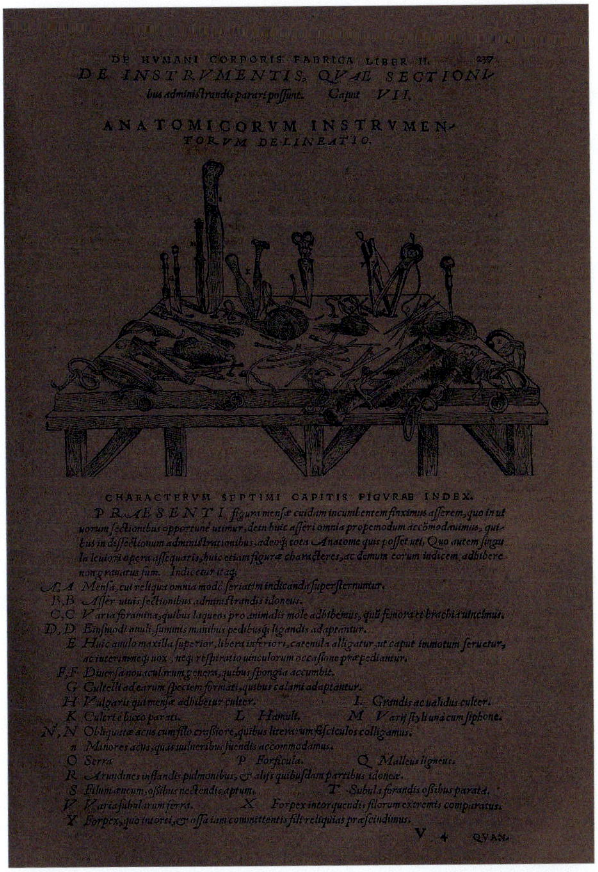

Fig. 1.23 The anatomical instruments of Vesalius shown in a page of his *Fabrica*. *Courtesy of Riccardo Mazzola, M.D., Milan*

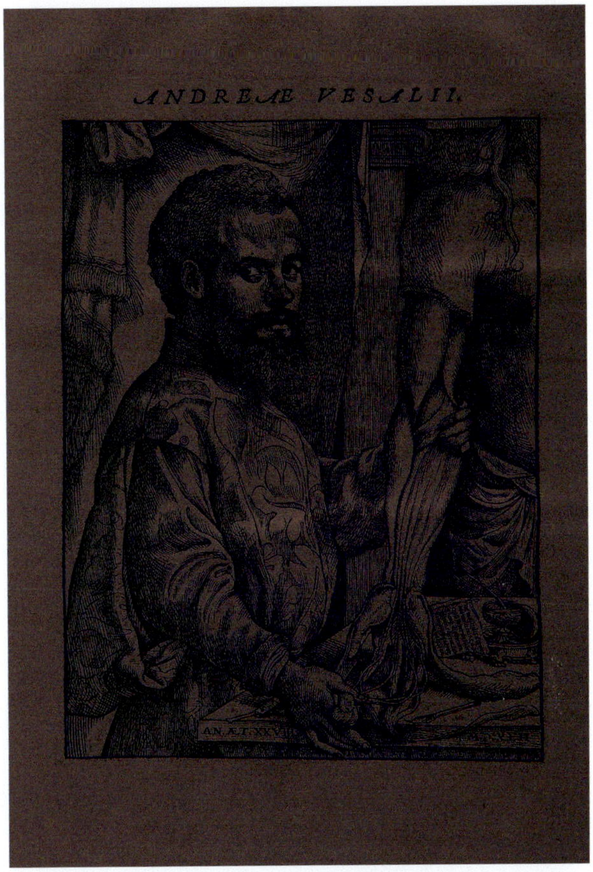

Fig. 1.24 Portrait of Vesalius taken from the second edition (1555) of the *Fabrica*. *Courtesy of Riccardo Mazzola, M.D., Milan*

age of 26 (Fig. 1.24). This remarkable work consisted of 659 pages with 203 anatomical illustrations, of which 19 were full-page plates and two were spread over two facing pages. On the title page we see Vesalius himself, surrounded by a crowd of students, conducting a dissection on a female cadaver (Fig. 1.20). Conscious of the substantial contribution that this book would make to the medical sciences, Vesalius chose both his publisher and his artists carefully and supervised the details of every step in its production. The work was dedicated to the Emperor Charles V and printed in Basel by Joannis Oporinus, who was a follower of Paracelsus. The woodblocks were prepared in Venice and Vesalius carried them to Basel himself in order to supervise the placement of the illustrations in the text and their final printing.

The artist responsible for the anatomical drawings on which the woodcuts were based is unknown and has formed the subject of considerable debate. There is general agreement that he must have been a follower of Titian and Giorgio Vasari (1511–1574) was probably correct in identifying him as the Flemish artist Stephan van Kalkar (c.1499–1550), who had studied under Titian, but this opinion has not been universally accepted, some experts retaining that van Kalkar merely supervised the preparation of the woodcuts (Figs 1.25, 1.26).

While he was in Basel overseeing the publication of his book Vesalius visited Charles V, who was so impressed by his gifts that he invited him to become his personal physician. Vesalius accepted and would hold this post for the remainder of his life, thus abandoning at

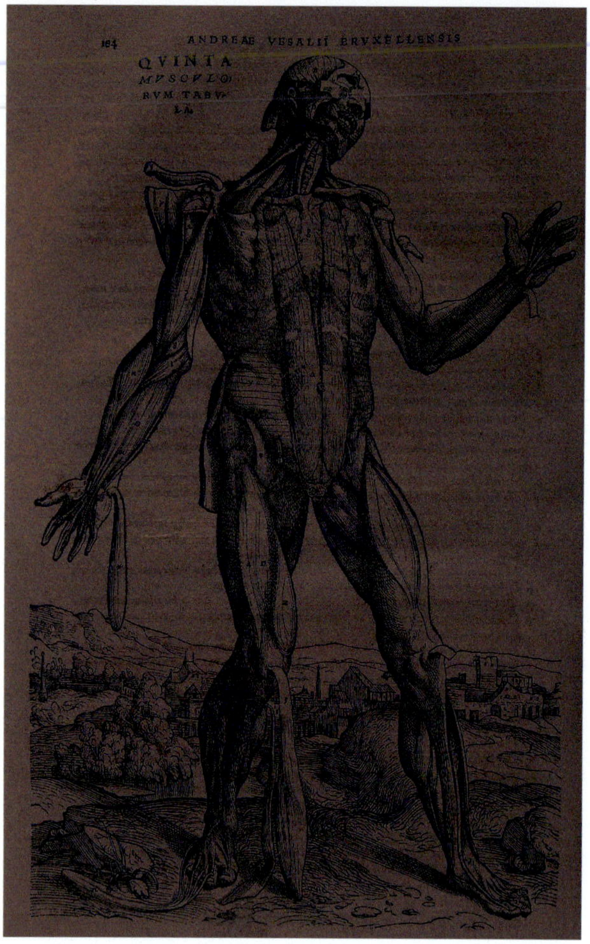

Fig. 1.25 Muscles in a *Tabula* from the *Fabrica* by Vesalius. *Courtesy of Riccardo Mazzola, M.D., Milan*

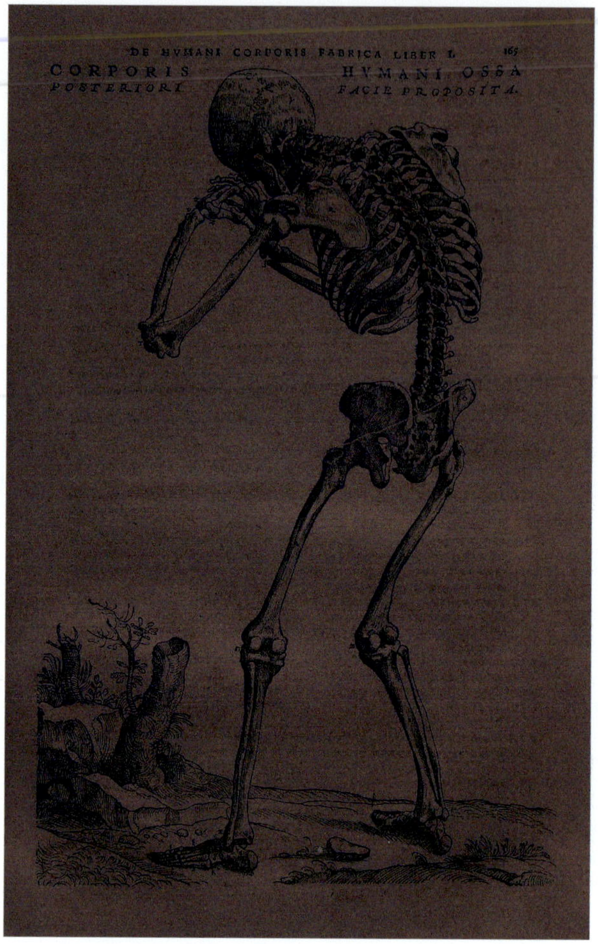

Fig. 1.26 Another skeleton by Vesalius. *Courtesy of Riccardo Mazzola, M.D., Milan*

the age of 28 a promising academic career for life at the imperial court. Destiny, however, had a less than happy fate in store for Vesalius. The physician, who had defied the Church's ban on dissections, was condemned by the Inquisition to make a pilgrimage to the Holy Land. This was a relatively clement sentence, but as Vesalius was returning from Jerusalem his ship sank off the coast of Zante. He perished and was buried on the Greek island at the age of 50.

Vesalius taught at the University of Padua for only four years, but during this period he literally revolutionized the study of anatomy. When documenting the results of his meticulous dissections, he devoted equal attention to the written descriptions and the illustrations to ensure their complete accuracy. The scientific precision and visual beauty of his anatomical drawings ensured the success of *Fabrica*, which inspired a new generation of anatomists (Figs. 1.27, 1.28). By applying his knowledge of embryology and comparative anatomy to the systematic study of the human organs, he was able to comprehend every aspect of their structure. Oddly enough the name of Vesalius is not linked to the discovery of any organs but there is no doubt that, despite the brevity of his career, he fully deserves the title of the "Reformer of Anatomy".

One merely has to compare his work with any of the texts, even the finest, that preceded it to realize the importance and originality of his contribution. Vesalius'

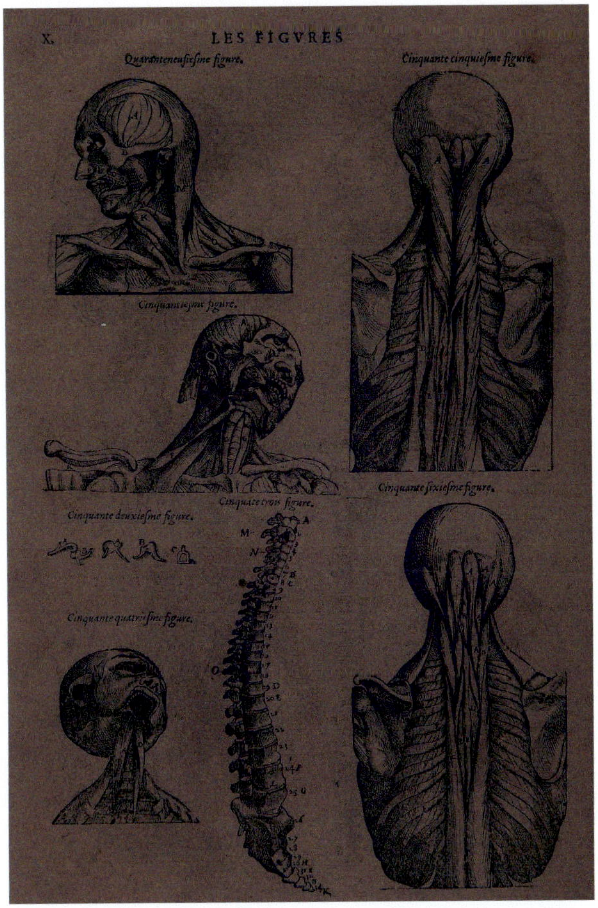

Fig. 1.27 Anatomical drawings from *Les Oeuvres* (1575) by Ambroise Paré. *Courtesy of Riccardo Mazzola, M.D., Milan*

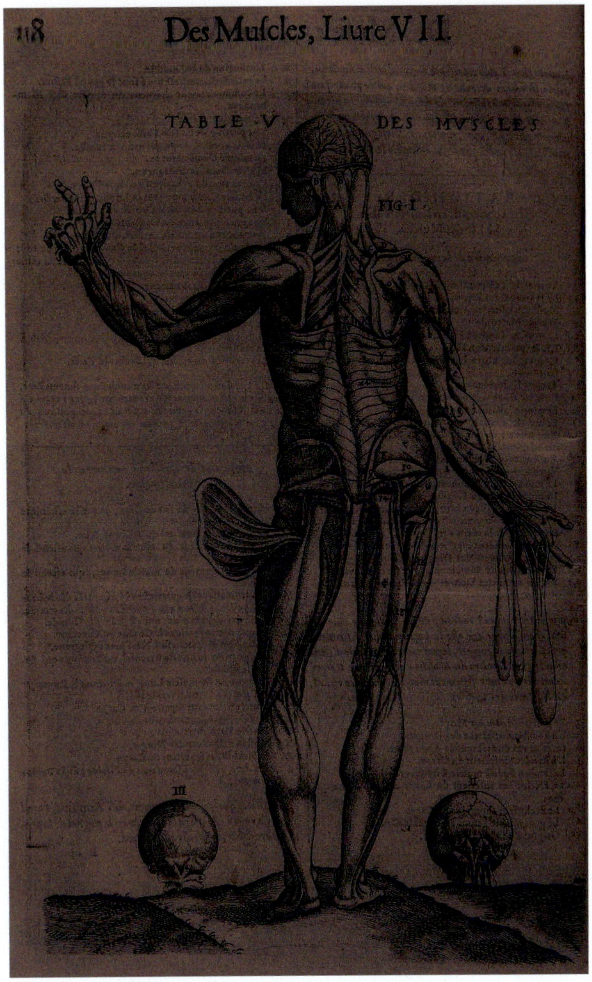

Fig. 1.28 Anatomical drawings from *Les Oeuvres de Chirurgie* (1598) by J. Guillemeau, a pupil of Paré. *Courtesy of Riccardo Mazzola, M.D., Milan*

achievements lay in the fact that he based his descriptions exclusively on his own observations, and thus was able to free himself from the bonds of Galen and the other authorities of Antiquity. When referring to Galen in his work *Epithome*[24] (1543), he noted: "Although easily chief of the masters, nevertheless he did not dissect the human body, and the fact is now evident that he described, not to say imposed on us, the fabric of the ape's body, although it differs in many respects [from that of humans]".

The Successors to Vesalius in Padua

When Vesalius gave up his position as professor of anatomy at Padua he did not leave a vacuum as in four years he had established an excellent school of anatomy that was able to continue his work. His immediate successor was Realdus Columbus (c.1516–1559), who later also taught in Pisa and Rome (Fig. 1.29). Columbus' book *De Re Anatomica*, published in the year of his death, is perhaps more readable and even better illustrated than

24 *Epithome* was an abridged version of *Fabrica* prepared by Vesalius and printed, according to Choulant [178], in the same year as the complete work by the same printer in Basel.

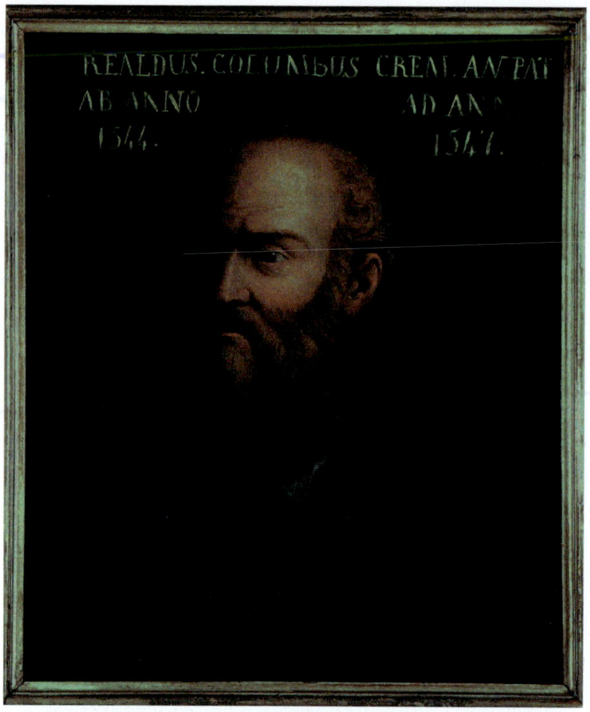

Fig. 1.29 Realdus Columbus (c.1516–1559) in a portrait hung in the hall of the Medical School of Padua. *Courtesy of the Rector of the University of Padua*

Vesalius' *Fabrica*, although it was less innovative [188]. The heart and aorta with their valves, for example, are described with great accuracy.

Columbus was however accused of stealing the ideas for his description of the lungs and pulmonary circulation, which laid the foundations for the discoveries of Harvey, from Michael Servetus (1511–1563), a Spanish physician and theologian who had been burned at the stake by a Catholic-Calvinist tribunal in Geneva called *Il Piccolo Concilio* for his opposition to the Catholic Church. All of his books were condemned to be burned, but it seems that some were pulled from the fire and saved, eventually reaching Colombus, who copied the sections on the pulmonary circulation.

In 1547 Colombus met the artist Michelangelo and attempted to persuade him to illustrate his book, but unfortunately for us, the famous artist showed no interest in the project.

One of Colombus' students was Jan de Valverde (c.1525–1587), the author of *Historia de la Composition del Corpo Humano*, a Spanish version of Vesalius' *Fabrica*. This work met with such a positive reception that it was soon translated into Latin, Italian and Flemish and published in several editions in Venice, Antwerp and Amsterdam [1003, 1004]. Its immense success lay perhaps in the fact that the book was printed in a smaller, more manageable and less costly format than Vesalius' tome, even though it included all of his illustrations as well as some new ones. Among these was a famous representation of the "flayed man",[25] an idea which Valverde may have borrowed from Michelangelo. Vesalius did not appreciate this brazen plagiarism of his work, however, and wrote: "Valverde who never set his own hand to a dissection and is ignorant of medicine as well as of the primary disciples, undertook to expound our art in the Spanish language only for the sake of shameful profit."

Gabriele Fallopius (1523–1565) also studied under Vesalius at Padua. After teaching anatomy at Ferrara and then Pisa, he returned to Padua where he published *Observationes Anatomicae* [296] and later *Tractatus de Decoratione* [298]. The books describes the results of his anatomical studies on various organs including the cranial nerves, the soft and hard palates, and the uterine tubes that bear his name. Fallopius' distinguished career was interrupted by his premature death at the age of 39.

Another illustrious anatomist in Bologna was Voicher Coiter (1534–1576), a contemporary of Fallopius who is considered to be the founder of modern embryology. Coiter studied the development of embryos up to and beyond the age of 20 days. Particularly interesting are his pioneering observations on the development of the skeletal system, which were based on the dissection of aborted fetuses and the cadavers of small children, *Tractatus Anatomicus de Ossibus Foetus Abortive* [187]. He completed his embryological studies with experiments conducted on 20-day chick embryos and published his results in the first systematic treatise on embryology to appear since the time of Aristotle. This includes *De Auditus Instrumento*, a remarkable chapter on the development of the ear.

---

25 In the Bargello Museum in Florence are two very fine statuettes of a "flayed man" by Ludovico Cardi, one carved in 1596 and the other in 1600. The artist's rendition of the muscles is remarkably accurate.

Coiter was the first of a series of post-Vesalian anatomists who have earned a place in the history of medicine for their studies of specific organs or organ systems; others include Fabricius ab Aquapendente, Giulio Casserio, Gaspare Aselli and William Harvey.

The opening decades of the seventeenth century were a most auspicious period for scientific research in Padua, as anatomists could benefit from the friendship and intellectual stimulus of colleagues working in other fields. The scientist Galileo Galilei was present in Padua around the same time as Gerolamo Fabricius ab Aquapendente (1533–1619) (Fig. 1.30) and William Harvey. He was said to be quite friendly with both of them. Harvey learned of the existence of the venous valves while studying anatomy under Fabricius and these structures would later provide him with the key to the mechanism of the pulmonary circulation.

Fabricius carried on his studies where Coiter left off and made a series of discoveries in comparative embryology that helped to lay the foundations for this branch of study as a separate science [293].[26] Among his many insights, he provided an explanation for various congenital malformations in humans (a subject which also greatly interested Harvey), retracing their origin back to the embryo [290]. Fabricius was the first to describe, in a text illustrated with copperplate engravings and published in Venice in 1600, the crystalline lens of the eye[27] and the structure of the ear [289].[28] He also grasped the close relationship that exists between the voice and the sense of hearing. As Richard Eimas [276] wrote, his anatomical illustrations remained "unsurpassed for many years". Fabricius also completed the construction of the anatomical theatre initiated a century earlier by Alessandro Benedetti.

Fabricius' studies of the organ of hearing were continued by his student Giulio Casserio (1581–1616), who in *De Vocis Auditusque* [159] provides a surprisingly modern description of the hearing and vocal apparatuses, illustrated with magnificent copperplate engravings. The book is divided into two parts. In the first we find anatomical drawings of the larynx and the sensory nerves, as well as the first recorded account of a tracheotomy. In the second part dissections of the organs of hearing in various species are presented and the ossicles are described for the first time. Casserio is also famous for his *Tabulae Anatomicae*, which was published posthumously in Venice in 1627 and contains detailed embryological studies. The copperplate engravings were the work of Francesco Valesio who, like van Kalkar, had studied under Titian. Among the last anatomists produced by the school of Vesalius we find the Belgian Adriaan van der Spieghel, known as Spigelius (1578–1625), whose son-in-law Antonicles van der Linden compiled and published after his death an excellent *Opera Omnia* containing a superb set of anatomical illustrations [948]. Van der Linden was also the author of a detailed work on embryology [563, 564].

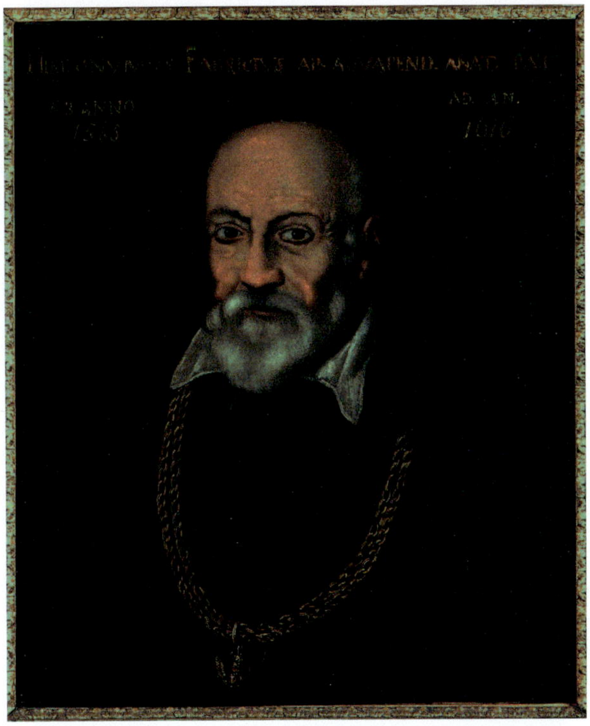

Fig. 1.30 Fabricius ab Aquapendente (1533–1619) who was professor of anatomy in Padua from 1565 to 1616 in a portrait hung in the hall of the Medical School of the University of Padua. *Courtesy of the Rector of the University of Padua*

26 See in particular, in Part I, the chapter *De Formatio Fetu*.

27 See *De Oculo, Visus Organo*.

28 See *De Visione, Voce Auditus*.

Other Schools of Anatomy in Italy

While Padua had perhaps the most outstanding school of anatomy in sixteenth century Europe, other universities made significant contributions. In Ferrara, for example, there was Giovanni Battista Canano (1515–1579), the author of an excellent work on the muscles entitled *Muscolorum Humani Corporis Picturata Dissectio* [154] which was illustrated by Girolamo da Carpi. Just after it was printed, however, Canano came across a copy of *Fabrica* and overcome with despair at how poorly his work compared with Vesalius' opus, he attempted to destroy every single copy of *Muscolorum*. Eleven exemplars survived, allowing Henry Cushing in 1925 to print a facsimile edition in Florence, and more recently Levi Robert Lindt to publish an English translation [562].

Perhaps the most important anatomist outside Padua in the sixteenth century was Bartolomeo Eustachius (1520–1574). Born in the town of San Severino Marche in the Papal State, he enrolled at the Faculty of Medicine in Rome and upon completion of his studies in 1539 was nominated *Physicus*[29] at the court of the Duke of Urbino. In 1549 he returned to Rome to take up the post of personal physician to Giulio Feltre della Rovere, the brother of the duke who later became Pope Paul III. Appointed professor of anatomy at the Università della Sapienza in Rome, he obtained permission to conduct dissections on human cadavers in an unusual concession by the Holy See.

A series of treatises by Eustachius, *De Auditus Organis*, *De Rerum Structure*, *De Vena Quae Azygos Graecis Dicitur* and *De Dentibus*, were brought together in a volume entitled *Opuscola Anatomica* [287, 288] and published in Venice by Vincenzo Luchino in 1563 in a limited edition with a small number of illustrations. These were among the few works by Eustachius to appear in print during his lifetime. Indeed the anatomist died before his most important book, *De Partibus Humani Corporis*, could be completed. The fifty-four woodcuts prepared for *De Partibus* in 1552 were delivered together with the manuscript to Matteo Pini, a student of Eustachius' who had been asked to supervise the publication of the work. Instead, for a variety of reasons this material ended up in the Vatican Library and much of it was lost. Some time later a descendent of Pini, the priest Andrea de Rossi, discovered the surviving text and, realizing its importance, asked the intercession of Giovanni Maria Lancisi, the physician to Pope Clement XI, to have *De Partibus*—or what remained of it—published. It finally appeared in Rome in 1714 (Fig. 1.31), but by this time the medical world's attention was entirely monopolized by Vesalius' *Fabrica*. Singer affirms that if *De Partibus* had been published when Eustachius was still alive, Vesalius would have had to share with him the title of "the founder of modern anatomy".

Eustachius' illustrations (Fig. 1.32), although less impressive, are certainly more accurate than Vesalius', and his text describes many significant discoveries. Furthermore, Eustachius was one of the first scientists to utilize the technique of copperplate engraving, which allowed the reproduction of far more minute detail. He also introduced the use of a grid along the margins of his illustrations to help the reader locate the different structures mentioned in the text.

Many anatomical discoveries can be attributed to Eustachius. He published the first work, *De Dentibus*, entirely dedicated to the teeth and describes their innervation in considerable detail. He also studied the structure of the ear: the ossicles, the tympanic membrane, the stapedius muscles, the valves and the tube that bears his name. Many of these discoveries are reported in *De Auditus Organis* (1562), which formed part of the small body of works published during his lifetime. Eustachius also deserves credit for having described the thoracic duct almost one hundred years before Pecquet.

Another Italian, Gaspare Aselli (1581–1625), who was born in Cremona and became professor of anatomy and surgery at the university in Pavia, was the author of a crucial discovery regarding the lymphatic system. During the dissection of a dog that had consumed a fatty meal just before its death, he observed a milky fluid emerge from an incision made in a lymphatic duct

29 Urbino had a most sophisticated public health service created primarily to care for those injured during the twenty or so wars conducted by Duke Federico during the course of two decades. The *Medicus publicus* or head of the Grand Duchy's medical service bore the imposing title of *Doctore Physicus et moderatore delle ossa* and was required to have a good knowledge of traumatology. This was considered so important that Costanzo Felici, perhaps the most renowned physician of the century, was not accepted for the position because he had no experience in this area [892].

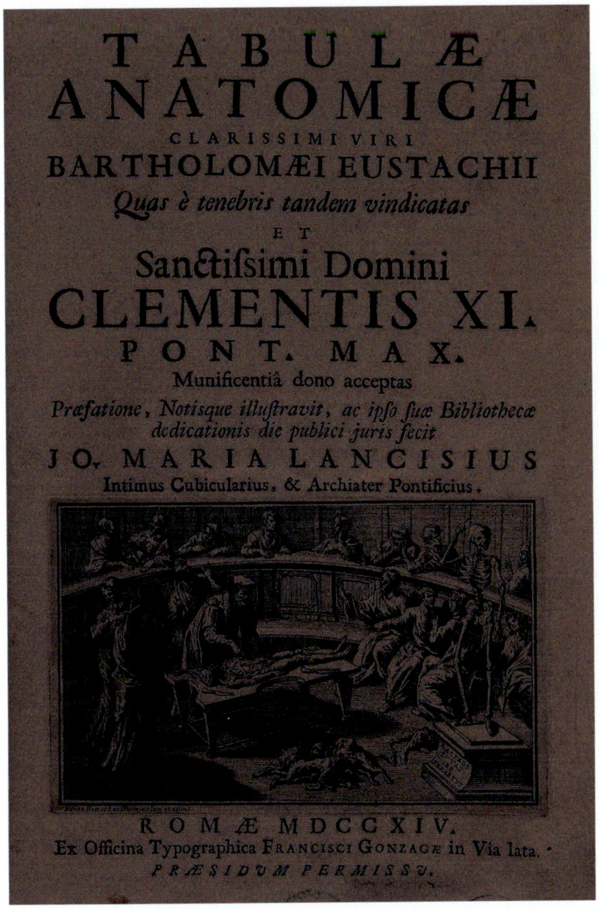

TABULÆ ANATOMICÆ
CLARISSIMI VIRI
BARTHOLOMÆI EUSTACHII
Quas è tenebris tandem vindicatas
ET
Sanctiſsimi Domini
CLEMENTIS XI.
PONT. MAX.
Munificentiâ dono acceptas
Præfatione, Notisque illuſtravit, ac ipſo ſuæ Bibliothecæ dedicationis die publici juris fecit
JO. MARIA LANCISIUS
Intimus Cubicularius, & Archiater Pontificius.

ROMÆ MDCCXIV.
Ex Officina Typographica FRANCISCI GONZAGÆ in Via lata.
PRÆSIDUM PERMISSU.

Fig. 1.31 Frontispiece of the book *Tabulae Anatomiacae* by Bartolomeo Eustachius (1520–1574). The book was published posthumously in 1714 in Rome. *Courtesy of Riccardo Mazzola, M.D., Milan*

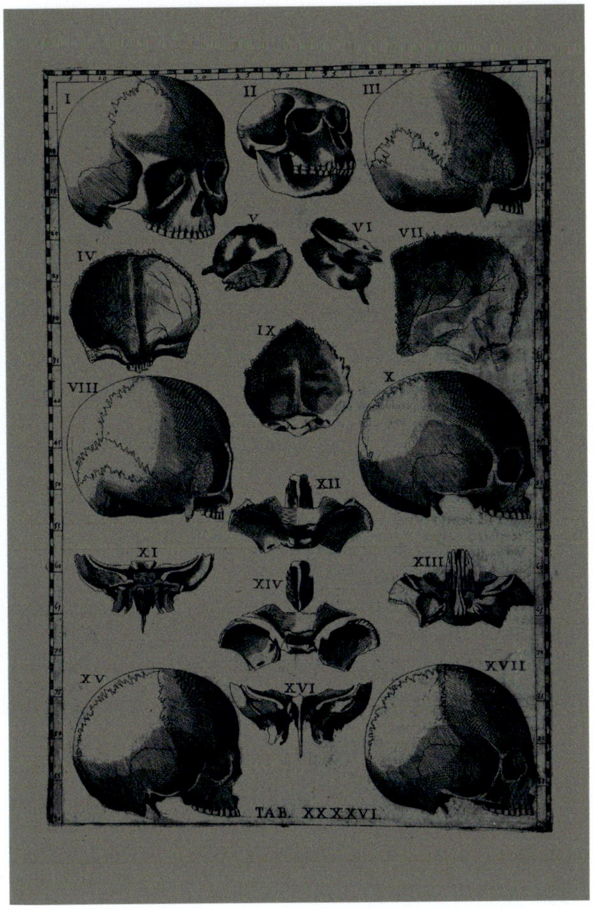

Fig. 1.32 An example of the high quality of Eustachius' anatomical drawings which have been judged better than those of Vesalius. *Courtesy of Riccardo Mazzola, M.D., Milan*

and realized that he must have severed one of the chyle vessels, structures described by the ancient Greek physicians Herophilus, Galen and Herasistratus but subsequently forgotten by anatomists. However, as we learn from a work published posthumously in Milan (1627) by his friend and colleague Tadino, who had been present at the dissection, Aselli believed that the chyle vessels emptied into the liver rather than the thoracic ducts. Some time later the French physiologist Jean Pecquet (1622–1674) rediscovered the thoracic ducts and described their function, publishing a book on the lymphatic circulation in 1651.

Anatomy Outside Italy After Vesalius

Although Italy was the centre for anatomical studies in the sixteenth century, important work was also being conducted elsewhere in Europe. For example in England, where anatomy, like the other arts and sciences, blossomed somewhat later than on the Continent and progress was slowed by restrictive legislation concerning the use of cadavers for teaching purposes, a license permitting dissections to be conducted by the Barber Surgeons Company in London was granted by Henry VIII in 1540.[30] We also know that during the mid-1560s anatomical demonstra-

30 At the Royal College of Surgeons in London is a very fine painting by Holbein commemorating the granting by King Henry VIII of a royal charter to Thomas Vicary of the Barber Surgeons. There is a similar painting in the Barber Surgeons' Hall.

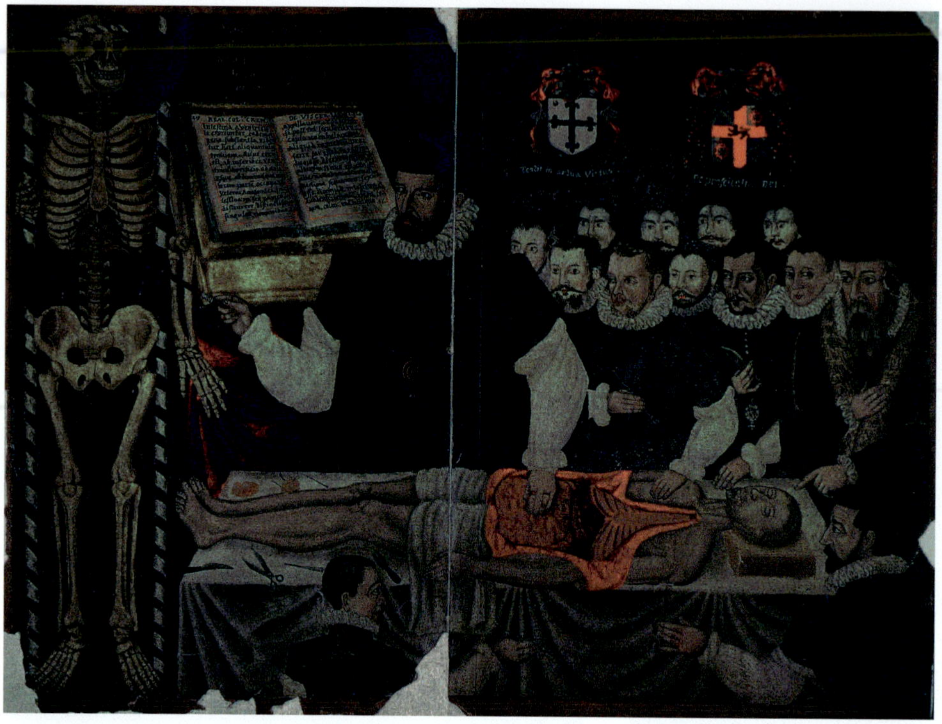

Fig. 1.33 John Bannister teaching students (oil on brown paper), sixteenth century English School, in William Hunter Collection. © *Glasgow University Library, Scotland – Bridgeman Art Library*

tions were given in the Company's hall by an Italian, Giulio Borgarucci, who had studied in Padua,[31] and that all members were required to attend these sessions.

Henry VIII's daughter, Queen Elizabeth, continued her father's policy and authorized dissections at the College of Physicians in 1565. Surgeons, or "barber surgeons" as they were called, were addressed as "Mr" rather than "Dr" and could only become affiliates (fellows), not members, of the College. This was the origin of the title "Fellow of the Royal College of Surgeons", which is still in use today to designate surgeons in the British Isles and the greater Commonwealth (FRCS). One of the first members of the Barber Surgeons Company was John Bannister (1533–1610), who was nominated Lecturer in Anatomy in 1572; his work was in large part inspired by Colombus and Vesalius (Fig. 1.33).

However, the English school of anatomy reached its peak with the discoveries of William Harvey (1578–1657)[415–418]. Born in Folkstone, Harvey studied medicine at Cambridge with John Caius and, after obtaining his degree, spent five years in Padua where he earned a second degree in 1602. In Italy he studied under Fabricius ab Aquapendente and became friends with Galileo Galilei. Harvey returned to England in 1615 and began teaching at the College of Physicians. During this same period he worked out the details of his revolutionary theory on the circulation of the blood.

In Padua Harvey had learned from Galileo how to apply the quantitative methodology of physics to the science of biology. If, as he estimated, every heartbeat sent two ounces of blood coursing round the body, it was a simple matter to calculate that at a rhythm of 72 beats per minute no less than 8,640 ounces of blood would circulate in the space of one hour. Anatomists were forced to ask themselves how it was possible that, in accordance with the generally accepted model of Galen, such an enormous volume of blood could pass in this amount of time from the right to the left side of the heart across the barrier presented by the interventricular septum, filtering through pores so small that no one had actually ever seen them. Harvey succeeded in demonstrating that this constant quantity of blood in reality travelled through

31 It is not known whether Giulio Borgarucci was related to the eminent Prospero Borgarucci who succeeded Vesalius as professor of anatomy at the university in Padua in 1564.

two complete circuits. The first was what he referred to as the "greater circle" that started from the left side of the heart and passed through the entire body by means of the arteries before returning to the right side of the heart through the veins. At this point the "lesser circle" brought the blood from the right side to the lungs and then back to the left side of the heart, where it began a fresh journey through the "greater circle". This hypothesis represented a bold challenge to concepts that had been accepted for centuries and Harvey had the greatest difficulty in persuading his colleagues to abandon the theories of Galen.

Naturally dissections of the heart and blood vessels contributed to the understanding and acceptance of his radical new idea, but definitive confirmation was obtained through *in vivo* studies on animals. Using the fundamental laws of hydrodynamics, Harvey applied ligatures at strategic points and conducted perfusion experiments, demonstrating for the first time that the heart acted exactly like a pump, pushing the blood through the two circles separately in a continuous cycle that lasted as long as life itself. These physiological principles are taken for granted today, but during the seventeenth century were anything but self-evident.

Harvey's complete description of the circulatory system took up seventy pages in his book and were a monumental event in the history of medicine [418]. An entirely new nomenclature had to be developed as a result of his discoveries, so that what were once called the "arterial veins" became the "pulmonary arteries" while the "venous arteries" became the "pulmonary veins". Before Harvey's studies, the distinction between these vessels was made solely on the basis of the colour of the blood contained in them, which was dark in the veins and lighter in the arteries.

Harvey also introduced the concept that different organs perform completely separate functions, a fundamental insight that would have enormous consequences for the study of medicine. It is therefore not surprising that R. Eimas [276] declared: "Probably no name is better known in the history of medicine than that of William Harvey."

As we have mentioned, Harvey's ideas met with great resistance. Distinguished scientists including Primerose attacked him for trying to overturn the theories of Galen. The opposition became so virulent that Harvey was obliged to move to Frankfurt in order to publish his book *De Motu Cordis* (1628) [415]. Only one hundred copies were printed in an abridged version that was described by Singer [932, 933] as "a pitifully small quarter [of the entire work]". We can imagine how difficult it was for Harvey's contemporaries to grasp a theory that was based purely on mathematical calculations—although for this very reason scientifically demonstrable—just as it was difficult for them to accept the notion that different organs might have separate functions and yet remain closely interconnected.

However, *De Motu Cordis* [415] eventually triumphed after the initially hostile reception and not only gained acceptance but was reprinted several times. In 1651 Harvey published another book, *De Generationem Animalium* which presented his theories on embryology. Rejecting the notion of "pre-formation", he demonstrated that all the various parts of the fetus gradually developed from the original egg [416, 417]. His embryology studies were the most important to be conducted since Aristotle, and all the more remarkable if one considers that the microscope was not yet available to him. All his works were included in *Opera Omnia* published in 1766, over a century after his death [418].

The anatomical studies conducted in England at the end of the seventeenth and during the first half of the eighteenth centuries focused on specific structures, many of which are of direct interest to plastic surgery. For example the maxillary sinus was described by Nathaniel Highmore (1613–1685) and named after him [431] although in reality the existence of this structure had already been reported by Casserio (1600) and it appears in a drawing by Leonardo dating from 1490. While at Oxford, Highmore collaborated with Harvey on his studies of chick embryos, arriving at results that Malpighi would confirm twenty years later [432].

William Cheselden (1688–1752) was an outstanding surgeon and anatomist[32] who worked at St Thomas' Hospital, London and then in Chelsea. He published two texts, *The Anatomy of the Human Body* [175] and *Osteographia of the Anatomy of the Bones* (1733). The second work was illustrated with engravings prepared

32 According to Garrison [360, 361]), Cheselden was probably the fastest surgeon who ever lived, known for being able to execute a lithotomy in 54 seconds!

by the Dutch artist Gerard van der Gucht (d.1776) from Cheselden's own anatomical drawings. A vignette on the cover shows us that the physician was aided in his task by a new invention, the camera obscura. The comparative anatomy illustrations were the work of another Dutch artist, Jacob Schijvoet, and show the skeletons of different species in curious attitudes. The human anatomical structures are depicted life-sized and each illustration is decorated with vignettes and osteological motifs.

The Dutch contribution to the study of anatomy in this period was significant and includes the work of artists such as Schijvoet and van der Gucht and the anatomists Bidloo and Albinus [408].[33]

Govard Bidloo (1649–1713) (Fig. 1.34) was a contemporary of Harvey and professor at the University of Leiden (after 1688). His *Anatomia Humani Corporis* [92], illustrated with one hundred and five engravings by Gerard de Lairesse (1640–1711) and published in Amsterdam in 1685, was called by Choulant [178] "a masterpiece of Dutch baroque art", although it was not very successful, perhaps due to its relatively poor text. In 1686 Bidloo received a visit from the English surgeon and anatomist William Cowper (1666–1711) who, aware of de Lairesse's fame as an artist (indeed he was considered to be Rembrandt's closest rival) and of the value of his illustrations, offered to publish an English edition of *Anatomia Humani Corporis*. In this way he obtained the 105 original copperplates and carried them off to London, where in 1689 he published an atlas entitled *The Anatomy of the Human Body, with figures drawn from life by some of the best masters in Europe* [205]. The book consisted of the engravings by de Lairesse plus nine of his own. He made no acknowledgement of Bidloo's authorship of the work, instead obliterating the name of the Dutchman on the title page and inserting his own in the cartouche. Victim of one of the most blatant cases of plagiarism in the history of medicine, Bidloo made a formal complaint to the Royal Society of London: *Gulielmus Cowper, criminis literari citatus…* [93] which included his correspondence with the English anatomist, but Cowper blandly denied that Bidloo held any rights over the illustrations and, despite the overwhelming evidence against him, the Royal Society took no action in the matter.

Setting aside this ignoble chapter in his career, William Cowper made some important contributions to the fields of anatomy and surgery, writing a book of his own (Fig. 1.35) and developing an innovative irrigation procedure to treat problems of the maxillary sinus. He contributed a chapter *On the Nose* to the anatomy treatise *Anthropologia Nova* (1707) by James Drake (1667–1707), in which Cowper proposed the extraction of the first permanent molar to gain access to the sinus through the alveolus. He also studied the musculature and compiled an atlas, *Myotomia Reformata*, published posthumously [206], which included descriptions of the action of individual muscles.

Another important figure was Bernard Sigfried Albinus (1697–1770), a physician born in Frankfurt-an-der-Oder who settled in Holland and wrote an excellent series of books illustrated with engravings of great quality that demonstrate the level of perfection reached in the art of anatomical illustration during the eighteenth century [10, 11, 13]. He also wrote on the osteology of the fetus [12].

During the seventeenth and eighteenth centuries anatomists focused on the study of single organs, many of which bear the names of the physicians who discovered them. *Observationes Anatomica* [895] by the Venetian Giovanni Domenico Santorini (1681–1737), who had studied in Bologna under Malpighi and was a close friend of Giovanni Battista Morgagni, contains descriptions that are of relevance to the plastic surgeon.[34] He concentrated with great detail on the anatomy of the face and discovered important details regarding its musculature, the tear

33 Dissection was a widespread and fully accepted practice in Holland in the seventeenth century, as is demonstrated by the large number of works of art depicting this activity. In *Anatomy* (1603) Arend Pietersz portrayed Dr Sebastian Egberts conducting a dissection; a similar work was executed by Thomas de Keyser in 1619. In Delft Hospital there is a superb painting by van Micrevelt (1717) of the anatomist Dr Van der Neer. Rembrandt was not only the author of the famous *Anatomy Lesson of Dr Nicolaes Tulp* (Mauritshuis, The Hague, 1632), in the Rijksmuseum in Amsterdam is another work by the old master, *Anatomy Lesson of Dr Jan Deyman* (1656), as well as a portrayal by an unknown artist of Dr Frederick Ruysch and a painting by Johan van Neck depicting an anatomy lesson being conducted on the viscera of a child.

34 The drawings for *Observationes Anatomica* were prepared by Marco Galli and engraved by Carlo Orsolini (1710–1780).

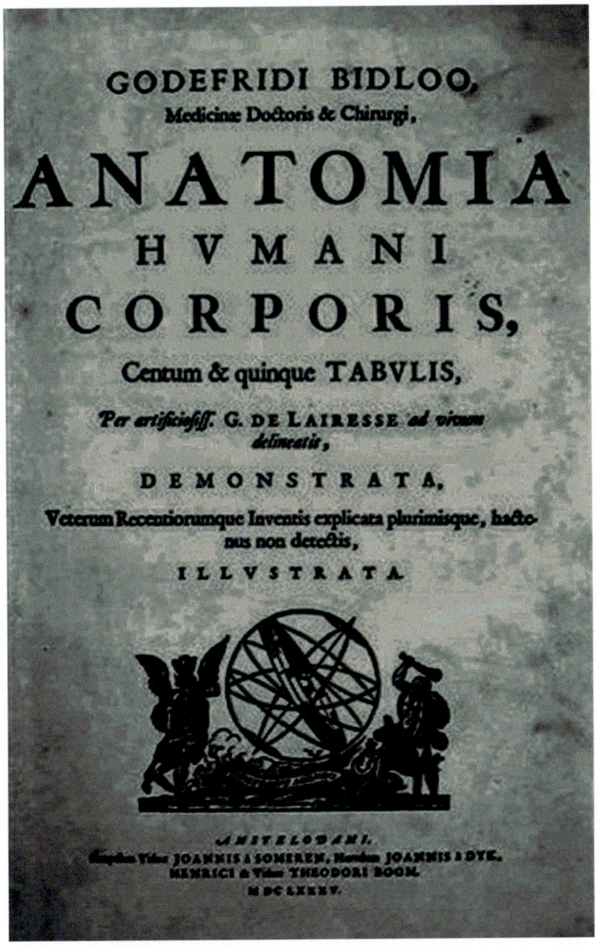

Fig. 1.34 Frontispiece of *Anatomia Humani Corporis* by G. Bidloo (1649–1713) considered by Chaulant as "a masterpiece of Dutch baroque art". *Courtesy of Riccardo Mazzola, M.D., Milan*

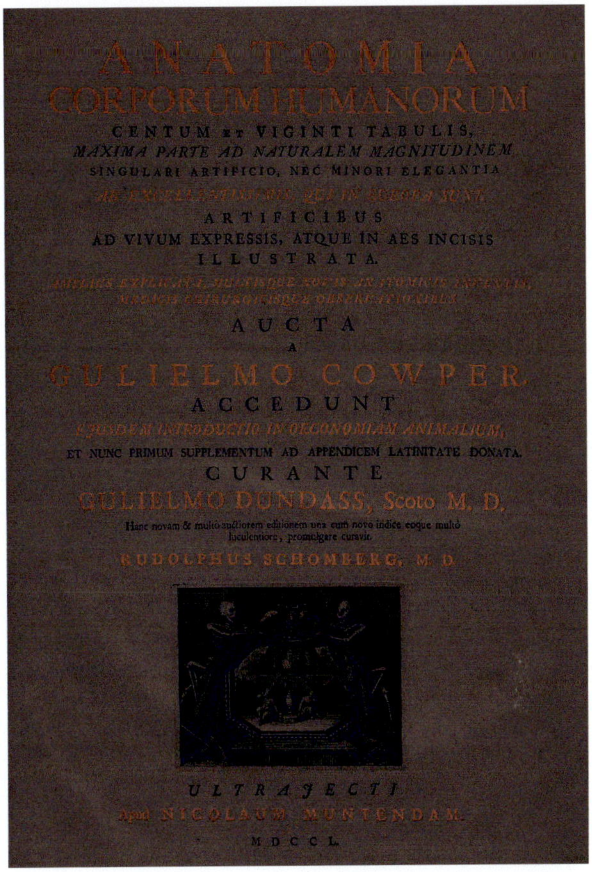

Fig. 1.35 *Anatomia Corporum Humanorum* (1750) by William Cowper. *Courtesy of Riccardo Mazzola, M.D., Milan*

ducts, the nasal cavity, the nasal concha and the ethmoidal sinuses, as well as describing the corniculate cartilage of the larynx, various facial nerves and the cranial veins. Santorini studied other parts of the human body and corrected many of the errors of previous anatomists, particularly with regard to the structure of the breast and the male and female reproductive organs. The splendid illustrations documenting these findings, prepared by the Venetian artist Battista Piazzetta (1682–1754), were published thirty-nine years after the anatomist's death in a work entitled *Septem Decim Tabulae* [896].

Santorini's friend Giovanni Battista Morgagni (1682–1771), who had studied under Valsalva in Padua, was arguably the founder of the science of pathological and microscopic anatomy. He received his degree in medicine and philosophy from the university of Bologna at the age of nineteen and then went to Padua, where in 1711 he was appointed to the first chair in theoretical medicine to be established in Europe. In his inaugural lecture he declared that the key to future advances in medicine lay in the experimental method. In 1715 he was nominated professor of anatomy in Padua, a position that he held until his death.

Morgagni's reputation was established by the publication of an early work, *Adversaria* [704], which shed important light on the disease process by correlating clinical manifestations with the organic lesions that caused them. A brilliant anatomist, he described in painstaking detail the form and function of many organs from the larynx and the kidney to the arteries and the testicles. In another monumental work, *De Sedibus et Causis Morborum per Anatomen Indagatis* (1761), which included pioneering studies on conditions such as hepatic cirrhosis, he laid the foundations for the study of pathological anatomy [705].

The physician and anatomist Paolo Mascagni (1755–1815), professor at the universities of Pisa and Florence, was the author of groundbreaking studies on the lymphatic system, whose course he was able to follow by injecting them with mercury. The results of his research were published in a paper *Prodrome d'un Ouvrage sur le Systeme des Vesseaux Lymphatiques* [613] which was awarded the prize of the Académie des Sciences de Paris in 1783. He received a second prize in 1787 for *Vasorum Lymphaticorum Corporis Humani Historiae Iconographia*, the same work in Latin, which was illustrated with twenty-seven engravings by Ciro Santi of Bologna. After his death the manuscript together with the illustrations by Santi were rediscovered in Pisa and published in Italian in 1816 [614].

When he died Mascagni was still working on a monumental atlas, *Anatomia per Uso Degli Studiosi e Pittori*, whose engravings were both magnificent works of art and unparalleled teaching instruments. They illustrate various parts of the body in their natural dimensions, in particular the first two show the human skeleton with its ligaments and joints, while engravings 3, 4 and 5 present life-sized frontal, lateral and dorsal views of a flayed man [615]. To cover the colossal expense of this project Mascagni was forced to cut costs wherever he could, and even to mortgage the family property, but unhappily did not live long enough to see the work to completion.

Anatomia per uso Scultori…, a book of anatomy for painters and sculptors was published posthumously in Florence in 1816. In 1823 three of Mascagni's colleagues at the University of Pisa prepared a new edition entitled *Anatomia Universa*, which is probably the largest medical text ever published (Fig. 1.36). It contains forty-four engravings printed on double folio sheets (each measuring 950 by 635 mm) which when unfolded present life-sized illustrations of the human body. The engravings were the work of the artist Antonio Serrantoni and are possibly the most remarkable anatomical illustrations in the history of medicine.[35]

Another Italian, Antonio Scarpa (1752–1832) [902] who studied together with Mascagni in Padua, went on to become professor of surgery at Modena and then Padua, where he played an important role in the development of the faculty of medicine. Scarpa concentrated his attention on the anatomy of the eye and plastic surgeons will certainly find much of interest in his work *De Oculi* (1801), whose success earned him the title of "The Father of Italian Ophthalmology". His studies of the other sensory organs such as *De Auditu et de Olfacto* [901][36] are also valuable. He was the first to describe the congenital club foot, the abdominal fascia and the triangle at the base of the femur (both of which were named after him).

Albrecht von Haller (1708–1777) was born in Bern and pursued his medical studies under Albinus in Leyden and Winslow in Paris before becoming a professor at Göttingen. He produced admirable descriptions of the anatomy of the face and in particular of the facial nerves, publishing the results of his research in the work *Icones Anatomicae* between 1743 and 1756 [409].

The anatomy of the head and face was also studied in detail by Jacques Gautier d'Agoty (1717–1785) who published two books with superb colour illustrations on the subject in 1748 [6].[37] He also published a work on the genitalia in 1773 [7] and a general anatomy with Fabian in 1752 [8]. Another French anatomist who is best known for his studies of the face, and in particular of the pan-

35 Only three copies of Mascagni's remarkable work are known to exist, one in Pisa (Museum of Human Anatomy, University of Pisa), one at the Accademia dei Fisiocritici in Siena, and one in a private collection in Pisa.

36 Up until the beginning of the twentieth century all lectures and publications from the departments of Pavia University had to be in Latin.

37 In reality, according to Ludwig Choulant, "The illustrations by D'Agoty cannot be recommended to students of anatomy for their faithfulness or accuracy, nor are they suitable in terms of fineness and exactness of detail, but rather as large and massive representations."

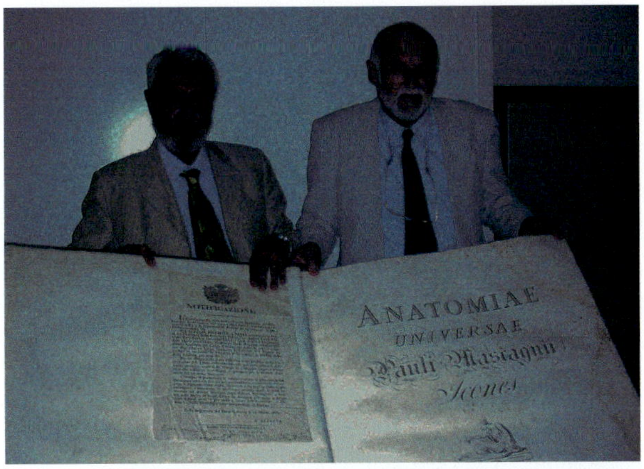

Fig. 1.36 The authors are holding *Anatomiae Universae* by Paolo Mascagni (1755–1815). *Courtesy of C. d. L. Flaminio Farnesi, Pisa*

niculus adiposus which was named after him, was Marie Francois Xavier Bichat (1771–1802), although he actually deserves to be remembered as the founder of pathological histology. Bichat conducted pioneering research, based on the careful correlation of findings from anatomical and clinical studies, that shed new light on many pathological processes. Indeed, while Morgagni demonstrated that a specific organ was often the seat of a disease, Bichat went further and showed that the disease might be associated with a specific tissue or structure within the organ. During the course of his research he identified and described no fewer than twenty-one different tissues. His book *Anatomie Génerale Appliquée* [91] is unusual in that it does not contain a single illustration.

The German, Samuel Thomas von Sömmering (1755–1830) was one of the most eminent anatomists of his day. He taught anatomy and surgery at the universities of Kassel, Munich and Frankfurt-am-Main, and wrote a text on human anatomy, *Vom Bau des menschlichen Körpers*, as well as several short but accurate treatises on the eye, the ear, the voice, the sense of taste, etc. Many structures were named after him and he was the first to describe the substantia nigra in the brain.

In Mainz during 1791 Sömmering published a study of the embryogenesis of various congenital malformations that is of immense relevance for plastic surgery. *Abbildungen und Beschreibungen einiger Missgeburten* [946][38] probably offered the first classification of the cranio-facial malformations in the medical literature [945]. In it Sömmering describes a series of malformations of the face and head, providing examples of cases of anencephaly, clefts of the face, hypertelorism and pterygium of the neck. A fascinating illustration showing different types of clefts appears on the title page. Sömmering's studies in this area were so complete and authoritative that the next significant advances would have to await the publication of Paul Tessier's work on the subject in 1974.

Abbildungen des menschliches Auges published in Frankfurt-am-Main in 1801, describes the microscopic structure of the eye. This publication was thought by Choulant [178] "the most perfect of the works of Sömmering", one which "after Zinn's monograph, become the foundation for all modern researches on the structure of this organ [the eye]. He aimed, like Albinus, at the discovery of the truth and of the beautiful in the form of every part of the human body and combined a perfect sense of artistic representation with the most exact perception of details." Sömmering continued his studies of the anatomy of the head, and published *De Basi Encephali et Originibus Nervorum Cranio Egredientium* in 1778. This work was illustrated by Carl Christian Glassbach Jr and contains descriptions of the skull base and cranial foramina. Choulant justly praised the anatomical works of Sömmering as a "combination of high anatomical truth and artistically beautiful reproductions".

The Modern Period

During the last two centuries detailed studies of specific organs and systems have greatly augmented our knowledge in every area of anatomy. However, since it will not be possible to discuss them all here we shall limit ourselves to a brief overview of those with a direct relevance to plastic surgery [384].

One of the founders of surgical anatomy was the Scottish surgeon and anatomist Charles Bell (1774–1842), the younger brother of the John Bell, also a surgeon and author. He was the first to describe the ligature of inac-

38 The manuscript of this work is conserved at the Anatomy Museum in Kassel.

cessible vessels such as the gluteal, common carotid and internal iliac arteries. He also conducted unprecedented research on the anatomy of facial movements in his work *Essay on the Anatomy of Expression in Painting* in 1806 [68]; in *Anatomy and Philosophy of the Expression* published in 1824 [69] he described the cranial nerves and suggested that they had two different functions, motor and sensitive (Fig. 1.37).

Bell succeeded in demonstrating the validity of his theory in a patient under the care of Sir Astley Cooper—a woman whose 7th cranial nerve had been accidentally severed during an ear operation. The patient exhibited a complete facial palsy, but retained all sensitivity to sensory stimuli on the face. His description of this case inaugurated the study of facial movements in normal subjects and in patients suffering from neurological and non-neurological diseases. His analysis of the effect of the emotions and character on facial gestures and expression make for fascinating reading even today. Probably his most important work was to distinguish between the distinct structure and function of the sensory and motor nerves in 1811.

In 1833, using money bequeathed by the Earl of Bridgewater, Bell published a monograph on the anatomy and physiology of the human hand entitled *The Hand: its mechanism and vital endowments as evincing design* which Eimas described as "unusual and perhaps unique" [276] because both the text and illustrations were prepared by the author himself, who was known for his artistic interests as well as his scientific work.

Another scientist who was fascinated by the physiological and psychological mechanisms underlying the expression of the emotions was Charles Darwin (1809–1882). In 1872 Darwin published a work entitled *The Expression of the Emotions in Man and Animals* in which he propounded his thesis that the chief expressive actions exhibited by man and by lower animals become innate and inherited, and that humans and non-human animals share such feelings as suffering, joy and anger. But he is mainly remembered for his seminal work *The Origin of the Species* published in 1859 [219].

In Italy Giuseppe Sterzi (1876–1919) conducted research on the superficial fascia and the subcutaneous tissues that, although not sufficiently appreciated by his contemporaries, would prove to be of fundamental importance to plastic surgery [958]. He published his findings in 1910 together with a study of the nervous system.[39] Four centuries earlier Vesalius had identified four cutaneous layers: the *cuticola* (epidermis), the *cutis* (dermis), the *pinguedo* (adipose tissue) and the *panniculus camosus*, a term which he used to refer to the muscles present in various regions of the dermis, such as the *platisma* of the neck. However, the existence of the superficial fascia was largely ignored until the nineteenth century, when surgeons such as Cooper, Scarpa and Lawrence described this fibrous sheet in the context of operations for inguinal hernias. Cooper, for example, demonstrated that the sheet might vary with the age, sex and degree of obesity of the subject.

Sterzi was the first anatomist to provide an accurate description of this neglected structure. He focused in particular on the fascia of the face and neck, but also made comparative observations on the fibrous envelope in other regions of the body and its close relationship

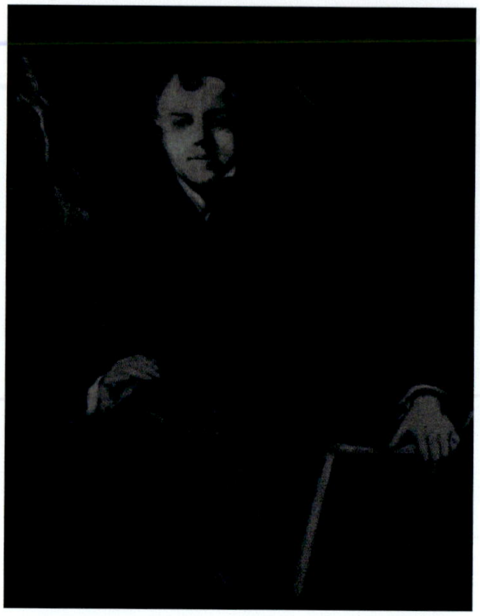

Fig. 1.37 Portrait of Charles Bell (1774–1842). *Courtesy of FMR Art.spa, Bologna*

39 Sterzi was a Pisan mathematician who developed an interest in medicine and became an anatomist. He taught in Sardinia and was about to transfer to the celebrated University of Padua when he died at the age of 43.

with the neurovascular system. For example, the association between the great auricular nerve and the superficial fascia in the parotid region, which plays such a central role in the facelift, was initially described by Sterzi. His work in this area would not be utilized until more than fifty years later with the studies of Tord Skoog [937, 938] and Mitz and Peyronie [680].

During the nineteenth century other studies appeared that could have had a significant influence on the development of plastic surgery were it not for the fact that most surgeons remained unaware of their existence for many decades.

One of these was undoubtedly Carl Manchot's (1866–1932) remarkable research on the anatomy of the cutaneous circulation [606] published in 1889. Its crucial importance to plastic surgery was not recognized until the last quarter of the twentieth century. Manchot was born in the town of Wipkingen, Switzerland on 30 April 1866 into a family with a long tradition of religious scholarship. His father was a Protestant minister and emigrated to Germany when Carl was just a few months old, settling in Hamburg. In 1885 Carl enrolled as a student at the University of Strasbourg, taking advantage of the scholarships that were being offered to attract students to this city recently annexed from France.

Gustav Schwalbe, a professor of anatomy at Strasbourg whose main area of interest was the sensory organs, recognized in the young Manchot the spirit of enquiry of the true researcher and assigned him the difficult task of researching the finely branching system of the cutaneous innervation. Aware that the nerves generally follow the same path as the body's arteries, Manchot succeeded in mapping out the course of their peripheral distribution. It is not known exactly what substance he injected into the arteries in order to follow their elusive trail, but the fact remains that within six months he was able to produce a complete map of the body showing all the cutaneous arteries and the regions that they fed. He only failed to detect the fine connections between adjacent cutaneous zones, which would be discovered fifty years later by M. Salmon [882, 883] as we will see in the chapter on the history of the skin flap.

Manchot received a prize of 300 Deutschmarks from the University of Strasbourg, plus another 300 DM which had not been awarded the previous year, in recognition of his achievement. Despite the encouragement of Professor Schwalbe, who realized the importance of his research, Manchot did not publish his results until three years later and in a very limited number of copies which were destined to languish on the dusty shelves of the library at the university's anatomy institute. If instead they had been brought to the attention of the international medical community, Manchot's work may have revolutionized all surgical procedure involving skin flaps.

Manchot completed his studies and returned to Hamburg, where he devoted the remainder of his life to the practice of his profession. He never published another article, and his remarkable research was completely forgotten until eighty-five years later, when W. Morain [692] came into possession of one of the rare copies of the original paper and translated it into English. Morain realized that Manchot's findings could resolve one of the greatest problems associated with the skin flap, whose use in reconstructive surgery had up to then been limited by the precarious and apparently random vascularization of the skin, surgeons being largely ignorant of the anatomy of the cutaneous circulation.

Before concluding our outlook on the Anatomy let us mention an similar story of a crucial discovery that might have had an immense impact on reconstructive surgery but instead remained completely ignored. This was the origin of the myocutaneous flap. Iginio Tansini of Pavia (1855–1943), as we will see in more detail in the chapter on skin flaps, had observed that the standard procedure for closing the defects left after radical mastectomies, which was to stretch large sections of skin from the lateral thoracic region, failed as often as it succeeded, ending in the partial or total necrosis of the flap. Investigating the possible causes together with Professor Sala an anatomist at the University of Pavia, Tansini succeeded in demonstrating that the blood supply to this area of the skin was derived in large part from the underlying latissimus dorsi muscle. It was therefore essential not to interrupt these vascular connections; indeed, the muscle offered the surgeon a broad, flexible area of tissue that could be exploited in breast reconstruction [970]. The concept of the myocutaneous graft therefore dates to 1906, but surgeons did not understand its importance until almost the end of the twentieth century, when Tansini's observations were rediscovered.

Modern plastic surgery is the result of innovations and techniques developed over the course of many centuries which would have been impossible without the anatomical discoveries described in this chapter.

Chapter 2

Healing of Wounds and the Development of Surgery

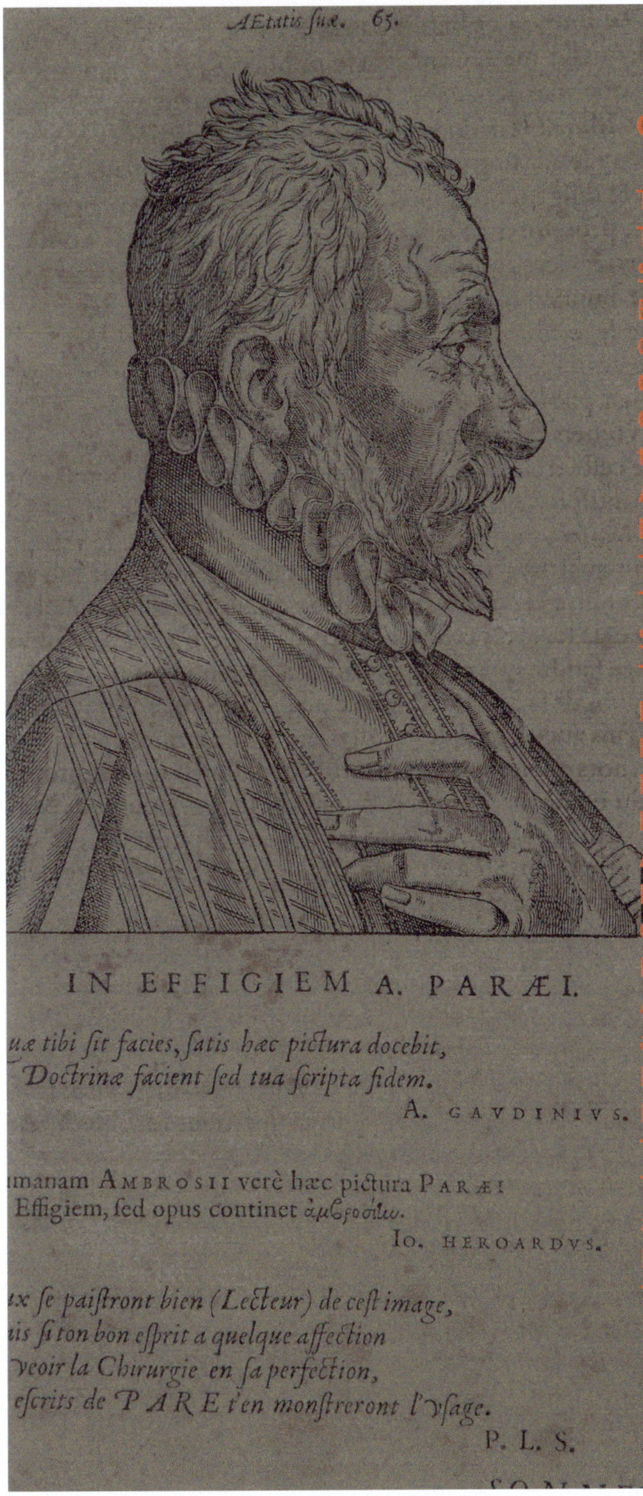

Contents

Two centuries ago James Garrich Moore (1763–1834) asked: "In what manner are cavities, whether formed by suppuration, wounds, or otherwise, filled up? What are the appearances of their filling up properly? In what manner is the new skin formed? What are the symptoms of its forming properly? In what case and in what manner are the parts, which are destroyed, restored?" [691].[1] The definitive answers to many of these questions were only discovered in recent times, but Moore did suggest ways to reduce pain during surgery [690].

There can be no doubt that our distant ancestors attempted by various means to speed the healing of wounds. Furthermore, they grasped the fundamental notion that the so-called *Vix Medicatrix Naturae* varied according to the type of wound in question. They observed that injuries whose margins were in direct contact adhered (*conglutinant* was the antique Latin term used) or mended in a process that later would be described as healing by *Primary Intention*. Those which did not follow this course—either because the necessary contact between the margins was lacking or else due to complications—mended in accordance with another process referred to as healing by *Secondary Intention*. The development of surgical procedures over the centuries for the treatment of wounds reflected the efforts of surgeons to induce healing by the first of these processes and remains the basis of reconstructive surgery [150].

The First Surgical Repairs

Just how far back do the earliest surgical operations date? It has been demonstrated that when faced with injuries caused by primitive weapons such as stones or clubs, and later arrows and lances, the first surgeons attempted to facilitate healing in different ways.

In ancient Egypt no distinction was made between the physician and the surgeon; instead, anyone engaged in the healing arts specialized in a specific group of diseases or injuries. The treatment of wounds was governed by the rules written by priests in the Sacred Books, which were kept in the temples but could be consulted by the public. Some idea of their practices may be gleaned from the images carved or painted on temple walls and various monuments, but our principal source remains an ancient document known as the Edwin Smith papyrus (Fig. 2.1).

In 1862 an American archeologist from the state of Connecticut, Edwin Smith (1822–1906), who wrote about ancient Egypt [939], acquired a papyrus from an Egyptian by the name of Mustapha Agha. When Smith died this papyrus was donated by his daughter to the New York Historical Society, which had it translated by James Henry Breasted, a professor at the Oriental Institute of Chicago. This translation [128] held many surprises for the medical community at the turn of the last century. The document, which was written sometime between 2600 and 2200 B.C., contains the descriptions of 48 surgical cases, each followed by a commentary that, most surprisingly, was based not on superstition but on concrete observation and logical reasoning. Only in one instance was a patient's recovery attributed to divine intervention rather than to the treatment administered.

In the papyrus we find, for example, instructions formulated in a somewhat empirical but quite practicable manner for making a rudimentary antiseptic based on incense and myrtle, substances known even today for their mild antiseptic action. These were mixed with oil and honey and applied to clean cotton bandages that could be placed on the wound to absorb its secretions. The author even recommended that copper salts be used to treat gangrenous ulcers.[2]

Another antique civilization which studied the treatment of injuries was that of Mesopotamia, the region lying between the Tigris and Euphrates Rivers.[3] The Babylonians, although better known for their discoveries in the areas of mathematics and astronomy, also reached quite a high level of achievement in the field of medicine. Despite the fact that illnesses were attributed by their re-

1 See the preface to James Garrich Moore's work *Dissertation on the Process of the Filling Up of Cavities*.

2 J.H. Breasted's translation of the *Edwin Smith Papyrus* (1600–1500 B.C.) was published by Chicago University Press in 1930. The original measures 4.68 × 0.35 m and the text occupies 28 × 30 cm. The title is in red with the text in black and describes 48 surgical cases.

3 The name *Mesopotamia* derives from the Greek words μεσο (between) and ροτομασ (river).

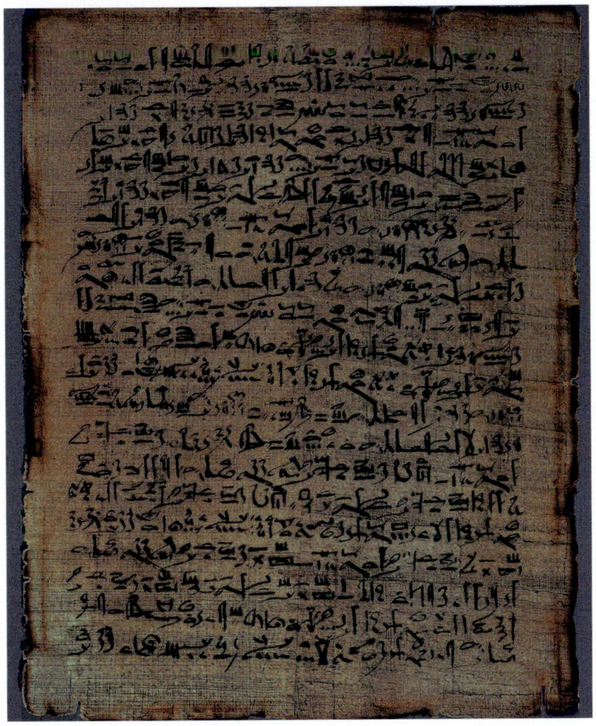

Fig. 2.1 Facsimile copy of The Edwin Smith papyrus dating from c.1600–1500 B.C., Egypt. It was bought in 1862 but only translated after Smith's death in 1906 by H. Breasted, Professor at the Oriental Institute in Chicago, for the New York Historical Society. It was published in 1930 in Chicago. *Private Collection, Archives Charmet – Bridgeman Art Library*

ligion to demonic influences, therapy was dictated by experience and logic rather than magic and superstition.

In 1849 the archeologist Sir Henry Layard found among the ruins of the Palace of Nineveh near the present city of Mosul in northern Iraq, which had been razed to the ground in 612 A.D., more than 20,000 clay tablets collected during the reign of King Ashurbanipal (668–626 B.C.). Some of these date to as far back as 1600 B.C. Among these, 660 are of medical interest and were studied by R.C. Thompson [989, 990]of the University of Oxford, who found the descriptions of treatments for many illnesses, including a limited number of surgical procedures. Two classes of healers existed: the *Ashipu* or magicians, whose approach was based primarily on religious faith and superstition, and the *Asu* or doctors, who were generally considered to be more reliable and who certainly followed principles that may be described as more *scientific*. For example, one of their remedies called for a variety of plant-based ingredients that could be "mixed with milk and beer in a small copper pan, strained, and then spread on the skin, [which was] bound until the patient recovered".

Another font of information is the Assyrian Code of King Hammurabi [4], a collection of Babylonian laws developed during his the reign (1792–1750 B.C.). The most complete version was carved on a stela discovered in 1901 by a French archeological expedition. It was studied by Rene Labat and today may be seen in the Louvre Museum in Paris [514, 515]. Certain of its provisions are of interest for the plastic surgeon because they codify the civil responsibility of the physician for the first time in history. For example: "If the physician shall make a severe wound with the bronze operating knife and kill [the patient] or shall open a growth with a bronze knife and destroy an eye, his hands shall be cut off." If such an injury was inflicted upon a slave, "he shall pay half of the value of the slave".[5]

The code included a list of prices for medical services, in which we discover that the bill always took into account and varied with the social status of the patient. In the case of a nobleman the charge was ten silver shekels for suturing a wound, whereas "if a physician has restored a broken nose in a patient [of ordinary rank], the owner of the nose must pay the Asu five shekels of silver".[6] If the patient was a slave, his master was responsible for settling the account.

Curiously, as Labat notes, in Mesopotamia the surgical scalpel was referred to as "the barber's razor", suggesting an interesting but unproven and perhaps somewhat unlikely connection with surgery as it came to be practised in Europe—generally by barbers—during the Middle Ages. Furthermore, according to the French scholar a separate category of doctors specializing in surgery did

4 Hammurabi is generally considered to have ruled from 1955 to 1913 B.C., although Allen Whipple dates his reign to around 2250 B.C.

5 Law no. 218.

6 Law no. 218.

not exist; it was the *Asu* himself who took up the scalpel when necessary.

The Closing of Wounds: Sutures and Bandages

Egyptians and Hindus

The transformation of a wound which was discharging blood or pus and whose edges were not in contact, into a different type of wound that would heal rapidly has always been the goal of surgeons. From the Edwin Smith papyrus we learn that the Egyptians employed strips of linen cloth, made adherent by the application of gum. These were used to close the margins of linear wounds. Such bandages were regularly used by embalmers after they had removed the organs. Indeed it is probable that the technique pre-dates the Egyptians since resins were already well known in 8000 B.C.

In addition, in four of the seven different cases of wounds described in the Edwin Smith papyrus it is stated that *sutures were used*. This is the first known mention of the technique and it should come as no surprise since embalmers routinely stitched up the incision after eviscerating the corpse. Such stitches are clearly visible along the abdomen of a mummy dating from the 21st dynasty (c.1100 B.C.) and described by Guido Majno [596]. The papyrus also discusses in considerable detail at least two cases involving surgery, and in one it is specified that the correct use of sutures could speed the healing process by preventing complications (case no. 10). Finally, the author of the papyrus writes: "Now after thou has stitched it, thou shouldst bind fresh meat upon [the wound] on the first day. If thou findst that the stitching of the wound is loose [and therefore there is the risk of infection or the breakdown of the tissue], thou shouldst draw it together for him with two crossed strips, and thou shouldst treat it with grease and honey every day until the patient recovers."

The Egyptians were also aware that when there was a risk of a haematoma it was necessary to allow the wound to drain. For example, in the case of facial trauma involving "discharging of blood from the nostrils but not the ears … [or] … when thou findest that the skull of a man is split, thou shouldst not bind it but leave it to moisten [i.e. allow the free flow of secretions], and moor him with mooring stakes until the period of injury has passed".

Pliny records that the Egyptians used powdered marble, which he called *menphites*, mixed with vinegar as a local anaesthetic; the application of this substance produced such marked swelling that the patient no longer felt the pain of his wound. It has also been suggested that the carbon dioxide produced by the chemical reaction may have had an analgesic effect.

What material was used for sutures? Unfortunately information on this point is scarce and confused, but silk thread appears to be one possibility. Instead, mention may be found of the use of the jaws of ants as a natural *staple* for small wounds. Possibly the Egyptians had observed that the formic acid seeping from the severed head of the ant might have a beneficial effect, even if they had little notion of the processes of infection or the disinfectant properties of acid [1043].

The hypothesis that the technique of suturing was first developed by the Egyptians has been challenged by Majno, who points out that the art of sewing was already known to the Neanderthals, as is demonstrated by the clothing which they fashioned, and it would be strange indeed if the first *Homo sapiens* had not thought of applying this technique to the closure of wounds. However Majno's thesis remains based on mere supposition for the moment.[7]

Although of less antiquity, the technique of suturing was also known in India. In his famous treatise *Samhita* written in Sanskrit (c.800–600 B.C., but which some experts date to as far back as 1000 B.C.) the Indian surgeon Susruta [90] suggested the use of cotton thread, hemp and even strips of leather, horsehair or animal tendons to draw the margins of wounds together, and advised apprentice surgeons to practise the technique on pieces of cloth. He distinguished four classes of wounds–*incised*, *contused*, *crushed*, or *torn*—and emphasized the importance of removing all foreign bodies and closing the wound as quickly as possible, although not "as long as the least bit of morbid matter, or pus remains in the wound".

7 Majno [596] also describes more recent examples of the use of the mandibles of ants to close wounds in both Africa and South America. Various insects (including *Atta cephalotes*, *Eciton burchelli*, *Eciton hyamatum*, *Labidue praedator* and *Oecophilla smaragdina*) have served as sutures in various parts of the world.

The sutured wound must then be bound with cotton and ashes to keep it dry. Susruta also suggested using the jaws of insects as staples: "Large black ants should be applied to the margins of the wound and their bodies then severed from their heads, after these have firmly bitten the part with their jaws."

The treatment of wounds described by Susruta anticipate the approaches used in modern medicine and, despite the differences in terminology, it is clear that he understood the fundamental mechanisms underlying the processes of healing by primary and secondary intention.

Susruta recognized the simple general principles necessary for uncomplicated healing in Chapter 19 of his *Samhita*. As well as recommending that the patient be nursed in a proper room on a comfortable bed with the head placed eastwards towards the gods, he advocated other basic rules. His sensible suggestions included "friendly company with affectionate friends able to dissipate pain … by amicable conversation" and to console him "in various ways". He also lists good and bad dietary measures, clean white clothing and rest for the injured part. He denies "sleep during the day" to ensure a restful night and says that "interview, conversation and contact with ladies should be avoided even at a distance". Furthermore, there should be complete "sexual abstinence". All these simple measures would make for uncomplicated wound healing without suppuration. Last, but not least, he says that healing will proceed smoothly if there are "priests and surgeons reciting texts from Rguada, Yajmueda and other benedictions". This general advice is accompanied by more specific information too detailed to list here, about dressings (Chapter 18), infection (Chapter 21), incurable lesions (Chapter 23), factors affecting prognosis (Chapter 28) and all the surgical procedures used to facilitate healing (Chapter 26).

The bleeding from a wound which could lead to grave or even mortal consequences was obviously a main concern and one of the earliest remedies discovered was cauterization. The Egyptians were the first to suggest the use of cautery, as is documented in another well-known medical papyrus acquired in 1873 by George Ebers (1837–1898) from a merchant who had discovered it preserved between the legs of a mummy in Thebes in 1863 [271]. Probably dating from the period of the 18th dynasty, the Ebers papyrus represents the longest existing ancient Egyptian document on the subject of medicine. In its 877 paragraphs covering 110 pages it offers a veritable encyclopedia on the medical arts of the period.

Considerable space is devoted to surgery, although many details regarding the techniques used and instructions for specific procedures are missing. Nevertheless, cauterization is mentioned for the first time as a means of controlling haemorrhage, the surgeon being advised "to cut and burn at the same time in order to check the bleeding", while later it is stated that if a larger vessel is involved and "the bleeding is very serious you must resort to burning with fire".[8]

In India cauterization was also a frequent procedure and Susruta tells students to practise using incandescent cauteries on fresh meat.

Greece and Rome

Although the first principle of the Greek physician Hippocrates (c.460 to c.355 B.C.) was that one should interfere as little as possible with the natural processes of healing, *primum non nocere* (first do no harm), the Greeks possessed considerable knowledge of how damaged tissues were repaired, which in turn suggested the best means of treating different types of diseases and injuries [467]. However, the fact is that while Hippocrates and his school at Cos introduced many important ideas in the area of medicine, as far as surgery was concerned they were much less innovative (Fig. 2.2).

For example, Hippocrates' position with regard to suturing was one of cautious reserve and there are very few references to the technique in the *Corpus Hippocraticum* (*Hippocratic Collection*) [434–437]. Indeed Allen W. Whipple [1044] declares that sutures are never mentioned in his work, but this statement is inaccurate. In the section *On Wounds* they are cited three times, in the context of injuries to the face, nose and lips. In case no. 5 for example, which describes a patient with a clean cut made by the edge of a broken pot, one may read: "Had there been any bruised flesh I would have helped the wound to produce pus, for pus makes the bruised flesh melt away. Since there is no bruise, I would make the

8 The Ebers papyrus is presently conserved at the University of Leipzig.

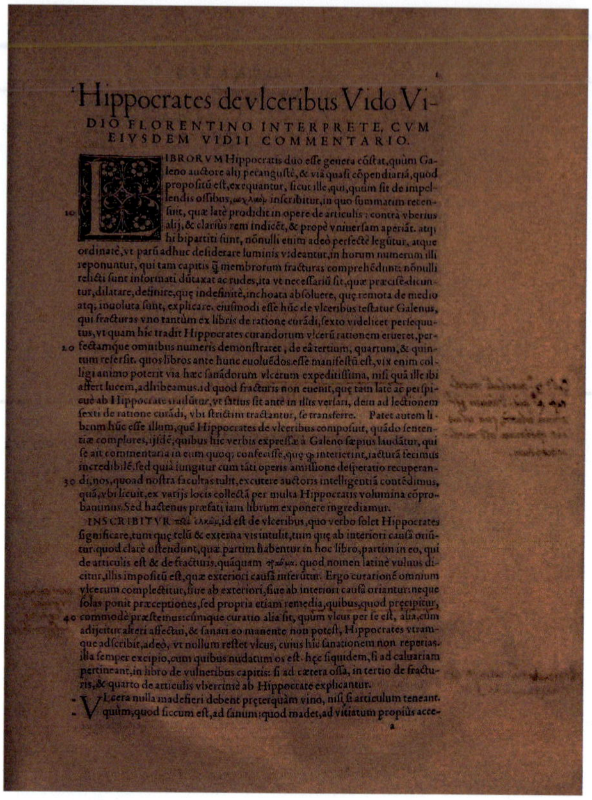

Hippocrates de vlceribus Vido Vidio Florentino interprete, cum eiusdem Vidii commentario.

LIBRORVM Hippocratis duo esse genera cōstat, quùm Galeno auctore alij perangustè, & viâ quasi cōpendiariâ, quod propositū est, exequantur, sicut ille, qui, quùm sit de impellendis ossibus, [illegible] inscribitur, in quo summatim recensuit, quæ latè prodidit in opere de articulis: contrà vberius alij, & clarius rem indicēt, & propè vniuersam aperiāt. atq; hi bipartiti sunt, nōnulli enim adeò perfectè legūtur, atque ordinatè, vt parū adhuc desiderare luminis videantur, in horum numerum illi reponuntur, qui tam capitis q̄ membrorum fracturas comprehēdunt: nōnulli relicti sunt informati dūtaxat ac rudes, ita vt necessariū sit, quæ præcisè dicuntur, dilatare, definire, quę indefinitè, inchoata absoluere, quę remota de medio atq; inuoluta sunt, explicare. eiusmodi esse hūc de vlceribus testatur Galenus, qui fracturas vno tantùm ex libris de ratione curādi, sexto videlicet persequutus, vt quam hîc tradit Hippocrates curandorum vlcerū rationem erueret, perfectamque omnibus numeris demonstraret, de eâ tertium, quartum, & quintum refersit. quos libros ante hunc euoluēdos esse manifestū est, vix enim colligi animo poterit via hæc sanādorum vlcerum expeditissima, nisi quā ille ibi affert lucem, adhibeamus. id quod fracturis non euenit, quę tam latè ac perspicuè ab Hippocrate traduntur, vt satius sit antè in illis versari, dein ad lectionem sexti de ratione curādi, vbi strictim tractantur, se transferre. Patet autem librum hūc esse illum, quē Hippocrates de vlceribus composuit, quādo sententiæ complures, ijsdē, quibus hîc verbis expressæ à Galeno sæpius laudātur, qui se ait commentaria in eum quoq; confecisse, quę quia interierint, iacturā fecimus incredibilē. sed quià iungitur cum tāti operis amissione desperatio recuperandi, nos, quoad nostra facultas tulit, excutere auctoris intelligentiā contēdimus, quā, vbi licuit, ex varijs locis collectā per multa Hippocratis volumina cōprobauimus. Sed hactenus præfati iam librum exponere ingrediamur.

INSCRIBITVR [illegible], id est de vlceribus, quo verbo solet Hippocrates significare, tum quę telū & externa vis intulit, tum quę ab interiori causā oriūtur. quod clarè ostendunt, quæ partim habentur in hoc libro, partim in eo, qui de articulis est & de fracturis. quāquam [illegible]. quod nomen latinè vulnus dicitur, illis impositū est, quæ exteriori causā inferūtur. Ergo curationē omnium vlcerum complectitur, siue ab exteriori, siue ab interiori causā oriantur: neque solas ponit præceptiones, sed propria etiam remedia, quibus, quod præcipitur, commodè præstemus: cùmque curatio alia sit, quùm vlcus per se est, alia, cùm adijcitur alteri affectui, & sanari eo manente non potest, Hippocrates vtramque adscribit, adeò, vt nullum restet vlcus, cuius hîc sanationem non reperias. illa semper excipio, cum quibus nudatum os est. hęc siquidem, si ad caluariam pertineant, in libro de vulneribus capitis: si ad cætera ossa, in tertio de fracturis, & quarto de articulis vberrimè ab Hippocrate explicantur.

VLcera nulla madefieri debent prętерquàm vino, nisi si articulum teneant. quùm, quod siccum est, ad sanum: quod madet, ad vitiatum propiùs acce-

a

Fig. 2.2 First page of *De Ulceribus* by Hippocrates (460–375 B.C.) translated by Vido Vidi who collected the works of the classical masters including Hippocrates, Galen and Oribasius in his *Chirurgia e Greco in Latinum Conversa, Vido Vidi Florentino Interprete* (Florence, 1544). *Courtesy of Riccardo Mazzola, M.D., Milan*

wound close quickly without waiting for the formation of pus." For the operation Hippocrates used a bronze needle which is carefully described in the text.

It has been suggested that the ancient Greeks were aware that wounds in which the surrounding tissue was not damaged (in particular, injuries to the face where the blood supply is particularly good) had a greater chance of healing and therefore reserved suturing for these types of injuries. In other cases they allowed suppuration to take place, a process which they had observed led to the elimination of the necroticized areas and stimulated the formation of granulating tissue. Suppuration did indeed contribute to the healing process, even if at the cost of a slower recovery and an additional degree of risk. This observation of Hippocrates gave rise to the principle *pus bonus et laudabile* which would endure for many centuries.

The Greeks' empirical understanding of the processes of healing is further illustrated by their principle that the wound must be kept dry. Although ignorant of the processes of infection, they deduced that secretions created a moist environment which favoured the development of complications, whereas dry wounds healed much faster. This simple observation had already been made by the Egyptians and the Hindus, but Greek physicians were the first to arrive at the conclusion that *astringents* should be applied before closing the edges of a wound. They furthermore grasped the importance of irrigating the wound and recommended wine mixed with boiling water for this purpose. Indeed, the Greeks understood that cleanliness was the first rule of medicine and Hippocrates insisted that the hands of the surgeon must be carefully washed and "the nails of the fingers should be trimmed in such a way that they do not surpass the fingertip, nor do they become too short". Bandages were considered an important aid to healing, as was the immobilization of injuries close to joints.

It is interesting to note that Homer's *Iliad* (460 B.C.)—in which the physicians of Olympus, Machaon and Polydorus were often called upon to remove arrows and other projectiles from wounds and to apply "soothing remedies for the pain"—contains, according to H. Froelich [341], no less than 147 descriptions of wounds sustained on the battlefield, of which 78% eventually proved fatal (Fig. 2.3). Homer gives a description of a bandage that was applied to the injured hand of Helen which would be accepted today "in the manner of a sling well wrapped in a cloth made of sheep's wool". These descriptions testify to the Greeks' considerable knowledge of injuries and their treatment. It is interesting to note that the term for surgery (χψρυργια) was coined on the island of Cos during the period that Hippocrates was teaching there.

The Greeks' approach to surgery was practical. They observed and applied treatments which were founded on clear evidence and not prejudice. In doing this they established basic pragmatic principles.

Controlling Bleeding

In the *Corpus Hippocraticum* there are no references to cautery for the control of bleeding, even though it is certain that this procedure was not only known but widely used. In fact, in the Collection's description of a typical

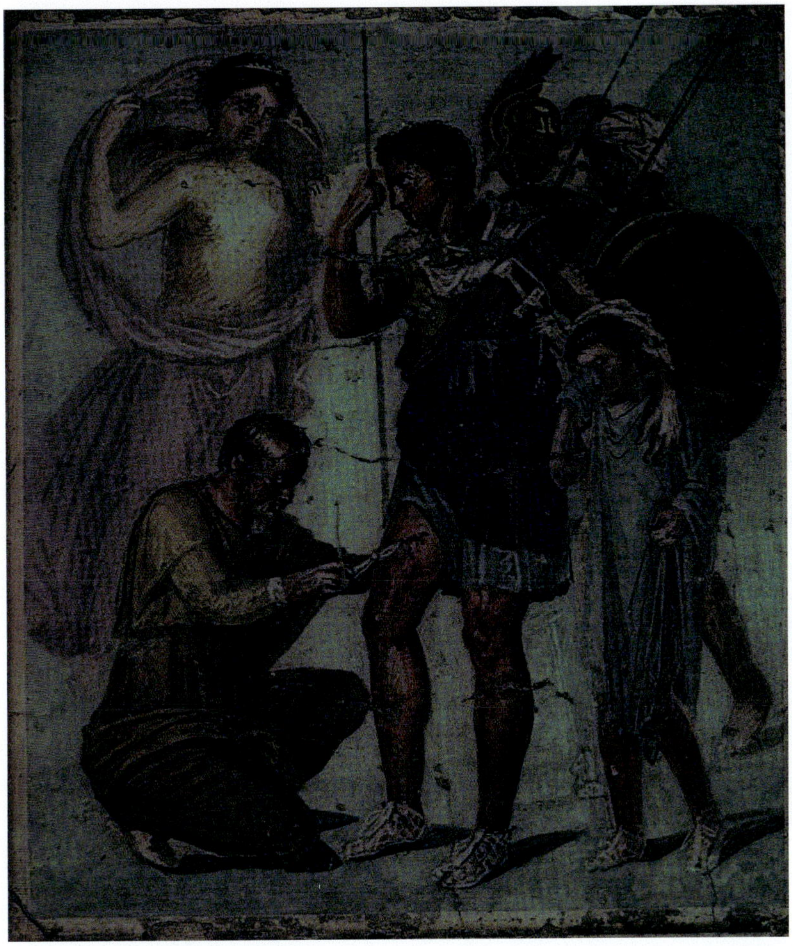

Fig. 2.3 Fresco from Pompeii showing the surgeon Japix extracting an arrow from Enea's thigh. Museo Archeologico of Naples. *By permission of the Sopraintendenza per i Beni Archeologici delle Province di Napoli e Caserta*

ιατρειον (or *medical clinic*), we read that "smoke was ever present from the brazier where the cauteries were kept red hot". Furthermore, there is at least one specific indication for cautery where the text recommends that ulcers be "burned with a caustic substance". Finally, Hippocrates employed the technique to treat cases of erysipelas and cauliflower ear, although he warned that in the latter case the ears could become reduced in size. Whether or not the ancient Greeks employed cautery in cases of bleeding remains unclear (Fig. 2.4).

The next important advance in the control of bleeding and the treatment of wounds comes from the Roman physician Aulus Cornelius Celsus (25 B.C. to 50 A.D.) Although aware of the efficacy of cautery in cases of bleeding, he did not place much importance to small losses of blood, instead he believed that bleeding was beneficial as it allowed noxious humors to be eliminated from the wound. In more serious cases of bleeding, however: "… the wound is to be filled with dry lint, and over that a sponge applied, squeezed out of cold water, and pressed down by the hand. If the bleeding is not checked thus, the lint must be changed several times, and if it is not effective when dry, it is to be soaked in vinegar. Vinegar is powerful in suppressing a flow of blood" [167, 168].[9] In the same paragraph Celsus suggests a completely new solution for bleeding, the use of ligatures "… the blood-vessels that are pouring out blood are to be seized, and round the wounded spot they are to be tied in two places …" Celsus was referring only to the veins here, probably because he believed that the arteries were filled with

9 See *De Medicina*, Book V, Chapter XXVI, 21 B and C.

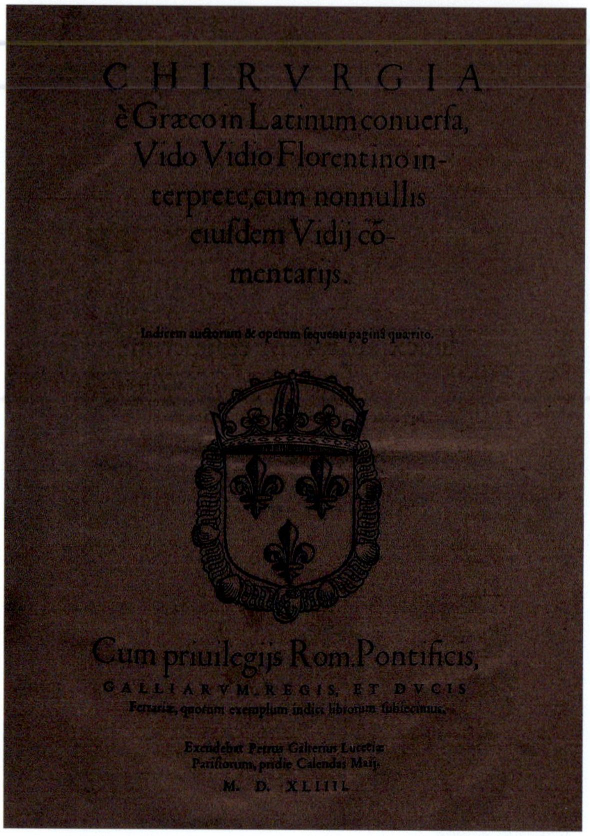

CHIRVRGIA
è Græco in Latinum conuersa,
Vido Vidio Florentino interprete, cum nonnullis
eiusdem Vidij cõmentarijs.

Indicem auctorum & operum sequenti pagina quærito.

Cum priuilegijs Rom. Pontificis,
GALLIARVM REGIS, ET DVCIS
Ferrariæ, quorum exemplum indici librorum subiecimus.

Excudebat Petrus Galterius Lutetiæ
Parisiorum, pridie Calendas Maij.
M. D. XLIIII.

Fig. 2.4 Frontispiece of *Chirurgia e Greco in Latinum Conversa, Vido Vidi Florentino Interprete*, Florence, 1544 by Vido Vidi (1508–1559) which includes the works of Hippocrates, Galen and Oribasius. *Courtesy of Riccardo Mazzola, M.D., Milan*

air, a concept that Claudius Galen (131–201 A.D.) would inherit and in his turn propagate [349, 351, 353, 354]. Celsus invented an instrument based on the same principle as the modern artery forceps, which he used to twist the vessels, thereby facilitating the tying of ligatures. He was also familiar with the principle of the tourniquet, but used it to treat snakebites, rather than bleeding, by binding the limb tightly to prevent the poison from passing into the general circulation.[10]

Other Contributions to Greco-Roman Medicine

It can be stated that the science of medicine for all practical purposes did not exist in Rome until the Greeks were defeated at Corinth in 146 B.C. and this holds all the more true for surgery. After that date, a gradual transfer of the entire Hellenic culture of the arts and sciences took place [1044]. Furthermore, skilled physicians were attracted to Rome by the prospect of establishing lucrative practices.

Celsus was certainly the most celebrated authority on medical subjects who was of Roman birth. His monumental eight-volume treatise *De Medicina* includes one volume devoted to surgery, which he defines as the branch of medicine "... which cures by the hand ... It does not emit medicaments and regulated diets, but does most by hand"[11]—certainly a most enlightened attitude for the period. Celsus also wrote on many other subjects including agriculture, the military arts, philosophy and law, and some have suggested that he was perhaps not actually a practising physician but an author with an encyclopaedic range of interests. Celsus' approach to medicine was in fact based on the teachings of Hippocrates, but he introduced a number of innovations which it is difficult to believe were not the fruit of his own experience (Fig. 2.5).[12]

For example, the use of suturing as a means of closing wounds is discussed at length: "If the wound is in a soft part, it should be stitched up, and particularly when the cut is in the tip of the ear or the point of the nose, or forehead, or cheeks, or eyelid, or lip, or on the skin over the abdomen."[13] Here Celsus appears to be referring to the same regions that his Greek predecessors considered most adapted to suturing and for the most delicate opera-

10 See *De Medicina*, Book V, Chapter XXVI, 21 B and C.

11 See *De Medicina*, Book VII, Proemium-.

12 Codex of Surgery in *Commentario* by Apollonio of Cizio (first century A.D.). Roland Capelluti from the *Scuola Salernitana* where the book was adopted as a text, wrote that "once the mandible has been grasped with one hand it should be moved repeatedly from left to right in order to allow the teeth to return to their original site" (*Apprenhendatur patients per mandibulam inferiorem et illam agitet huc et illuc dones dentes inferiorer superioribus adequentur*).

13 See *De Medicina*, Book V, Chapter XXVI, 23.

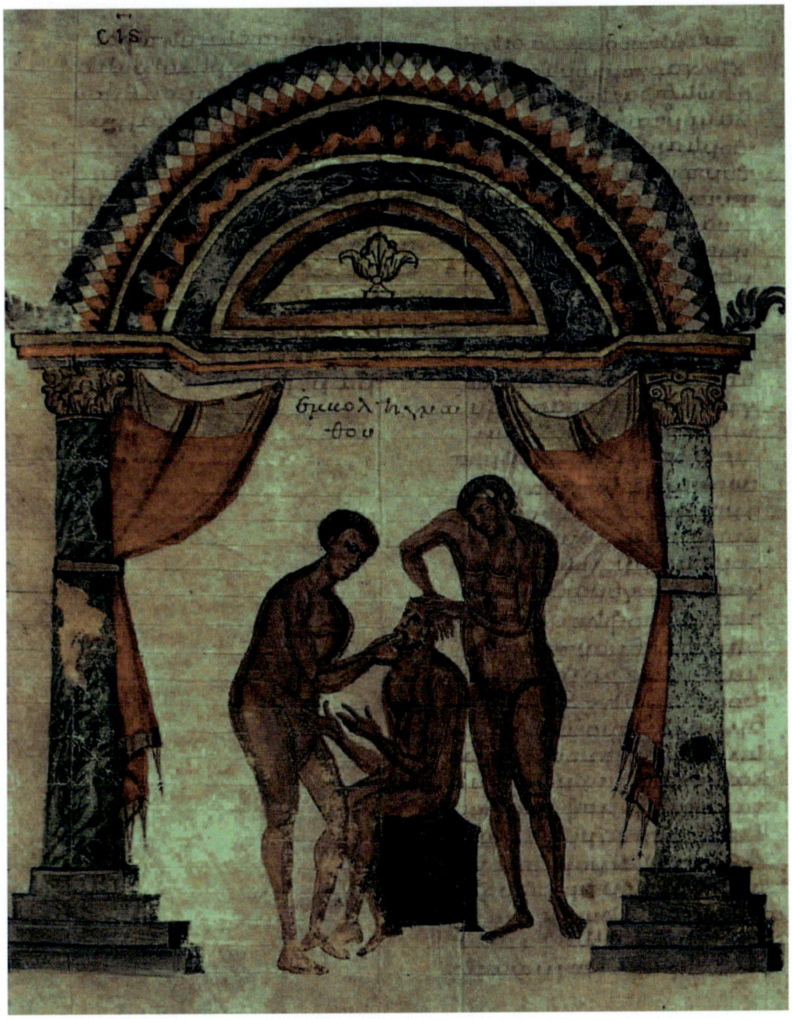

Fig. 2.5 Reduction of a dislocated mandible, a miniature from the Codex of Surgery in the Commentario of Apollonio from Cizio (first century A.D.) who wrote this book about Hippocrates. (ms.Laur.Plut.74.7, c.198v) *By permission of the Biblioteca Medicea Laurenziana, Florence, Ministero per i Beni e le Attivita Culturali*

tions he recommended using "women's hair".[14] However, Celsus recognized that this procedure was not always effective and in some cases: "… if the wound is in the flesh, and gapes, and its margins are not easily drawn together, then stitching is unsuitable, and fibulae [pins] are to be inserted, which draw together the margins to some extent and so render the subsequent scar less broad."

He reiterated the importance of cleaning the wound and removing all extraneous matter before suturing: "But neither [sutures nor fibulae] should be inserted until the interior of the wound has been cleansed, lest some blood-clot be left in it. For the blood clot turns into pus, and excites inflammation, and prevents agglutination of the wound. Not even lint which has been inserted to arrest bleeding should be left in, for this also inflames the wound. The sutures or fibulae should take up not only skin, but also some of the underlying flesh …".[15]

Celsus fully recognized the problems associated with tight wound closure, which had already been recorded by the Egyptians in the Smith papyrus. As he observed: "Generally, however, fibulae leave the wound wider open, [while] a suture joins the margins together, but these

14 It is interesting to note that the surgeons at the Ophthalmologic Clinic of the University of Geneve used the hair of the nuns who worked as nurses at the hospital for their minute corneal sutures up until the end of the nineteenth century [596].

15 See *De Medicina*, Book V, Chapter XXI, Par 23.

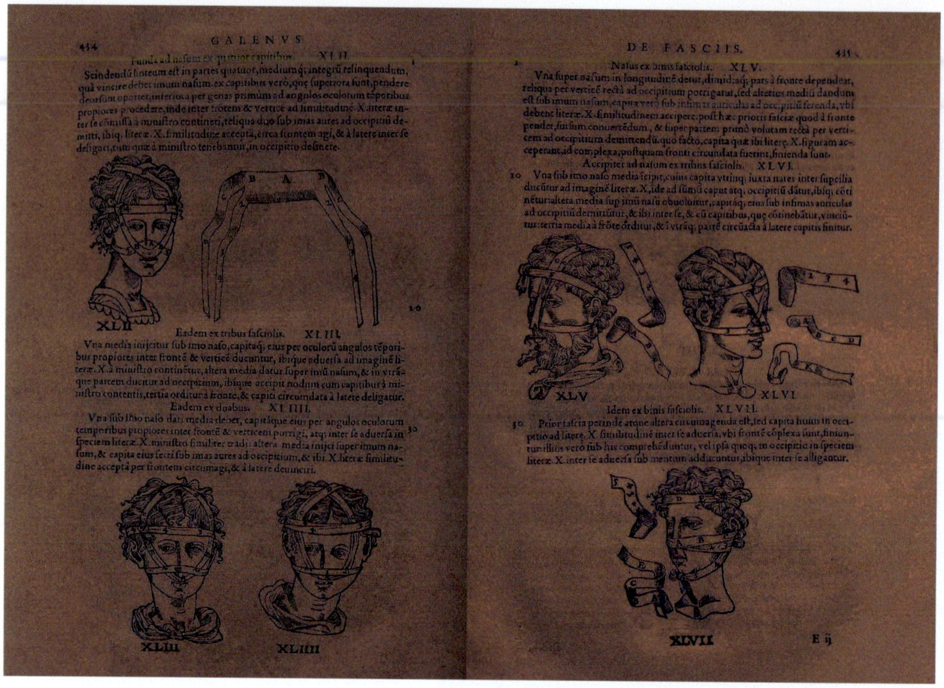

Fig. 2.6 Pages from *De Fasciis* by Galen (ca. 131–201 A.D.) translated by Vido Vidi and included in his *Chirurgia e Greco in Latinum Conversa, Vido Vidi Florentino Interprete* (Florence in 1544). *Courtesy of Riccardo Mazzola, M.D., Milan*

should not be brought actually into contact throughout the whole length of the wound, in order that there may be an outlet for any humour collecting within." He described the classic quartet of symptoms *rubor, tumor, calor et dolor* (redness, swelling, heat and pain),[16] which are still taught to first-year medical students today as the infallible warning signals of inflammation.

In addition to describing wounds to the face and neck, Celsus was perhaps the first author to treat the subject of penetrating abdominal wounds with extrusion of the viscera. He described how the organs should be repositioned, and recommended that the omentum be drawn over them and the suture be carried out layer by layer beginning with the peritoneum.

Another key figure in Roman medicine was Claudius Galen (129 to c.199 A.D.) [351, 353, 354]. Galen was actually born in Pergamon in Anatolia where he studied at a renowned Greek school, the Asklepieion (Ασκλεπιειον). After completing his medical studies at Smyrna, he spent five years in Alexandria. We know that Galen carried out his first operations in Pergamon where he served as the surgeon to a troop of gladiators. It was based on this first-hand experience that he formulated his approach to the treatment of wounds, recommending—like Hippocrates and Celsus—the removal of all extraneous bodies, the washing of the wound with wine, and early suturing (Fig. 2.6).

Curiously enough, after following this practice for some time Galen reversed his position and become an advocate of unguents and medications applied to induce suppuration and thus healing by the second intention. Although the reason for this about-turn is unknown, he had probably observed that many patients whose wounds were treated by immediate suturing developed infections and gangrene, particularly in the living quarters of the gladiators which were not the cleanest. An open and festering wound might take longer to heal, but was preferable to death from septicemia. Once again

16 See *De Medicina*, Book III, Par 10, 11.

confirmation was provided for the Hippocratic maxim *pus bonus et laudabile*.

At the age of 33 Galen moved to Rome where he became a highly successful physician, counting no less than three Roman emperors among his patients. Galen wrote 129 texts on the subject of medicine, of which 86 have survived. It is not surprising therefore that he became the undisputed authority for physicians and philosophers and remained so for a long time—some would say for much too long because his influence lasted more than ten centuries and become an obstacle to progress and the acceptance of new approaches to treatment. In particular, his notion that suppuration was beneficial and indeed indispensable to the healing of wounds prevailed until the thirteenth century, when Theodoric of Cervia and Henry de Mondeville finally dared to question the idea. Some of his other ideas would not be overturned until the discovery of antisepsis by Lister in the nineteenth century.

It is interesting to compare the very different personalities of Hippocrates and Galen. Hippocrates was motivated by rigorous intellectual honesty and a profound scientific curiosity, which led to the assimilation of concrete facts. From these he acquired an understanding of the symptoms of particular diseases and the nature of the body's pathological and healing processes. All of his treatments were guided by this knowledge. Galen, whom we must remember was not only a physician but also a philosopher, based his teachings on theoretical notions which, brilliant and convincing though they might appear, were sometimes erroneous. He adjusted his facts to fit these theories and never mentioned his failures, no doubt convinced that his ideas could not be challenged. As a consequence, although he made some noteworthy contributions to medicine and in particular to surgery, his teachings later became a serious hindrance because, as Whipple [1044] wrote: "… to question his authority was anathema except for some brave and independent individuals".

Our knowledge of Galen, like that of Hippocrates and Oribasius [821] whom we will meet shortly, is in large part based on the work of Vido Vidi (1508–1559) who collected all of the writings that he could find by these authors and published them in a monumental work, *Chirurgia e Greco in Latinum Conversa, Vido Vidi Florentino Interprete* (Florence, 1544) [1018, 1019]. This was illustrated by Primaticcio (1504–1570), an artist influenced by the Byzantine school of painting. The book contains all of the surviving works by these classical authorities, and certain sections are of particular interest to the plastic surgeon (Fig. 2.7a, b). For example, Galen wrote what amounted to a systematic and exhaustive treatise on cranio-facial surgery, an entirely new and unexplored subject for his time.[17] In it he describes various types of trauma to the face and head, together with their diagnosis, specific treatment and prognosis. He includes a discussion of cerebral concussion, with a description of the technique of trephining the skull and its possible complications. Galen placed great importance on the bandaging of wounds and provides instructions on how to bandage every region of the body, including no less than 59 methods of bandaging cranial lesions which are particularly interesting [790].[18]

After the Decline of the Roman Empire

Four centuries would pass before any advances worth mentioning were made in the treatment of wounds and head trauma. In fact, with the exception of the use of grafts for injuries to the face, a procedure introduced by Oribasius of Alexandria (c.325) which we will discuss in our chapter on flaps [754–757, 821], no significant contributions can be found until the studies of trauma by Paulus Aegineta (624–690) in the seventh century [3–5]. Aegineta was the author of a seven-volume treatise [19] which not only contains a detailed description of the ligature of vessels in cases of refractory bleeding, but also a remarkably sophisticated discussion of the treatment of facial trauma. He examines the problems of reduction

17 *De Vulneris Capitis.*

18 The original manuscript by Vido Vidi is conserved in the Bibliothèque Nationale de Paris (cat. no. 6866).

19 In the same work Paulus Aegineta describes a treatment for hypospadias and another for nose fractures. The author also deserves to be mentioned for having introduced the tracheostomy and surgery of the lips, which he carried out using a special scalpel which he called "the knife for plastic operations".

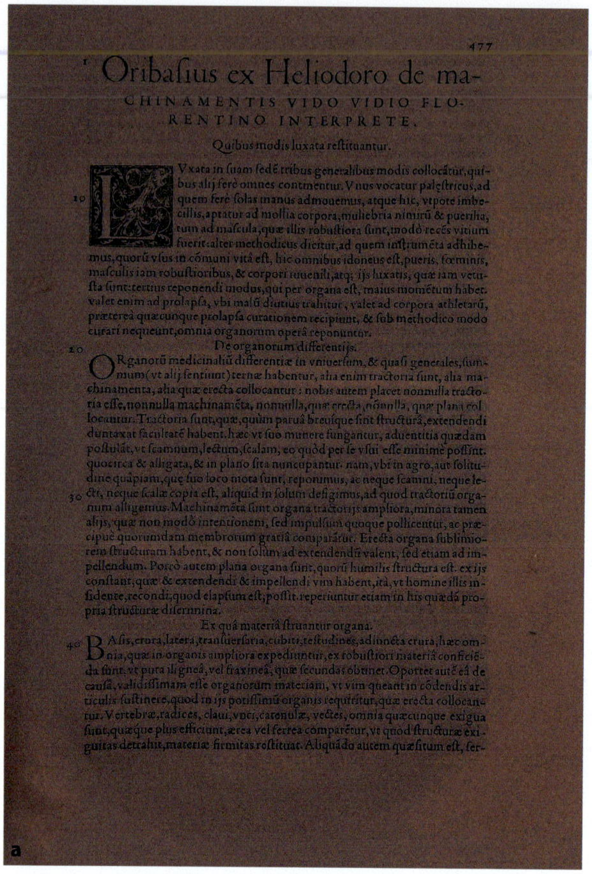

Oribasius ex Heliodoro de ma-
CHINAMENTIS VIDO VIDIO FLORENTINO INTERPRETE.
Quibus modis luxata restituantur.

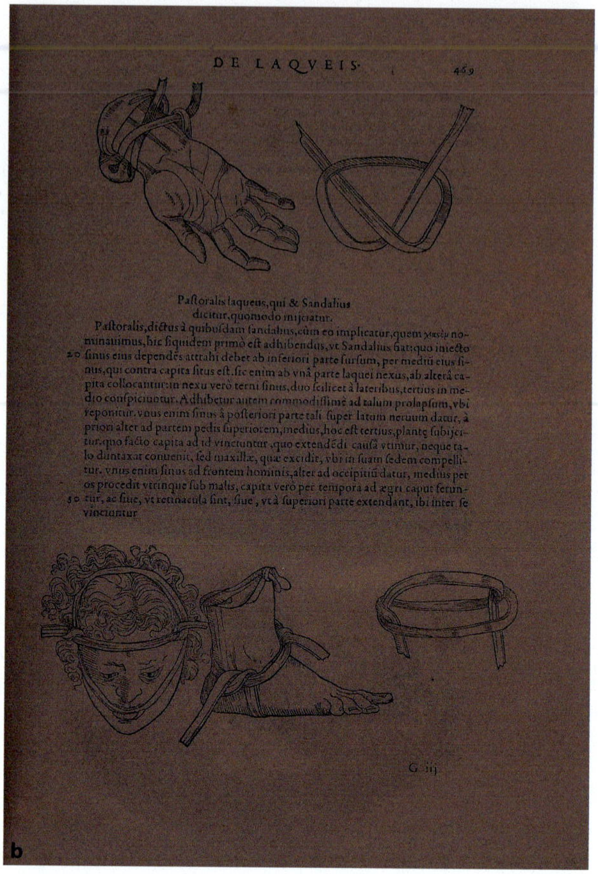

DE LAQVEIS.
Pastoralis laqueus, qui & Sandalius dicitur, quomodo iniiciatur.

Fig. 2.7a,b *De Laqueis* by Oribasius (c.325 A.D.) translated by Vido Vidi and included in his *Chirurgia e Greco in Latinum Conversa, Vido Vidi Florentino Interprete* (Florence in 1544). The illustrations show the type of bindings he used to try to stabilize fractures and dislocations. *Courtesy of Riccardo Mazzola, M.D., Milan*

and fixation of fractures and presents the first description of the technique for fixing the segments of a broken jaw by wiring the teeth, in his case with threads of gold.[20] He thus made significant contributions to the origins of Plastic Surgery [403].

The Contributions of the Arabs

It is well known that in the Middle Ages the monasteries preserved and passed on knowledge from classical times. This included medical texts from Greece and Rome. It is often forgotten however that the Arabs were responsible for preventing much of the well known medical practices from antiquity being lost. This is especially true of surgery which was neglected by the church.

In the fifth century A.D. a group of Aramaeans belonging to the Nestorian sect emigrated from Syria to Persia for religious reasons. Having inherited a large portion of the legendary library of Alexandria, they founded the Gandi-Sopor, the world's first teaching hospital. This institution formed a pathway which transmitted the greater part of their medical knowledge, in particular the translations of the works of Galen, to the Arabs. In addition to Galenic medicine, the Arabs adopted the Nestorian system of teaching and established their own hospitals in Bagdad, Cairo, Aleppo and Damascus, where for the

20 See *Chirurgie*, Book VI, Chapter 19.

first time the medical specialties of psychiatry and ophthalmology were taught.

The Arabs profited from the knowledge they had received from the Nestorians, and the science of medicine made immense strides, reaching its peak with Abul Quazim Halaf Ibn'Abbas az-Zahrawi, better known as Albucasis (936–1013 A.D.) [540]. Born in Cordoba during the golden age of Arab rule, he became the greatest Arab surgeon in history and wrote *El Tariff* (*The Method*) [14–18], an encyclopaedic work on medicine and surgery that even included a history of medicine [360, 361].[21] He is considered to be one of the moving spirits behind the rebirth of surgery, because it was through his teachings that the practice spread from Cordoba across western Europe (Fig. 2.8).

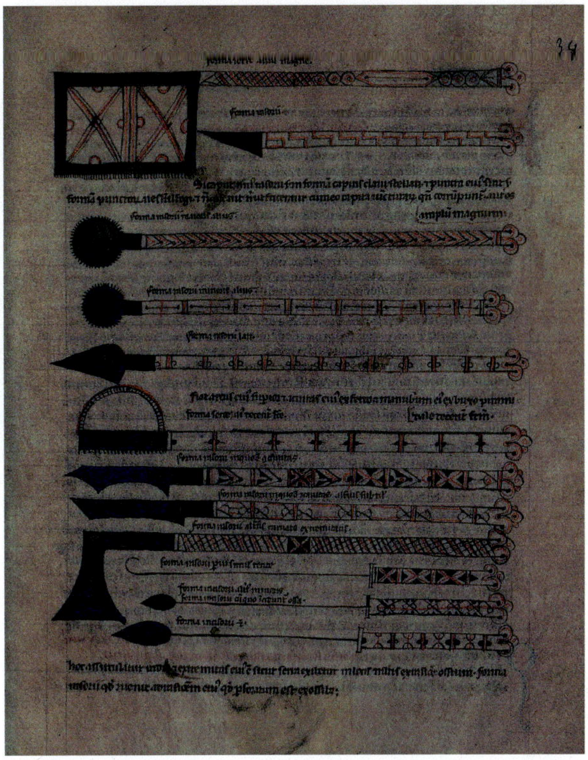

Fig. 2.8 Arabic surgical instruments from *Methodus Medendi* by Albucasis (936–1013). Thirteenth century translation into Latin of his *Altasrif* which was probably the first treatise dealing only with surgery. *By permission of the Biblioteque Nationale de France, Paris*

Albucasis perhaps more than anyone else was responsible for the acceptance and diffusion of the technique of cautery in the West. He taught that this procedure was of great value and furnished detailed instructions regarding its use in 57 chapters of his treatise. Cauterization was widely employed by Arab physicians to control bleeding and treat wounds of every type for they were convinced that it would speed healing, prevent infections and facilitate hyperemia.

According to Garrison, cautery was such a diffuse practice that the Arabs "practically set aside the knife" and suturing was rarely carried out. This is not entirely true, because Albucasis does describe various surgical operations that involved the use of the scalpel, such as one already described by Aegineta for hypospadias. We also find descriptions of delicate sutures to the nose, lips and ears which would generally, although not always, preclude the use of cautery.

Cauterization was practised using either "incandescent instruments" or natural "revulsive" methods. According to Albucasis, "Those parts treated with [cauteries in] gold do not develop infections." He further wrote: "What is usually said of cauterization, that it is an extreme method, is true. But only in the sense that it works even when other methods have failed." Nevertheless he advocated caution in its routine use: "He who uses cautery must exercise solid judgement, with a certain foresight which is not so easily described … Never perform an operation without first watching it performed by others and without having experience of the technique."[22]

Like Hippocrates he employed deep cauterization to stabilize cases of chronic dislocation of the shoulder. Where less invasive procedures were called for, as in the repair of the ectropion or lacrimal fistulae, he recommended the use of natural *revulsives*. His description of a gentle cautery carried out in a patient with a lip defect is quite celebrated. The area that was to be closed by su-

21 *El Tariff* was included by Guy de Chauliac in his collection of the works of the ten most important surgeons of the period, *Cyrurgia Magna*, published in Venice in 1531. A separate edition of *El Tariff* entitled *Methodus Medendi* was also published independently in Venice in 1541.

22 *El Tariff* contains an entire chapter dedicated to *De sutura nasii, et labii et auris.*

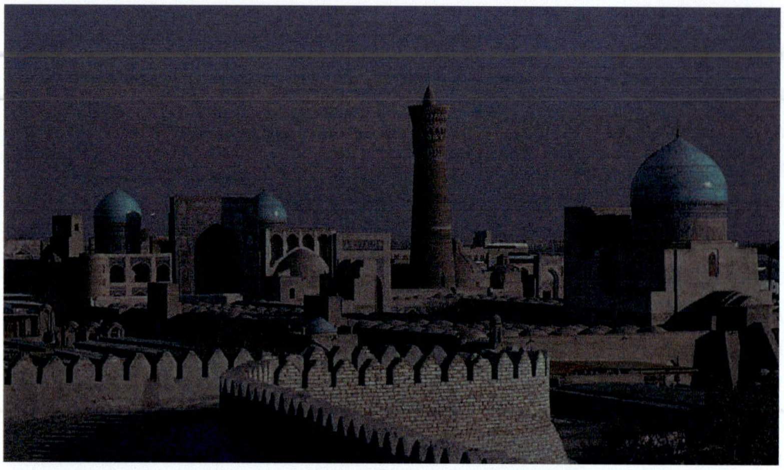

Fig. 2.9 View of Bukhara where Avicenna studied at the Royal Library of the Samanids. In his youth he learnt philosophy, geometry and the logic of Porfirius but at the age of 16 years medicine became his main interest. *PJS*

turing was prepared by inserting a clove of garlic into a pocket of skin created for the purpose, and on the following day the garlic was removed before the suturing commenced. Cauterization was almost always followed by suppuration, a natural process which Albucasis, like his predecessors Hippocrates and Aegineta, generally favoured.

In our discussion of the Arab contribution to medicine we cannot neglect to mention Rhazes (860–932), the author of the most important medical treatise in the Arab language according to Albrecht von Haller [409]. However, Rhazes' interest in surgery, and the specific problem of the healing of wounds, was limited.

Another Arab author who, although primarily a physician, introduced important advances in surgery was Avicenna [41, 42]. Born in 980 in the village of Afshaneh in Turkestan, he demonstrated a precocious interest in philosophy, law and medicine, pursuing his studies first under teachers and then on his own, frequenting the Royal library of the Samanids in Bukhara (Fig. 2.9). He embraced the Hippocratic principle that natural forces were the most important factor in the healing of wounds, [23] writing that: "When the ulcer is so large that the two margins cannot be brought into contact and there remains a gap that is full of foreign matter, there already being a loss of substance, then healing will necessarily be by cicatrization. … If the loss of substance be of flesh … we cannot hasten the process."

The basic principles which Avicenna set out for the treatment of "the continual loss of soft tissues" were to splint the unstable parts, arrest the bleeding, immobilize the involved part and prevent sepsis as far as possible. To achieve the latter he soaked his bandages in wine before applying them to the wound. He used cautery but warned his readers of the risk of exposing the underlying nerves, fasciae and ligaments. Avicenna's writings on the subject of anaesthetics are also of interest. He discusses the properties of the poppy, mandrake, hemlock, white and black henbane, and even considers the analgesic effect of cold temperatures induced by snow or ice.

The Contribution of the Scuola Salernitana

In Europe the influence of Arab medicine waned after the re-conquest of Spain by the Christians, but re-established itself in a certain sense with the creation of the *Scuola Salernitana*. In reality, while this school made a fundamental contribution to the development of anatomy and medicine, at least initially it dedicated much less attention to surgery. Nevertheless, during the thirteenth century a shift was seen as the teachers at Salerno began to re-evaluate the role of surgery in the practice of medicine. This change came about thanks to the influence of such figures as Ruggero of Salerno and Rolando of Parma

23 See *Canon*, Book I.

(late twelfth century), who adhered to the Galenic principles of suppuration and healing by second intention. Ruggero proposed the application of a somewhat curious material—lard—to the wound in order to stimulate suppuration. They each taught their students the techniques of ligating bleeding vessels, draining wounds, and suturing.[24]

Although the *Scuola Salernitana* remained active until the Napoleonic age, its importance declined after 1200 with the establishment of the rival institution at the University of Naples.

The Late Middle Ages and the Renaissance

During the Middle Ages monasteries served as the last remaining fortress of medicine, for it was here that the monks translated, copied and transmitted the classical texts of antiquity. In addition to their teachings, however, prayer, Christian faith, and the promise of eternal life came to be considered as indispensable to the healing of illnesses.

Naturally, whatever their possible effects, these spiritual elements certainly contributed little to the results of surgery. Furthermore, while monks were allowed to exercise their skills as physicians, the rights to practise surgery and anatomy were strictly prohibited because these were considered manual activities and, worse still, associated with the shedding of blood. As a result, the surgeon John Thomson [991] observed in 1813, "So degraded indeed was the practice of surgery that a principal part of it, the care of the wounds, was commonly entrusted to women and ignorant pretenders." The situation was slow to improve, even after the establishment of the first universities (Bologna 1088, Montpellier 1181, Padua in 1222, Naples in 1240),[25] because the primary scope of these institutions was to teach philosophy and theology, and they remained under the dominion of the Church. In 1215 Pope Honorius III decreed that "… no cleric must practice blood-letting or indeed any surgical operation or even watch them, and no subdeacon, deacon or priest should exercise any type of surgery". This interdict was confirmed by Pope Boniface VI at the end of the thirteenth century and again by Pope Clement V in Avignon at the beginning of the fourteenth century. They each formally separated medicine from surgery on the grounds that *Ecclesia abhorret a sanguine* (The Church abhors blood), and forbade members of the clergy from practising the latter. During this period the Faculty of Medicine of Paris refused to admit any student who did not reject surgery.

Operations were therefore left in the hands of *cerusici* or barber-surgeons. It became commonplace for monks who practised medicine to send those patients in need of minor surgery such as blood-letting or the lancing of abscesses to the barbers who came regularly to the monastery to cut their tonsures. They were at least skilled in the use of the razor! The most able and intelligent of these managed by dint of much practice to reach such high levels of competence—given the standards of the period—as to be considered genuine surgeons. The famous "barber-surgeons" of England can trace their origins back to this time when, from necessity, a path had to be found between the sacred and the profane.

The Galenic theory favouring the processes of suppuration found its first opponent in Theodoric Borgognoni (1205–1296), the bishop of Cervia, who wrote: "… it is not necessary, as Roland and Roger of Salerno have written, as many of their disciples teach, and as all the modern surgeons profess, that pus must be generated in wounds. No error could be greater than this. Such a practice is indeed to hinder nature, prolong the disease, and prevent the conglutination and consolidation of the wound." He instead recommended that the physician cleanse the wound with wine, remove all foreign bodies, and then suture it without the application of any ointments, unguents or other substances [122].

During the thirteenth century, university students began to rebel against the severe monastic rules to which they were subjected, in particular the vow of celibacy. Some therefore—especially those interested in surgery, which was still banned at the universities—left the priest-

24 See *La chirurgia di Teodorico*, Book II, Chapter 27.

25 Tho Quoc Tu Giuam (Temple of Literature) which was practically a University for literature and philosophy as well as what could be called today, Political Sciences was started in Hanoi, Vietnam by the Emperor Ly Thanh Tong in honour of Confucius, seven years before Bologna University was founded.

hood in order to be able to exercise their profession more freely. In this way a class of surgeons with formal training in medicine emerged, some of whom became quite expert although for a long time they remained controversial figures due to the lingering opposition to surgery.

One of them was Lanfranchi da Milano (d.1315) who, although he was an ordained priest, had an acknowledged son by the name of Mastro Bonnet who practised surgery in Montpellier. In his work *Cyrurgia Parva* [520], written in 1295, Lanfranchi described how he treated ulcers and wounds (Fig. 2.10). He must have been gifted in reconstruction, as he describes in his book the successful re-implantation of an amputated nose. It is not surprising that a surgeon capable of such an exploit would underline the importance of accurate suturing, particularly when treating injuries to the face, because "this is a part that is constantly exposed to view". He also emphasized that the stitches must be sufficiently deep and that the creation of any "dead spaces" was to be avoided. Lanfranchi described the U-suture and the mattress suture many centuries before Lexer, who is generally credited with these innovations. He was an advocate of cauterization to control bleeding, but also explained the principles of ligation, torsion and compression of the vessels, which was to be applied as necessary, depending on the gravity of the haemorrhage.

Lanfranchi was convinced of the shared origins of medicine and surgery, and believed that every surgeon should have medical training: "Omnia practicus est teoricus, omnis cyrurgicus est practicus: ergo omnis cyrurgicus est theoricus" ("Every practical exercise is [also] theoretical, every surgeon is a practitioner and therefore every surgeon is [also] a theoretician").

With increasing numbers of students and physicians leaving for the reasons described above, the universities, particularly in Italy, finally began to admit lay students who were accorded the same privileges as the clergy. This change in policy led to the rise of a new figure—the academic surgeon—and as a consequence, according to John Thomson: "The Italian physicians ought to be regarded as the restorers of Surgery in Modern Europe" [989, 990].

One of this new breed of surgeons was Henry de Mondeville (1260–1320), who achieved considerable fame as a professor at the universities of Bologna and Montpellier. Born in the village of Mandeville or Mondeville[26] close to Caen in Normandy, he studied at Montpellier under Lanfranchi and like him became a priest. He developed an interest in cutaneous defects of the face and introduced a number of revolutionary concepts for the treatment of wounds. To begin with, in his treatise *Chirurgie* [682] written between 1306 and 1320, but published in 1478 and then only in a fragmented version,[27] de Mondeville declared his opposition to the practice of cauterization and the subsequent process of suppuration. He recommended instead cleaning the

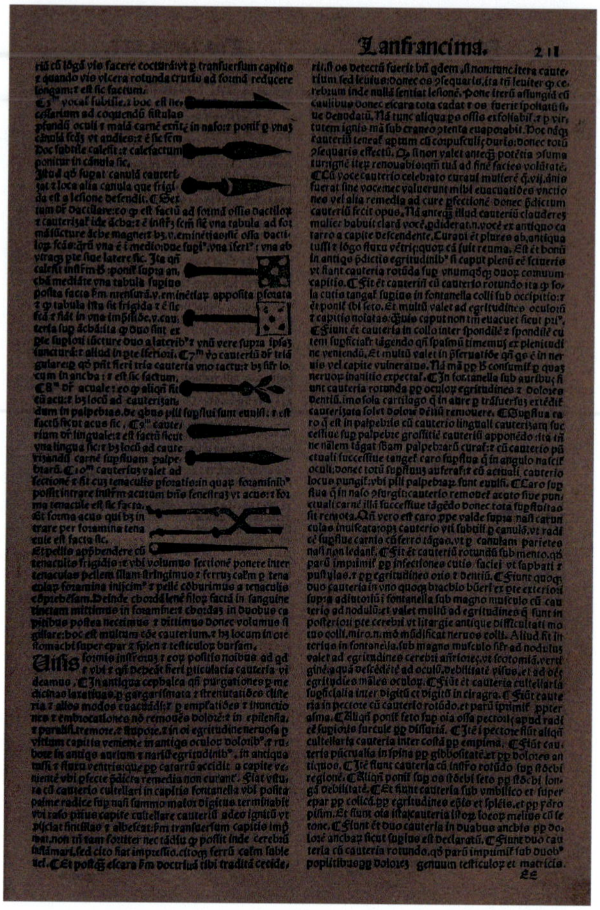

Fig. 2.10 Surgical instruments by Lanfranchi da Milano. Taken from the *Cyrurgia Parva* which in turn is part of Guy de Chauliac's *Cyrurgia Magna* published in 1363. *Courtesy of Riccardo Mazzola, M.D., Milan*

26 The names Emandeville, Hermandeville and others have also been proposed.

27 The manuscript of the first edition is conserved in the Karolinska Biblioteket at the University of Uppsala, Sweden.

injury thoroughly with "wine as hot as the patient can bear" (thus anticipating the use of antiseptics), the application of dry bandages (which should not be changed too often in order to avoid further trauma to the injury) and, in the case of ulcers, a strong antiseptic in a balsam of verdigris. He also experimented with the techniques for controlling bleeding that he had learned from his professor, Lanfranchi.

During his time in Bologna, Henry de Mondeville had the opportunity to study *Spongia Soporifera*, a text on anaesthesia written by Ugo Borgognoni and his son Theodoric of Cervia. He would henceforth use these techniques routinely to induce analgesia during his operations.

A subsequent treatise, *Deuxième Traité des Plaies*, is of interest because it shows de Mondeville's remarkably advanced interest in the aesthetic problems caused by scarring, particularly in the case of the face and breasts. Indeed, he advised surgeons to exercise particular care in treating the injuries of patients to whom, because of their social or professional position, an unsightly scar would be a particular handicap.

De Mondeville also studied the problem of haemorrhaging from larger vessels, for which he suggested an incision of the dermis in order to expose the bleeding stump. This could then be pulled out with a specially designed hook and twisted around itself. If this measure was insufficient the surgeon could apply a ligature, the ends of which should be left protruding from the margins of the sutured wound so that they might easily be "fished out again" if there was a recurrence of bleeding. This twisting approach, which he called in Latin *torcere* or *contorcere*, was also adopted by Jehan Yperman (1295–1351) who used the Dutch term *verdreyen* 1055].

Henry de Mondeville became so well known for his skill as a surgeon that he was appointed *Chirugien du Roi* by Philippe le Belle in 1301. His work was included together with others in *Cyrurgia Magna* by Guy de Chauliac.

As we approach the Renaissance, noteworthy contributions to surgery and the art of healing were made by Guy de Chauliac (1300–1368), whom we have already had occasion to cite as the editor of the famous treatise *Cyrurgia Magna*, a collection of the works of the ten most famous surgeons of the period (Fig. 2.11a,b).[28] Born in Chauliac in Auvergne, he joined a religious order and studied medicine at Toulouse, Montpellier and finally Paris, also spending a short time practising anatomy in Bologna. In Avignon, de Chauliac became the personal physician to three successive popes (Clement VI, Innocent VI and Urban I)[29] and earned a reputation as the most gifted surgeon of his time. He was perhaps the last in a long and illustrious line of cleric-surgeons who included Lanfranchi and de Mondeville.

De Chauliac maintained that the surgeon must above all promote the natural process of healing by carefully cleaning the wound, staunching the bleeding and drawing together the margins using sutures. He reports his suturing technique in careful detail, emphasizing the importance of using sharp polished needles. He also provided a description of the mattress suture, which he explained was designed to reduce the tension and create an accurate approximation of the wound margins. For ulcers and cutaneous defects, whatever their cause, he recommended a conservative approach, being quite opposed to the use of cautery, ointments or bandages. De Chauliac was also probably the first physician to suggest the early excision of cancerous lesions [295].

Cyrurgia Magna was compiled around 1363 and published in Lyon in French in 1478, while a more complete edition was printed by Gregorio de Gregori in Venice in 1513. For more than a century it remained the most widely used surgical text in Europe.

An important contribution to the treatment of wounds was made by Pietro d'Argelata (d.1423), who studied under de Chauliac and later became a professor in Bologna. In his work *Chirurgia*, published in Venice in 1480, in addition to recommending dry bandages

28 Guy de Chauliac (c.1300–1368): *Cyrurgia Magna* was started in 1363 under the title *Inventorium Seu Collectorium Cyrurgie* and completed in 1378 when it was published in French. At that time Guy was in Avignon, where he had been called as personal doctor by Pope Clemente VI. The book is divided into seven parts of which the first is devoted to anatomy, all the others deal with surgery with the exception of the last which is a practical manual about blood letting, application of leeches, cupping and various other medical performances.

29 Guy de Chauliac advised Pope Clement VI to flee from Avignon to escape the Black Death in 1348 but stayed behind to care for the sick. Miraculously, having caught the plague he survived and recovered after 6 weeks.

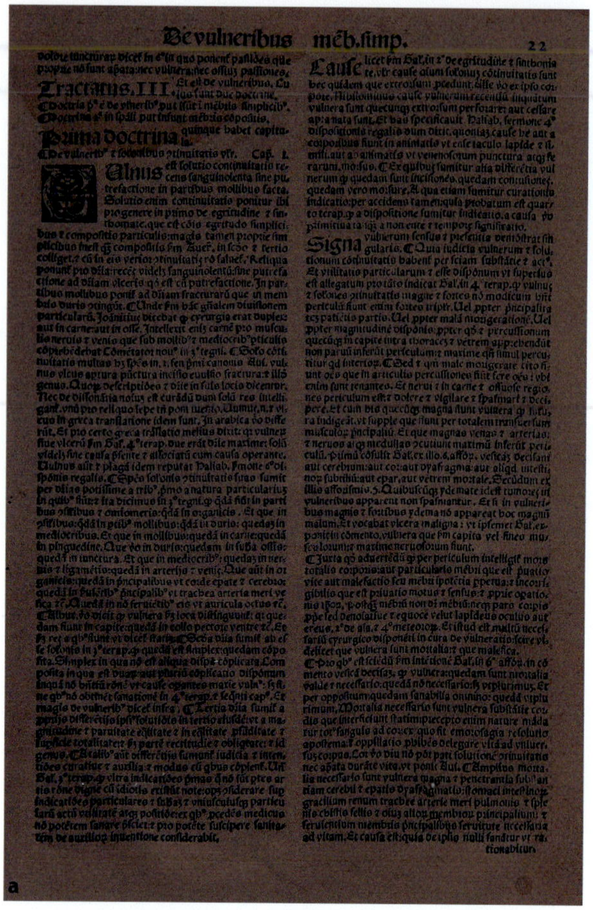

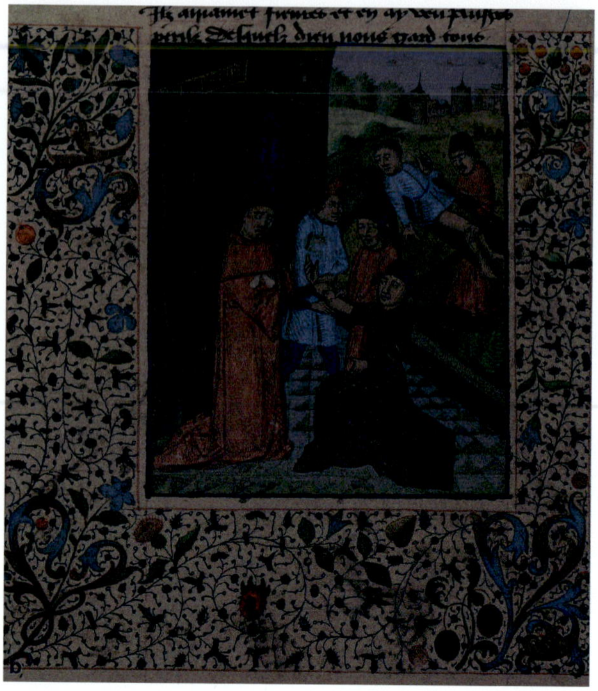

Fig. 2.11 **a** First page of the *Cyrurgia Magna* by Guy de Chauliac, a collection of the ten foremost authors of the time compiled in 1363. *Courtesy of Riccardo Mazzola, M.D., Milan.* **b** Fifteenth century manuscript showing Guy reducing a dislocated elbow. *By permission of the Biblioteque National de France, Paris*

he proposed a genuine innovation—the use of tubes to drain the wound [30].

Faith in the principles of Galen began to vacillate with the teachings of Henry de Mondeville and Guy de Chauliac and, in particular, the positive effects of suppuration which were still accepted without question in the fifteenth century began to be questioned. Their revolutionary school of thought found an advocate in the somewhat controversial but undeniably brilliant physician Théophraste Bombard von Hohenheim (1493–1541) (Fig. 2.12), better known as Paracelsus [764, 765]. His doctrine with regard to the treatment of wounds may be summed up in one of his famous pronouncements: "Keep the wound clean and distinct and preserve it from outside enemies. The fundamental treatment that I would suggest for the healing of wounds is that medicines be applied to protect the infected injury from external factors." In this passage it is suggested for the first time that an irregular process of healing might be caused by external agents and not the imaginary and endogenous humors of Antiquity. Paracelsus also wrote: "It is nature that prepares the destruction of the disease. The physician is merely an instrument to assist nature in its work. The therapy for wounds is therefore a defensive one, to ensure that no mishaps occur and no limitations are posed on nature's effects"—certainly not a widely accepted concept in 1536! Nonetheless even Paracelsus, who was decidedly opposed to any concept not supported by logic and concrete facts, sometimes mingled elements of magic and alchemy with his science.

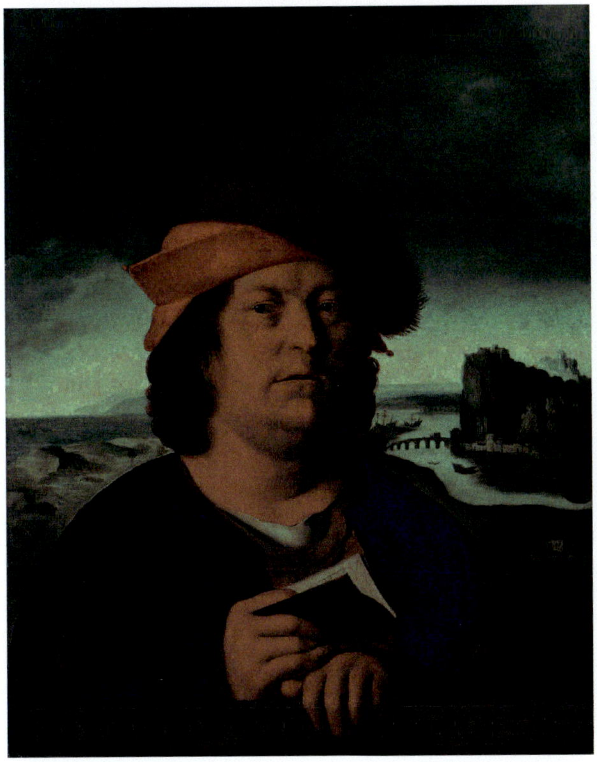

Fig. 2.12 Portrait of Aureolus Theophrateus Bombatus alias Paracelsus by Metysys Quentin (1465–1530). Louvre Museum, Paris. *By permission © Photo RMN / © Hervé Lewandowski*

The treatment of wounds made further progress with the work of Fabricius ab Acquapendente (1537–1619), who dedicated the second volume of his work *Opera Chirurgica* to the subject [291–293]. Like de Mondeville he realized the importance of the aesthetic outcome in the healing of face wounds and observed that, while a depressed scar might be inevitable, particularly if suppuration has taken place, protruding or inverted margins could only be the effect of careless surgery or a failed effort to cauterize the *camis luxurians*, his term for excessive granulation.

Professional Societies and Their Role in the Development of Surgery

The introduction of surgery into the curriculum led to the rise of a new figure who practised both medicine and surgery at the university. His background was based on the scientific foundations of the period which were admittedly meager. This change was not sufficient to overcome a lingering aversion to surgeons. Distrust arose in large part from the presence of unqualified practitioners or, worse still, charlatans with no scientific or medical preparation at all. They did much to discredit the medical arts. Furthermore, surgery itself had always been associated with risks and failures could be severely punished, as we have already seen from the Code of Hammurabi. In the sixth century the king of Burgundy executed two *Phisici* on the tomb of his beloved wife Austrichildes, whom they had failed to save from the plague. Later, in 1337 an itinerant physician incautiously offered to treat Johannes of Bohemia who had been struck blind. When it was found that he could not restore the king's sight he was thrown into the Oder River [360, 361]. Such events were not rare, although it must be admitted that some form of punishment was justified because in many cases operations were conducted by unscrupulous or foolhardy individuals entirely lacking in education, training or experience, with disastrous results.

This situation motivated the more qualified and responsibly minded surgeons to unite in organizations which, like the guilds formed by craftsmen and merchants, sought to regulate the standards of their profession. The members established specific criteria with regard to knowledge and technical skill, and as a consequence the general level of competence improved and patients became more willing to place themselves in the surgeons' hands.

The codes established by these organizations varied from country to country but their basic principles were quite similar. In Sicily King Ruggero issued an edict in 1140 requiring aspiring surgeons to undergo examination by the teachers at the *Scuola Salernitana*. The candidates also had to furnish proof of their technical ability and their knowledge of human anatomy. The physicians of Florence, one of the first cities to establish guilds for its artisans and merchants, founded a medical association in 1349 which had remarkably strict standards for its time, requiring members to follow regular courses and to attend the dissections conducted at its school of medicine [89].

In France the teaching of surgery was banned at the faculty of medicine of Paris, but students could receive instruction at the Ecole de St. Côme in the capital. This school, established in 1200, was divided into two sec-

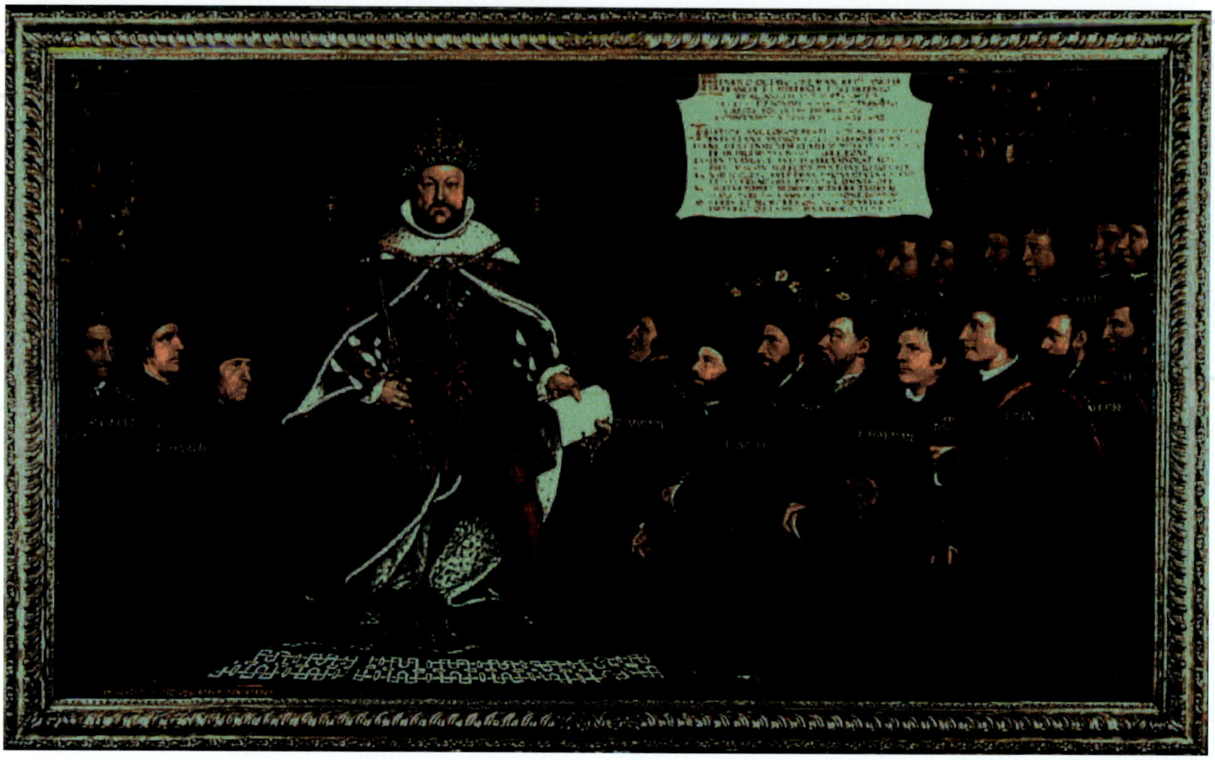

Fig. 2.13 King Henry VIII handing the charter to Thomas Vicary at the time of the Union in 1540 between the Company of Barbers and the Guild of Surgeons. The painting is by Hans Holbein the Younger (1497–1543) and is kept in the Barbers Surgeon Hall in London. *Courtesy of the Worshipful Company of Barbers, London*

tions: one reserved for the cleric-surgeons (*the doctors of the long robe*) and the other for lay surgeons (*the doctors of the short robe*) and graduates had to pass an examination before they were allowed to practise. Later a similar institution run by barber-surgeons was created in Toulouse and became quite famous.

However, it was in England that professional associations developed most fully and perhaps played an important role in transforming surgery into a genuine profession, equal in prestige to medicine. An organization was first mention in 1308 when Richard the Barber was ordered to keep order among the barbers. A group was formed to discourage conduct that might bring discredit upon the profession. In reality barber-surgeons had already organized their own society by the time of the papal bull of 1163 forbidding the members of religious orders from shedding blood and hence from practising surgery or even dentistry. These functions were taken up by the barbers of this association. The company also included surgeons in their number, the first being recorded in a list of members in1312. Those practising in London in 1368 were licensed to form a guild and after eight years the Lord Mayor and Aldermen allowed them to exercise some control over the surgeons. Despite including some surgeons in there number a power struggle arose between the Barbers Company and the Guild of Surgeons. This ended when Edward IV granted the Barbers a charter of incorporation in 1462. This made their long standing practices legal. In 1493 the Company and the Guild agreed to follow the same rules and to grant diplomas allowing successful participants to carry out surgery. But in 1511, early in the reign of Henry VIII, an act of Parliament was passed which placed the licensing of surgeons in the hands of Bishops (Fig. 2.13).

During this period surgeons began to demand full recognition for their profession and to have the word "barber" removed from their title. In 1745 another schism took place between the barbers and the barber-surgeons in the company. Finally, the Royal College of Surgeons was created as a parallel institution to the Royal College of Physicians. Since initially its members did not possess a university degree in medicine, they were referred to as Master (colloquially "Mister"), a title which British surgeons still retain with a certain pride today.

Battlefield Surgery

Surgery originally developed as the art of wound repair and therefore during the course of history frequent wars provided surgeons opportunities to exercise their skills. We have already seen how Galen developed his surgical principles based on his experience in the treatment of the wounds of gladiators.

At the beginning of the second millennium, with the invention of gunpowder and the introduction of the harquebus on the battlefield, the surgeon was forced to confront a large number of problems hitherto unknown to him. These challenges led directly to significant advances in the art of surgery. In the past armies sometimes travelled with an itinerate surgeon in their midst, but by the fourteenth century his presence had become an absolute necessity.

One of the first military surgeons to be recruited was J. Yperman (1295–1351), a Fleming who had studied with Lanfranchi. He was placed in charge of treating the wounded in the French army during the course of one of the battles of Ypres,[30] where it appears that the harquebus was used for the first time, although some historians date this innovation to the battle of Crecy en Ponthieu in western France. It was at Crecy during the Hundred Years' War that the battle between Edward III of England and Philip VI of France took place in 1346. Twenty-five thousand men lost their lives including a large portion of the nobility of France. Yperman recounts his experiences in his book *La Chirurgie* [1055], which contains new concepts and techniques developed in an attempt to mend the terrible ravages of these novel weapons. Unlike traditional arms with their sharp points, cutting edges or crushing power for which there existed codified treatments tested by centuries of experience, these explosive arms not only caused fearsome losses of body fluids and tissue, but also the entry into the wound of extraneous material such as soil, fragments of clothing, and debris, often causing fatal contamination.

The frequency of infection and gangrene increased drastically and one of the first remedies introduced, at least for the limbs, was the hitherto almost unknown practice of amputation. The ligation of the large arteries and veins became a routine procedure, although it was not always practised because haemostasis was generally achieved by cauterization. Furthermore, since the idea had taken root that gunpowder was poisonous and constituted the principal danger of gun shot wounds (whereas in reality it was the extent of the injury and necrosis of the tissue which led to infection, gangrene and death), the barbarous practice of pouring boiling oil on the involved site was adopted. This was meant to serve as a haemostat, an antidote to the poison of the gunpowder, and a cautery the injured tissue, but in reality it probably only added another trauma to those already present. The practice persisted until the reign of Charles IX (1550–1574), when it was prohibited in France and ligatures become the accepted technique to stop bleeding.

Another surgeon who contributed to the development of reconstructive surgery for battlefield injuries was Heinrich von Pfolsprundt (or Pfolspreundt) (born c.1435) [796], a *Bruder* (Brother) of the Teutonic Order he served as a military surgeon with the Prussian army during the Polish campaign. He described in great detail the treatment of gunshot injuries, which he referred to as "new wounds". His work was not particularly original, merely presenting a compendium of well-established concepts.

The surgeon who most vigorously promoted the theory that the devastating effects of harquebus wounds were

30 Ypres was the theatre of many historic battles, particularly during the interminable wars between France and England. In 1302 Flanders confronted Philippe IV le Belle on this battlefield, and then in 1383 Ypres was besieged by the English, who destroyed a large part of the city. The walls were rebuilt in three years, but were once again destroyed in 1560 by Charles V. It is likely that the harquebus was first used on the battlefield during the English siege of 1383. In support of this hypothesis we may cite the interesting fact that the word *harquebus* probably derives from the Flemish word *hakebus*, which was used to refer to a particular type of cannon that was mounted on a tripod.

to be attributed to gunpowder poisoning was Hieronimus Brunschwig (1450 to c.1512), an Alsatian who wrote extensively on the subject of gun injuries in his work *Dis ist das Buch du Chirurgia Hautwirchung* [138–140].[31] To eliminate the poison, he adopted the suggestion of Ruggero of Parma and used lard to drain the wound but also "to absorb the poison".[32] He also recommended inserting animal bristles into fistulae and agitating them briskly in order to cleanse the wound and induce suppuration (Fig. 2.14).

His preferred solution for bleeding was the ligature of single vessels rather than cauterization, particularly during amputations. Interestingly, he attributed great importance to the *imaginativum*, or the psychology of the patient, who had to be persuaded to believe that the haemorrhaging had stopped.

Considering the cruelty of the methods generally used in this period, the care devoted by Brunschwig to the treatment of wounds is noteworthy. In fact, he did his best to achieve inconspicuous and cosmetically acceptable scars.[33] On this subject he wrote: "Human beauty is expressed in the face and a well-formed body. Therefore, oh Physician, be careful and diligent in caring for facial wounds. Wherever possible make very fine stitches. In wounds of the mouth start with the first stitch in one corner and then put in stitch after stitch, very close to one another—below, above, and on the side—so that the mouth will maintain its pleasant form even when the person is about to speak"—recommendations that we might only expect to find in a modern treatise on cosmetic surgery. He understood that the cleanliness of the operating area and of the wound itself were of fundamental importance. The section of his book on narcotic preparations, which demonstrates his familiarity with work of the thirteenth century physician Ugo Borgognoni,[34] and one describing his technique for wiring the fractured jaw to the teeth just as Aegineta did centuries earlier,[35] show his depth of knowledge. Also significant is the fact that *Das ist das Buch du Chirurgia* was written

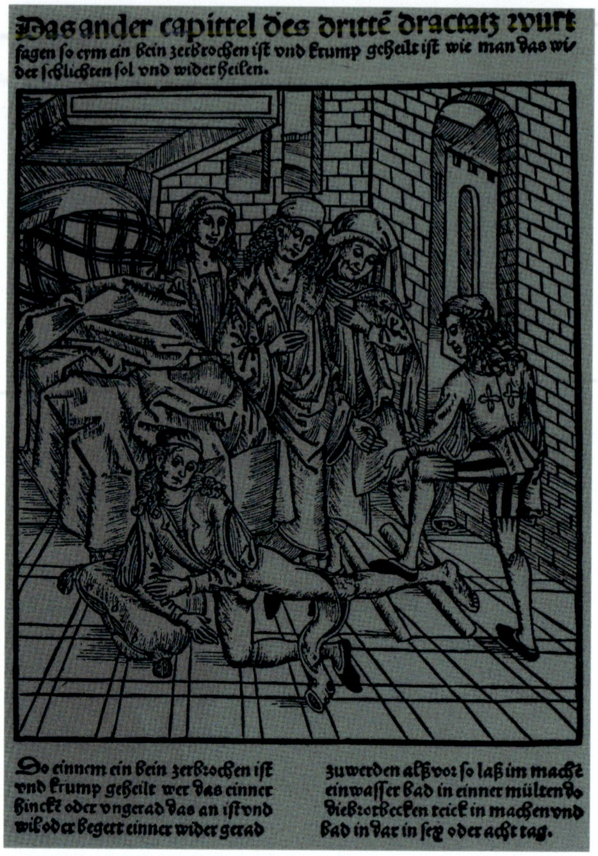

Fig. 2.14 A woodcut from Brunschwig's, *Dis ist das Buch der Chirurgia Hautwirkung der Wundartsney* (1497), probably the first illustrated treatise on surgery. The surgeon is re-breaking a leg to treat a fracture malunion. Brunschwig supported Pfolsprund's view that gunshot wounds were poisoned by gun powder and had to be treated with boiling oil. *Reprinted from* Surgery an Illustrated History *by Ira M Rutkov © 1993 with permission of Elsevier*

31 Brunschwig's work *Das ist das Chirurgia*, which appeared in Strasbourg in 1497, was among the first books to be published in Germany.

32 See the chapter *Das Zehende Capitel.*

33 See the chapter *Das Fecht Capitel.*

34 See the chapter *Das Capitel XI.*

35 See the chapter *Das Fiyerd Capitel.*

not for academic surgeons, but for the "barber-surgeons practicing in walled villages far from any assistance".

The belief in the toxicity of gunpowder was continued in Italy by Giovanni da Vigo (1460–1525), who stated that harquebus wounds "must be burned with cautery or with boiling oil. At the very least they should be treated with Egyptian ointment." Da Vigo was born in Rapallo in 1460. It is not known where he pursued his medical studies, although it seems probable that his only teacher was his godfather, Mastro Battista. He eventually moved to Rome where he entered into the service of Cardinal della Rovere, who would later become Pope Julius II. This redoubtable ecclesiastic preferred, as Da Vigo wrote, to don "the helmet more often than the tiara", and therefore the surgeon accompanying him did not lack for occasions to exercise his skill. The third book in his nine-volume work *Practica in Arte Chirurgica Copiosa*, published in Rome in 1514 [222], is entirely devoted to the healing of wounds (Fig. 2.15).[36] *Practica* was so successful that no less than 52 editions including translations into German, French, English and Spanish saw the light, even if Garrison [360, 361] judged this reception to be "out of all proportion to its value". Among the supporters of da Vigo's school of thought was Jean de Gerdsdorff (c.1551), who not only advocated pouring hot oil on wounds, but insisted that the operation be repeated at least two or three times a day, using fresh oil each time [364]. After this treatment he suggested applying to the wound an infusion of lime bark—a meagre consolation to the patient![37]

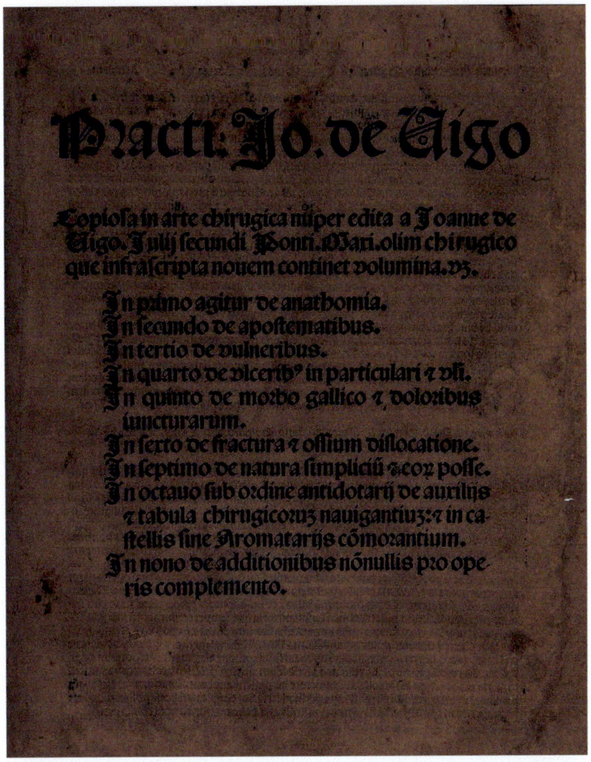
Practi. Jo. de Vigo

Copiosa in arte chirugica nuper edita a Joanne de Vigo. Julij secundi Ponti. Mari. olim chirugico que infrascripta nouem continet volumina. vz.

In primo agitur de anathomia.
In secundo de apostematibus.
In tertio de vulneribus.
In quarto de vlceribus in particulari et vli.
In quinto de morbo gallico et doloribus iuncturarum.
In sexto de fractura et ossium dislocatione.
In septimo de natura simpliciu et eorum posse.
In octauo sub ordine antidotarij de auxilijs et tabula chirugicorum nauigantium: et in castellis sine Aromatarijs cōmorantium.
In nono de additionibus nōnullis pro operis complemento.

Fig. 2.15 Frontispiece of *Practica in Arte Chirurgiuca Copiosa* by Giovanni da Vigo (1460–1525) published in Rome in 1514. It includes the treatment of gunshot wounds and ulcers. Part of the success of this book was due to the report of the "new" disease, syphilis. *Courtesy of Riccardo Mazzola, M.D., Milan*

Ambroise Paré and His Revolutionary Treatment of Wounds

Notwithstanding the fanatical enthusiasm with which the surgeons of the period inundated wounds with boiling oil, some signs of reason began to appear among them [588]. The first to question the theory of poisoning by gunpowder was Leonardo Botallo (1519–1587), who demonstrated that the powder contained neither poisonous nor caustic substances.[38] He also seems to have guessed that the real reason why gun wounds behaved differently from incised wounds was because of contamination by foreign bodies, and therefore scalding them with boiling oil was a useless practice that should be abandoned [123].

The first true revolution in the treatment of gun wounds was brought about by Ambroise Paré (1510–1590) (Fig. 2.16) who, approaching the problem from a purely scientific standpoint, argued that there did not exist any valid presuppositions or concrete evidence to

36 See *Liber Tertius. De Vulneribus.*

37 Jean de Gerdsdorff invented various instruments for battlefield surgery, including a *tireballes* to remove projectiles and fragments of metal.

38 See Botallo's *De curandis Vulnersi sclopetorum*, published in 1580.

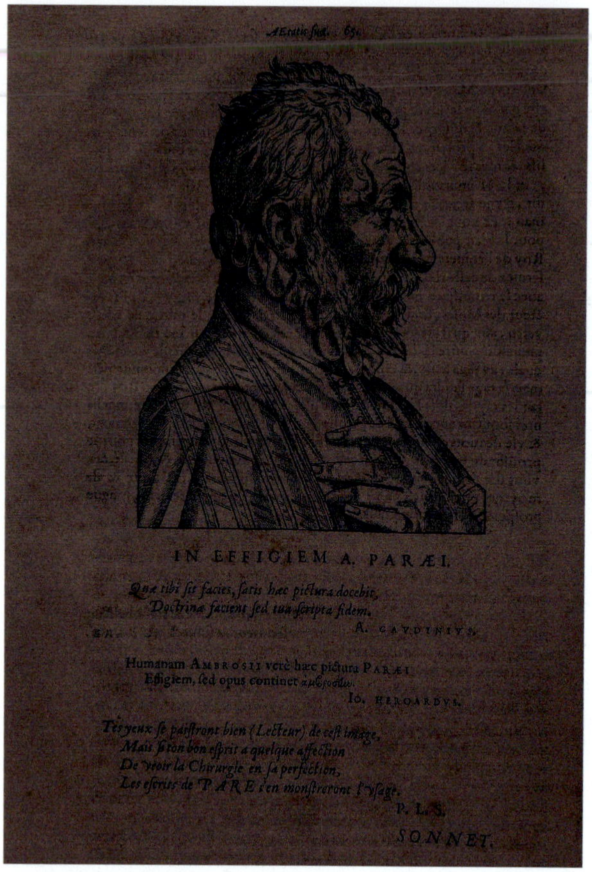
IN EFFIGIEM A. PARÆI.
Quæ tibi ſit facies, ſatis hæc pictura docebit,
Doctrinæ facient ſed tua ſcripta fidem.
A. GAVDINIVS.
Humanam AMBROSII verè hæc pictura PARÆI
Effigiem, ſed opus continet
IO. HEROARDVS.
Tes yeux ſe paiſtront bien (Lecteur) de ceſt image,
Mais ſi ton bon eſprit a quelque affection
De veoir la Chirurgie en ſa perfection,
Les eſcrits de PARE t'en monſtreront l'vſage.
P. L. S.
SONNET.

Fig. 2.16 This portrait of Ambroise Paré (1510–1590), probably the greatest surgeon of the sixteenth century, is taken from his famous work *Les Oeuvres* (1575). *Courtesy of Riccardo Mazzola, M.D., Milan*

support the theory that these types of wounds were poisoned.

Paré was born in Laval near Mayenne to a family of Huguenots and received a modest education, learning neither Latin nor Greek. He arrived in Paris in 1529 and became a barber-surgeon at the Hospital of the Hotel de Dieu. Despite his lack of classical knowledge, the professors at the College de St. Côme allowed him to study with them; indeed, he was such a brilliant student that they waived the usual fees and granted him a diploma without requiring him to take the qualifying exam. In his commentary on Paré's career and works, J.F. Malgaigne [600, 601] wrote that the names of his professors were unknown but, having recognized the unusual gifts of the young man, they most laudably: "... instructed him in the theories and methods of Lanfranchi, Guy de Chauliac and Vigo and on the views of Galen concerning surgery".

In 1537 Paré became a military surgeon. At this time France was not only engaged in an internal conflict with the Huguenots which would soon assume the proportions of a genuine war, but had also embarked on a series of confrontations with the English, as well as in Italy, Germany and the Low Countries. This offered the young surgeon innumerable opportunities to prove himself on the battlefield, and Paré earned a high reputation during the course of many campaigns for his valor and technical skill. Initially he was snubbed by the Parisian medical establishment, one of the reasons being that, ignorant of Latin, he wrote his medical works in the vernacular, but despite this his reputation grew and during his long career he served as surgeon to four of the kings of France (Henry II, 1509–1555; Francois II, 1543–1560; Charles IX 1550–1574;[39] and finally Henry III, 1551–1589).

A prolific author [768–770], at the age of 26 while he was in the service of M. de Montejan, Paré wrote his first treatise on wounds (Fig. 2.17), in which he expressed his opposition to the use of boiling oil and suggested instead bandaging the wound with egg yolk, turpentine and rose oil.[40] Although it would only be published in 1575, with this work Paré revolutionized the treatment of gunshot wounds. In fact, he himself said "I was not any expert at that time in matter of chirurgey: neither was I used to dresse wounds made by gunshot. Now I had read in Jean de Vigo that wounds made by gunshot were venenate or poisoned and that by the reason of the gunpowder: wherefore, for their cure, it was expedient to burn or cauterize them with oely ceders scalding hot, with a little treacle mixed therewith. I knew that caustic could not be powdered into wounds without excessive pain. I, before I would runne a hazard, determined to see whether the chirurgions used any other maner of dressing to these wounds. I observed that all of them used the method of

39 Although King Charles IX took active part in the massacre of the Huguenots, firing upon the fleeing Protestant nobles from his palace, he took care to protect his surgeon, on one occasion (it is said) by hiding him under his bed.

40 See *Discours sur le Livre des Plaies par Harcquebutes & Autres Baston à Feu.*

dressing which Vigo prescribed. I found that such as I dressed with a digestive oely, made of yolk of an egg, oil of roses and terpentine, free from vehemence of pain to have a good rest and that their wounds were not inflamed, nor tumified; but on the contrary the others that were burnt with the scalding oely were feverish tormented with much pain and the parts about their wounds were slow … [He concluded] I now invite all young surgeons to abandon this cruelty and inhumanity."

Paré described in painstaking detail the procedure of tying of blood vessels which had been conceived by Celsus, advocated by de Mondeville, and which he employed during amputations. Introduced almost *ex novo*, ligation quickly became routine during the siege of Denvillers in 1552. The first case of amputation described by Paré was that of an unfortunate postilion by the name of Piron Garbier whose leg had to be removed through the thigh.

In Paris during the intervals between his numerous military campaigns he conducted dissections and, according to Malgaigne, became *prosector* for the illustrious professor of anatomy Sylvius. With his friend Thierry de Hery, Paré carried out a series of dissections, reporting the results of his studies in 1550.[41] In 1545 he published his masterly treatise on wounds, *La Mèthode de Traiter les Playes Faictes par Hacquebutes et Aultres Bastons a Feu*, considered to be the first scientific text published in France. The fruit of more than a decade of experience as a military surgeon, it offers a complete exposition on battlefield injuries; the section on burns is particularly authoritative. *La Mèthode* immediately attracted the attention of the entire profession and was translated into many languages.

Not content with this achievement, in 1572 Paré produced his masterpiece, *Cinq Livres de Chirurgie* (*Five Books on Surgery*),[42] a handbook that provided everything the surgeon needed to know about war wounds. Printed in a small format by André Wechel so that it could be easily packed and carried, it includes sections not only on gun wounds, but also on the treatment of fractures, dislocations, gout, poisonous insect and animal bites with instructions on bandaging, and illustrations of many surgical instruments of his own invention (Fig. 2.18a–c).

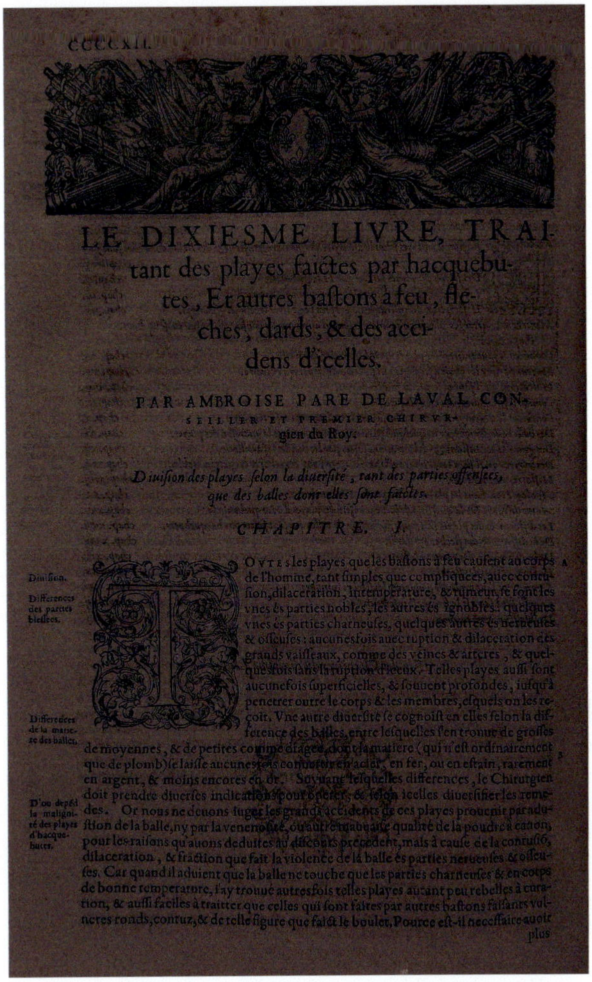

Fig. 2.17 The section of Paré's book *Les Oeuvres* where he deals with gunshot wounds. He forbade the use of boiling oil while campaigning in Italy, instead using egg and turpentine with immediate improvement. *Courtesy of Riccardo Mazzola, M.D., Milan*

In 1575 Paré published a complete edition of his works in 27 volumes entitled *Les Oeuvres* [769] containing a large number of anatomical drawings illustrating surgical procedures. The work sold out in a very short

41 The title of this work, published in 1550, was *Briefve Collection de l'Administration Anatomique*.

42 *Cinq Livres* was published after *Dix Livres* which appeared in 1564 [768] possibly because it was condensed and made more portable for the surgeon in the field.

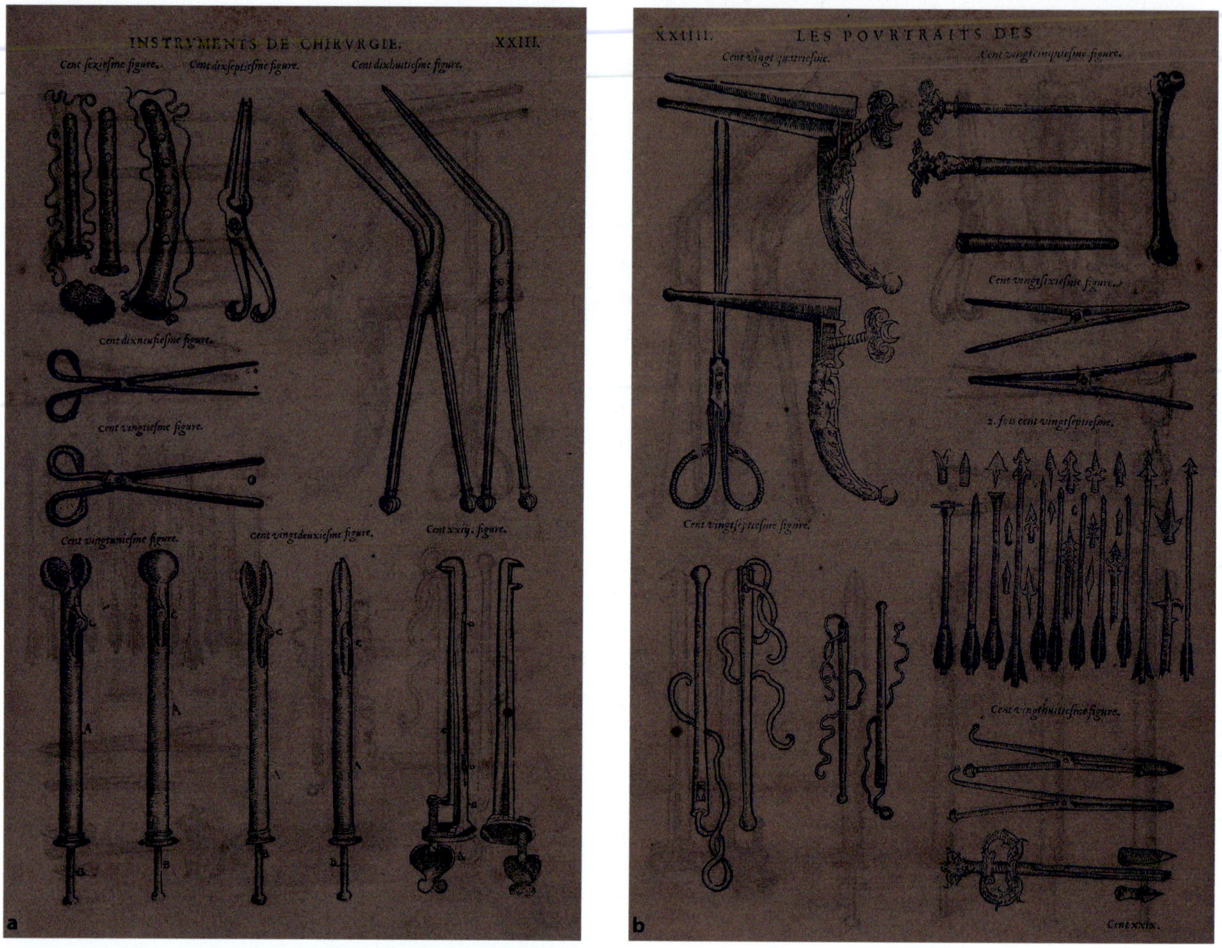

Fig. 2.18a–c Some of Paré's instruments described in *Les Oeuvres*. *Courtesy of Riccardo Mazzola, M.D., Milan*

time and a second edition with an even larger number of illustrations was prepared by Paré three years later. In this remarkable work of more than 2,000 pages, Paré set the canons for the treatment of wounds which would provide the foundations for all subsequent developments in the area. *Les Oeuvres* covers all the branches of surgery in a comprehensive fashion and the plastic surgeon today will find innumerable points of interest regarding not only the treatment of wounds, but also congenital malformations, surgery of the genitalia, and descriptions of an endless array of instruments, prostheses, false teeth, etc. with imaginative suggestions for their application (Fig. 2.19a, b).

In recent years Paré has been rediscovered as a pioneer who established the five principles of surgery, i.e. (1) to take away what is superfluous, (2) to reset in their original places parts which are displaced, (3) to separate tissues that have been fused together (4) to join those which have been separated and finally (5) to repair the defects of nature. In the twentieth century Gillies also adopted similar principles for plastic surgeons and Millard added to these to produce the ten commandments of plastic surgery (see recommended reading).

A true man of science, Paré was also a deeply religious man and on a statue erected in his honor we find these words inscribed in French: *I treated them, God healed them.*

Other Contributions During the Sixteenth Century

One of the most significant and far-reaching developments to take place in plastic surgery between the sixteenth century and the modern era was the rediscovery

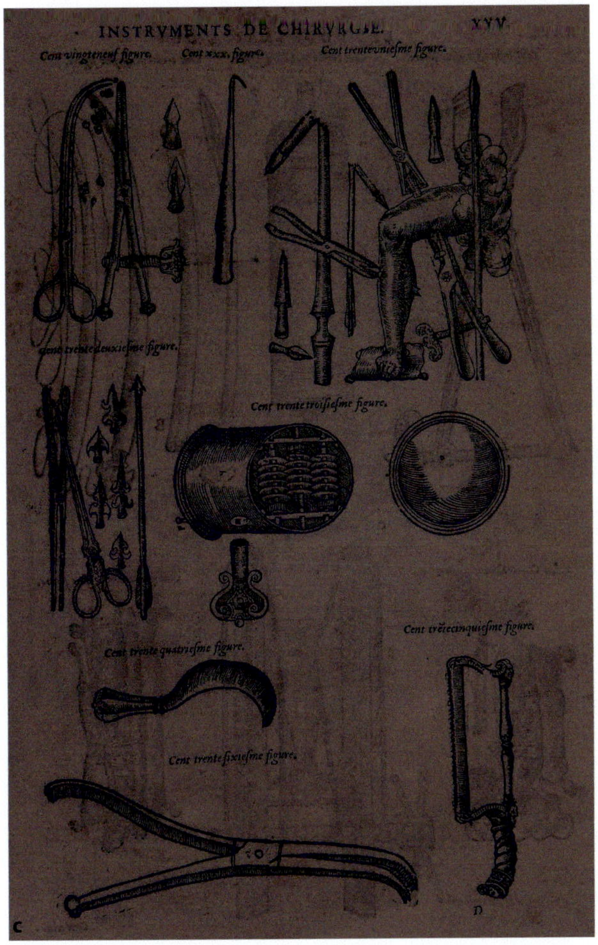

Fig. 2.18a–c *(continued)* Some of Paré's instruments described in *Les Oeuvres. Courtesy of Riccardo Mazzola, M.D., Milan*

of the skin flap. In reality, skin flaps had already been used for the reconstruction of the nose, lips and ears millennia ago in India by Susruta, during the period of the Roman Empire by Celsus and Oribasius, and in the fifteenth century by the Branca family in Sicily and the Vianeo family in Calabria. However, the Italians left no written descriptions of their procedures, and therefore it was only in the sixteenth century that this technique came to be regularly used and described accurately, objectively and scientifically from both a biological and a clinical standpoint by Gaspare Tagliacozzi (1545–1599) [969]. This new advance will be discussed in more detail in the chapters on flaps and nasal reconstruction. But its use was destined to transform the techniques for the closure of cutaneous defects, even if its application would remain limited to the face for many years. Tagliacozzi also deserves credit for developing a method for moving the flap from its original site in the arm to a recipient site on the face. This "distant flap" would find many applications in plastic surgery.

In the sixteenth century surgeons continued to study the problem of facial trauma. In his seven volume work *Chirurgiae Libri Septem,* Giovanni Andrea della Croce (1514–1575) devoted considerable space to the treatment of fractures and trauma to the head, introducing some new topics, such as lesions of nerves, that had been completely ignored until then [231, 232].

Wilhelm Fabry von Hilden (1560–1624) was another notable surgeon. As a child von Hilden wanted to become a physician, but the death of his father when he was ten years old and of his godfather three years later made this impossible. He therefore chose surgery, which offered the advantages of a shorter and less expensive course of study than the traditional curriculum in medicine (which included rhetoric, philosophy and other academic subjects). Even though he did not have the advantages of a classical education, he could write respectable Latin and published a useful surgical text, *Observationes et Curationum Chirurgicarum Centuriae* [433].[43]

Von Hilden introduced several new ideas, including what was perhaps the first classification system for burns, which he called *Traumi Termici*. He divided them into three classes: *levissime*, with redness and moderate pain; *mediocrem*, with marked pain, swelling and blisters; and finally *insignam*, with necrosis of the skin (in his words, "black skin which, if it is pricked with a scalpel, falls through"). He suggested various remedies to avoid the problems that could develop during the healing of burns, such as the application of splints to minimize the contraction of scarred skin and the insertion of pieces of linen cloth or lead foil to avoid the adherence of delicate parts such as the lips or eyelids.

He studied the processes of infection and employed the term "inflamation" in the same sense that it is used today. With exceptional intuition he deduced that infec-

43 *Observationes et Curationum Chirurgicarum Centuriae* was published in Basle between 1606 and 1641.

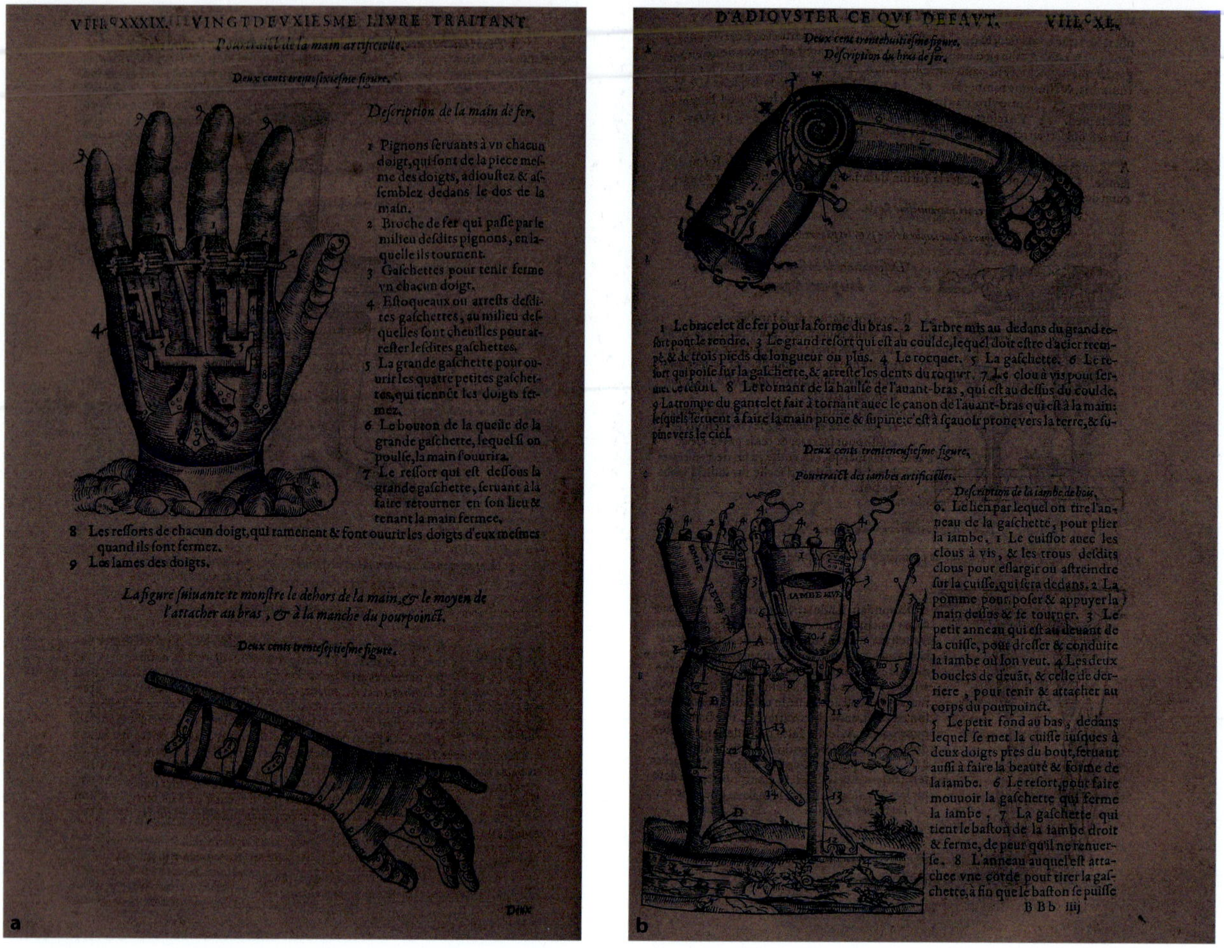

Fig. 2.19a,b Paré's prostheses. He devised an obturator for the palate, false noses, limb prostheses, hernia trusses and even an artificial penis. *Courtesy of Riccardo Mazzola, M.D., Milan*

tions were not carried by the humors of the body, but rather spread along specific anatomical paths. His descriptions of gangrene and other phenomena are models of lucidity and logical reasoning.[44]

During the course of the sixteenth century some techniques were refined (Fig. 2.20a, b)[45] and surgical instruments became increasingly sophisticated and functional. Many of these were designed by Johannes Schultes, also known as Scultetus (1595–1645), who had studied under Fabricius ab Aquapendente in Padua and later with Adrian von Speigel. He describes them, together with a series of bandages, splints and other medical equipment in *Armamentarium Chirurgicum* [908, 909].[46] He also gives an account of different surgical operations, includ-

44 Wilhelm Fabry von Hilden was probably the first surgeon to use a magnet, apparently at the suggestion of his wife, to remove metal fragments from the eye.

45 Antonio Philippo Ciucci, a citizen of Arezzo, published his book *Promptuarium Chirurgicum* in 1679 describing several techniques one of which was a repair of cleft lip.

46 *Armamentarium Chirurgicum* was published posthumously in 1655 by a nephew who bore the same name as his uncle, Johannes Schultes.

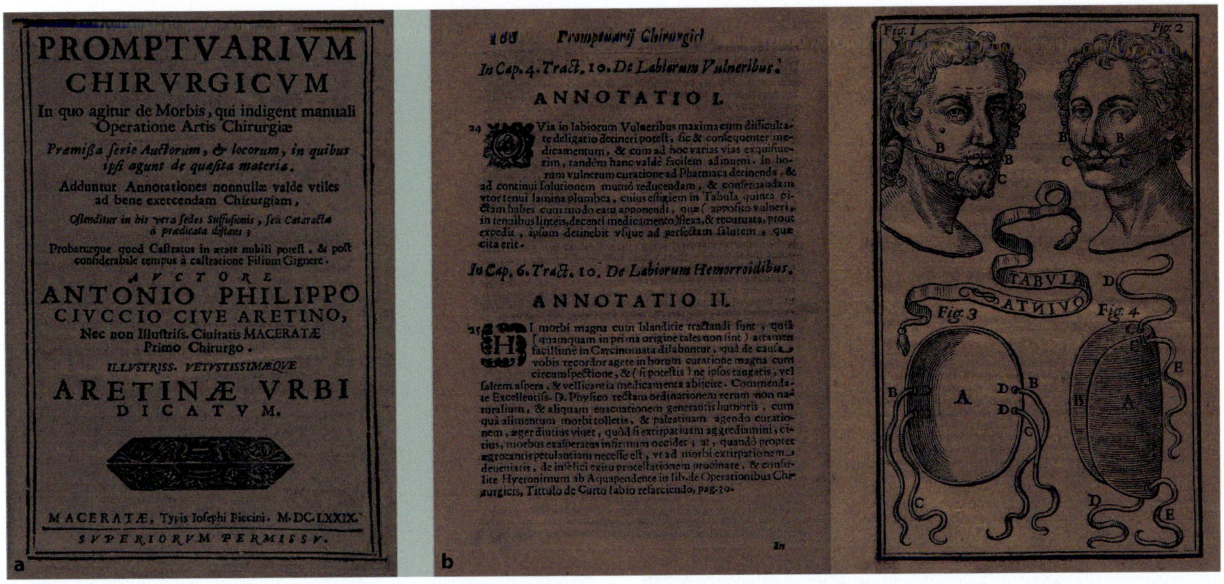

Fig. 2.20a,b An interesting book *Promptuarion Chirurgicum* published by Ciucci in 1679 in which he describes lip repair. *Courtesy of Riccardo Mazzola, M.D, Milan*

ing procedures involving the ear (Figs. 2.21, 2.22) and the breast.[47]

Another Italian who, according to Garrison deserves mention for his contributions to the development of surgery was Cesare Magati (1579–1647) of Scandiano near Modena, who taught that gunpowder was not poisonous and spurned the application of ointments and other substances. He used moistened bandages, trusting to the natural processes of healing to do the rest [589]. "It has been demonstrated that what heals wounds is nature and not the physician or his medicines. It is true that pus moves, and it does so naturally. If new flesh must be made or the broken nose held in place by the skin that pulls upon it, these are all works wrought by nature. If something has to be cemented she attends to it … nature correctly performs her duties as long as the physician is merely her servant, and it will be his office to increase the strength of healing nature and to avoid or remove every thing that may oppose or hinder her work."

Astrology, Alchemy, Magnetism and Other Novelties

Progress was slow despite these contributions and after the advances of the sixteenth century a certain regression took place. Indeed it transpired that in the sphere of wound healing other schools of thought led to the search for "the squaring of the circle, the multiplication of the cube, so that astrology, alchemy and magic were rampant" [360, 361]. In this unscientific atmosphere empiricism and overt magical practices flourished.

For example, in 1658 Sir Kenelm Digby (1603–1665) (Fig. 2.23) described with utmost seriousness at the University of Montpellier his *Sympathetic Powder* [247] to which he attributed wonderful healing powers. In reality it consisted merely of vitriol dissolved in water, recrystallized and dried in the sun. Its efficacy was vouched for by no less a personage than the Duke of Buckingham, who claimed that his personal secretary had been cured of a gangrenous ulcer by the application of a bandage

47 The chapter *De Abscissione mammae carcinomata exulceratio affectae* in Scultetus' *Armamentarium Chirurgicum* contains an illustration (no. XXXVII) showing a technique for breast excision; the blood supply has been cut off by a tourniquet applied to the base of the breast.

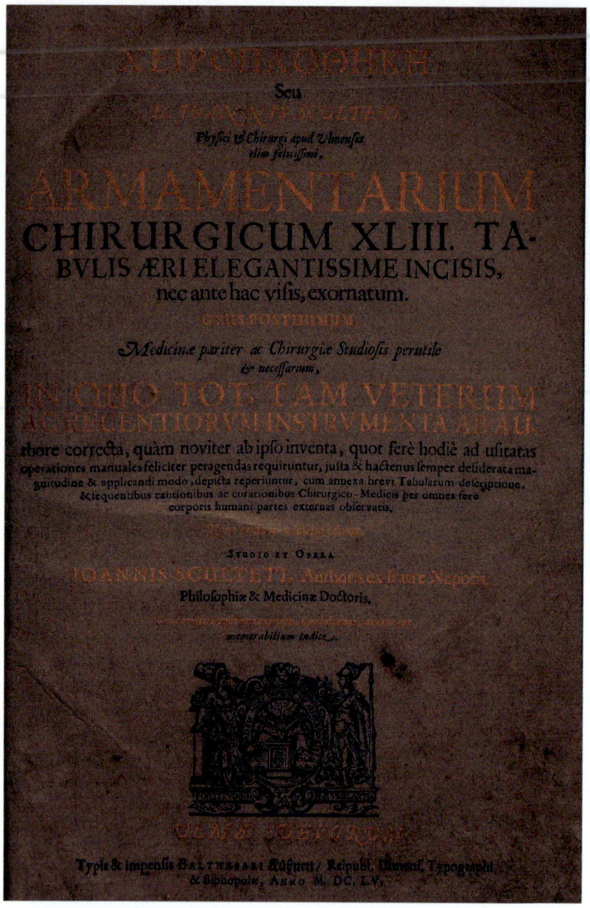
Seu
ARMAMENTARIUM
CHIRURGICUM XLIII. TA-
BVLIS ÆRI ELEGANTISSIME INCISIS,
nec ante hac visis, exornatum.
Medicinæ pariter ac Chirurgiæ Studiosis perutile
& necessarium,
IN QUO TOT, TAM VETERUM
AC RECENTIORVM INSTRVMENTA AB AU-
thore correcta, quàm noviter ab ipso inventa, quot ferè hodiè ad usitatas
operationes manuales feliciter peragendas requiruntur, justa & hactenus semper desiderata ma-
gnitudine & applicandi modo, depicta reperiuntur, cum annexa brevi Tabularum descriptione,
& sequentibus cautionibus ac curationibus Chirurgico-Medicis per omnes ferè
corporis humani partes externas observatis.
STUDIO ET OPERA
JOANNIS SCULTETI,
Philosophiæ & Medicinæ Doctoris,
memorabilium indice.

Fig. 2.21 Frontispiece of the *Armamentarium Chirurgicum* by Johannes Schultes, also known as Scultetus (1595–1645). The book was published posthumously in 1653 by his nephew. It is contains a catalogue of all his ingenious devices and 20 of the 40 plates show accurate illustrations of his instruments. *Courtesy of Riccardo Mazzola, M.D., Milan*

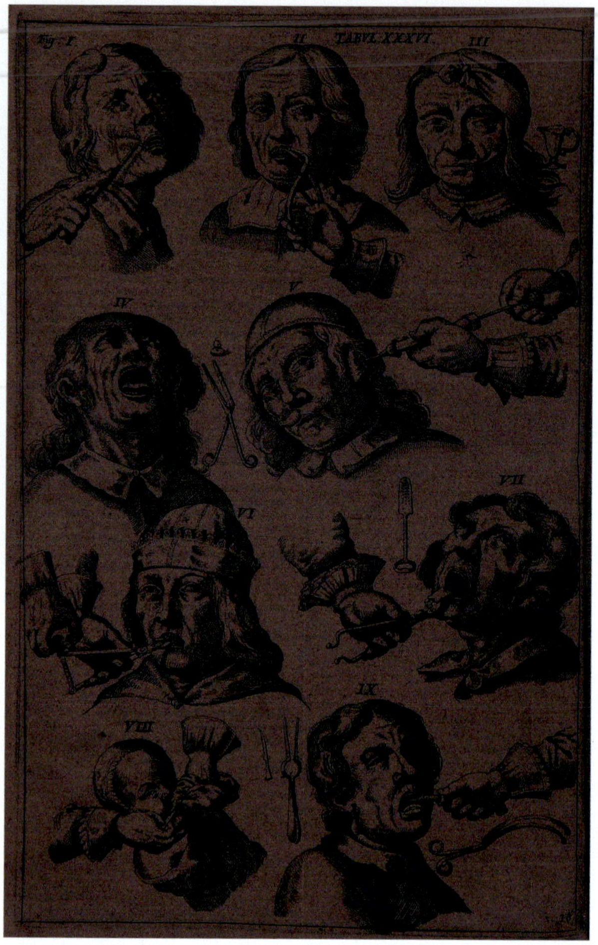

Fig. 2.22 A page of Scultetus' book where he describes the treatment of facial wounds including skull fractures. *Courtesy of Riccardo Mazzola, M.D., Milan*

impregnated with a solution of this powder. The interest in Sir Kenelm's medicine faded quickly, but the spirit of quackery that fueled it may be considered a sign of the times.

Rather more deserving of our attention are the studies on magnetism pursued by William Gilbert (1544–1603) who, after completing his studies at St. John's College in Cambridge, set up practice in London and earned such reputation that he was eventually appointed personal physician to Queen Elizabeth I. In 1600 he published *De Magnete, Magnetiticisque Corporis et de Magro Magnete Tellure, Physiologia Nova* (*On the Magnet, Magnetism of the Body and the Great Magnet of the Earth, New Physiology*) [372], reporting the results of experiments which he claimed demonstrated that magnetism possesses an invisible force capable of facilitating the healing of tissues.[48] Magnetism and its supposed healing properties would find an illustrious advocate in Athanasius Kircher (1602–1680), [495, 496] a Jesuit priest from Fulda. His theory that magnetism was a vital force emanating from

48 William Gilbert is credited with the discovery of the polar axis, the principle on which the modern compass is based.

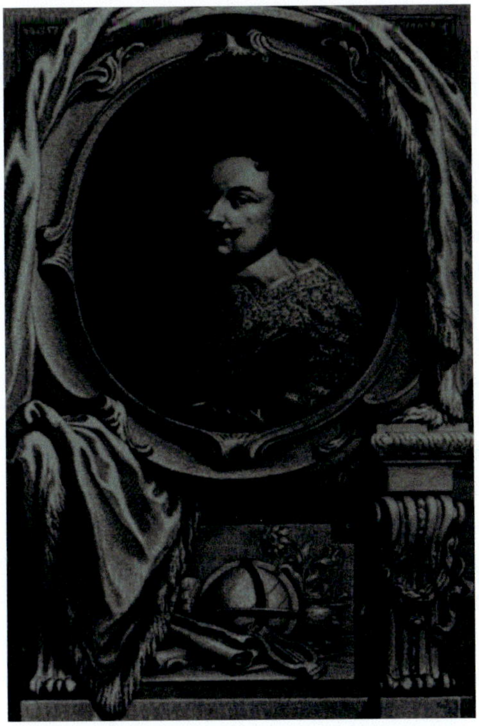

Fig. 2.23 Portrait of Sir Kenelm Digby (1603–1665) the inventor of the "sympathetic powder" to which wonderful healing powers were attributed. *Courtesy of FMR Art.spa, Bologna*

both the stars and the human body, capable of mysterious phenomena that could act positively on the healing process, was enthusiastically supported by R. Fudd (1574–1637), R. Goclemius (1572–1621) and von Helmont (1577–1644).

Kircher also conducted experiments in hypnotism and catalepsy, but his fame as a scientist is based on the results of his original microscopic studies, which demonstrated the presence in decaying tissues of "worms" not visible to the naked eye and led him to formulate the hypothesis that disease spread by "contagium animatum". During the plague which ravaged the city of Rome in 1656, he examined blood taken from a victim under the microscope and was surprised to observe "innumerable swarms of worms", which he thought were animated corpuscles which acted as carriers of the disease. With the relatively low magnifying power of his instrument, it is doubtful that Kircher was actually able to see bacteria, but he nevertheless developed a firm belief in the existence of living parasites that were responsible for the spread of disease, the very basis of modern bacteriology. His intuition went even further for he wrote: "Flies feeding on the juices of the diseased and dying, hurry off and deposit their excretions on food, so that the persons who eat it are infected."

The pseudo-science of magnetism reached its peak with Franz Anton Mesmer (1734–1815), who studied medicine in his native city of Vienna and presented a dissertation on the influence of the planets on human physiology and pathology. He believed firmly in the existence of a "distant power" [662] circulating through the universe that could be captured and used to heal wounds. This doctrine, which he presented in Paris in 1778, sustained considerable interest and controversy in academic circles.

Blood Transfusions and Other Developments

Despite the temporary success of such esoteric notions, which were mere deviations from the true path of scientific progress, by the end of the sixteenth century other, more solidly based discoveries were leading to genuine advances in surgery and the healing of wounds. It was in this period that Harvey worked out his revolutionary theories concerning the circulation of the blood which, combined with Malpighi's discovery of the capillary system, led to a genuine understanding of the human circulatory system. The first attempts at blood transfusions soon followed.

Robert Boyle conducted practical experiments to test the hypothesis proposed in 1656 by Christopher Wren that medicines might be administered by intravenous injection and then carried throughout the body by the blood. Wren had done this to give wine and beer intravenously to a dog. The experiment was repeated by other scientists and Johann Elsholtz (1623–1688) published his experiences in a book *Clysmatica Nova* in 1665 (Fig. 2.24). Giovanni Colle da Belluno, professor of medicine at the University of Padua and physician to the Grand Duke of Tuscany, declared that this procedure could be used to transfer blood, although it is unclear whether he actually carried out a transfusion or had simply conceived the idea. Francesco Folli (c.1623–1685) a well known physician practising in Florence announced that he had thought of the idea in 1654 and attempted it using a slender silver tube introduced into the artery of

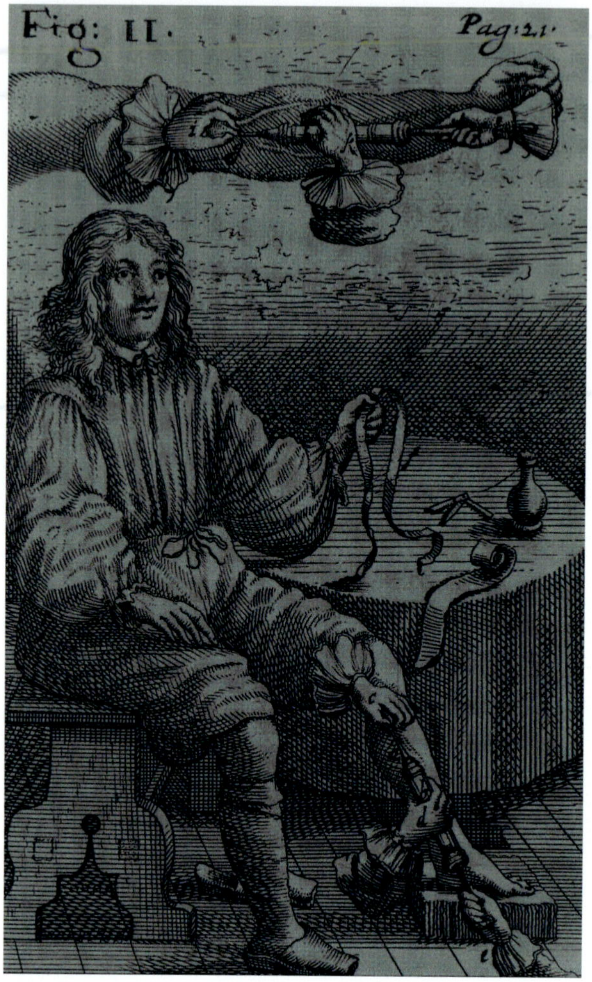

Fig. 2.24 An early attempt at blood transfusion from *Clysmatica Nova* by Johann Elsholt (1667). The first edition was published in Berlin in 1665 and did not include this picture which was added in the second edition published by Danielis Reichellii with the prints of Geirgi Schultzi of Brandeburg in 1667. This was after the first documented attempt at blood transfusion by Robert Lower (1631–1692) of Cornwall in 1665. *From* Surgery an Illustrated History *by Ira M Rutkov, 1993 by permission of Elsevier*

the donor and a wooden cannula inserted into the vein of the recipient. However, more precise information on this experiment is lacking.

The first reliably documented attempt was that of Robert Lower (1631–1692), a physician living in Cornwall, who in 1665 demonstrated an actual blood transfusion between two dogs at the Royal Society of London and for the first time provided a written report recording his experiments [580, 581]. This was by uniting the cervical artery of one animal to the jugular vein of the other; both dogs survived. In November of the same year he announced a second breakthrough when he administered the blood of a lamb to the ailing Reverend Arthur Coga. The patient survived and declared that after this treatment his condition was much improved.

These experiments generated much interest and reports of other successful attempts followed suit, although the claims and their purported consequences were subject to exaggeration.[49] For example, one may read the account of a transfusion of blood from a sheep to a dog which resulted in a copious growth of wool on the back of the latter!

The very first therapeutic transfusion appears to have been attempted in France by Jean Baptiste Denis (or Denys) (c.1625–1704), who reported that he, encouraged by Lower's attempts, transfused the blood of a lamb into a boy in 1667 and repeated the procedure one year later [235]. However, he was prohibited from continuing his experiments after the death of a patient was attributed to his novel procedure. Obviously physicians were entirely ignorant of the immunological consequences of this medical procedure. Nevertheless, thanks to such studies the feasibility of blood transfusions had been demonstrated, although almost two centuries would pass before government and Church restrictions (including an edict in France and a papal bull) were lifted and therapeutic transfusions became legally admissible. It was only on the threshold of the twentieth century, when George H.F. Nuttall (1862–1937)[50] described the precipitation test [741] and H. Hymen, E. Brown-Sequard and K. Lendsteiner discovered and identified the human blood groups, that transfusions could become a routine procedure.

49 In a letter written from Rome, where she was living in exile after her abdication, Queen Christina of Sweden declared that she was not disposed to accept a transfusion of blood from a lamb, preferring to receive blood from a lion should it be possible.

50 George Nuttall was born in San Francisco and became professor of biology at the University of Cambridge at the beginning of the twentieth century.

John Thomson (1765–1846) studied the various factors that play a role in the healing of wounds and in the processes of regeneration in general. He published a systematic and exhaustive work on the subject which underlined the most important approaches to treatment [991].

The Role of Scientific Societies

In the eighteenth century significant impetus was given to the development of surgery and to the recognition of its parity with the other branches of medicine thanks to scientific organizations such as the Royal Society, founded in London in 1660 and the *Académie Royale de Chirurgie*, which merged with the *Académie Nationale de Médecine* after the French Revolution. The *Académie Nationale de Médecine* was founded in 1730, recognized by a royal decree in 1743, and charged with nominating the professors of surgery in France. It also collected and published scientific work in the area of surgery, granting recognition to those of special interest. In the area of healing, for example, an award was conferred in 1738 on Le Chat [538] for his study of gun wounds and another to Bordenave [121] for his research on the treatment of ulcers and infected bone cavities.

The Revival of the Skin Flap and the Discovery of Grafts

As we will see, the skin flap was introduced for the first time by Susruta many centuries before the birth of Christ, and then re-popularized in the sixteenth century by Gaspare Tagliacozzi. Nonetheless, for reasons that we will discuss in the appropriate chapter, the technique fell into almost complete disuse during the seventeenth and eighteenth centuries. On the threshold of the nineteenth century, a report by François Chopart [177] was published. He had employed a pedicle flap in 1799 to close a defective lip. Like the news appearing in the *Gentleman's Magazine* in 1794 on the regular use of a flap in India for the reconstruction of the nose, this did not substantially change the surgical practice of the time.

Against this backdrop of almost complete indifference, an enterprising young English surgeon, Joseph C. Carpue (1764–1846), took an interest in the technique. He spent nearly two decades researching the subject before he attempted the operation himself, publishing *An Account of Two Successful Operations for Restoring a Lost Nose* in 1816 [157]. With this, the attention of the scientific world was finally awakened and such eminent surgeons as von Graefe in Germany and Delpech in France began to study the technique, introducing various improvements and becoming new pioneers of the method. As we will see in the next chapter, the skin flap revolutionized the approach to the repair of cutaneous defects, and rapidly became a routine procedure. It permitted surgeons to reconstruct areas where a significant amount of tissue had been removed, thus allowing them to carry out operations, such as the excision of tumours that previously would not have been possible.

The literature before 1800 contains reports of only isolated and for the most part unsuccessful attempts to carry out free skin grafts. After exhaustive studies by Giuseppe Baronio (1758–1811) [53, 54] proved that such operations were feasible, the way was opened for the development of this new and remarkably effective technique for the repair of cutaneous defects. Many surgeons adopted it, particularly in France, and their experience confirmed the utility of the method. Among these were Frederic Blandin (1798–1849), Michel Serre (1799–1849) and Antoine Jobert de Lamballe (1799–1867). De Lamballe published the results of his research in Paris in 1849 in a two-volume work, *Traité de Chirurgie Plastique* [464] which, with its 1,200 pages and 18 clear colour illustrations, contributed significantly to the spread of this technique.[51] His text was so well received that an English edition was published in London in 1849.

Infection

Of all the problems that have plagued surgeons down the centuries, infection was the most troublesome, especially

51 J.B. Ballière was the official publisher for the *Academie Nationale de Medicine* in Paris. The fame of both the author, Antoine Jobert de Lamballe, and the printer ensured the success of the work.

as little was understood about its aetiology. Death was the result in more than 60% of patients and this could reach 75% in those wounded on the battlefield. Even if, as we have seen, some authors as far back as Hippocrates had guessed on empirical grounds that cleanliness was crucial to the successful healing of wounds, it was only in the nineteenth century that a scientific explanation for the origins of the complication, which eventually came to be called "infection" began to emerge.

One of the trailblazers in this field was Ignaz Philip Semmelweis (1818–1865) who, after studying under Skoda and Rokitanski in Hungary, came to Vienna and, while working in the Gynaecology Clinic at the University, made a brilliant discovery on the basis of a series of elementary observations [915, 916]. The clinic had two wards and he noticed that patients consistently asked to be assigned a bed in one of these wards, using every excuse to avoid the other. Upon investigation it emerged that in one of the wards there was an extremely high rate of puerperal fever while in the other the incidence of this complication was well within the norm. Semmelweis then noted that the patients in the ill-reputed ward were followed by medical students, who examined them immediately after their morning anatomy class. In the other ward the patients were cared for by nursing students who were required to adhere to the strictest standards of hygiene and to wash their hands after each gynaecological examination, both for their own protection and that of their patient.

The death of a colleague from an infection contracted when he accidentally cut himself during an autopsy led Semmelweis to connect the two sets of facts. When he imposed stricter rules for hygiene in the second ward the mortality from puerperal fever fell from its previous rate of more than 10% to 3%, and the average fell even further to 1.27% when the staff of both wards began using a solution of calcium chlorate to wash their hands. The conclusions drawn by Semmelweis were confirmed by the American physician, author and poet Oliver Wendell Holmes (1809–1894) [447].

The association of these facts shed light on the causes of infection, but the actual mechanism remained a mystery until the discoveries of Louis Pasteur (1822–1895) (Fig. 2.25) and his "theory of germs", in what may be considered the earliest studies in bacteriology, made it possible to reach a complete understanding of the phenomenon [777]. It is fascinating to retrace the steps by which Pasteur made his revolutionary discovery.

Pasteur was actually a chemist who had graduated in 1847 from the prestigious *Ecole Normale Supérieure* in Paris. His initial area of interest was crystallography and it was only in 1855, when he became a professor at the Faculty of Science of the University of Lille, that he began to study the processes of fermentation at the request of the rich and influential beer producers of the region. Up to this time, fermentation had been regarded as a purely chemical process based on a theory developed by the German chemist Justus von Liebig (1803–1873). In 1857 Pasteur demonstrated instead that alcoholic fermentation was a biological phenomenon,[52] and that the presence of various microscopic but living entities was necessary to trigger the chemical reactions involved.

This led him to the true explanation for the mechanism underlying the phenomenon of "spontaneous generation" which had fascinated but mystified scientists since the time of Aristotle. In 1858, after a long scientific dispute with F.A. Pouchet, Pasteur demonstrated before the *Académie des Sciences* that the liquids used for experiments on spontaneous generation, if sterilized beforehand, showed no signs of organic reproduction. For example, sterilized grape juice would never turn to wine. The existence of micro-organisms had finally been discovered![53] For the scientific community it was just a short step from the theory of the spontaneous generation to the discovery of the bacteria that were its cause. This step led directly to the fundamental concepts that physicians and even more particularly surgeons, needed to be able to understand the processes of infection.

One of the first to grasp the practical implications of Pasteur's discoveries was the surgeon Sir Joseph Lister (1827–1912) (Fig. 2.26), who dedicated his career to the study and prevention of infection in the operating room. Born in Essex, Lister studied medicine in London and then moved to Scotland for seven years, where he worked with the orthopedic surgeon James Symes and married his daughter Agnes. Lister soon noted that ex-

52 See *Memoires sur la fermentation appelée lactique*, published in 1857.

53 Of great interest, if somewhat extraneous to the subject of plastic surgery, are Pasteur's studies of the alcoholic fermentation of wine.

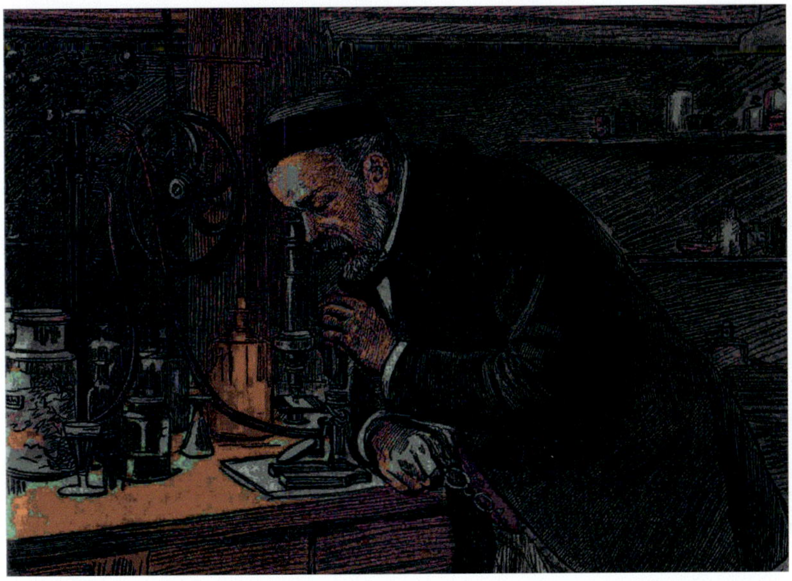

Fig. 2.25 Portrait of Pasteur by Adrien Marie (1890)

posed fractures tended to develop septicemia whereas closed fractures did not and drew the logical conclusion that exposure to air led to decay and sepsis.

However, it soon also became clear to him that air itself was not directly responsible for the contamination of these fractures, but rather the microscopic particles floating in it. He had furthermore grasped the fact that not only air, but any object that came into contact with the wound might contaminate it: instruments, sutures, bandages, even the hands of the surgeon. He wrote: "The septic properties of the atmosphere depended not on oxygen, or any gaseous constituent, but on minute organisms suspended in it. … It occurred to me that decomposition in injured parts might be avoided without excluding the air by applying, as a dressing, some material capable of destroying the life of the floating particles."

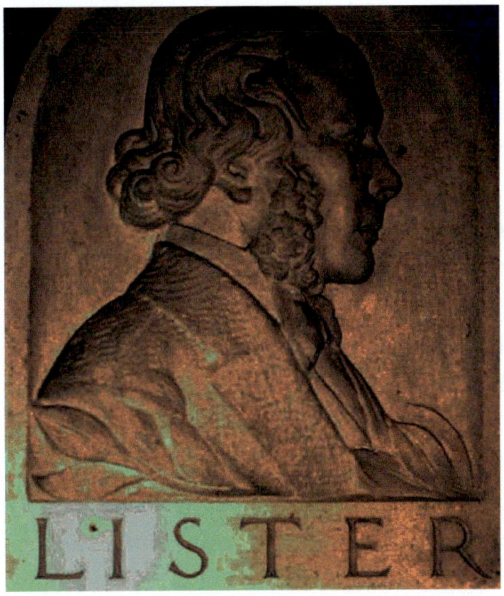

Fig. 2.26 Joseph Lister (1827–1912) from a relief at the Royal College of Surgeons in London. *Reproduced by kind permission of the President and Council of the Royal College of Surgeons of England*

Pasteur had already demonstrated that the process of fermentation could be stopped in a liquid simply by boiling it, because heating destroyed the "particles" that triggered the process. Naturally a wound could not be "boiled" and therefore Lister began to investigate whether chemical substances might be capable of extinguishing these living organisms. He experimented with zinc chlorate and various sulphides with less than satisfactory results before turning his attention to carbolic acid, which he discovered was quite effective mixed in a ratio of 1:20 with water. He henceforth demanded that his assistants wash their hands with this solution both before and after each operation, and even sprayed it in the air of the operating room (Fig. 2.27). He used it mixed with oil to dress wounds and fill the cavities of abscesses. As an added precaution the members of his surgical team were required to change their operating gowns, which were

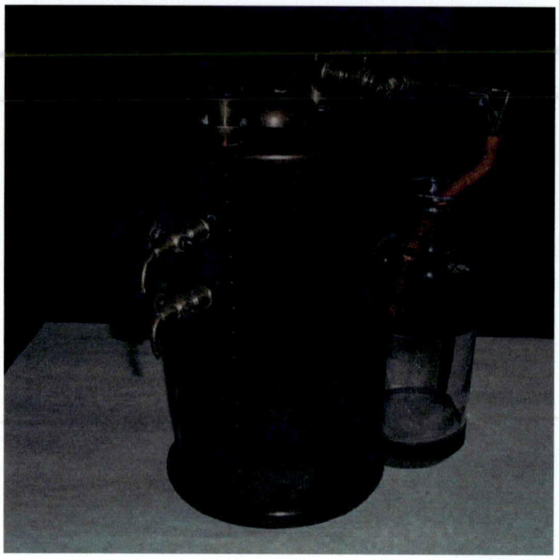

Fig. 2.27 Lister's carbolizer. *By permission of the Museum of Medicine, Institut for Sundheedsviddenskab, University of Copenhagen*

usually impregnated with blood and pus from the previous patient, before beginning a new operation.

Lister believed that the suture could also present a source of infection [566] and in 1861 published a paper elucidating his theory and recommending that surgeons first "carbolize" their catgut, that is, leave it to soak for a long period of time in carbolic acid. He was so convinced that in 1873 he published a second paper reiterating his method. This work was summarized in 1818 [568]. Lister became professor of surgery at Glasgow and invited Pasteur to visit him. When the eminent French scientist arrived he welcomed him with the words, "I must show you just how deeply surgery is indebted to you."

The Franco-Prussian War served Lister as a testing ground for his theories and he published his results in the *British Medical Journal* in 1870 [567]. The reduction in the rate of infection was impressive, and the practice of antisepsis was born. This breakthrough contributed dramatically to the development of surgery, which up to this time had been associated with such high risks that no operation was even considered unless truly a matter of life or death. Nonetheless, as so often happens in the scientific world, the revolutionary discoveries of Pasteur and Lister were not universally accepted and when Lister returned to London in 1877 he had to face the hostile scepticism of older surgeons. Billroth in Germany, for example, snorted that he refused to: "operate in a rain of carbolic acid!"

Lister found a staunch supporter on the other side of the Atlantic, however, in James Marion Sims (1813–1883), who like all gynaecologists was encountering great difficulties in treating certain vesico-vaginal fistulae. The relapse rate was unacceptably high in his view, and he attributed the problem to the suture. After experimenting with a variety of materials including silver wire [930], he found that the best result could be obtained with carbolized catgut; indeed so successful was this technique that he was invited to Europe by Nélaton, Velpeau and Larry to lecture on the subject.[54]

The new understanding of infection together with the discovery of anaesthesia and improvements in surgical techniques opened up new possibilities for the surgeon. Safer painless surgery broadened the indications for operative treatment. Furthermore, with improvements in the use of flaps and skin grafts, reconstructions that had previously not seemed possible become routine. For example, the surgical treatment of tumours, especially those of the face, increased markedly because the defect caused by the excision could be closed. The prognosis for cancer victims improved as wider surgical excision became possible. The new methods which came about will be discussed in later chapters.

The Role of Surgical Instruments

Surgery could not have advanced far without the development of special instruments. In the early days these were simple and often modifications of everyday tools–knife, fork and spoon! As man's ingenuity and knowledge increased, surgeons designed more complex instruments to allow them to achieve their goals. Sometimes the reverse happened and new technical developments brought the realization that an operation, previously considered out of the question, was now possible. One has only to

54 J. M. Sims is known for having invented the vaginal speculum and the standard position for gynaecological operations.

think of the development of operating microscopes and fine sutures in modern times. Over previous centuries many devices we now consider everyday, were invented because of the ingenuity of both surgeons and artisans when looking for a solution to a difficult problem.

By contrast many complex tools are no longer used, having been replaced by new technology. Some became obsolete as the surgical repertoire changed. The history of surgical instruments is a topic in itself and we can only touch on a few landmarks from the past in this brief account. Readers are recommended to comprehensive works on the subject [494, 987].

The Smith papyrus [939] describes closure of skin wounds with strips of linen coated with an adhesive gum not unlike present day butterfly tapes or Steristrips™. Sutures were also discussed in this text and used for the same purpose. The needles were large and traumatic by comparison to those of the present day. The use of various threads such as cotton, hemp, horsehair, animal skin and tendon were well known around 800 B.C. when Susruta wrote his *Samitha*.

Hippocrates (460–375 B.C.) devised an instrument to replace nasal fractures, called a *Shalak* as we will see in the chapter on nasal reconstruction.

One of the earliest records of an instrument being devised specifically for surgery is probably by Celsus (25 B.C. to 50 A.D.) around the time of Christ. In his *De Medicina* he conceived an instrument very similar to our artery forceps, which he used to stop bleeding and assist vascular ligation. Galen introduced special bandages for every area of the body in the second century and those described by the Greek master for skull and facial fractures are surprisingly similar to the ones used in later years.

Aegineta (624–690) also attempted to stabilize broken facial bones in the seventh century by using interdental wires. However it was not until Johannes Schultes (1595–1645), who was a pupil of Fabricius ab Aquapendente and later von Spiegel, do we find a treatise devoted to surgical instruments. In the early seventeenth century he wrote his *Armamentarum Chirigicae* which also describes a wide variety of bandages, "ferulae", splints and other supports [908].

Before this Ambroise Paré (1510–1590) devised a large number of surgical instruments which he described in his *Cinq Livres de Chirurgie* in 1572 [855]. He later also reported a variety of prostheses in *Les Oeuvres* including palatal obturators and false metal noses. The later were alternatives to the nasal reconstruction which became popular across the Alps in the various schools of Italian nasal reconstructions described in detail in that chapter. Gaspare Tagliacozzi for example used a selection of specifically designed instruments. When one considers the prevalent environment of academic and commercial competition each surgeon must have guarded details of his operation and the tools he used very carefully. Although once established the likes of Tagliacozzi were very happy to publish their methods and thus advertised their prowess.

It is easy to forget injection needles which despite being very simple, contributed disproportionately to the successful care of sick patients. Robert Boyle, Christopher Wren, Giovanni Cole and Francesco Folli in the seventeenth century all played a part.

Early crude suture material always carried the risk of infection and wound suppuration. We have seen how this was reduced by the introduction of carbolized catgut by Joseph Lister in the nineteenth century.

Instruments, sutures and bandages were common to all branches of surgery and it was not until the late nineteenth and early twentieth centuries that surgical specialization stimulated the need for different instruments for such fields as eye surgery, orthopaedics and urology.

These disciplines include plastic surgery. However, a list of special instruments frequently bearing eponymous names, invented in the past 150 years is too long to record here. They were frequently introduced when a new operation appeared. Examples include Joseph's nasal saws which were used routinely in rhinoplasty operations in Europe in the early twentieth century. Likewise, special instruments for holding the jaws apart while repairing a cleft palate made surgery easier and they were initially "borrowed" from dentists. These were modified to allow easier access and surgeons had their own preferences. Eventually these important instruments were designed in several parts to allow the jaws to be "jacked" open and the anaesthetic tube to be was held securely in the tongue depressor. The type much used in the UK in recent times was the Kilner-Dot gag, which also incorporated a suture holding device, while in America the Dingman gag gained popularity (Fig. 2.28a,b).

The advent of anaesthesia made operations previously impossible a reality. Although quick surgery was still a necessity the patient did not suffer the pain that was inevitable in bygone days. But operations on the upper air-

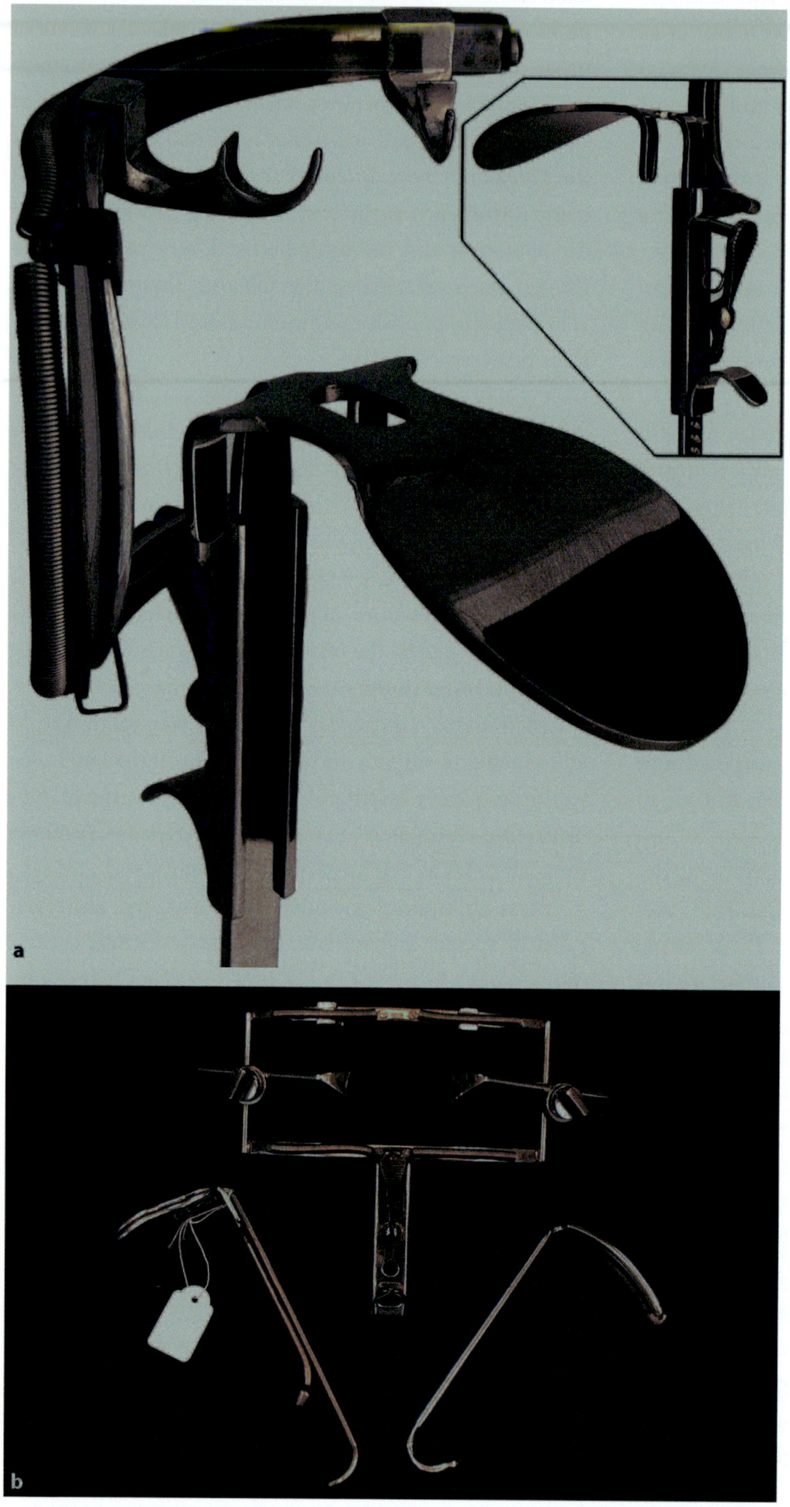

Fig. 2.28 **a** Kilner-Dott gag. **b** Dingman gag. *Photographic Dept., Morriston Hospital, Swansea*

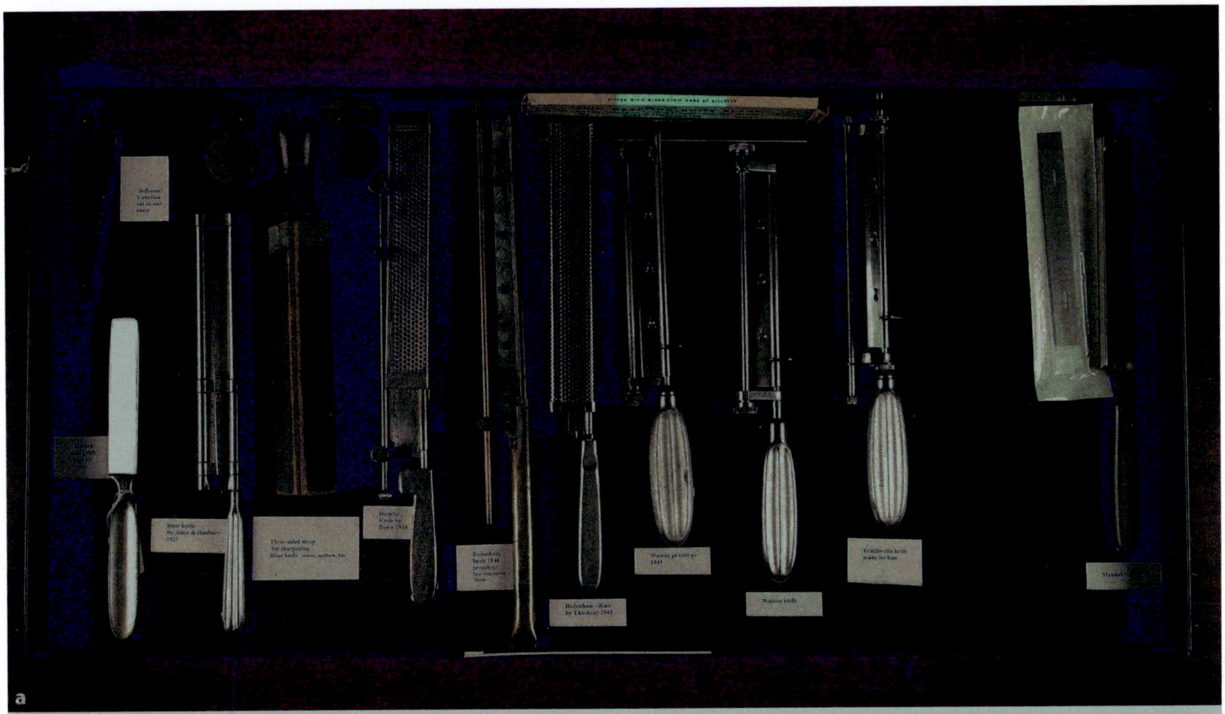

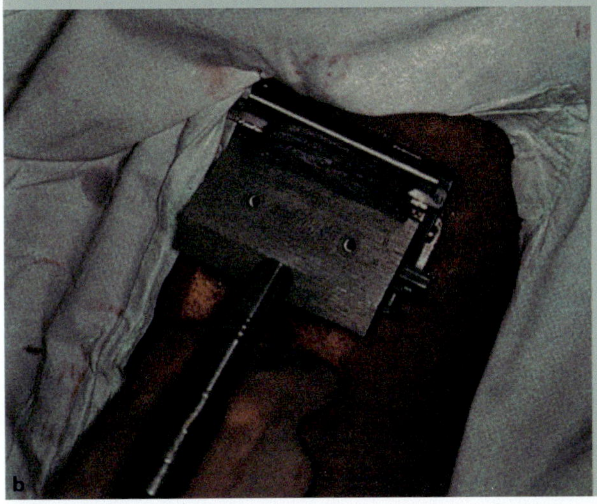

Fig. 2.29 **a** A collection of graft knifes. *Left to right* Thiersch Razor (below a cut-throat razor); Blair with strop 1927; Humby 1938; Bodenham prototype with first disposable blade 1944; Bodenham-Blair 1949; Watson prototype 1949; Watson production model; Braithwaite; Mandal from Norway. It seems that the first to conceive a calibrated hand knife for harvesting skin was an Argentine surgeon, Finocchietto in 1920 but it was Graham Humby from Great Ormond Street Hospital in London who refined and popularized its use. *From the Antony Wallace Archive by courtesy of the British Association of Plastic Reconstructive and Aesthetic Surgeons.* **b** A pneumatic dermatome, a later alternative to the hand knife. *PSR*

way remained difficult using inhalation anaesthesia until the advent of special airways and the endotracheal tube. These combined with the specialized gags allowed the palate and the oral cavity to be approached safely.

Around the same time the importance of delicate atraumatic surgery was recognized and surgeons like Gilles and McIndoe introduced hooks and fine forceps for handling the skin. Their introduction helped sustain the whole ethos of atraumatic technique. It would be necessary to devote a whole chapter to give an adequate description of the evolution of skin-graft knives. The early instruments were initially unguarded and resembled large "cut-throat" razors. They required regular sharpening. Disposable blades were a godsend when they arrived on the scene around 50 years ago. The guarded Humby graft knife with an adjustable blade [453, 454] was later modified in turn by Bodenham, Braithwaite and Watson and they are still in use today. Others have added their own designs and there are many variations of this indispensable instrument. Pneumatic dermatomes never became popular as they were cumbersome and hard to use but lighter more reliable electric dermatomes allowed skin grafts to be taken easily with a uniform thickness and shape (Fig. 2.29a,b) [72]. These transatlantic developments are now widely accepted and consequently the skills used with the free graft knife are being lost. But the small reliable graft knife invariably proves to be a good traveling companion when venturing into developing countries.

Drum dermatomes of the type designed by Padgett (Fig. 2.30) and used for cutting large rectangles of full thickness graft have had their day and are now mainly museum pieces (Fig. 2.31). This is also true of the Gibson-Tuff knife devised for the grafting of lymphoedema patients using thick grafts taken from the large pieces of excised tissue. They and other tools are fascinating reminders of the past.

Nowadays it is hard to imagine that the many advances which have occurred in the last quarter of a century could have come about without the ingenuity of instrument makers and suture manufacturers. One has only to look at a routine operating schedule to see what a wide variety of atraumatic sutures and instruments will be used and to note that the operating microscope will be wheeled into theatre every day. The advances in surgical technique which have come about over the years could not have been happened without these tools of the trade.

All the discoveries mentioned here contributed to advances in reconstructive techniques which will be discussed in future chapters.

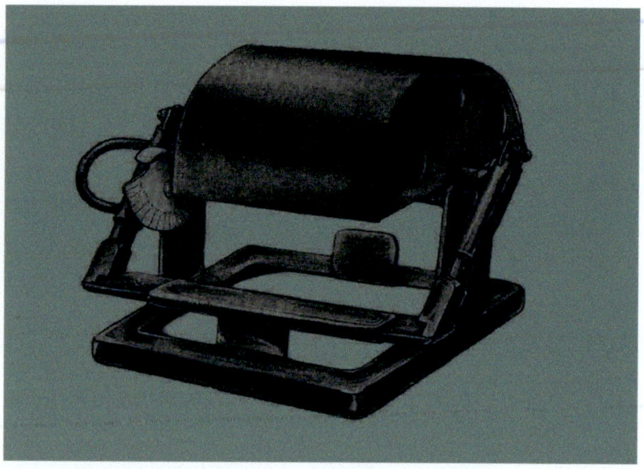

Fig. 2.30 Padgett dermatome used for cutting large rectangles of thick skin grafts. *PSR*

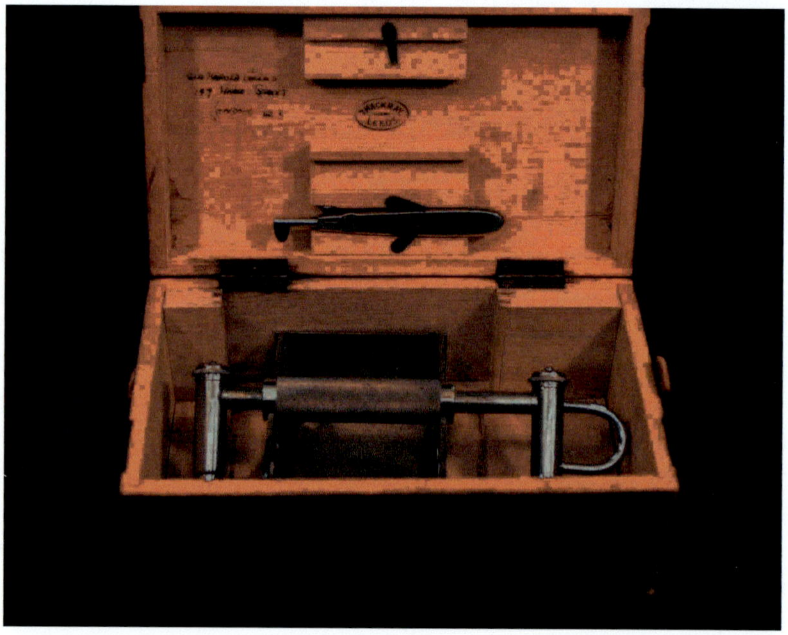

Fig. 2.31 The personal drum dermatome used by Sir Harold Gillies. *From the Antony Wallace Archive by Courtesy of the British Association of Plastic, Reconstructive and Aesthetic Surgeons*

Chapter 3

Skin Flaps

Contents

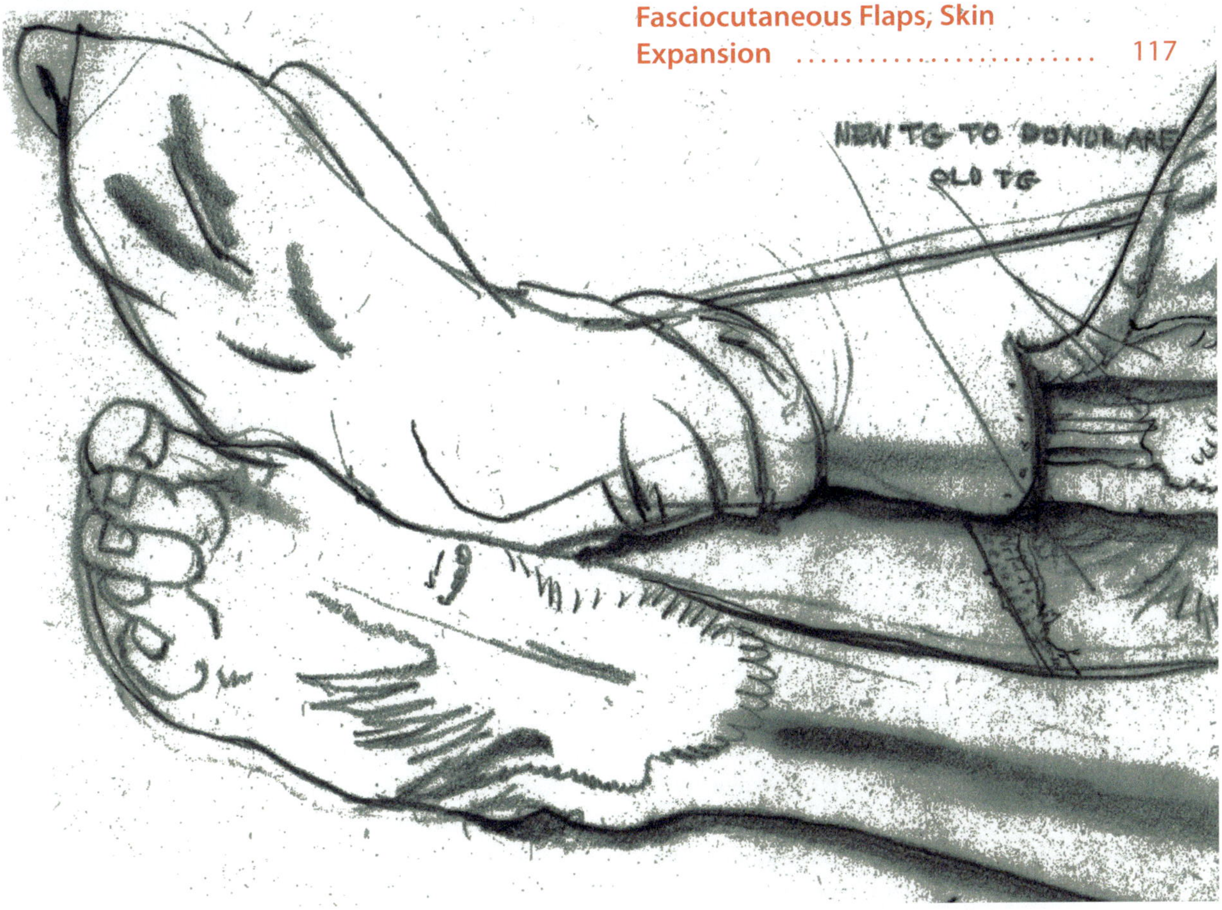

As we have seen, our ancestors understood the difference between healing by primary and secondary intention and devised various procedures to induce the most favourable process possible given the means and knowledge at their disposal. One important breakthrough was, without question, the invention of the skin flap although the initial flaps were quite different from those in use today, particularly those developed in the last 50 years (Fig. 3.1).

For beginners it may be helpful to start by distinguishing between the skin flap and the graft. In the latter the tissue is completely detached from its original donor site and will only take root and thrive if it receives an adequate blood supply from the vascular bed upon which it is placed. The skin flap instead remains connected by at least one of its sides (at first they were usually quadrangular in shape) to its original site. It is this base that guarantees the blood supply needed for the flap to survive.

Surgeons first experimented with variations of the local flap. This is a portion of skin from the area next to the defect that is moved directly into the area where the skin is missing. Over time this procedure was improved, refined and finally, with the technical advances of the last century, completely revolutionized. This chapter will discuss the history of the skin flap, from its inception as a means of closing simple cutaneous defects to the vast range of flaps in use today, and the various solutions that were devised to assure its vascularization.

The skin flap was used for centuries to cover and facilitate the healing of different types of cutaneous defects. Through experience surgeons found that the flap could be manipulated and positioned in different ways, giving rise to the principles of *advancement* (Fig. 3.2), *transposition* (Fig. 3.3a–c) and *rotation* (Fig. 3.4a–c). They also learned about the limits of these repairs. For example, the size of the defect naturally could not exceed the amount of skin available from the donor region. Furthermore, they realized that the survival of the skin flap depended above all upon whether or not it was sufficiently vascularized. In particular, if a flap was too long in relation to the width of its base, the risk of necrosis increased significantly. Hence, the axiomatic *length-breadth ratio* was established, and only recently have solutions been found to overcome this constraint. With the simple flap the only source of vascularization that the surgeon could count upon was the network of capillaries originating from its base. This network is denser in certain regions, such as the face or areas covered with hair, where there is a greater leeway in the interpretation of the length-breadth ratio, but the principle remained inviolable. These flaps came to be referred to as *random pattern flaps* because of the precariousness of their blood supply.

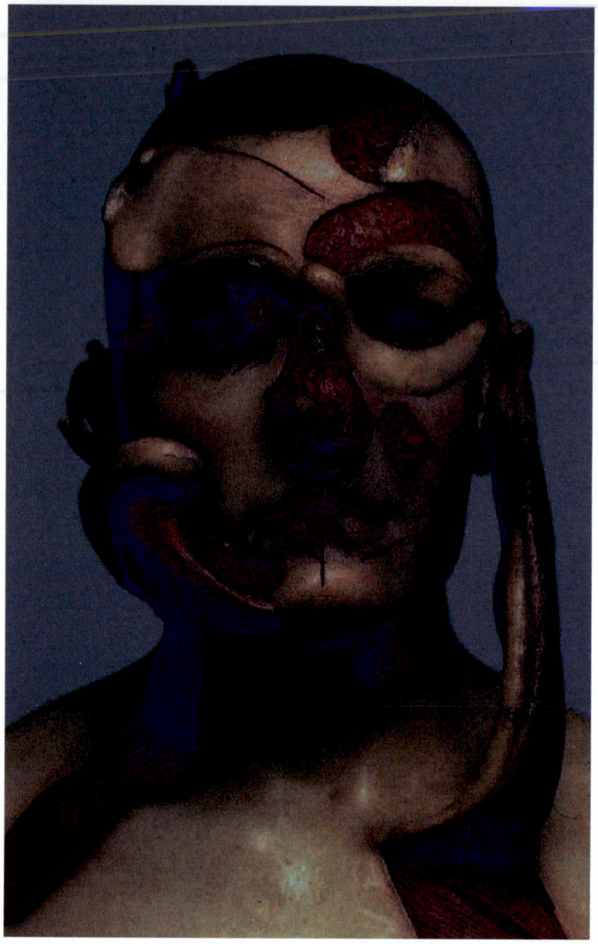

Fig. 3.1 Wax model of facial flaps used at the Queen's Hospital in Sidcup during World War I for instructing new surgeons. *Reproduced by permission of the Gillies Archives, Queen Mary's Hospital, Sidcup, UK – authors photograph*

Local flaps had limitations. Skin in the adjacent area may be insufficient in size, too valuable or difficult to move. In this case *distant flaps* of skin became necessary and these were used from very early times (see nasal reconstruction). Their blood supply was still random in nature although by chance or design surgeons learned that flaps in certain areas were more reliable. These *distant flaps* did not come from adjacent areas of skin and

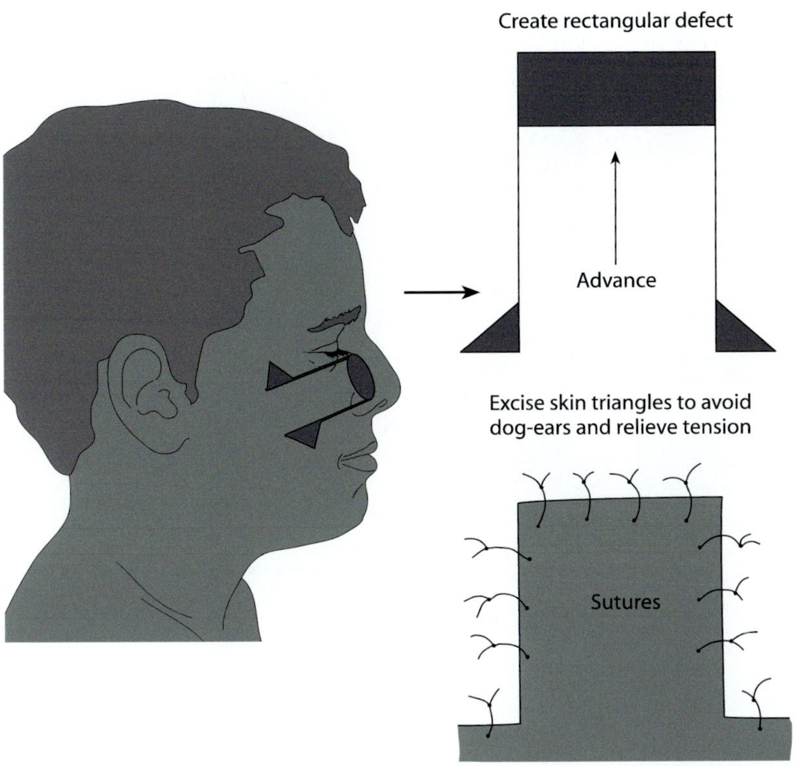

Fig. 3.2 Diagram showing a simple advancement flap of the type probably first used in India and by Celsus. *PJS*

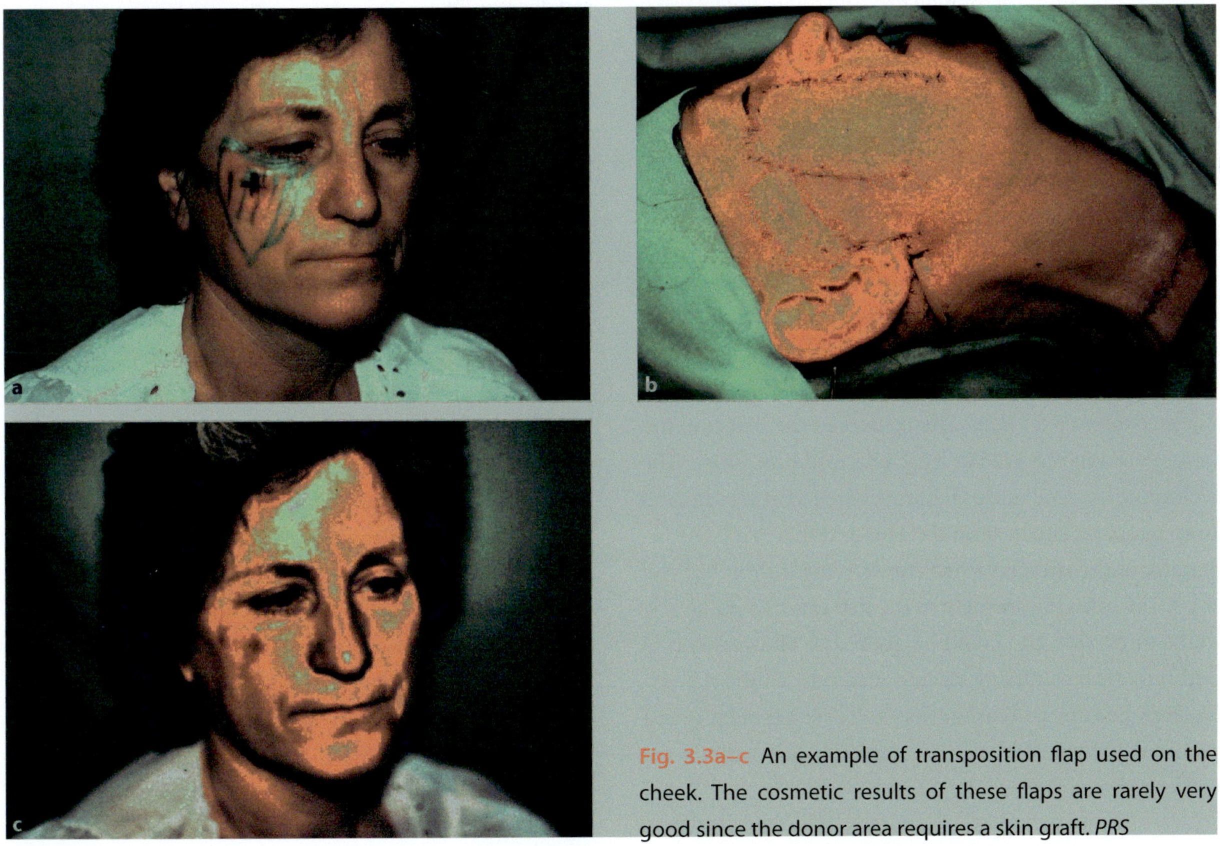

Fig. 3.3a–c An example of transposition flap used on the cheek. The cosmetic results of these flaps are rarely very good since the donor area requires a skin graft. *PRS*

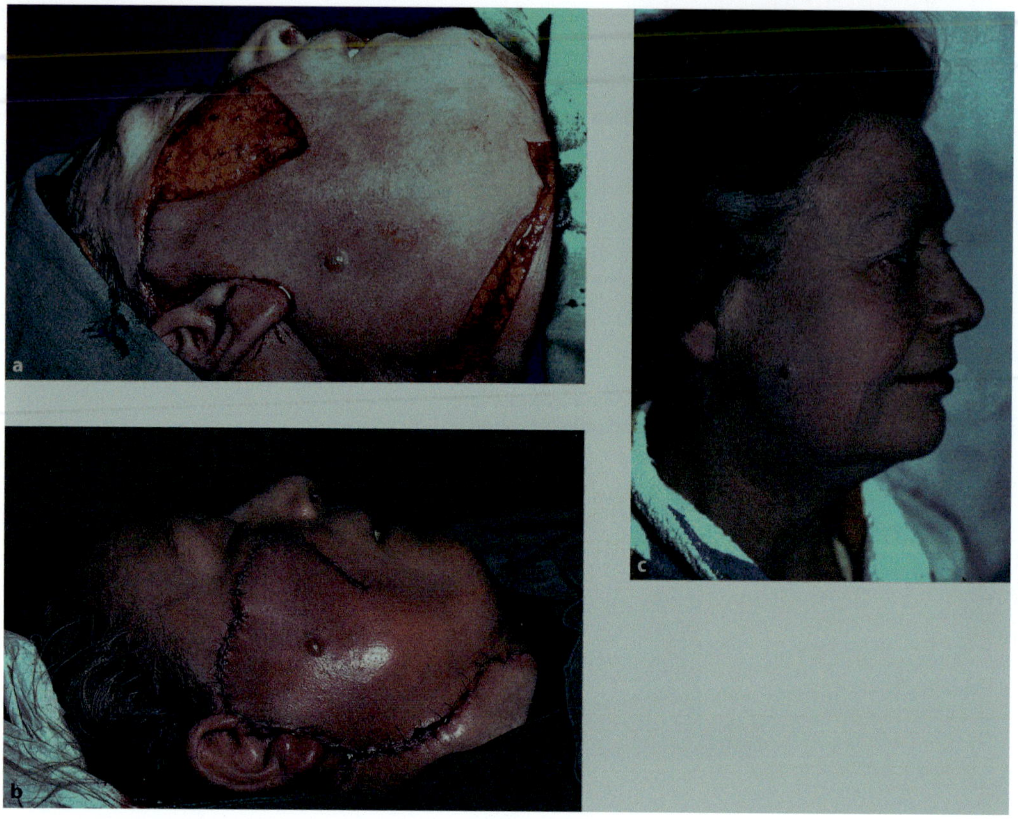

Fig. 3.4a–c Example of rotation flap. The donor defect can be closed directly. *PJS*

of necessity were designed with a temporary bridging segment, the pedicle, through which the blood supply nourished the flap (Fig. 3.5). When it had acquired a new blood supply from the bed of the defect this pedicle was divided and could be returned to the donor area. These *distant direct flaps* which covered the defect at the first operation required at least a second procedure. The technique became more elaborate when skin was moved from a remote site in several stages and this taxed the ingenuity of the surgeon when transferring *distant indirect flaps*. The bridging segment of the flap was inevitable raw on its underside and could be grafted or allowed to role naturally or by suturing its margins, into a tube. Cross-leg flaps became a common way to cover leg defects and required patients to lie in uncomfortable positions for weeks between stages (Fig. 3.6a,b).

Surgeons also discovered that the *random pattern flap* could be "trained" to survive on a relatively narrow base before transfer. This involved incising the sides of the flap in stages to allow the capillary circulation to re-establish and to nourish a larger section of skin than would have been possible if all three sides had been detached at once. This procedure came to be known as *delaying* the flap. A classic example is the *tubed pedicle flap*. The initial operation of tubing a piece of skin in a suitably lax part of the body left the skin attached at both ends and was said to allow its blood supply to become orientated in a longitudinal fashion allowing a larger piece of tissue to be moved safely at a later stage either directly to the defect or by a suitable carrier (Fig. 3.7a–d).

These techniques date from very different periods and some which were refined over the years, particularly

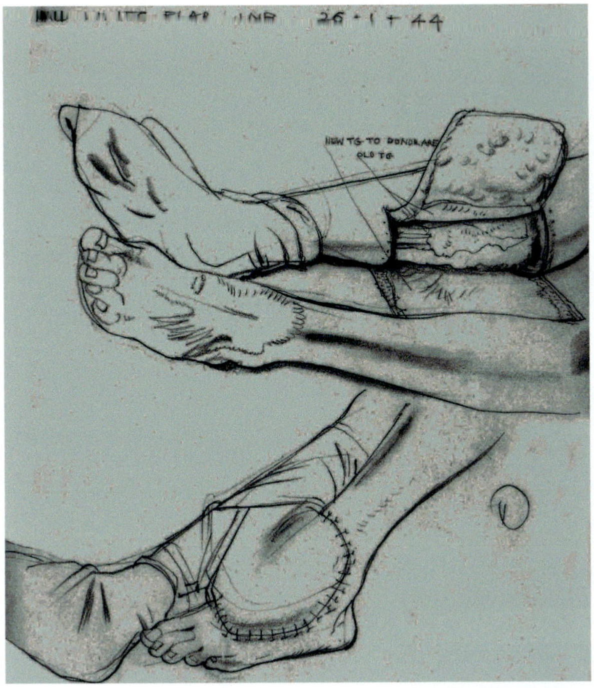

Fig. 3.5 A drawing of a cross-leg flap made by the medical artist and daughter of Sir William Orpen RA. She worked with Rainsford Mowlem at Hill End Hospital, St Albans and Mount Vernon Hospital, Northwood. *From the Antony Wallace Archive, courtesy of the British Association of Plastic Reconstructive and Aesthetic Surgeons*

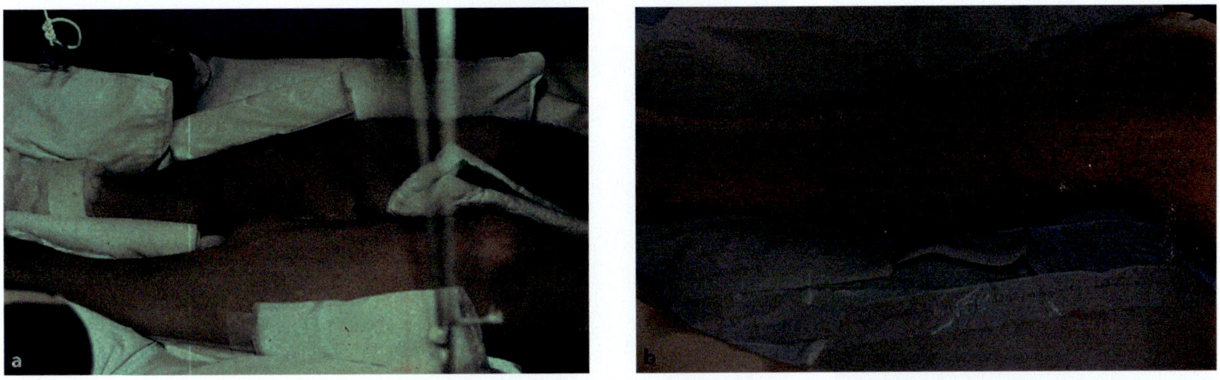

Fig. 3.6a,b Pre- and post-operative views of a cross-leg flap for trauma, separated after three weeks. *PJS*

during the two world wars, are still in use today although this has become infrequent because of new discoveries.

The rules were completely rewritten and traditional notions such as *random circulation* and the *length-breadth ratio* were abandoned as knowledge of the skin circulation improved and the *axial pattern flap* was invented. This flap was supplied by a predictable artery and vein that entered at its base and ran for its entire length, supplying a well-defined area of skin referred to as the cutaneous vascular territory. This enabling its survival *in toto* as long as the artery and vein were preserved and the territory was not exceeded. At long last, survival was no longer exclusively dependent on the capillary circulation, the length-breadth ratio became irrelevant, and theoretically there was no limit to the size of the flap that might be transposed as long as it remained in the territory of the named blood vessels (Figs. 3.8, 3.9).

With the advent of microsurgery and the successful replantation of amputated fingers, surgeons realized that these flaps could be transferred in a similar fashion

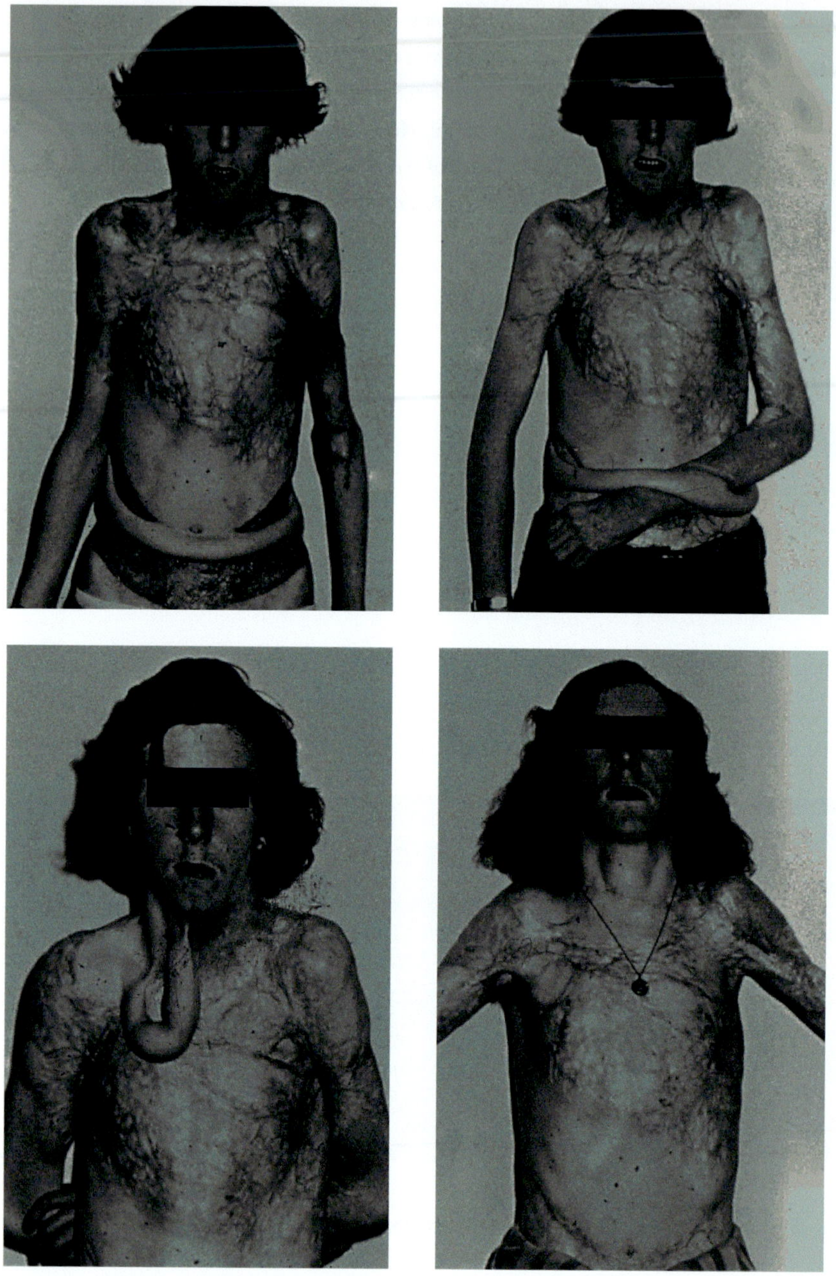

Fig. 3.7 **a** Example of a tube pedicle flap from the abdomen to the neck via the wrist used to treat a burn contracture of the neck. *PJS*. **b** *see next page*

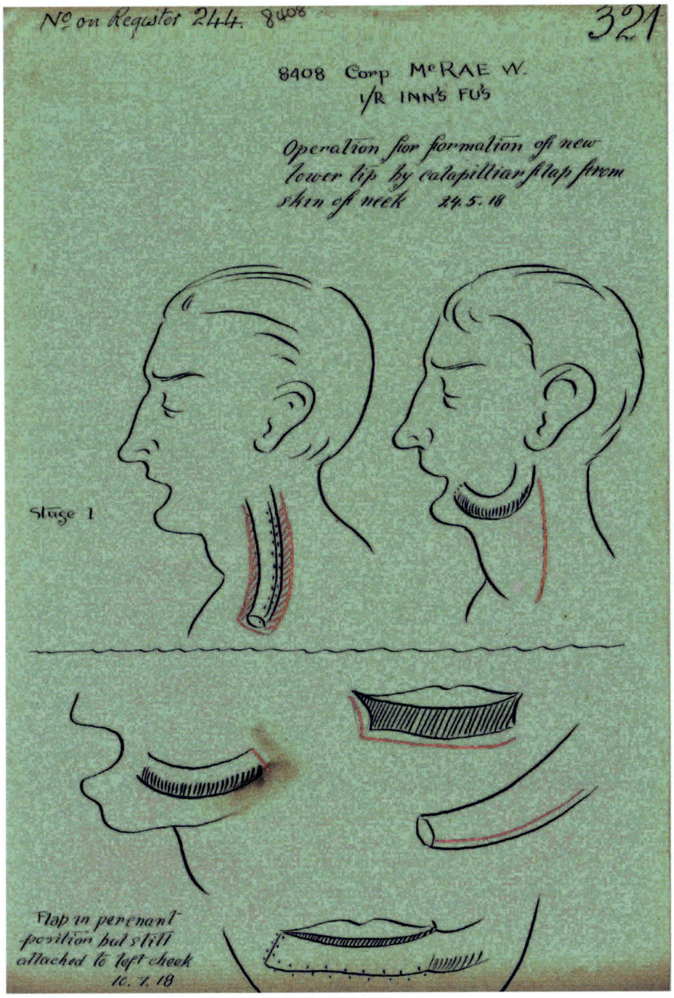

Fig. 3.7 *(continued)* **b** Gillies' diagram of a tube from the neck to reconstruct the lip of a soldier treated in his unit at Sidcup. *Reproduced by permission of the Gillies Archives, Queen Mary's Hospital, Sidcup, UK*

by re-anastomosing the donor vessels to other recipient vessels of a similar diameter in the area of the defect. The *free flap* was invented and the reconstruction was achieved in one operation. This success simulated the search for other *axial flaps*. Surgeons painstakingly re-examined the blood supply of every square inch of skin and a number of new donor regions were identified. Some of the new flaps were vascularized by axial skin vessels and others through muscle or facia. As well as skin other tissues such as bone were included and composite flaps became a reality.

The *axial flap* is remarkably versatile as it can be used in the form of either a local, distant or free flap. Today the surgeon's armamentarium for the repair of skin defects is much larger than could have been imagined 50 years ago, and we will describe its evolution here.

Local Flaps

It is not known exactly when the first skin flap was used. The earliest description is contained in the *Samhita* of Susruta (c.800–600 B.C.), although some date this to 1000 B.C. In ancient India physicians became adept at using flaps to reconstruct entire sections of the face, as will be discussed in the chapter on nasal reconstruction. Based on the same principle as the modern *advancement flap*, a quadrangular section of skin was incised along three of its sides with the fourth side left intact to ensure the blood supply to the flap, and then the skin was undermined and advanced to cover the adjacent defect.

Elsewhere similar cutaneous flaps were described in the works of Aulus Cornelius Celsus (25 B.C. to 50 A.D.) who, according to Edward Zeis [1059, 1060]

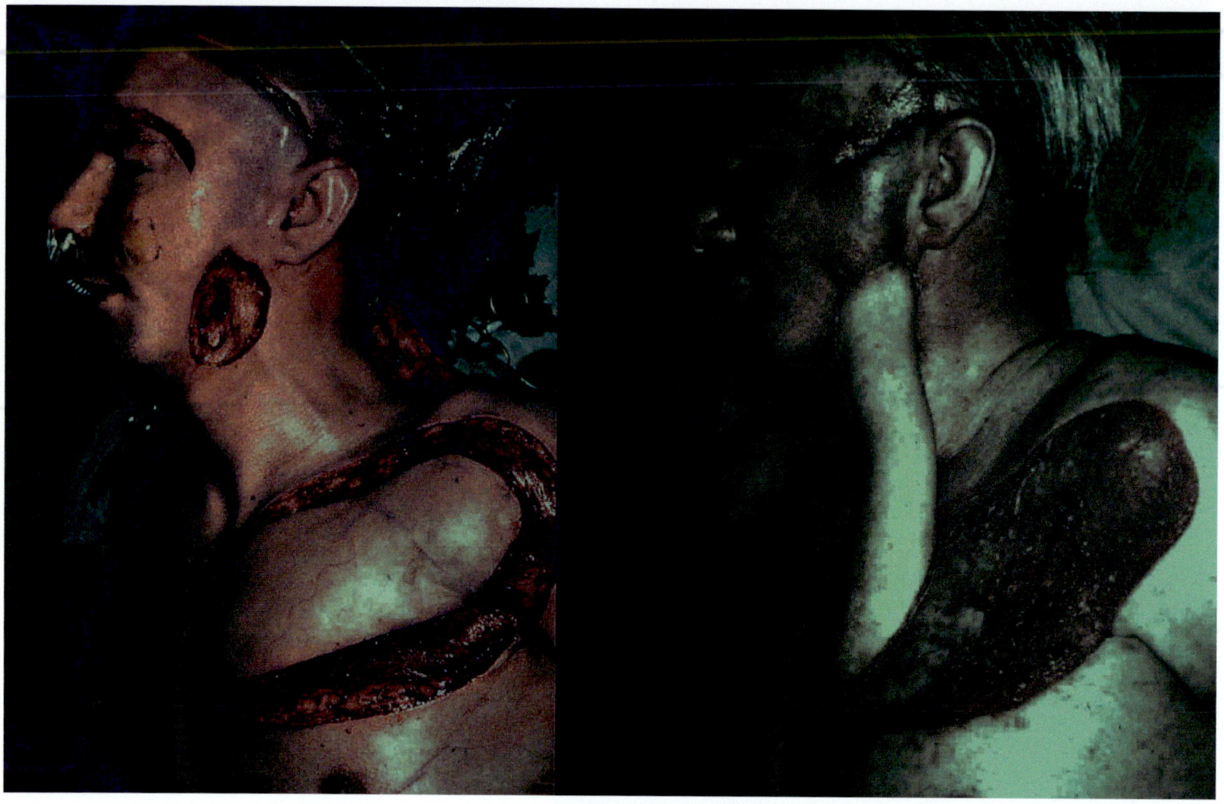

Fig. 3.8 Example of two axial pattern flaps used to provide lining and cover after resection of oral cancer. The deltopectoral flap as described by Bakamjian and the forehead flap were standard techniques before the advent of microsurgery. *PJS*

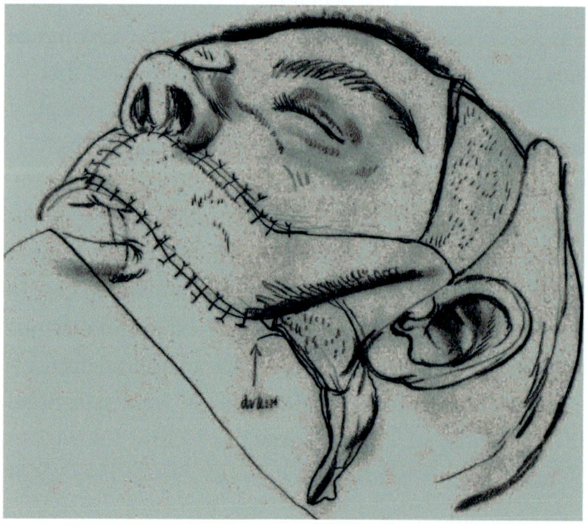

Fig. 3.9 Another drawing by 'Dickie' Orpen of a forehead axial pattern flap. *From the Antony Wallace Archive, courtesy of the British Association of Plastic Reconstructive and Aesthetic Surgeons*

may be considered the founder of plastic surgery in the West. Despite the claims of some historians, it does not appear that Celsus carried out nose reconstructions using skin flaps. However, the detailed descriptions in *De Medicina* (Fig. 3.10) leave no doubt that he successfully repaired lips and ears after trauma by surgical means [167, 168]. As the Roman physician correctly observed, if a patient presented with a new defect the tissue would not grow spontaneously and therefore the physician had to import it from adjacent regions. "In the case of the lips, if these have become too much contracted, there is also a loss of necessary function, because it becomes less easy both to take food and to speak plainly. Now new substance is not produced at the place itself, but is drawn from the neighbourhood and when the change is small this hardly robs any other part and may pass unnoticed, but when large, it cannot be so. And again, this procedure is unsuited to the aged, to those in bad bodily condition and to those whose wounds heal with difficulty."[1] The advancement flap described so clearly by Celsus did not greatly differ from Susruta's procedure.

Celsus introduced one important improvement to the procedure, recommending that the surgeon modify the defect whenever possible, imposing a geometric (preferably quadrangular or triangular) outline so that it could be more easily covered by a matching flap. "The method of treatment is as follows: the mutilation is enclosed in a square; from the inner angles of this, incisions are made across, so that the part on one side of the quadrilateral is completely separated from that on the opposite side. Then the two flaps, which we have freed, are brought together."[2]

After Celsus nothing more seems to have been written on the subject of skin flaps until Oribasius (325–403 A.D.) of Alexandria suggested their use in *colobomata* (the Greek word for "defect") of the ear, nose, lips and forehead [754–757].[3] The geometric forms adopted by Oribasius in his flap operations were similar to those recommended by Celsus. Recently Lascarotos, Mimis and Voros [531] suggested that Oribasius passed on this surgical procedure to the Arabs, and hence indirectly to Europe. If this is confirmed, Oribasius must be acknowledged to have played a key role in the development of plastic surgery in Western medicine.

Another important contribution was made in the middle of the seventh century by Paolus Aegineta, in whose works we find the first description of a fundamental concept in flap surgery, the undermining of the skin [427]. Although Aegineta does not appear to have used flaps in the modern sense, in his discussion of the repair of *colobomata* he wrote: "First the skin is freed on the under side, then the edges of the wound are drawn together and the calloused part is removed. Then the stitches holding them in place have to be applied." This technique would greatly improve the results of flap surgery.

After Oribasius the skin flap fell into disuse for a period of many centuries. The next reference is probably in the works of Theodoric of Cervia (1205–1298) [979–981]. Abraham J. van Heekeren wrote in his thesis on the history of rhinoplasty in1853 [421] that Theodoric proposed their use for the reconstruction of the nose: "Theodoricus cervianus licere desectum nasum in suo loco repare credidi" ("Theodoric from Cervia thought that it was possible to repair the nose with tissue drawn from its own site").[4] In reality we have been unable to identify any mention of elective cutaneous flaps by Theodoric. It is possible that van Heekeren misinterpreted the repositioning of a traumatic flap of skin left partially attached at the time of an injury, as in this passage from *Cyrurgia* Theodoric says "Sutura perfecta facta cum multa cautela in suo loco reponas" ("A perfect suture [must be carried out on the partially raised parts] after replacing them with great care …").[5]

1 *De Medicina*, Book VII, Chapter IX.

2 See Part II of this book, chapter on *Facial cleft*.

3 See *Collectionum Medicorum Reliqui*, Volume 3, Chapter 26.

4 See *Cyrurgia*, Book I, as well as Book II, *De Vulnere Nasi*. Here Theodoric discusses in detail the treatment of nasal trauma. In neither chapter, however, does he mention a procedure that might be interpreted as a surgical flap.

5 Theodoric's *Cyrurgia* was published in French in Lyon in 1478, in Latin in Venice in 1498 and again in 1513. It was included in the collection of surgical works compiled by Guy de Chauliac and published under the title *Cyrurgia*. Other authors appearing in this collection were Bonaventura da Castello, Bruno da Longoburgo, Rolando da Parma, Ruggero, Lanfranchi, Leonardo da Battipaglia, Jesus Hali and Canamusalo di Baldach.

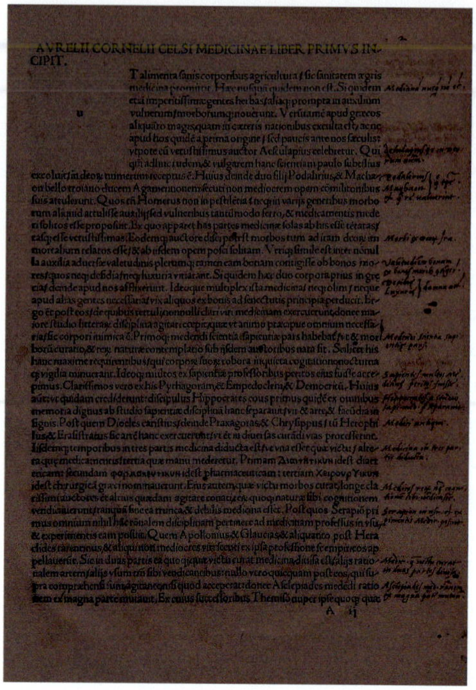
AVRELII CORNELII CELSI MEDICINAE LIBER PRIMVS INCIPIT.

Fig. 3.10 The first page of Celsus' second edition of *De Medicina*. The first edition was published in Florence in 1478 and was probably the first medical book to be printed. *Courtesy of Riccardo Mazzola, M.D., Milan*

Distant Flaps

All of the techniques discussed thus far have been *local flaps* drawn from a donor site adjacent to the recipient defect. However, the fifteenth century witnessed a revolutionary development: the invention of the *distant flap*. It is not clear exactly why the Sicilian Antonio Branca felt impelled to attempt with new techniques when his father Gustavo Branca had so brilliantly mastered the use of the local flap for nose reconstructions. Perhaps the aesthetic sensibility of the Renaissance played a role, making the conspicuous scars left by the *local skin flap*, particularly on the face, less acceptable. Furthermore, in Sicily a succession of invaders, each with his own highly refined culture and innate appreciation of beauty, left their mark—from the Phoenicians, to the Greeks and Romans, and finally the Arabs.

The fact remains that Antonio Branca, as we will see in the chapter on nasal reconstructions, began incising flaps from the inner arm rather than the face, and transferring them to the region of the nose. The patient then had to wait until the flap had established itself before the pedicle uniting it to the arm could be detached. Branca probably applied this new type of flap exclusively to nasal reconstructions, but the underlying notion that a flap could originate from a region other than that of the defect itself was new. Soon the *distant flap* was being applied by other surgeons, first to the nose by the Vianeo brothers in Calabria, and then to other parts of the body by Alessandro Benedetti (1460–1525), professor of surgery at Padua [70, 71], and Heinrich von Pfolsprundt (c.1450) in Germany [796]. The distant flap would become one of the principal techniques of plastic surgery in post-Renaissance Europe.

The practising members of the Branca and Vianeo families were all barber surgeons and therefore not only did they refuse to publish any accounts of their procedures, they did their best to keep them secret in order to discourage competitors. Another Italian, Gaspare Tagliacozzi (1545–1599), professor of anatomy and surgery at the University of Bologna, sought instead to teach the latest techniques and encourage their dissemination. He described with painstaking scientific detail the procedures that were being carried out empirically by the Branca and Vianeo families, provided full details of the clinical and surgical techniques involved, discussed the possible complications and their treatment, and even attempted to explain the underlying biology of the skin flap. By adopting this modern, objective approach he helped to pave the way for the surgeons of the future (Fig. 3.11).

Tagliacozzi's work *De Curtorum Chirurgia per Insitionem* [969] did not limit itself to a discussion of nose reconstructions, but also described the use of flaps for the repair of ears[6] and lips.[7] It is interesting to note that, although he certainly possessed considerable experience in the use of arm flaps, for a variety of operations on ear defects Tagliacozzi preferred the local flap which was more

6 See the chapter *De Curtorum Aurium Chirurgia* (*On the Restoration of Mutilated Ears*) in *De Curtorum Chirurgia per Inscritionem*.

7 See the chapter *De Labiorum Restaurationem* (*Lip Repairs*) in *De Curtorum Chirurgia per Inscritionem*.

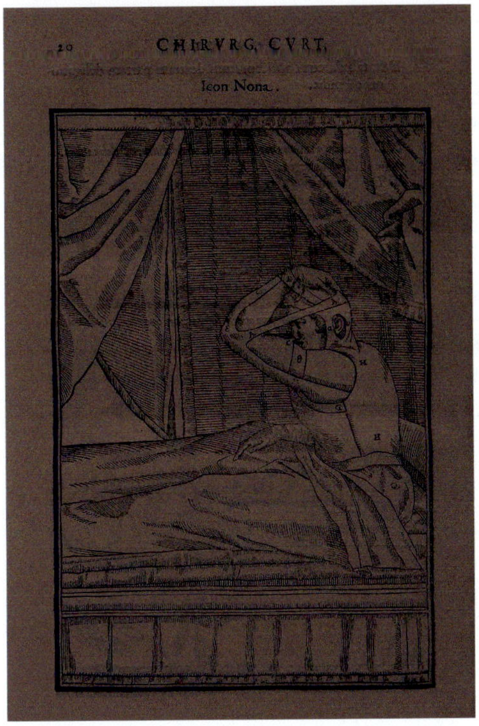

Fig. 3.11 An example of a distant flap from the arm as described by Tagliacozzi to reconstruct the nose. *Courtesy of Riccardo Mazzola, M.D., Milan*

convenient, "Caeterum non ex brachio sed ex regione post auriculam proxima" ("Not in the upper portion of the arm but from the post-auricular region nearby"). He warned his readers that this particular region was more densely vascularized than the arm and provided additional instructions on how to stop the bleeding.

Although the importance of Tagliacozzi's work was universally acknowledged when it appeared in print, his procedure failed to win many adherents and was eventually forgotten. Various factors contributed to this, including the opposition and perhaps envy of a number of highly placed colleagues who criticized his method on various grounds, often based on inaccurate information. In any case, this was a period of general recession in all branches of surgery, with isolated exceptions. One surgeon who made a genuine contribution was Jacques Guillemeau (1550–1613) who closed a large defect due to a congenital facial cleft. He suggested using bilateral relaxing incisions [400, 401], a technique that was revived by H.F. Le Dran [541], and became the basis for the bipedicle flap.

The Rebirth of the Skin Flap

With few exceptions, the flap was not exploited again until the very end of the eighteenth century, when two events helped to revive interest in the procedure.

The first of these was the publication of eyewitness accounts by visitors returning from India. They had watched native surgeons reconstructing noses using skin flaps in what was clearly considered to be a perfectly routine operation. Galvanized by these remarkable reports, Joseph C. Carpue (1764–1846) gathered as much information as he could by interviewing witnesses and after conducting some practice dissections, attempted the operation himself on two patients with gratifying results. The monograph on this exploit, published in 1816, *An Account of Successful Operations for Restoring a Lost Nose*, generated a veritable sensation [157].

The *frontal flap* adopted by Carpue was identical to the procedure that had been employed in India for centuries, although it is not mentioned in the *Samhita*. Historians disagree as to who was the first to use the *frontal flap*. Some attribute its invention to the Kandra family of Poona (c.1400 A.D.) although Hakin Dina Nath Kamgihiara, the last descendent of this family, affirmed that it was being practised by his ancestors as far back as 1000 A.D. In any case, this procedure was unknown in Europe and excited intense interest among surgeons in England and on the Continent when they learned of it.

For example, the illustrious German surgeon Carl Ferdinand von Graefe (1787–1840) carried out a comparative study on nose reconstructions using the Indian local flap and Tagliacozzi's distant flap, which he had rediscovered [390, 391, 393]. Following his recommendation, the German school re-introduced the use of flaps in reconstructive surgery. Colleagues in other European countries followed suit[8] and the practice soon gained ad-

8 Among the many authors who wrote about facial reconstruction in the nineteenth century we may mention Jacques Mathieu Delpech (1777–1832) in 1821; L. Labat in 1834; Johan Friedrick Dieffenback (1794–1847) in the same year; Ernst Blasius (1802–1875) in 1842; and Charles Emanuel Sedillot (1804–1883) in 1848 [914]. Sedillot was from Strasbourg and wrote on many plastic surgery topics. He is better known for performing the first gastrostomy and popularizing the use of inhalation anaesthesia.

herents in the United States with the work of Thomas D. Mutter (1811–1867) [720].

By the end of the nineteenth century the interest raised by Carpue in 1816 had led to a veritable rebirth of the skin flap, above all for reconstructions of the face. Progress was accelerated by a second factor, which was the growing importance of surgery in two different areas; the treatment of cancer and the repair of wounds received on the battlefield during the wars of the nineteenth century.

For many centuries surgeons were convinced that skin cancer was incurable. The Venetian Filippo Masiero wrote in 1688 [616] that there was little to be done and that the phrase spoken by Jesus to Mary Magdalene after his resurrection "Noli me tangere" could be applied to patients with cancer of the face (Fig. 3.12).[9] In recent times J.P. Bennett has used the term when writing about rodent ulcer [73]. Happily, by the middle of the eighteenth century a series of enterprising surgeons demonstrated that this pessimism was unjustified. In a paper presented in 1755 before the *Royal Society* [220] Jacques Daviel (1693–1762) reported on the successful treatment of ten cases of "ulcus rodens". Later Martinet de la Creause wrote that the prognosis could be improved by excising a large amount of the tissue surrounding the cancer [207]. This was feasible because surgeons now knew the defect could be closed by means of a flap. De la Creause described three cases of recurrent cancer of the face which he treated in this way. After these reports surgeons proceeded with more confidence to operate on tumours, using flaps to repair the defects left by the excision (Figs. 3.13, 3.14) [664].

In 1830 Romand reviewed 30 cases of reconstructions of the lower lip and the different techniques that were used, including skin flaps [856, 857] and in 1907 Charles Nélaton (1852–1911) and Louis Ombrédanne (1871–1956) counted 94 papers in the literature reporting the use of skin flaps to reconstruct the lower lip [727]. According to an exhaustive study by Riccardo F. Mazzola and Gabriella Lupo a total of 280 articles describing cases of flap reconstructions were published during the course of the nineteenth century [627]. It may be said that T.J.S. Patterson was entirely justified in describing this period as "the era of flaps" [782].

The success of the procedure and hence its acceptance, was probably related to the fact that most of these flaps were on the face where the blood supply made them a reliable proposition. Repairs made in other regions of the body, where failure and the resulting bad scars were more acceptable, may have been less satisfactory.

Developments Before and During the Nineteenth Century

Given this period of intense activity, it is no simple matter to provide an exact chronology of developments in skin flap surgery. Nevertheless, technical improvements led to advances which we will attempt to retrace.

Before the invention of the skin flap, surgeons could only close skin defects by suturing them directly and they tried with different methods to reduce the tension of the wound. The papers published by Antoine Louis [579] in 1768, P. Bouisson [124] in 1826 and M. Serre [917] in 1842 emphasize this point. They were not actually working with flaps, but were nevertheless seeking to resolve the dilemma facing all surgeons. The first priority was to remove all the tumour tissue necessary to ensure the survival of the patient, no matter how large a defect it might create, but they were then left with the problem of how to close this defect.

Twenty years before the *Indian flap* arrived in Europe, in 1779, Francois Chopart (1743–1795) employed an *advancement flap* from the chin of a patient to close a defect in his lower lip [177]. Carpue heralded this as "the first plastic surgery operation of modern times" although, as was perhaps to be expected, the final result was disappointing. The tendency of the flap to retract toward the donor region and perhaps also the tightening of the scar drew the lip down and greatly altered the line of the mouth. Notwithstanding these drawbacks, Chopart's *procedée du tiroir* was widely adopted in France and within a short space of time various modifications had been introduced, a clear sign of its acceptance.

Chopart's patient had a cancer involving the entire lower lip as well as the right commissure and a small portion of the upper lip. Such a defect could certainly not

9 See *La Chirurgia Compendiata*, Venice, 1702, p 41. This book was a treatise on oncology *ante litteram*.

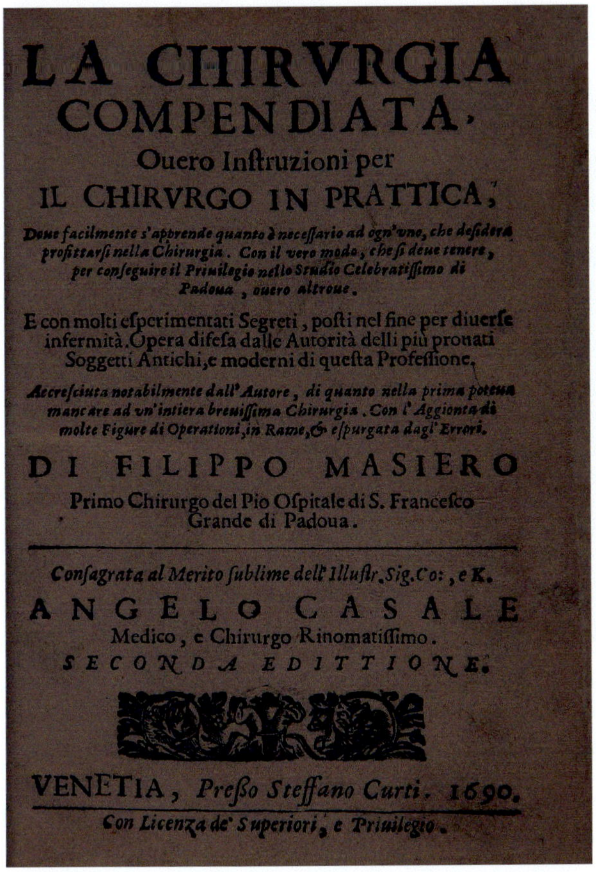

LA CHIRVRGIA COMPENDIATA.

Ouero Inſtruzioni per

IL CHIRVRGO IN PRATTICA;

Doue facilmente s'apprende quanto è neceſſario ad ogn'vno, che deſidera profittarſi nella Chirurgia. Con il vero modo, che ſi deue tenere, per conſeguire il Priuilegio nello Studio Celebratiſſimo di Padoua, ouero altroue.

E con molti eſperimentati Segreti, poſti nel fine per diuerſe infermità. Opera difeſa dalle Autorità delli più prouati Soggetti Antichi, e moderni di queſta Profeſſione.

Accreſciuta notabilmente dall'Autore, di quanto nella prima poteua mancare ad vn'intiera breuiſſima Chirurgia. Con l'Aggionta di molte Figure di Operationi, in Rame, & eſpurgata dagl'Errori.

DI FILIPPO MASIERO

Primo Chirurgo del Pio Oſpitale di S. Franceſco Grande di Padoua.

Conſagrata al Merito ſublime dell'Illuſtr. Sig. Co:, e K.

ANGELO CASALE

Medico, e Chirurgo Rinomatiſſimo.

SECONDA EDITTIONE.

VENETIA, *Preſſo Steffano Curti.* 1690.

Con Licenza de' Superiori, e Priuilegio.

Fig. 3.12 Frontispiece of Filippo Masiero's *La Chirurgia Compendiata* where he claimed that skin cancer was best left alone and could not be successfully treated by surgery. He used the phrase *Noli me tangere* from St. John's Gospel (Chap. 20 v. 17) to emphasize his opinion. *Courtesy of Riccardo Mazzola, M.D., Milan*

have been closed with a direct suture. Chopart made two vertical incisions, one on either side of the chin, and advanced the flap upward to cover the defect. He may not have been aware that Celsus nineteen centuries earlier and the Hindus in an even more ancient epoch had used very similar flaps. It should come as no surprise therefore that Aristide A.S. Verneuil (1823–1895) described the *tiroir* as a completely new and entirely French procedure [1013]. In 1824 Charles Francois Lallemand (1790–1854) moved the base of the flap to beneath the mandible [519], while in 1828 Philibert Joseph Roux (1780–1854) emphasized the importance of radically undermining the flap [865, 871]. In 1829 J. Morgan [706–708] and C. Viguerie [1020] used a bipedicle flap to advance skin from the margins of the defect.

One serious drawback of Chopart's *advancement flap* was that folds of redundant skin tended to form dog-ears. These folds were not only unsightly; they also hindered the movement of the flap and its placement over the defect. A brilliant solution to this problem was presented by Camille Bernard [79] to the *Societé de Chirurgie de Paris* in 1852, although Karl von Burow (1809–1864) published a paper in 1855 describing a similar technique that he claimed he had been using for several years [147]. Both surgeons proposed that a triangle of skin be excised from each side of the flap's base in order to facilitate its advancement and improve the final appearance of the repair. This modification came to be known as the *Burow-Bernard technique*, and in England as *Burow's triangle*.

Despite these improvements the *advancement flap* presented serious drawbacks, forcing surgeons to look for other solutions. The lower lip was one of the preferred sites for experimentation. Lallemand was followed by Bernard Rudoph von Langenbeck (1810–1887), who in 1839 raised two *transposition flaps* from beneath the mandible [522]. This left an interposed island of skin on the chin beneath the flap that prevented its downward displacement. The disadvantage of von Langenbeck's procedure was that it left no tissue to close the donor region.[10] Conversely, the bilateral flaps were broadly undermined and could be easily transposed to achieve closure with minimal tension.

The nasolabial sulcus has always served as a source of skin flaps, because the donor region can be closed quite easily by direct suture. Blasius [115, 116], Dieffenbach [242, 244–246] (Fig. 3.15) and later Viktor von Bruns (1812–1883) [137] used this as a donor site for lip constructions. The skin around the eyes was also exploited. In 1829 Johan Karl Fricke (1790–1841) raised an inferiorly based flap from the lax skin around the patient's eye to reconstruct an eyelid [338] and in 1855 redundant tissue from the upper eyelid was used by Louis de

10 Skin flaps were commonly used in this period. The practice of anaesthesia was not yet widespread and therefore the harvesting and grafting of a suitable piece of skin would merely have caused the patient further suffering.

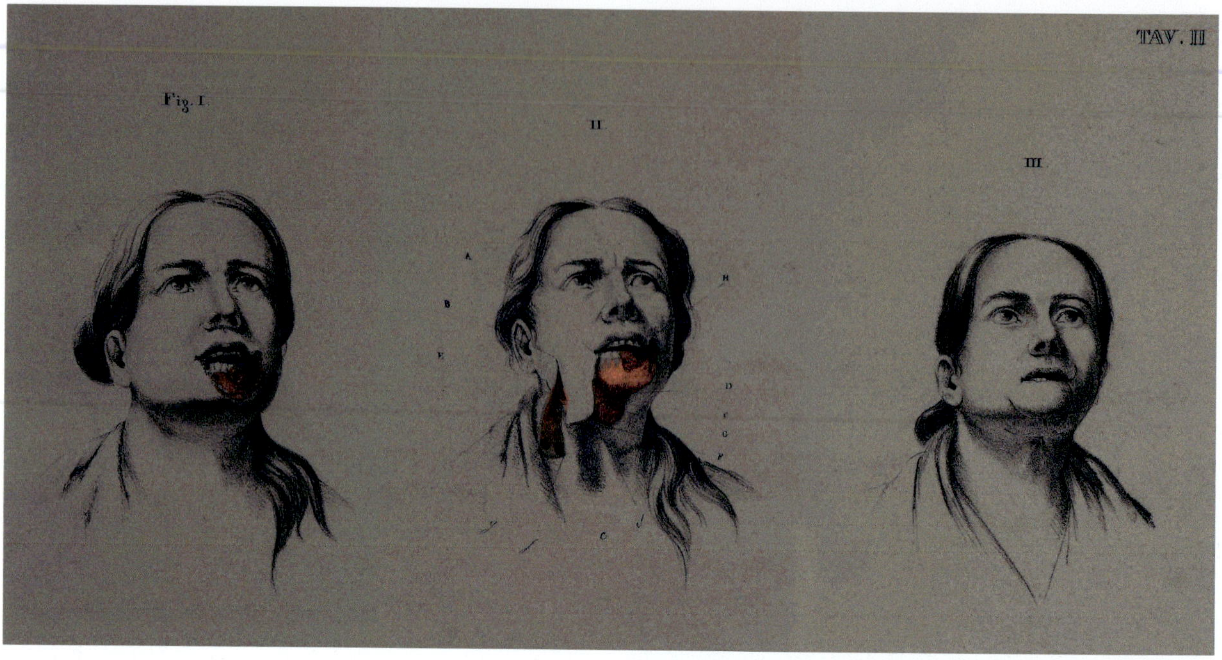

Fig. 3.13 An example of how skin flaps made it possible to excise large lesions on the face, from Paolo Baroni's *Operazioni Chirurgiche Fatte* 1857 Rome. The book was responsible for the spread of facial flaps to treat skin cancer in Italy. *Courtesy of Riccardo Mazzola, M.D., Milan*

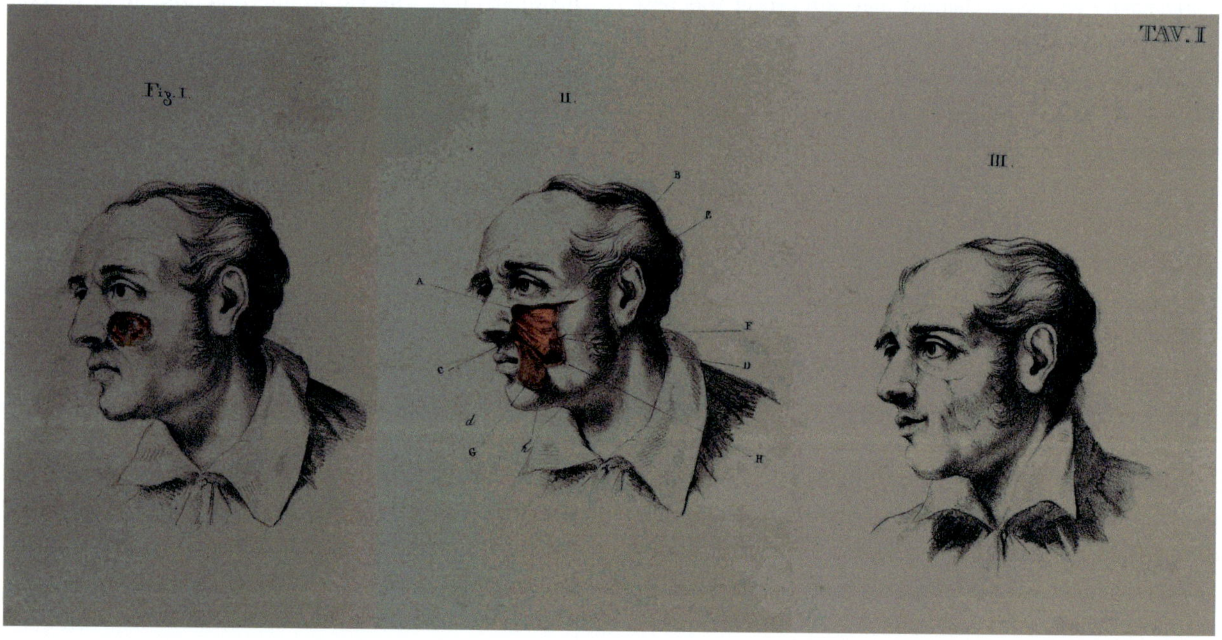

Fig. 3.14 Another example from Paolo Baroni's *Operazioni Chirurgiche Fatte* 1857 Rome. *Courtesy of Riccardo Mazzola, M.D., Milan*

Wecker (1832–1883) and Edmond Landolt (1845–1926) [1039] to make a pedicle flap for the reconstruction of the lower eyelid. Fritze and Reich [340] also described flaps for eyelid reconstruction in 1845 (Fig. 3.16a,b) and other surgeons had their own solutions to defects of the lower lip and chin (Figs. 3.17, 3.18).[11]

The success of these operations encouraged surgeons to explore other means of reconstructing lips and eyelids. Thus W.E. Horner [448] in the United States in 1837, Serre [917] in 1842 and C.P. Dénonvilliers [236] in 1854 suggested the use of multiple small *transposition flaps* to correct ectropion. Although they bear certain similarities, these cannot be considered as forerunners of the Z-plasty which, according to McCarthy [628] was invented by O. Berger in 1887 [78]. Berger described his ingenious procedure, which was designed to relax the tension of a scar by raising triangular flaps at its two ends and transposing them, in 1904. In 1849 in Finland Lars Henrik Törnroth described a similar method used to treat an axillary contracture [994] and much later in 1914 Hippolyte Morestin recommended multiple Z-plasties to correct all types of contracted linear scars which subsequently became the method of choice [699, 700].

After its revival, perhaps the first surgeons to apply a flap in a region other than the face were Sir Astley Cooper (1769–1832) and B. Travers (1783–1858) [196, 197], who used a flap for urethral reconstructions in 1819. Sir Astley had earlier attempted to use nitric acid to close "small unnatural apertures of the urethra", but realized that larger defects required a different approach, "similar in principle to that which has been performed from time immemorial in India for making a new nose". He and Travers prepared a superiorly based scrotal flap, rotated it over the defect, and fixed it in place with four stitches. They then introduced a catheter into the urethra and kept it there for three months until healing was established. Other flaps in the genital area were used by Delpech [233, 234] in France and Langenbeck [522] in Germany to treat hypospadias.

Delpech went on to propose new designs for the flap, including a folded, superiorly based *rotation flap* which he claimed allowed the surgeon to reconstruct both the cover and lining of the lower lip in a single operation. Although this procedure was only partially successful, probably due to the kinking of vessels within the fold, it was adopted by many surgeons.

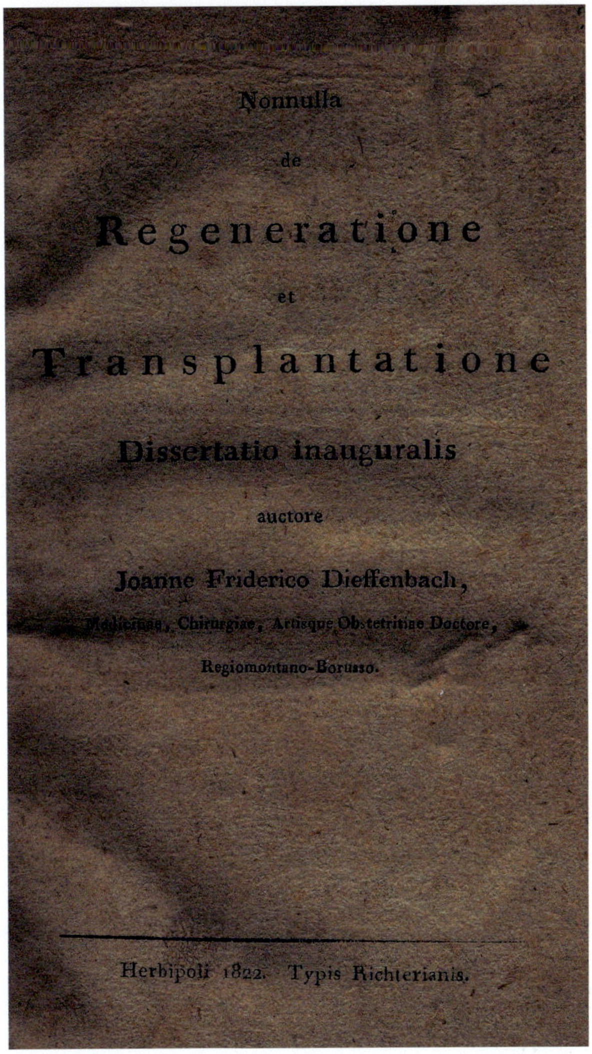
Nonnulla
de
Regeneratione
et
Transplantatione
Dissertatio inauguralis
auctore
Joanne Friderico Dieffenbach,
Medicinae, Chirurgiae, Artisque Obstetritiae Doctore,
Regiomontano-Borusso.
Herbipoli 1822. Typis Richterianis.

Fig. 3.15 Frontispiece of Johan Frederick Dieffenbach's thesis *Regeneratione et Transplantatione* published in 1822. Dieffenbach's interest in transplantation stimulated others in the early nineteenth century. *Courtesy of Riccardo Mazzola, M.D., Milan*

The well-known drawbacks of the *local flap* had been partly resolved by Antonio Branca, whose nasal reconstruction technique was recorded and used by Tagliacozzi for his own operation in the sixteenth century. *Distant flaps* fell into disuse until the nineteenth century

11 See Rogers BO (1979) Julius von Szymanowski (1829–1868). His life and times. *Plast Reconstr Surg* 64:465.

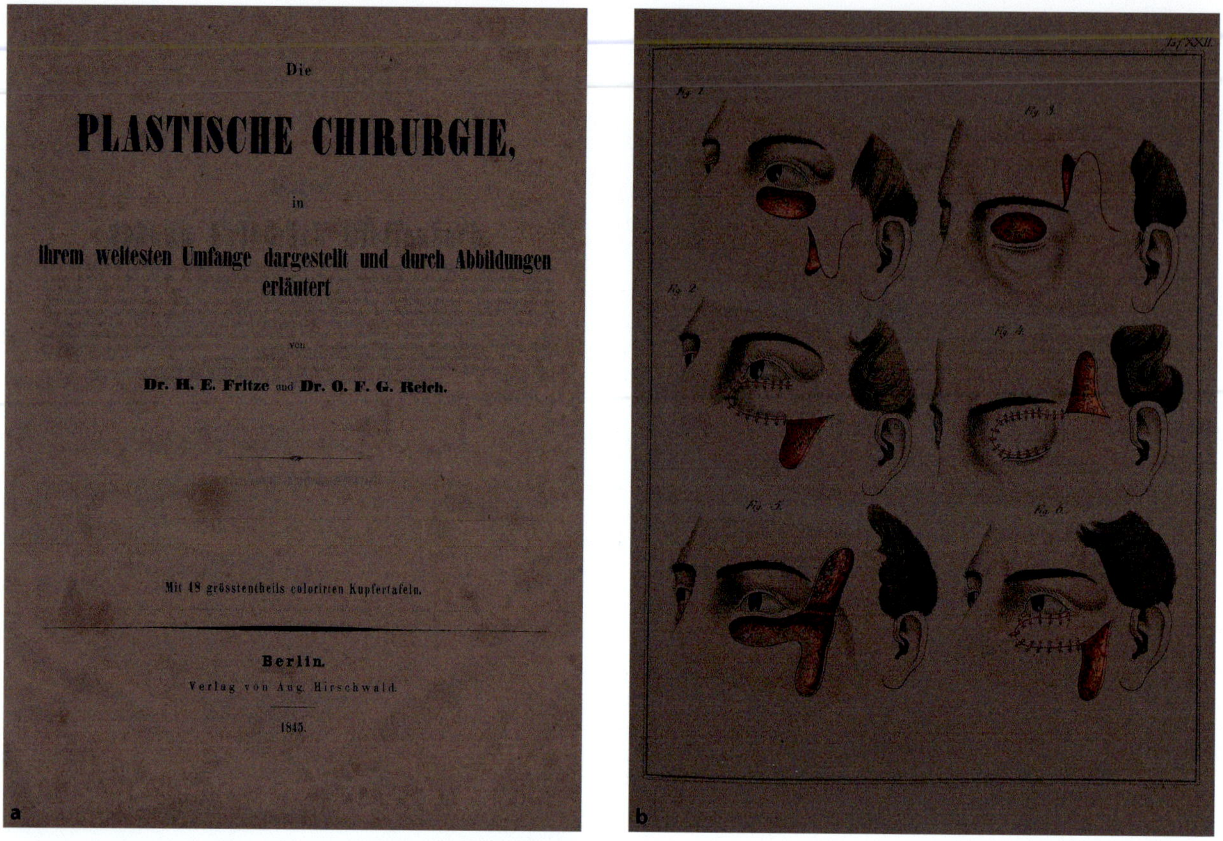

Fig. 3.16 **a** Frontispiece of the book *Die Plastische Chirurgie.* **b** Diagrams showing flaps for eyelid reconstruction from Fritze and Reich (1845). This was one of the earliest books dealing entirely with reconstructive surgery. *Courtesy of Riccardo Mazzola, M.D., Milan*

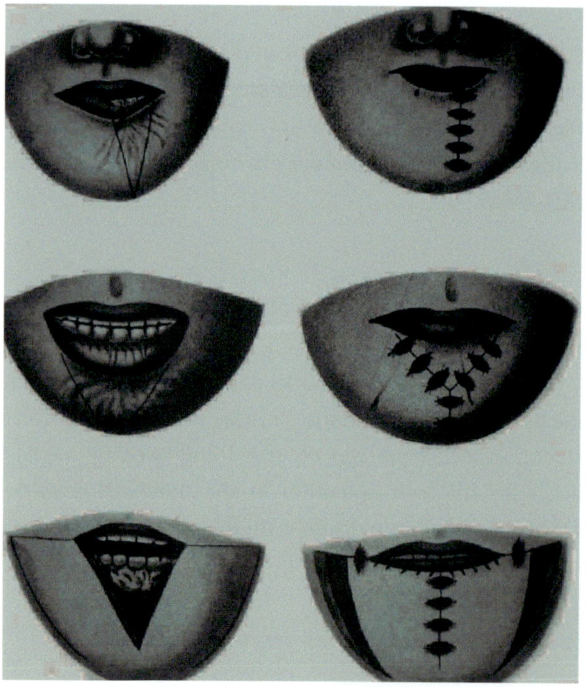

Fig. 3.17 Methods for reconstructing the lower lip, including a V-Y flap, as conceived by Dieffenbach and quoted by Fritze and Reich in 1845 [340]. *Courtesy of Riccardo Mazzola, M.D., Milan*

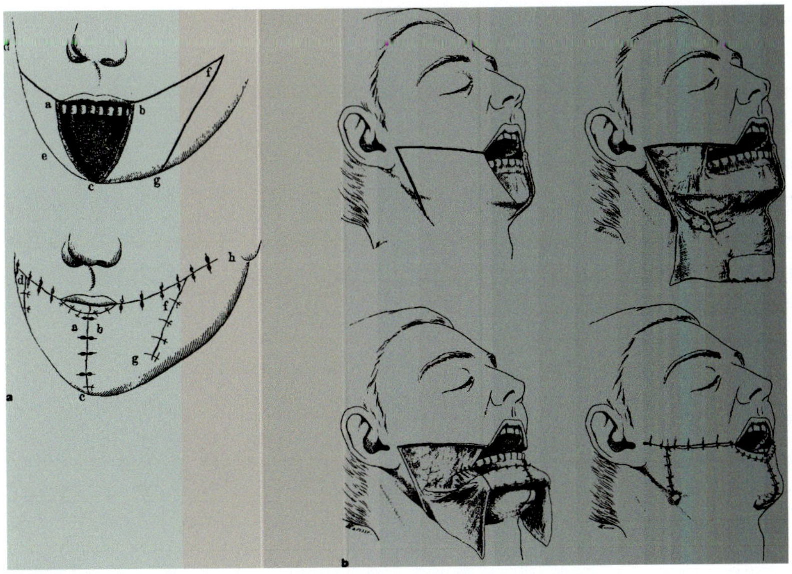

Fig. 3.18 Two large transposition flaps designed by Julius von Szymanowki (1829–1868) for reconstruction of the chin, taken from his book *Handbuch der Operativen Chirurgie* (1870). *Courtesy of Riccardo Mazzola, M.D., Milan*

when, as we have already noted, knowledge of the Indian flap arrived in Europe and from there spread to the rest of the world. In the United States, Jonathan Mason Warren (1811–1867) modified Tagliacozzi's method in 1840, raising a flap on the forearm rather than the upper arm and, in his first case, dividing the pedicle on the fifth day, which allowed the patient to convalesce in a less uncomfortable position [1032]. The premature separation of the flap, however, probably led to its partial necrosis which prevented him from reconstructing the alar of the nose. Von Graefe also reported good results with the Italian method [391].

In this period *distant flaps* began to be used elsewhere than the face. The legs of those suffering from disease or trauma were a frequent area. Frank H. Hamilton (1813–1886) was the inventor of the famous *cross-leg flap*, which he carried out for the first time in 1856 to cure a chronic ulcer [410]. He had attempted the same procedure in another case 12 years earlier but the patient refused, no doubt put off by the prospect of a long period of immobility with his legs bound together. The operation was successfully repeated by G.O. Lange [521] and soon, with various improvements and modifications, the cross-leg flap became the method of choice for the repair of large defects in the lower limbs.

The Tubed Flap

Up to this time, the portion of tissue forming the bridge between the donor region and the recipient site in all *distant flaps* remained uncovered and this raw surface almost invariably became infected. The problem was particularly serious in military hospitals at a time when antibiotics were not yet available. A Russian ophthalmologist, Vladimir P. Filatov[12] of Odessa (1874–1956), came up with an ingenious solution. By making two parallel incisions and suturing their margins to cover the exposed segment, he succeeded in creating a protective "suitcase handle" of the bridge that greatly reduced the risk of infection. It is worth noting that he was working in difficult conditions because of the First World War at a time when the Russian revolution had reached Odessa. The tubed flap he invented proved to have many benefits and greatly influenced developments over the next 50 years, particularly in battlefield surgery.

Filatov conducted many experiments on rabbits before attempting his flap repair on a patient for the first time in 1916. He raised a tubed flap on the neck to close a defect following the excision of a tumour from the lower eyelid. He wrote, the tube consisted of "a strip

12 The son of an ophthalmologist, Vladimir P. Filatov studied medicine in Moscow and joined the staff of the city's Ophthalmology Hospital in 1899. He moved to Odessa in 1903 to take up the position of "Ordinator", becoming an assistant in 1906 and finally succeeding to the chair held by Prof. Golvin as director of the Ophthalmology Clinic.

of skin, with the layer of subcutaneous adipose tissue, which remained connected to the upper part of the neck at the mastoid process and to the lower end at the [upper part of the] sternum." Filatov observed that "… the skin pedicle would adjust itself to the new condition of blood circulation and the necessary anastomoses would develop, [thus creating] a solid nutritional base for the flap." Two weeks later he placed a free graft of buccal mucosa measuring 3.5 × 3.5 cm under the distal portion of the flap. After waiting another four days, he carried out the total excision of the lower eyelid. He then transferred the flap and proceeded to reconstruct the eyelid complete with lining and cover. The transposed tube was left in place for four weeks. Once he was certain that the new eyelid would survive the tube was divided, trimmed and returned to the donor site (Fig. 3.19) [312].

Filatov wrote enthusiastically: "The formation of a stalk-like, round nutrient pedicle for the flap … guarantees almost normal nourishment." He admitted that he had conceived his idea after reading the work of E.F. Snydacker who described an open (although not tubed) flap for the reconstruction of the eyelid in 1907 [944]. However, the Russian was quick to underline one of the principal advantages of his tube: "The round stalk flap gives protection against infection." As he observed: "The formation of the round stalk nutrient pedicle in plastic operations is not to be regarded merely as a variation of Snydacker's method. There is a matter of a new principle that guarantees the nourishment of the transplanted flap." Filatov foresaw that his method could be applied in other regions of the body, "irrespective of the type of plastic procedure and its location," and even suggested that a pedicled tube flap might be applied to a distant site if moved in successive stages.[13]

It seems that H. Ganzer was not aware of Filatov's work when in March 1917 he reported to the *Berlin Laryngology Society* the results of an operation carried out to reconstruct the mouth and mandibular region in a patient by means of a series of *tubed flaps* raised from his chest, shoulder and upper arm [356]. In the same year he used a *tubed flap* from the arm of a patient to close a large palate defect.

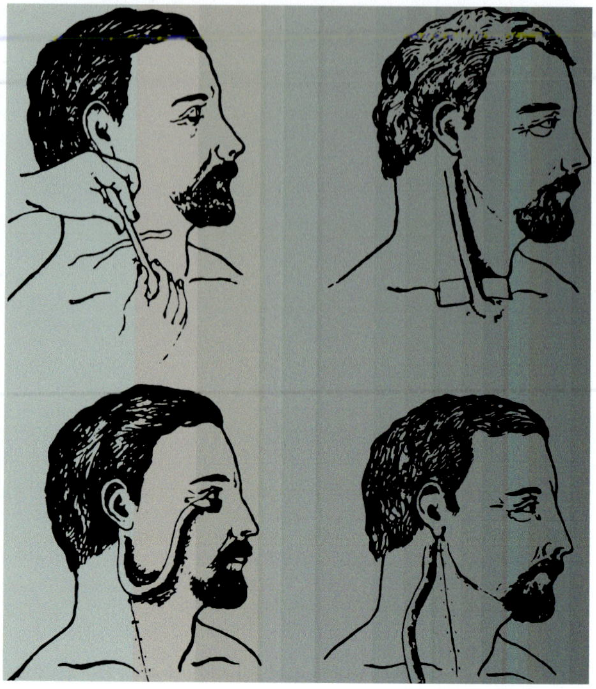

Fig. 3.19 Diagram taken from the original article of Vladimir P. Filatov in *Vestnik Olftalmologii* in 1917 showing the stages of his *round pedicle* flap to reconstruct the eyelid [312]

Another pioneer who used tubed flaps was Victor Morax (1866–1935). He employed the procedure in 1919 to close a large forehead defect following the removal of a naevus. Earlier he had demonstrated his bravura by executing a bilateral lower lid reconstruction using a flap raised from the upper part of the patient's neck. After one lid had been reconstructed and its circulation appeared to be well established, the flap was detached from its base and swung over to complete the second repair [693, 694].

13 Before the outbreak of the First World War, Filatov was able to take a trip to Western Europe and visit many of the most important universities in Germany, Austria, France and Czechoslovakia. In 1912 he carried out his first corneal transplant. Despite the chaos caused by war and revolution (Odessa was ruled by a local government that was opposed to the Bolsheviks until 1916, and was occupied in March 1918 by the Austro-Hungarian Army) Filatov managed to continue his research and invent the tube flap.

The surgeon primarily responsible for popularizing the *tubed flap* technique was Sir Harold Gillies (1882–1960). Indeed, his name is so closely associated with the technique that many assume he was its inventor (Fig. 3.20). It is certainly possible that when he began using the *tubed flap* he was unaware of the achievements of Filatov, due firstly to all the confusion generated by the First World War and the Russian Revolution, and secondly to the fact that he would probably not have come across Filatov's work as it was published in a Russian journal of ophthalmology. In any case, in October 1917 Gillies carried out his first *tubed flap* repair as a surgeon in the British Army. The patient was an Able Seaman who had suffered severe facial burns when his ship, HMS Malaya, exploded at the battle of Jutland in 1916. He arrived at the military unit 18 months later and Gillies reconstructed his face with *tube pedicle flaps*. The flaps were inset on 17 October 1917 a date that was to became important in a controversy that arose later (Fig. 3.21a–d). Gillies did not report the case at the time but in 1919 wrote an exhaustive account of a series of similar operations, which was published in the following year [373]. In the same year he published his book *Plastic Surgery of the Face* based on his wartime experiences [374].

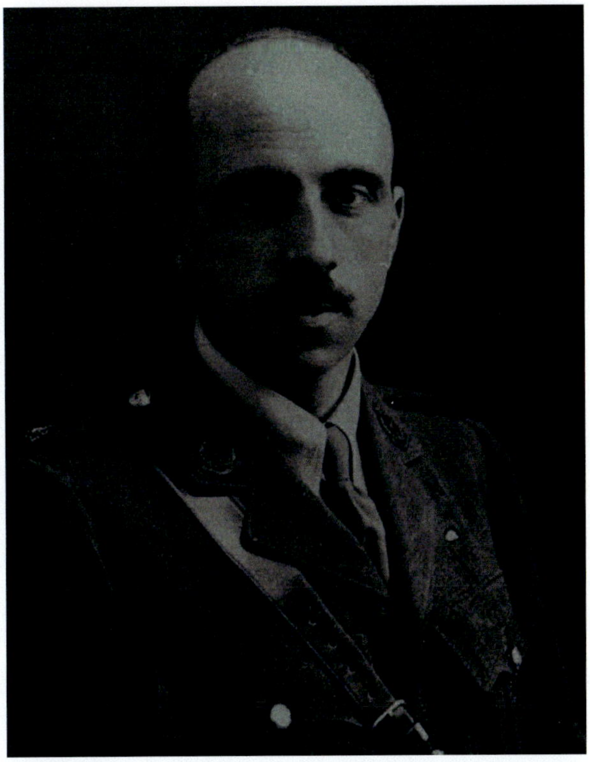

Fig. 3.20 Portrait of Major Gillies (later to become Sir Harold) when he was working at Sidcup during World War II. *Reproduced by permission of the Gillies Archives, Queen Mary's Hospital, Sidcup, UK*

Harold Gillies was 32 when the war started and in February 1915 he volunteered to join the Red Cross. Already interested in reconstructive surgery of the face, he was appointed to the unit of Charles Valadier, a French-American dental surgeon who had successfully established a hospital for the treatment of jaw wounds at Wimereux, near Boulogne. During this time Gillies had the opportunity to visit Morestin[14] in Paris. He had already acquired a reputation as a brilliant reconstructive surgeon. Gillies' report to the British Army Medical Services was so convincing that Sir Alfred Keogh, the director and Mr Arbuthnot Lane, army chief surgeon, ordered Gillies to report to Cambridge Military Hospital at Aldershot "for special duty in connection with Plastic Surgery".

From that day all facial injuries were sent to this hospital but unfortunately the numbers were so many that a new Unit was required. Gillies was supported by two dental surgeons named Fraser and King, but soon teams from the rest of the Commonwealth come to learn the new techniques and to help. Kelsey Fry, a British dental surgeon became an important member of the team (Fig. 3.22).

In July 1916 when the Allies started the great offensive on the Somme the hospital was overwhelmed by thousands of wounded. On the first day of the battle alone some 60,000 soldiers were killed. Despite the fact that the surgeons worked day and night and the unit was enlarged it was clear that new facilities and a bigger team were needed. Early in 1917, inspired by the experience from Queen Mary's Hospital in Roehampton, which offered excellent results for amputees, a similar institution for facial injuries was established at Sidcup, Kent in a large

14 See Lalardie JP (1972) Hippolyte Morestin (1869–1918). *Br J Plast Surg* 25:39. Morestin took charge of the Plastic Surgery Unit at Hôpital Val de Grace, Paris in 1915.

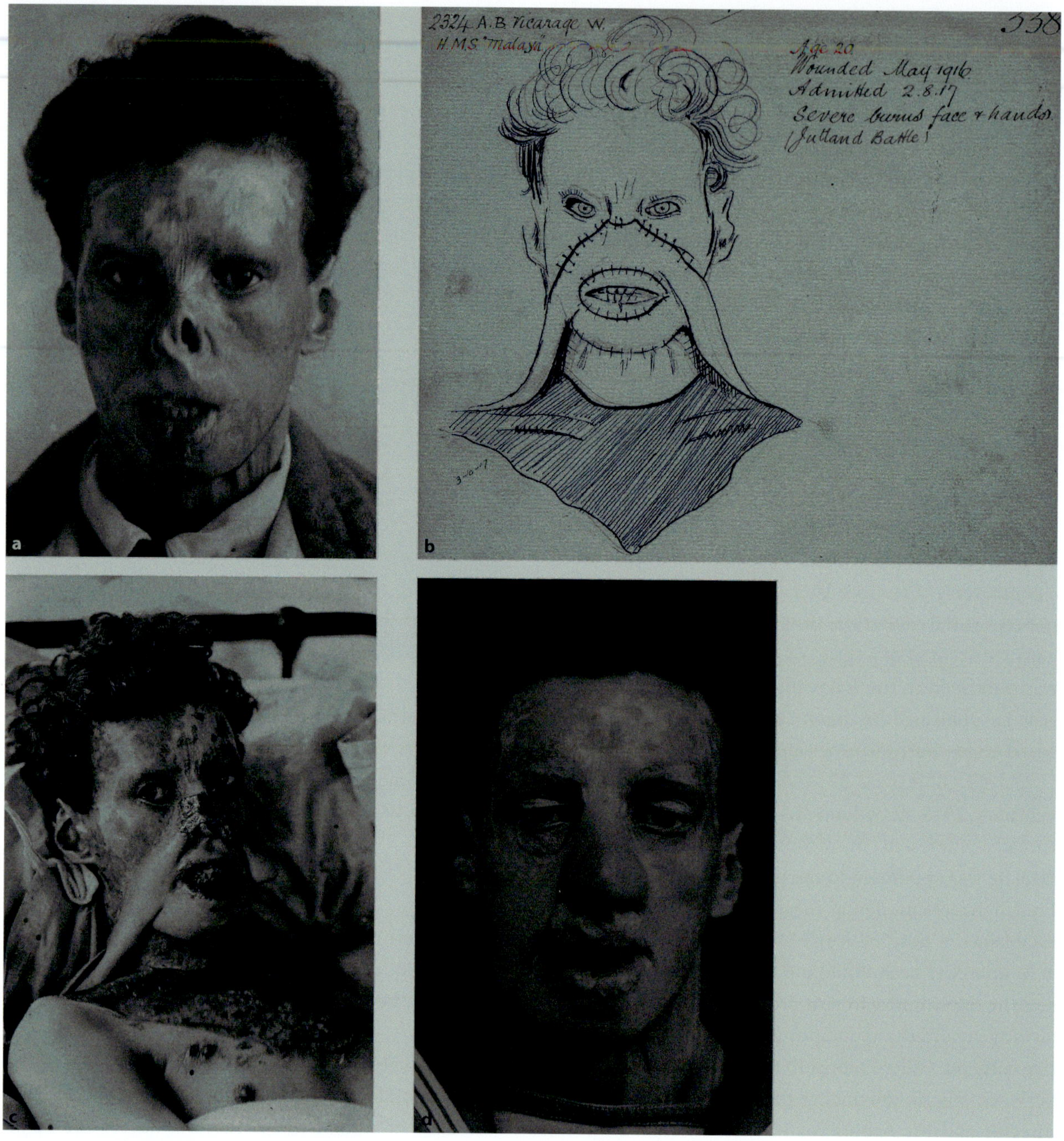

Fig. 3.21a–d Stages of the very first tubed pedicle flap performed by Harold Gilllies in 1917. *Reproduced by permission of the Gillies Archives, Queen Mary's Hospital, Sidcup, UK*

mansion called Frognal House. It became known as the Queen's Hospital because of the support of King George V's wife Queen Mary and is now officially Queen Mary's Hospital Sidcup. This was the first Unit dealing only with Facial Plastic Surgery anywhere in the world. Surgeons from the British Isles and the overseas Dominions joined the team and, when news reached the United States, surgeons came from America to learn the new techniques. Among them was Vilray Blair from Missouri. When he returned home his experience helped the creation of the new speciality of plastic surgery in America.

Among the doctors who worked at Sidcup a special mention should be made of Ivan Magill. He came to Sidcup as an anaesthetist to join Eade who had already developed the technique of giving an anaesthetic in the sitting position. Rowbotham was another member of the anaesthetic team. Under the difficult conditions of facial reconstructions it was hard to maintain the airway and maintain clean aseptic conditions. Magill developed many new techniques among them the endotracheal tube.

Gillies also insisted that all operations should be carefully recorded with drawings and illustrations. This improved planning and assisted the development of new methods. Henry Tonks, a surgeon with a gift for art provided many sketches and water colour paintings which were not only used for recording but eventually became pieces of art in their own right (Fig. 3.23a–c). Most of them are still kept in the *Royal College of Surgeons* in London. Tonks became Professor of Fine Art at the Slade School in London (Fig. 3.24a,b).[15] Other artists worked at Sidcup and a new photographic department flourished. Wallace has written a valuable account of the history of clinical photography in plastic surgery and burns [1026]. Technicians were also on hand to help make equipment and facial prostheses (Fig. 3.25a–c).

If one remembers that until a few years before the war, plastic surgical operations had been performed relatively infrequently by general surgeons the experience of this unit helped establishing Plastic Surgery as a new speciality. Around 5,000 patients were treated and about 15,000 reconstructive operations performed. After the unit closed in 1925, civilian plastic surgery hospitals led by surgeons who had gained vital experience in the war were established around London (Fig. 3.26)[16] and during World War II the services of plastic surgeons was needed once again. McIndoe was one of them and treated pilots

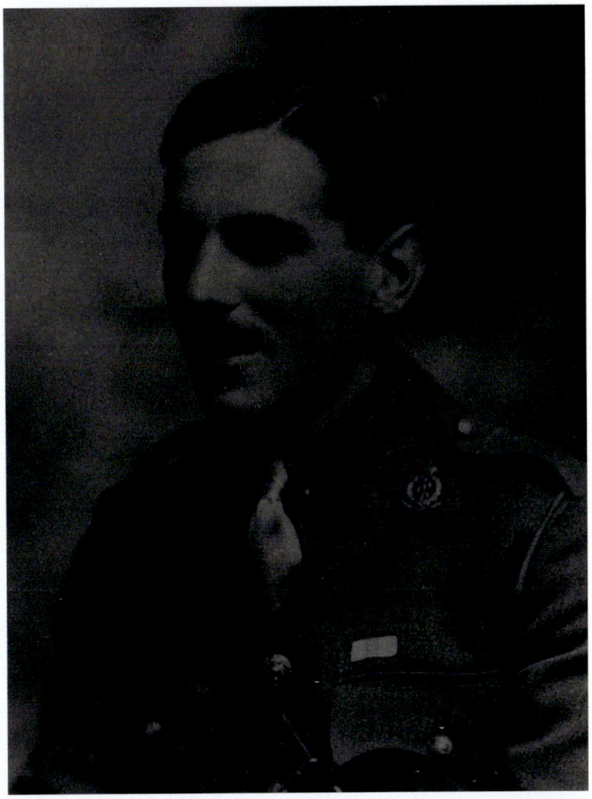

Fig. 3.22 Portrait of Major Kelsey Fry who worked with Gillies at Sidcup. His dental skills were of paramount importance in the treatment of facial injuries. *Reproduced by kind permission of Dr Ian Kelsey Fry*

15 J.P. Bennett has written a beautifully illustrated monograph as a supplement to the *British Journal of Plastic Surgery* entitled *Henry Tonks and his Contemporaries*. This contains excellent reproductions of the Tonks pastels from this period. *Br J Plast Surg* (1986) 39: 1–34.

16 Hill End, St Albans were Mowlem worked (the unit move to Mount Vernon in 1953), Nuffield Hospital, Oxford and Stoke Mandeville, Aylesbury under Kilner, East Grinstead with McIndoe and Rooksdown House, Basingstoke where Gillies continued. This unit subsequently moved to Roehampton.

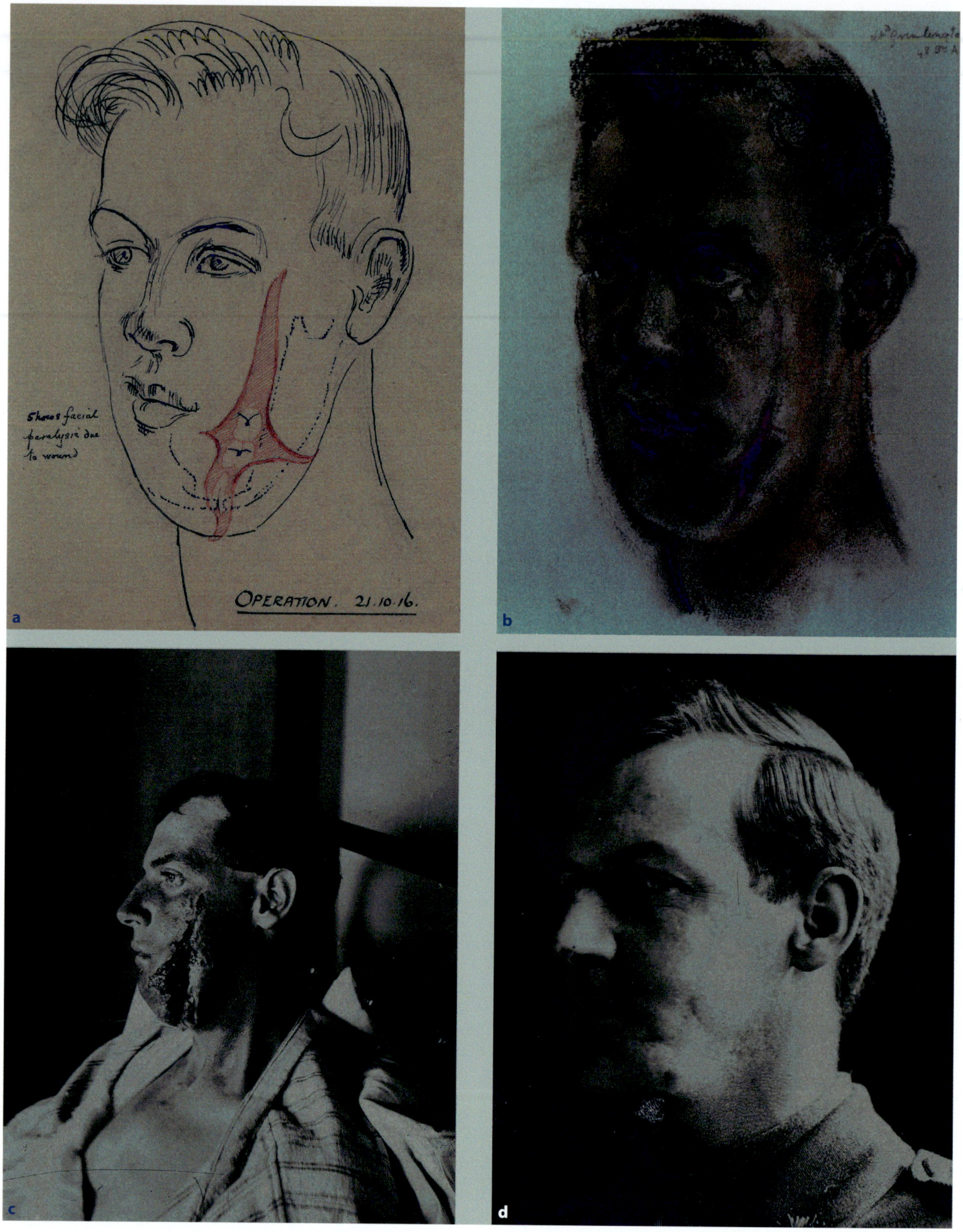

Fig. 3.23a–d An example of a drawing and a pastel made by Henry Tonks with photographs of the patient before and after treatment. *Reproduced by permission of the Gillies Archives, Queen Mary's Hospital, Sidcup, UK and The Royal College of Surgeons of England*

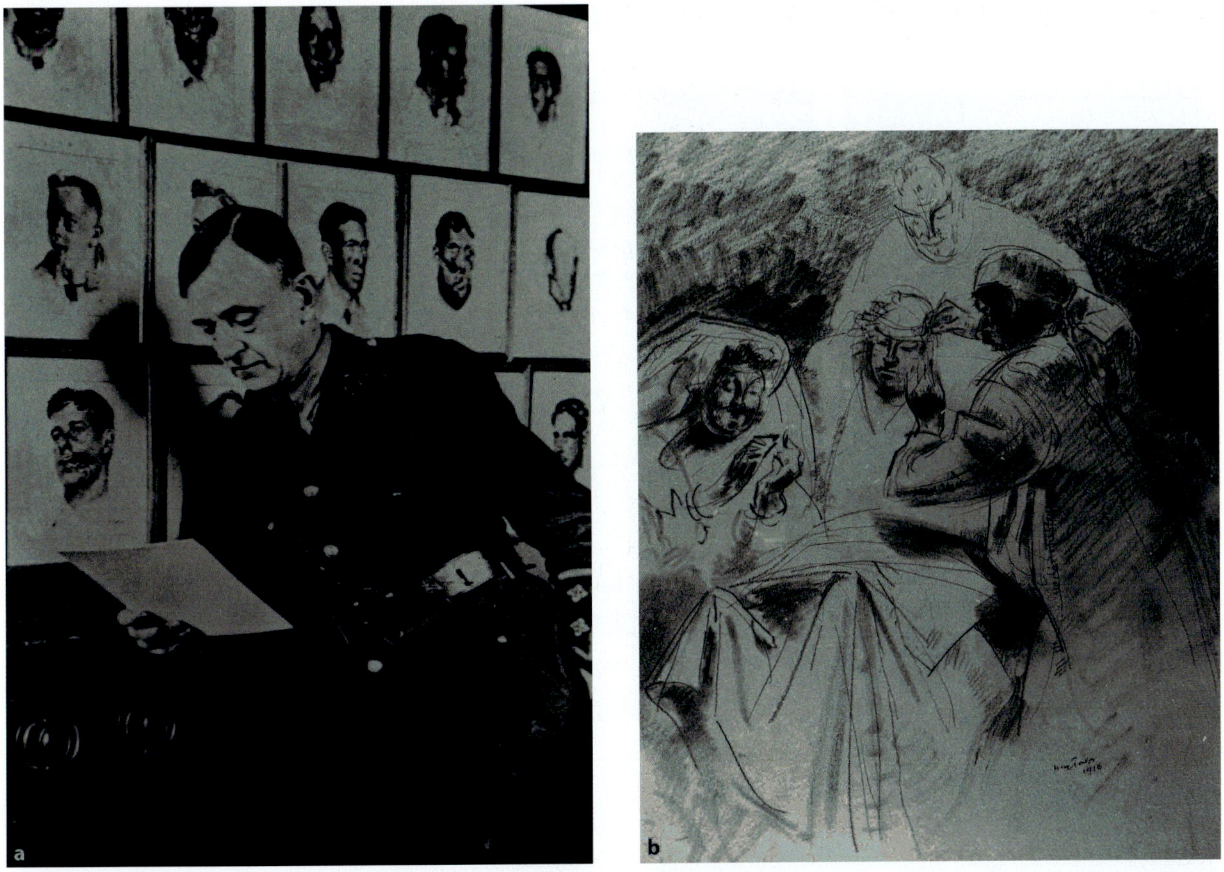

Fig. 3.24 **a** Photograph of Tonks in his room at Sidcup and **b** his drawing of surgeons in theatre. *By permission of The Royal College of Surgeons of England*

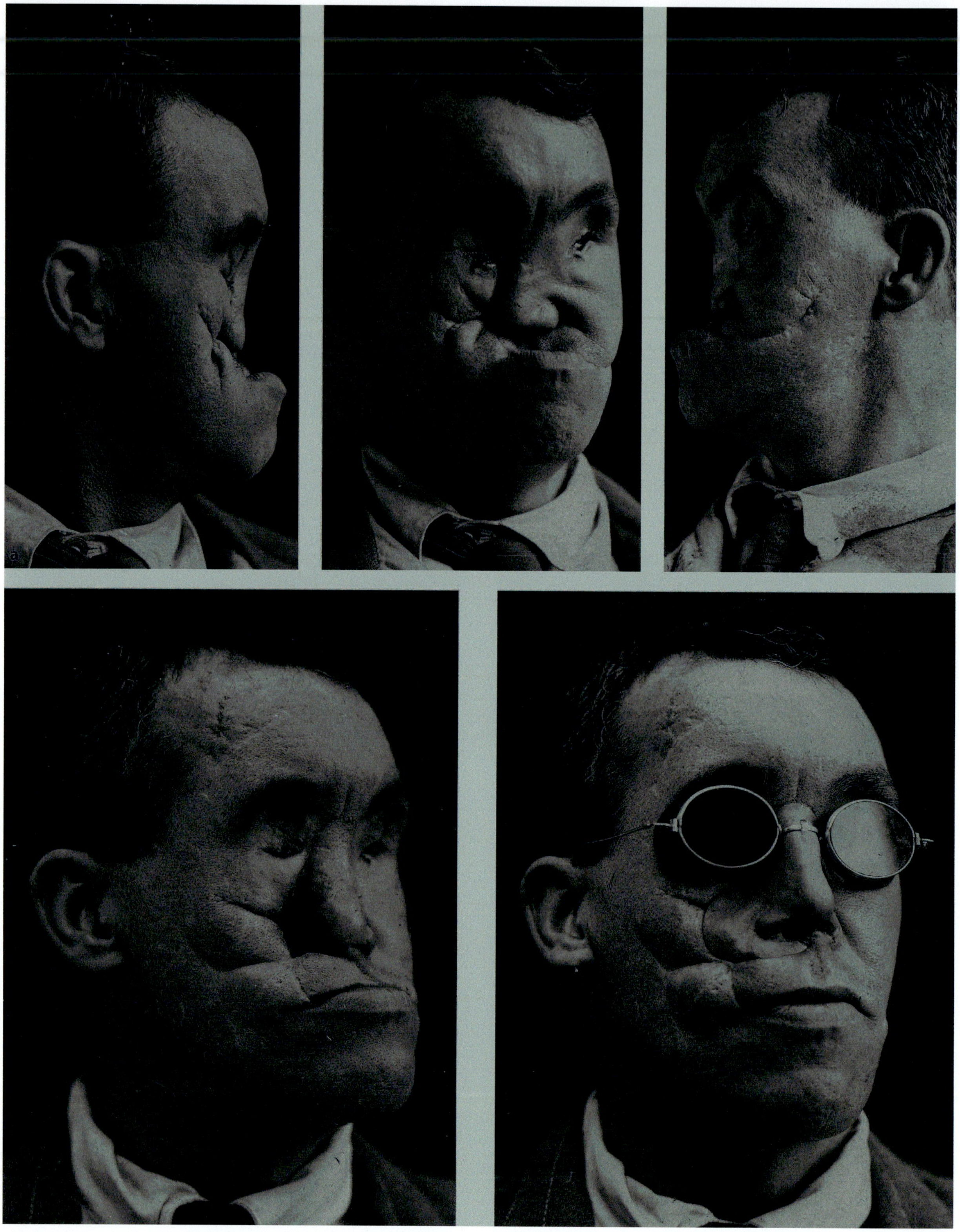

Fig. 3.25a–c Soldiers with severe facial wounds frequently required custom-made prostheses combined with surgery as part of their rehabilitation. This patient had numerous operations and an obturator, nasal prosthesis and spectacles to hide his missing eyes. *Reproduced by permission of the Gillies Archives, Queen Mary's Hospital, Sidcup, UK*

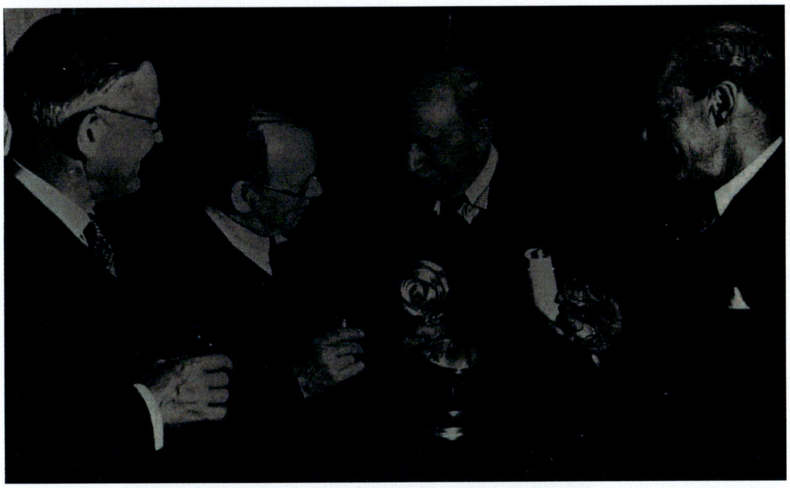

Fig. 3.26 The four great men of British Plastic Surgery: *left to right* McIndoe, Kilner, Gillies and Mowlem. *Courtesy of the British Association of Plastic Reconstructive and Aesthetic Surgeons*

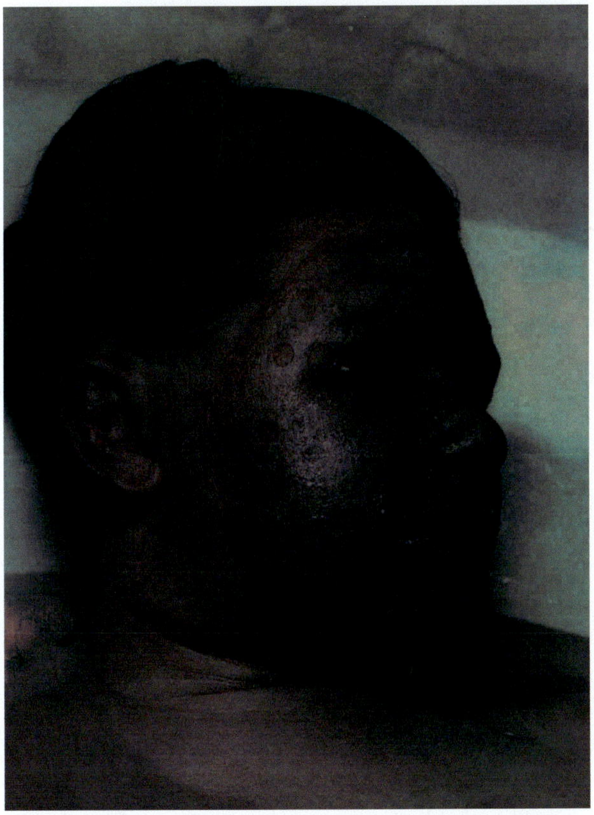

Fig. 3.27 Pilot with a facial burn typical of those treated during the Battle of Britain in World War II by McIndoe and his team at East Grinstead Hospital. They formed the "Guinea Pig Club" after the War. *Photograph by Percy Hennell from the Antony Wallace Archive, courtesy of the British Association of Plastic Reconstructive and Aesthetic Surgeons*

injured in the Battle of Britain at East Grinstead Hospital (Fig. 3.27).[17]

Fortunately most of the detailed records afrom Queen Mary's Hospital have been collected into the *Gillies Archive* and form a very valuable source for research.[18]

Among the many new innovations that came out of the necessities of war were the new techniques in plastic surgery and anaesthesia first pioneered at Sidcup. The tube pedicle practised by Gillies and his team is the one that is remembered today.

Like many cases before and since, controversy arose about the first *tube pedicle* to be performed. J.L. Aymard, a South African surgeon and member of Gillies team at Sidcup, successfully transferred a *tube pedicle flap* on 18 October 1917 to reconstruct a facial defect. He immediately published an account of his feat and claimed it to be the first [45]. This gave rise to an acrimonious dispute, but it was finally established that, although Aymard published his results first, Gillies had performed his operation two weeks before his rival who, the story goes, actually witnessed the second stage of this operation (Fig. 3.28).

While Aymard returned to South Africa to nurse his grievances, Gillies continued with his work and between the wars demonstrated that his new technique could be used with confidence in every part of the body. The vast experience from the war was applied in civilian practice. *Tubed flaps* became a standard method of reconstruction and were moved over distances. These procedures, with names such as the *jump flap* (moved via an intermediate carrier such as the wrist) and the *waltzed* or *caterpillar flap* (transferred end-over-end from the donor area to a distant recipient area), demanded a skilful hand and a thorough knowledge of the biology of flaps in order to minimize the loss of tissue at each stage many of which were performed under local anaesthetic.

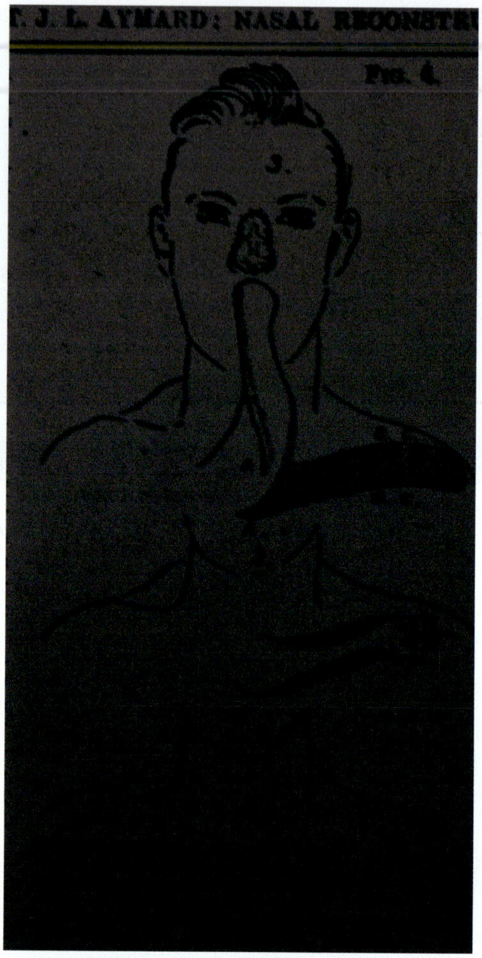

Fig. 3.28 Diagram of Aymard's tube pedicle from his article in the Lancet of 1917 which led to the controversy about who performed the first flap [45]

The Vascular Flap

Most of the flaps described above were based on a "random" and hence somewhat precarious blood supply, the only certain source being the capillary circulation in the subdermal plexus. It is probable that the flaps raised in some areas such as the face may have included an artery and a vein entering at the base, but when this occurred it was usually by chance and not by design, for the surgeon was still probably unaware of its importance. They learnt from experience that some flaps did better than others. This was possibly the case in the Indian rhinoplasty. Later

17 Percy Hennell who was advisor to the Royal Society and an eminent practitioner of his art was a war photographer in WW II and recorded patients in the four plastic surgery units round London. His rare technique of using three permanent dyes has ensured the longevity of his colour prints.

18 A short but comprehensive report on the activities of Queen Mary's Hospital Sidcup during the war and in following years was published in 1994 by Andrew Bamji, curator of the Gillies Archive at the hospital.

there were also claims that by tubing the flap the vascular network was encouraged to reorientate itself along the axis of the tube over the course of several weeks. But the specific network of vessels in the donor area was never studied before a flap was planned.

Pietro Sabattini (1810–1864) probably deserves the credit for the first flap that made specific provision for a recognized vascular supply (Fig. 3.29). In 1838 he reconstructed an upper lip defect using a full thickness flap from the lower lip that was vascularized by means of a narrow pedicle containing labial vessels [875]. The advantages of this flap in terms of mobility were obvious, and its potential applications must have been equally evident. Unfortunately, few surgeons learned of Sabattini's discovery, probably because it was published in Italian and hence was not read by the greater part of the scientific community (Fig. 3.30) [626].[19]

Nevertheless, the underlying principle slowly gained ground. In 1848 Sophus August Vilhelm Stein (1797–1868), without any knowledge of Sabattini's work, published an account in Danish in the local medical journal of the use of two triangular flaps raised from the upper lip and transposed to repair a central defect in his lower lip [952]. Due to their small size, the flaps were safer and the tension of the closed defect was distributed more evenly. The pedicle could be sectioned after three weeks. Stein also used single *vascular flaps*, but never published a paper on this method.[20] Unfortunately his technique failed to reach the attention of the international community for the same reasons that had prevented the spread of Sabattini's discovery [792, 793].

Thus, when the American surgeon Robert Abbe (1859–1928) published his report of the transposition of a vascular flap between the upper and lower lip, 60 years after Sabattini in a well-known medical journal in English, his name became forever linked with the procedure

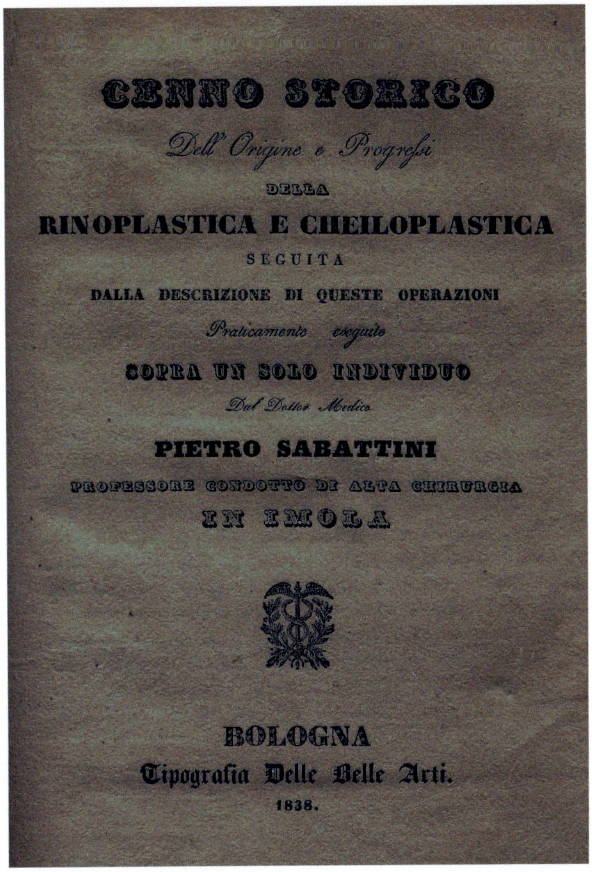
CENNO STORICO
Dell' Origine e Progressi
DELLA
RINOPLASTICA E CHEILOPLASTICA
SEGUITA
DALLA DESCRIZIONE DI QUESTE OPERAZIONI
Praticamente eseguite
SOPRA UN SOLO INDIVIDUO
Dal Dottor Medico
PIETRO SABATTINI
PROFESSORE CONDOTTO DI ALTA CHIRURGIA
IN IMOLA
BOLOGNA
Tipografia Delle Belle Arti.
1838.

Fig. 3.29 Frontispiece of Sabattini's book *Cenno Storico dell'Origine e Progressi dell Rinoplastica e Cheiloplastica* published in Bologna in 1838. *Courtesy of Riccardo Mazzola, M.D., Milan*

19 According to John B. McCraw [629], Pietro Sabbatini's flap may be the first myocutaneous, as well as the first vascular flap ever executed.

20 Sophus August Vilhelm Stein's biography is most interesting and serves to shed some light on the practice of surgery in Scandinavia a mere 150 years ago. Stein learned his trade from his father, who was a barber surgeon. At that time in Denmark, there still existed a clear distinction between the fields of medicine and surgery; medicine was taught at the University of Copenhagen while aspiring surgeons received instruction at the Academy of Surgery. The standard of teaching at the academy was so high that many medical students attended courses there to learn something of surgery. Stein's career followed an unusual course in that he first practiced for many years as an unskilled surgeon, before being accepted as a student at the university at the age of 34. However, like Tagliacozzi his outstanding gifts were soon recognized and in 1835 he received an appointment to teach anatomy. Ten years later Stein was appointed to the first chair of surgery at the University of Copenhagen without a medical degree.

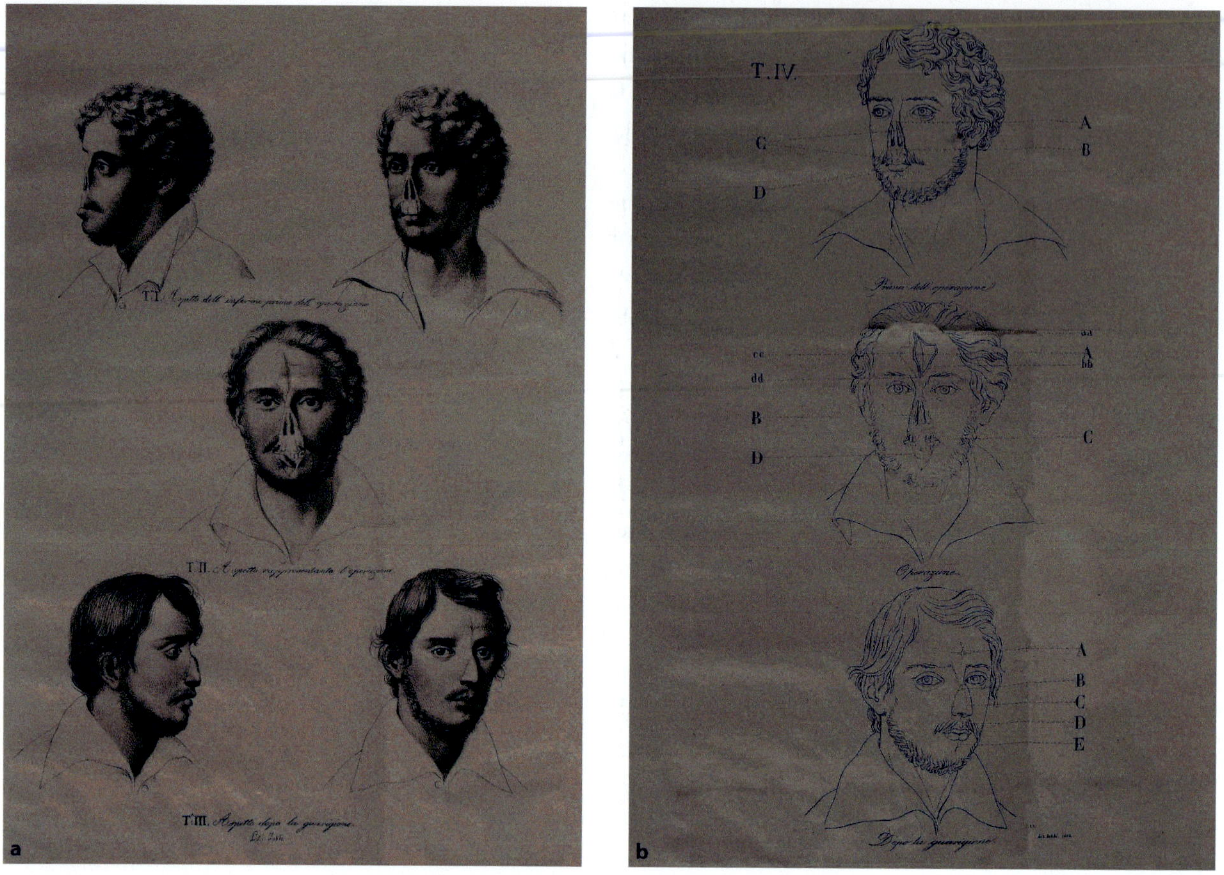

Fig. 3.30a,b Diagrams of Sabattini's first case in which he used a flap from the lower lip to reconstruct an upper lip defect with a forehead flap for the nose. This predated Abbe's flap by about 40 years. *Courtesy of Riccardo Mazzola, M.D., Milan*

despite the protests of many who asserted that the honour should go to Sabattini [2].[21] In Finland, Jacob August Estlander (1851–1881) conceived a method to reconstruct defects of the lip near the commissures that yielded excellent results [284, 285].[22] This approach, although often requiring a second operation to reconstruct the commissure and restore the size of the mouth, allowed the surgeon to avoid the awkward situation of a vascular pedicle crossing the mouth in a vulnerable position, and the necessity of a second operation to section this base. Estlander could have become a surgeon of great stature, but his career was cut short most tragically by his death at the age of 30.

Vascularized flaps based on anatomically identifiable vessels were subsequently used by other surgeons to design more secure flaps in different regions of the

21 See Martha T. Gnudi and Jerome Webster; Riccardo Mazzola and John T. Hueston; N.C. Petersen; and Paolo Santoni-Rugiu and Riccardo Mazzola.

22 Jacob August Estlander stated that he had never come across any reference in the literature to the use of vascular flaps for labial reconstructions and therefore could not have known about the discoveries by Sabbatini and Stein, both of which were published in the authors' native languages. The question as to whether Robert Abbe was aware of the work of Estlander is an entirely different matter, because the Finnish surgeon published his findings in German, a language that was certainly current in the scientific community, 26 years before Abbe used his vascular flap. Furthermore, in 1876 Estlander was invited by many American medical institutions to lecture on this subject in a well-publicized tour.

body. For example, in 1887 Robert Gersuny of Vienna (1844–1924) employed a submandibular flap to repair the mucosal defect in a cheek created by the excision of a tumour [365], and in 1893 the American Theodore Dunham closed a similar cheek defect with a forehead flap provided with a narrow pedicle that included branches of the superficial temporal vessels [263]. He waited three months before sectioning the pedicle and returning the bridging skin to the donor site in the forehead, which had been temporarily covered with a free skin graft. In 1898 George Howard Monks (1853–1933) devised a flap based on the same principle, but introduced a significant modification. He use it for the reconstruction of an entire eyelid following cancer surgery. To avoid the necessity of a second operation he created an island of forehead skin sustained by a subcutaneous vascular pedicle, which was then tunnelled across the temple [686]. The replacement of the lining of the oral cavity following excision of extensive oral cancer had always taxed reconstructive surgeons [274] and the temporal flap subsequently became the treatment of choice for many years [640]. It was simple to raise, reliable and provided ample tissue when turned into the mouth either above or beneath the zygomatic arch. Its bulk was a drawback which was eventually overcome with the advent of microvascular surgery and the "Chinese Flap" (see later). This heralded its fall from favour.

These were sporadic and isolated clinical cases, but concurrently the problem of the vascularization of specific areas of the skin was being studied in depth. In our chapter on anatomy we discussed the remarkable work of Carl Manchot (1866–1932) [606],[23] whose thesis on the cutaneous arteries and the regions they fed was published in German in 1889 in a limited number of copies that never circulated outside Strasbourg and therefore did not come to the attention of surgeons for many decades (Fig. 3.31).[24]

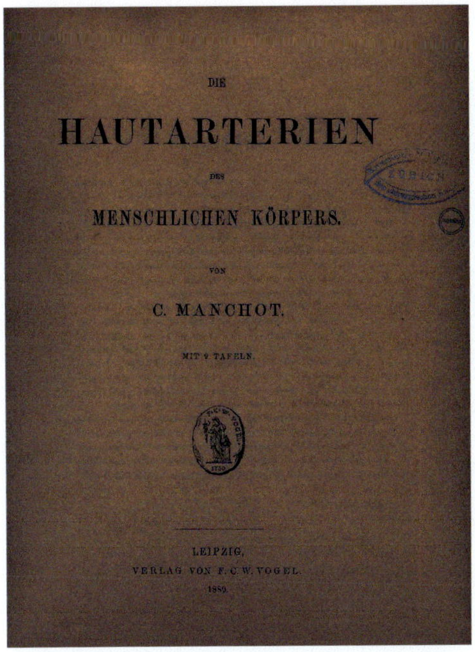
DIE

HAUTARTERIEN

DES

MENSCHLICHEN KÖRPERS.

VON

C. MANCHOT.

MIT 9 TAFELN.

LEIPZIG,

VERLAG VON F. C. W. VOGEL.

1889.

Fig. 3.31 Frontispiece of Manchot's book *Die Hautarterien des Menschlichen Körpers* published in 1889. *Courtesy of Riccardo Mazzola, M.D., Milan*

Almost half a century later in 1936, M. Salmon [882–884], without any knowledge of Manchot's work, studied the blood supply to the skin in fifteen cadavers by injecting their arteries with ink. Through careful dissection and x-ray studies he managed to chart many arterial areas, showing the density of their vascular input, the anastomotic links between them, and how adjacent territories were fed by these networks. The territories described by Salmon did not correspond exactly with those delineated by Manchot, but both contributed to define the vascular areas supplied by single vessels (Fig. 3.32a,b).

Unfortunately the clinical implications were completely ignored. For example, when Jacques Joseph [724] raised a large chest flap to reconstruct the defect left after the excision of a retracted scar in the neck of a burn patient, it included one of the charted territories but he was probably unaware of Manchot's work and Salmon's had not yet been published. Jerome P. Webster was probably also ignorant of Manchot's discoveries when he devised his thoraco-abdominal tubed pedicle flaps [1037]. We will never know whether their selection of these vascularized territories was deliberate or pure serendipity.

23 Carl Manchot was born in Switzerland to a poor family that would never have been able to send him to medical school. The ambitious young man therefore moved to Alsace, which had recently been annexed by Germany, in order to take advantage of the special conditions being offered by the German government to attract students to the University of Strasbourg.

24 See Chapter 1, p 48.

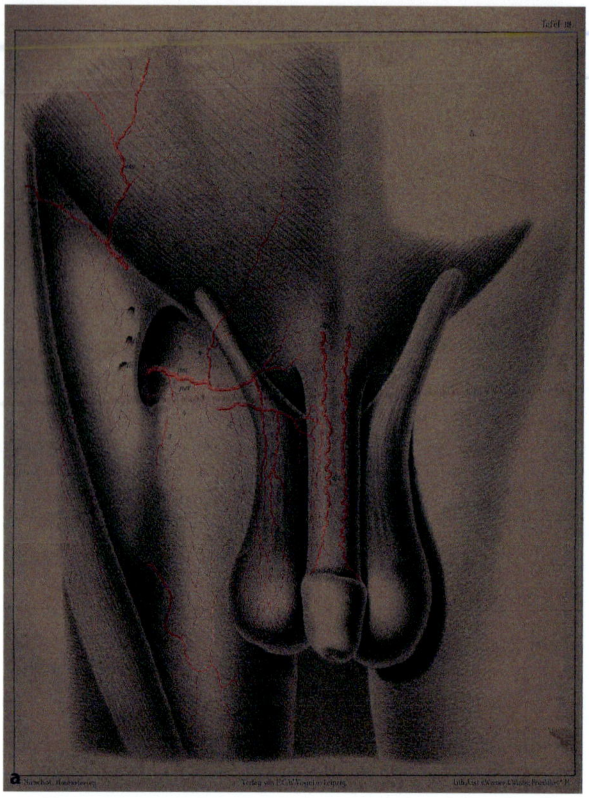

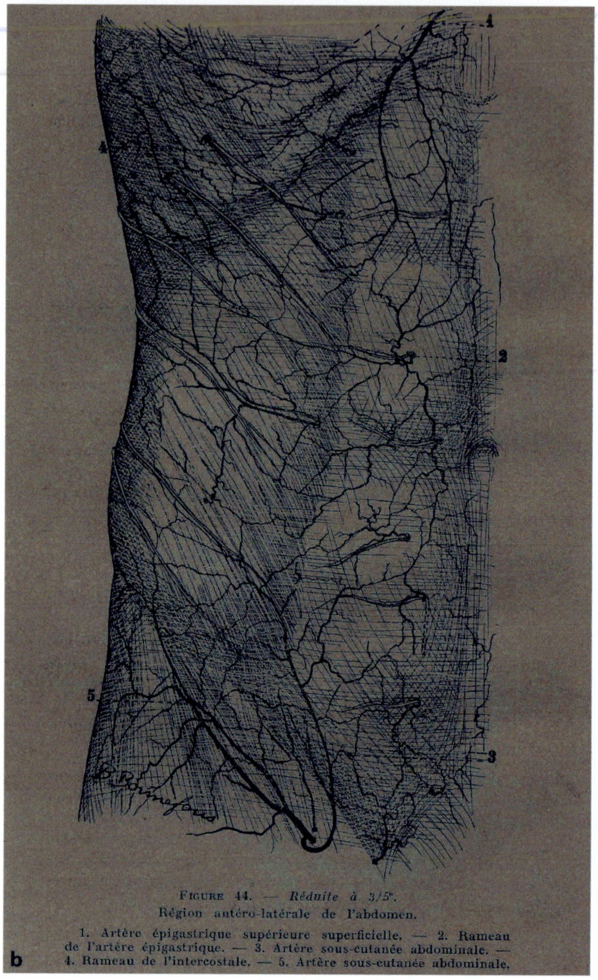

Fig. 3.32 Diagrams of the groin to compare the vascular territories outlined by **a** Manchot and **b** Salmon. *Courtesy of Riccardo Mazzola, M.D., Milan*

It was only in 1969 that Milton, while working on the blood supply of skin flaps in pigs, came across a copy of Manchot's thesis in Strasbourg and translated it, although he never succeeded in finding a publisher. His experiments on skin flaps in pigs were of vital importance and debunked several of the old maxims. One important conclusion was that the "length breadth" ratio was unsound if a cutaneous artery was included in the base of a flap [673–677]. The diffusion of the historic studies had to await the appearance of Jovanka and Ristic in 1983, [483] of Morain in 1985 [692] and for their translations of Manchot's *The Cutaneous Arteries of the Human Body*. Taylor and Palmer brought the subject up to date with their description of "angiosomes" in 1987 [975] and Taylor and Tempest produced a translation of Salmon's *Arteries of the Skin* with a commentary and additional experimental information in 1988.[25] We can only speculate on how different the evolution of plastic surgery might have been had the discoveries of Sabattini, Manchot and Salmon received the attention they deserved at the outset. Instead, their full consequences were only felt a century later when the blood supply to territories of the skin was re-examined and John McCraw and his collaborators looked deeper and systematically applied the concept of vascular territories to their work on musculocutaneous flaps [629, 630].

Even if surgeons remained unaware of these fundamental studies, the realization was spreading that the crucial factor determining the survival of a flap was not the *length-breadth ratio*, but whether the flap was suffi-

25 Michel Salmon (1988) *Arteries of the Skin*. Edited by GI Taylor and M Tempest, Churchill Livingstone.

ciently vascularized by vessels passing across the pedicle. The importance of this fact had already been noted by the work of surgeons such as Johannes F.S. Esser (1877–1946),[26] who in 1909 used a double pedicle flap raised from the scalp as a visor for staged mandibular reconstructions [282]. In 1946 this was modified into a single pedicle flap by V.H. Kazanjian, who observed that the vessels from a single pedicle were sufficient to feed the entire flap [487]. He based his conclusion on his experience with the Indian technique, which he used to elevate a frontal flap based solely on the supratrochleal vessels, passing it through a cutaneous tunnel to repair a nasal defect. We will meet Kazanjian later. On his return to America after the First World War he became well known for his important work on the treatment of facial injuries [488].

These flaps proved extremely versatile. The forehead flap was vascularized by the superficial temporal vessels. During World War I, Esser had already employed flaps that he referred to as "biological", because they were nourished through a thin pedicle that included vessels and possibly nerves, in facial reconstructions. He deserves credit for having demonstrated, long before the concept won general acceptance, that a flap could survive on the circulation of a narrow pedicle as long as it included blood vessels.[27] His wartime experience led him to devise many flaps, especially around the face [280, 281] and his contributions to plastic surgery are expertly covered in Haeseker's Doctoral Thesis of 1983 [404].

Once the importance of vascularization had been established, surgeons devised other flaps supplied by vessels crossing their base, which led to the resolution of some difficult reconstruction problems particularly in areas of the body with a limited cutaneous blood supply. One of the first was probably the *hypogastric flap* fed by the superficial inferior epigastric arteries, described by the English surgeon J.B. Wood in 1863 [1049]. He used this flap to cover a defect on the upper limb of a young female patient (Fig. 3.33). Although the vessels on this occasion seem to have been included by chance, Wood immediately grasped their importance. He went on to use his flap in other reconstructions, and eventually described several different cases, including some of bladder ectopia.

Despite its potential, the groin area would not be fully exploited for more than a century. In 1946 Shaw and Payne [921] revived the technique, using a *tubed flap* to cover the defect on the back of a hand, but a full appreciation of the technique had to await the work of Smith, Foley and McGregor, who provided a detailed anatomical description of axial pattern flaps in general and the groin flap in particular in 1972–1973 [941, 942]. Eventually the groin area became an important source of reliable flaps, especially following the development of microsurgery and the free flap.

We have already mentioned Aymard in 1917. His tubed flap was raised in the deltopectoral region. This area was re-explored 50 years later by Bakamjian [49] and became one of the cornerstones of head and neck reconstructions. Bakamjian demonstrated that the perforating vessels from the internal mammary artery in the second, third and fourth intercostal spaces supply an area of skin extending laterally across the chest as far as the deltopectoral groove, and that a flap elevated in this region receives an additional supply of blood from the thoraco-acromial artery (Fig. 3.8). Littlewood [571] further improved the flap by adding a skin paddle, although he emphasized it had to be delayed. Necrosis in this area was common since the axial blood supply only extended as far as the deltopectoral groove, and division of the thoraco-acromial artery could act as the "delay".

By now the frontal, deltopectoral and groin areas were accepted as reliable sources of flap tissue, even if their dimensions did not respect the time-honoured length-breadth ratio. Taylor et al. laid the groundwork for another important development in 1975 [974]. They demonstrated that the deep circumflex iliac artery supplied a portion of the iliac crest and the skin overlying it. In the age of microsurgical free flaps this provide a source of

26 Johannes F.S. Esser was born in Leiden in 1877. He began his medical studies in Holland and then transferred to Paris to study under the eminent surgeon Hippolyte Morestin. When the First World War broke out, Esser offered his services to both the French and British armies but was refused, and eventually signed on as a "civilian war surgeon" in the Austro-Hungarian army. According to Haeseker [404], between 1915 and 1921 Esser operated on more than 10,000 injured soldiers.

27 Esser's contributions to the development of modern plastic surgery include the introduction of the epithelial inlay for the oral cavity, the transplantation of a toe to the hand (an operation already carried out by Carl Nicoladoni) and the invention of a large number of flaps for various clinical situations.

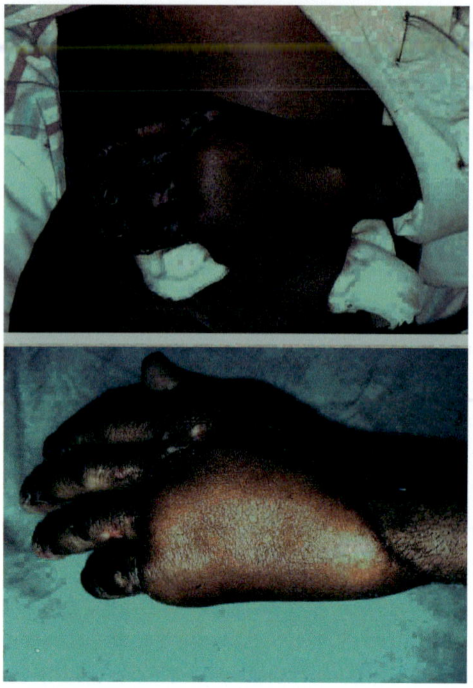

Fig. 3.33 Axial pattern hypogastric flap as described by Wood in 1863. *PJS*

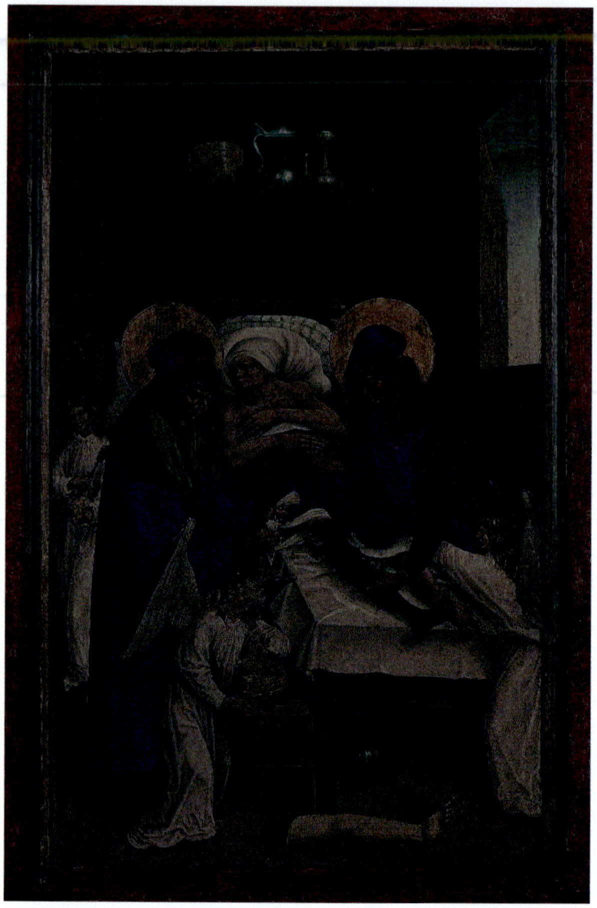

Fig. 3.34 The transplant of a leg from a black donor to a white recipient according to the legend of Saints Cosmas and Damian as represented in a painting from the *Schwäbische Malerei* of the *Schnaiter Alter* in Stuttgart dated from the second half of fifteenth century. *By permission of the Württenbergisches Landesmuseum, Stuttgart*

skin and bone for composite reconstruction of bone and skin defects. Free joint transfers had already been investigated experimentally by Buncke et al. in 1967 [141].

In our review of the history of flaps, we have used the name "axial" in various contexts. Credit for defining this term should be extended to McGregor and Morgan who clarified its use in several territories previously used in reconstructive surgery [641]. A limited number of *axial flaps* were known at the time, and their paper on axial and random blood supply explained why these were successful. The vessels that supported these flaps were predictable, supplied well-defined skin territories and were usually around 2–3 mm in diameter.

The Advent of Vascular Microsurgery and the Free Flap

The revived interest in axial flaps coincided with breakthroughs in microsurgery (Fig. 3.34). The use of magnification and fine sutures made it possible to repair very small vessels, and surgeons in America (Kleinert and Kasdan [500]) and Japan (Komatsu and Tamai [505]) demonstrated that amputated digits and hands could be successfully replanted using this technique (Figs. 3.35a,b, 3.36a,b).

It followed that one should be able to anastomose the vessels of axial flaps with those of the recipient region in the same way. This hypothesis received support when Cobbett [180] reported that he had carried out the first free digital transfer at Queen Victoria Hospital, East Grinstead in 1969, reconstructing a thumb by transfer-

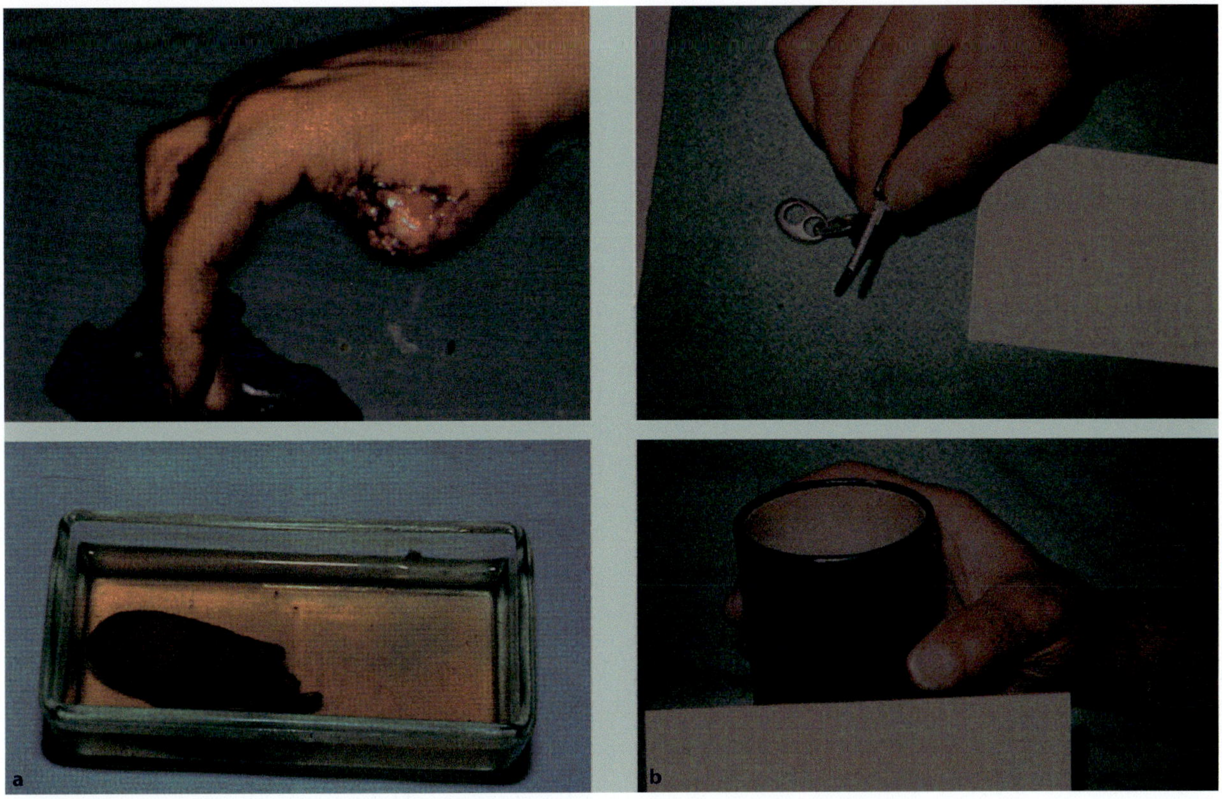

Fig. 3.35a,b A case of thumb re-implantation from 1975 with the result at eight months. *PSR*

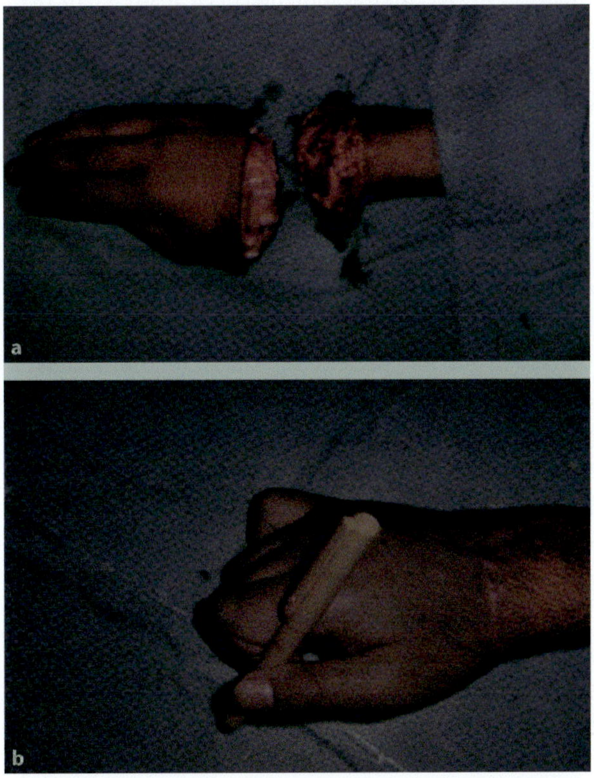

Fig. 3.36a,b A hand re-implant with the result at six months. *PSR*

ring the patient's big toe using microsurgical techniques. While this did not constitute a free skin flap in the strict sense of the term, the operation demonstrated that it was possible to transfer tissues from one site to another in a single operation. It also confirmed the validity of the principles underlying the new field of reconstructive microsurgery.

In this way the *free flap* was born. There is still disagreement concerning who actually coined the term and who carried out the first *free flap* procedure. Surgeons in many hospitals around the world had already experimented with *free flaps* in animals, but it is possible that the first successful operation in a human was performed to Harii, Ohmori and Ohmori [413]. They used a *free flap* taken from the scalp and vascularized by the superficial temporal vessels to resolve a problem of alopecia. The case was reported in 1974. However in the literature the case published in 1973 by Daniel and Taylor [212] describing a *free groin flap* transferred to the leg to repair a compound injury takes priority. The difference between operation and publication date is pedantic! These two reports were followed by a wave of papers by many authors describing similar successes. They included O'Brien et al. [745] and Ikuta et al. [460] (Fig. 3.37a–c).

Microsurgical free tissue transfers became a reality due to the ingenuity and skill of modern surgeons, but would not have been possible without the development of sophisticated operating microscopes, which first came into use in 1928 [742, 743], needles and sutures of remarkably slender calibre and specialized instruments and clamps which were initially "borrowed" from other specialists.[28] Around this time studies on nerve suture confirmed that the use of magnification and fine sutures were essential for a good result and microneural repairs became routine. The early pioneers such as Seddon and Sunderland set the scene for the likes of Millesi and Narakas in peripheral nerve surgery and improvements in facial palsy soon followed (Fig. 3.38) [26]. Free muscle transfer added to the success of what was formerly an unrewarding area (Fig. 3.39a–c).

In these early days of microsurgery the *groin flap* was used more frequently than the other known *axial pattern flaps*. It was difficult because of the short vascular pedicle and invariably gave a poor cosmetic result because of its thickness. It was evident that a greater choice of donor flaps was needed and this stimulated a closer look at the blood supply of the skin which had been started by Manchot and Salmon.

The vascularization of the skin has now been thoroughly studied and the ways by which it receives its blood supply have been reviewed and reclassified. An excellent presentation of the subject may be found in Cormack and Lamberty's *The Arterial Anatomy of Skin Flaps* published in 1994 [198]. They also classified skin flaps on the basis of anatomy rather than chronology.

Myocutaneous Flaps

Up until this time efforts had concentrated on defining the blood supply that came to the skin randomly or by specific named vessels in an axial pattern. Several workers began to look at a deeper layer and asked if the skin received a blood supply through the underlying muscles? In fact this question had been answered in 1896 by Iginio Tansini (1855–1943), whom we have already encountered in our chapter on anatomy (Fig. 3.40). He described a large flap elevated from the axillary region that he used to reconstruct chest wall defects after radical mastectomies [970]. Based on his experience with this procedure he suggested that in certain parts of the body, the cutaneous circulation derived from the underlying muscles. In his clinical case, he demonstrated that the circulation to a broad posterolateral area of the chest derived from the underlying latissimus dorsi muscle (Fig. 3.41a–c). Much later the *latissimus dorsi flap* would provide the key to reliable breast reconstruction.

Regrettably, his revolutionary work passed unnoticed and the few surgeons outside of Italy who heard of his work dismissed it out of hand. For example, Davis [225]

28 O'Brien, Henderson and Crock of Melbourne made an important contribution with their invention of the metalized microsuture (*Med J Aust* 1970, 17:17). This technique, which consists of making a very slender needle at the end of a nylon suture 19 microns in diameter by electrolysis, provided an ingenious solution to the difficult problem of designing a needle and thread fine enough to suture a vessel whose lumen was often less than 1 mm in diameter.

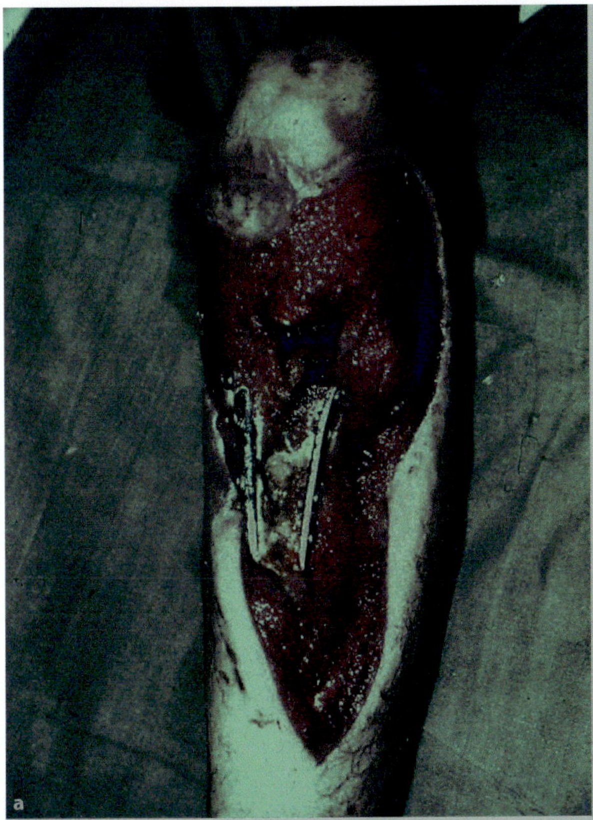

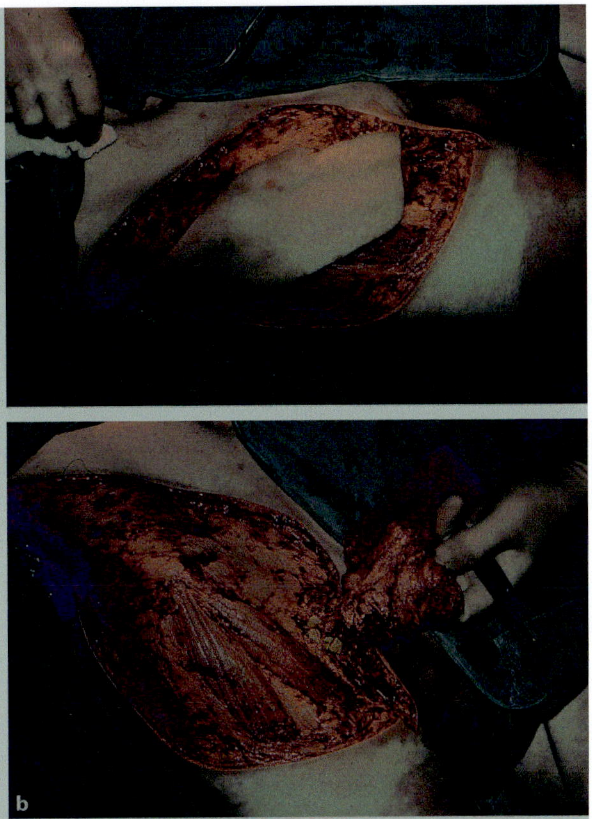

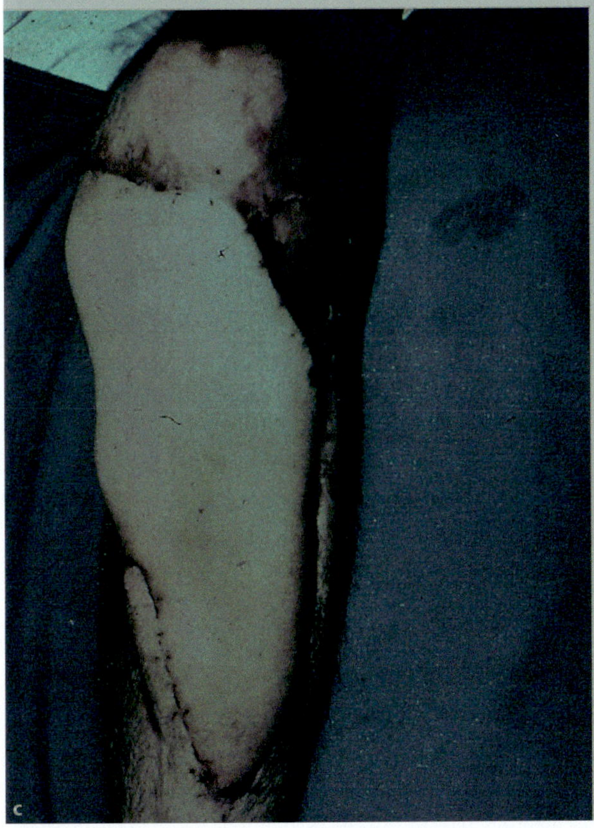

Fig. 3.37a–c A free groin flap from the early days in 1975. *PJS*

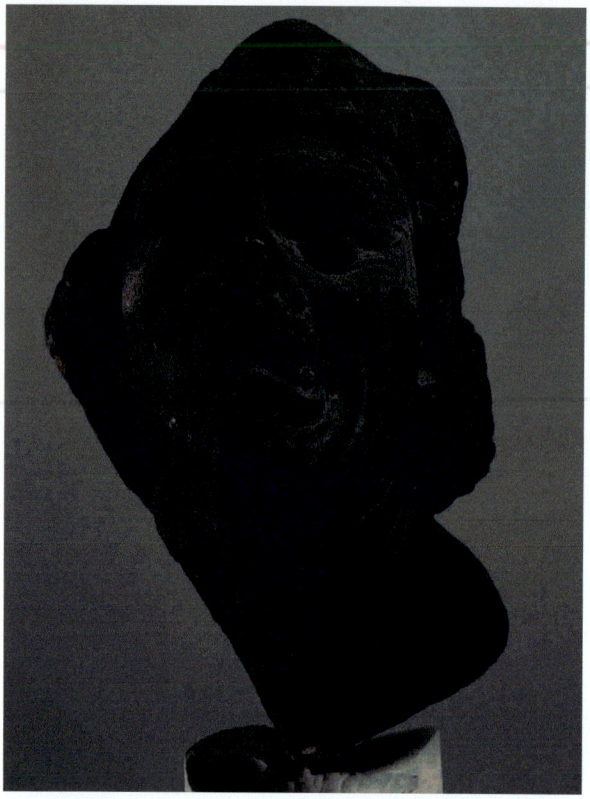

Fig. 3.38 A stone carving with facial palsy entitled *La face grimacant* by the school of Nicolas de Leyde (1460–1525) from the Museum de Notre Dame at Strasbourg. *By permission of the Musée de l'oeuvre Notre Dame de Strasbourg. Photo Musées de Strasbourg, A Plisson*

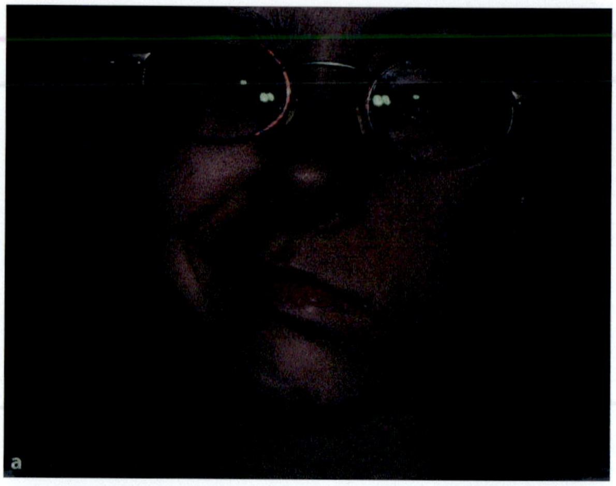

Fig. 3.39a–c A case of facial palsy treated by staged free microvascular latissimus dorsi muscle transplantation preceded by cross-facial nerve graft in a teenager. *Courtesy of Grazia Salimbeni Ughi, M.D., Pisa*

of the Johns Hopkins University in Baltimore wrote: "Unfortunately a glance at the diagram will show the impossibility of carrying out this method successfully … For these reasons, in many instances we must depend on skin grafts." McCraw [629] attributes this negative reception to "… the inefficient transfer of medical information, the rigid professional hierarchy of that day, and the relentless protagonism of one's personal method of surgical practice … Tansini did use a unique method to repair a massive anterior chest defect [which] escaped the surgical consciousness and the imagination of that time."

The rediscovery of the *myocutaneous flap* would have to wait another 50 years, but then progress was rapid. Apparently unaware of Tansini's work, Owens used a sternomastoid *myocutaneous flap* in 1955 to augment the circulation of the overlying skin [762]. Successively other muscles were studied and the pattern of their blood supply and the area of skin they supported were defined. *Muscle flaps*, i.e. flaps without skin that were subsequently covered with a free skin graft, were used in cases of compound fractures of the lower limb with good results as long as the defect was small and located in the upper two-thirds of the tibia.[29] Among the muscles studied, the gastrocnemius muscle was found to be extremely versatile, both alone and as a *myocutaneous flap*.

During the decade from 1968 to 1978 the *myocutaneous flap* continued to evolve, and at this juncture the school of surgery in Atlanta, Georgia made a particularly significant contribution. McCraw et al. [631] conducted a series of injection studies on the vascularization of various muscles and their overlying skin and in a remarkably short period of time developed a whole range of *myocutaneous flaps* that were put into practice, often

29 The Finnish surgeon Maximus Videkin of Schulten [907] deserves mention here; in 1897 he used muscle tissue to fill an osteomyelitic cavity.

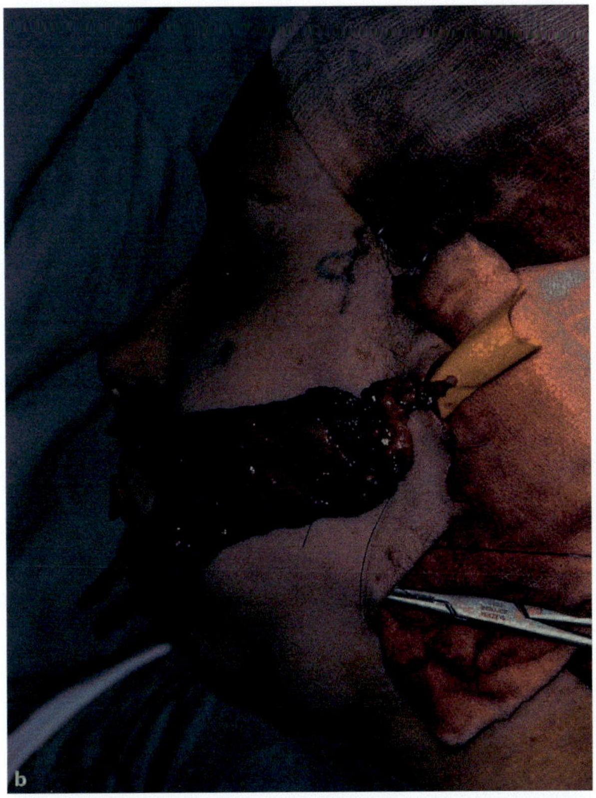

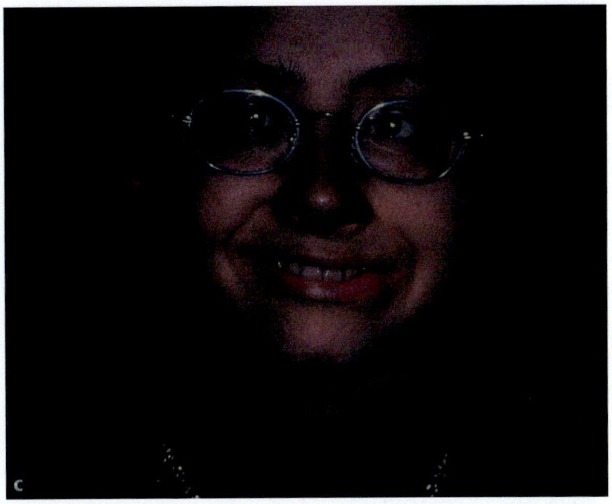

Fig. 3.39a–c *(continued)* A case of facial palsy treated by staged free microvascular latissimus dorsi muscle transplantation preceded by cross-facial nerve graft in a teenager. There is a pleasing result nine months after the second stage and microneural repair. *Courtesy of Grazia Salimbeni Ughi, M.D., Pisa*

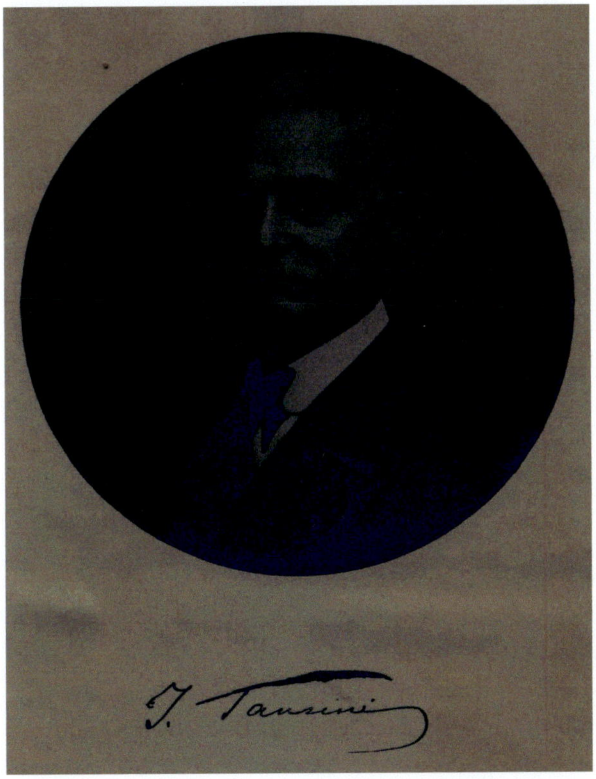

Fig. 3.40 Portrait of Iginio Tansini. In 1896 he used the first myocutaneous flap to repair a large skin defect resulting from a mastectomy. *Courtesy of Riccardo Mazzola, M.D., Milan*

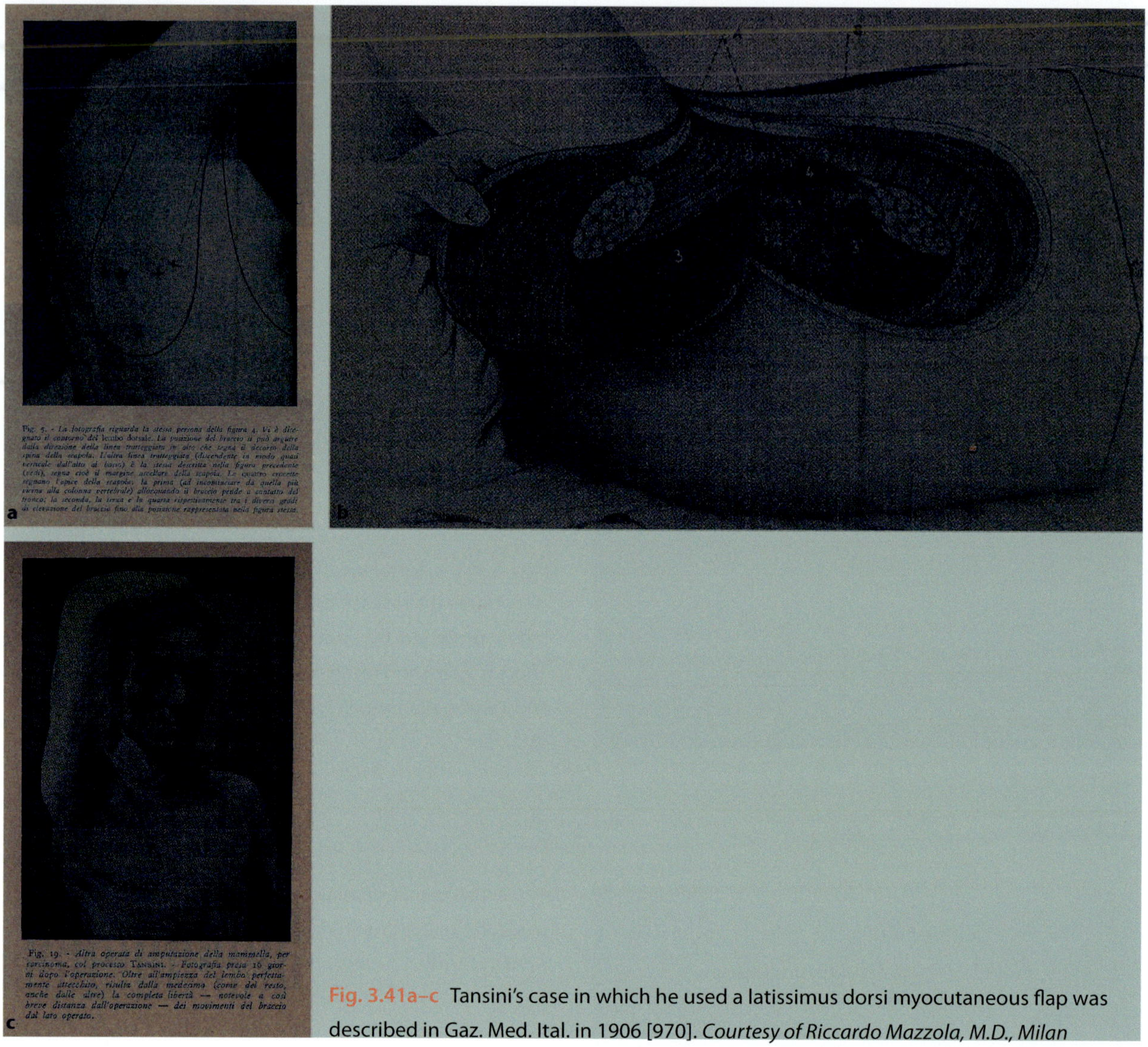

Fig. 3.41a–c Tansini's case in which he used a latissimus dorsi myocutaneous flap was described in Gaz. Med. Ital. in 1906 [970]. *Courtesy of Riccardo Mazzola, M.D., Milan*

with spectacular results. Muscles defined according to their different types of vascular pedicles were shown to support the skin overlying them (Fig. 3.42a,b).[30]

The invention of the muscle flap and the *myocutaneous flap* added new and highly versatile options as they could also be used as free flaps. This added to the very limited number of axial flaps then available to the plastic surgeon. The *latissimus dorsi flap* and the *rectus abdominis flap* became widely used for breast reconstructions.

The development of free muscle transfer with microneural repair also made it possible to treat such difficult problems as facial palsy which we have already mentioned. Microlymphatic repairs for cases of lymphoe-

30 One of these patients was a 62-year-old woman who underwent an operation for the reconstruction of her vagina by means of two myocutaneous flaps drawn from the femoral biceps muscle. In another case where the gracilis muscles were used, the sensitivity of the posterior cutaneous nerve of the thigh was preserved, and ten months after the vaginoectomy the patient was able to resume normal sexual activity. This and other triumphs were reported by McCraw, Massy and Shangling [632] and in another paper by Dibbell [238].

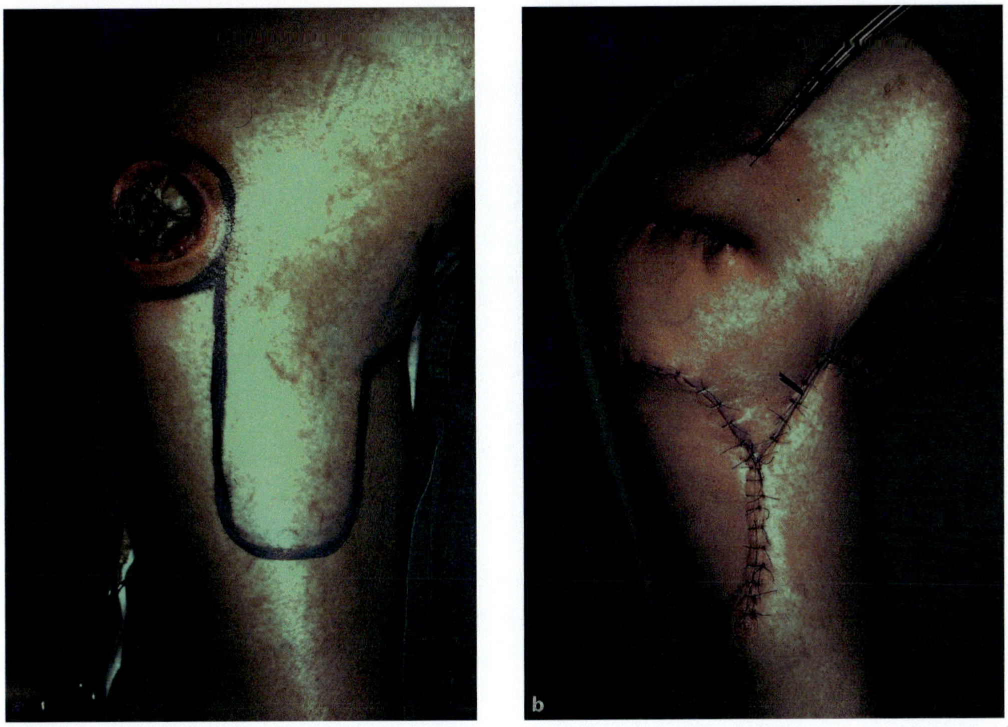

Fig. 3.42a,b Myocutaneous tensor fascia lata flap used to cover a bed sore. *PJS*

dema also had a brief period of popularity but proved unsuccessful [744].[31]

There are many situations, however, where muscle flaps transferred on a pedicle or by microvascular anastomosis are too thick. In 1978 Song et al. [947] and Yang et al. [1054] described the radial artery *forearm flap*, now known as the *Chinese flap*, which has proved useful both as a reverse pedicle flap on the hand and as a free flap for intra-oral reconstructions. This *fasciocutaneous flap* gave an extra impetus to flap design.

Further Developments: Fasciocutaneous Flaps, Skin Expansion

As surgeons learned more about the cutaneous blood supply, other flaps were developed. The discovery that the cutaneous tissue vascularized by the radial artery is fed by perforating vessels passing to the skin along the intramuscular fascial septum, and analogous findings in other regions, led to the creation of a new class of flaps called *fasciocutaneous flaps*. Such a flap on the lower leg had already been described by Bengt Pontén in 1981 [812]. These flaps were subsequently reclassified by Cormack and Lamberty (Fig. 3.43a–c).

All of the experimental and clinical data from the last three decades of the twentieth century demonstrate that, far from being based on a random blood supply, the skin receives blood through specific modalities which, once identified and studied, can lead to a successful outcome in a wide range of flap procedures.

We cannot close this chapter without mentioning briefly, the introduction of the technique of skin expansion. One hundred years ago, in 1905 Alessandro Codivilla (1861–1912) noted that limb lengthening operations

31 Gilbert, O'Brien, Vorrath and Sykes described the experimental technique in 1976 and in 1977 O'Brien, Sykes, Threlfall and Browning published clinical work but the method did not have lasting benefit in lymphoedema patients. *Br J Plast Surg* 29:355; *Plast Reconstr Surg* 60:197.

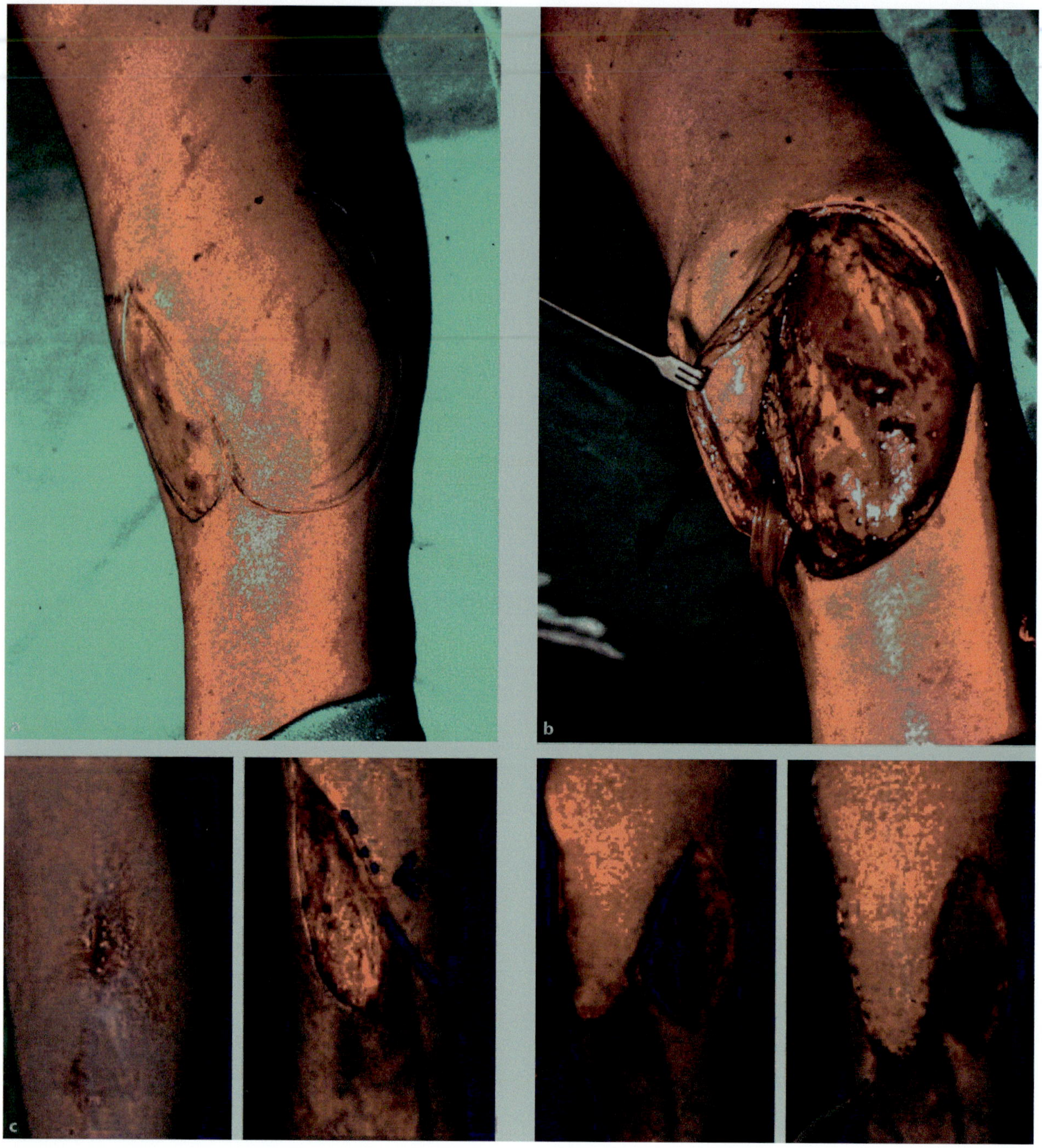

Fig. 3.43a–c Fasciocutaneous flap used for a traumatic defect in the leg. *PSR*

were accompanied by an extension of the skin and other soft tissues, which adapted themselves painlessly to the new length [184]. Although this observation was in a sense redundant, the elasticity of the skin in pregnant women being a natural phenomenon, the first to draw the logical inference and attempt to exploit this elastic capacity was Neumann in 1957 [730]. He implanted a rubber balloon under the skin of a patient in the post-auricular area and expanded it until there was enough skin to carry out a reconstruction of the ear.

Twenty-five years later Radovan [822, 823] and Austad [39] took up where Neumann had left off, each proposing a different method to stretch the skin. Radovan invented an expander made of silicone rubber that could be inflated in stages through a valve implanted under the skin, while Austad developed a self-expanding device. Radovan's method won general acceptance and since then skin expansion has become a routine procedure in breast reconstructions, to treat alopecia and in a whole range of face reconstructions. Many of the possible applications of skin expansion are described in a useful handbook by Sasaki [899].

As we have seen the development of skin flaps was slow and hesitant in the early years but in recent times it has gained such momentum that it has been hard to keep abreast of new developments. Each time one opens a journal there is frequently another new flap which provides a better solution to a difficult clinical problem. Some of these flaps have not stood the test of time but many have and we are perhaps entering a new period of consolidation awaiting the next important discovery.

Chapter 4

Skin Grafts

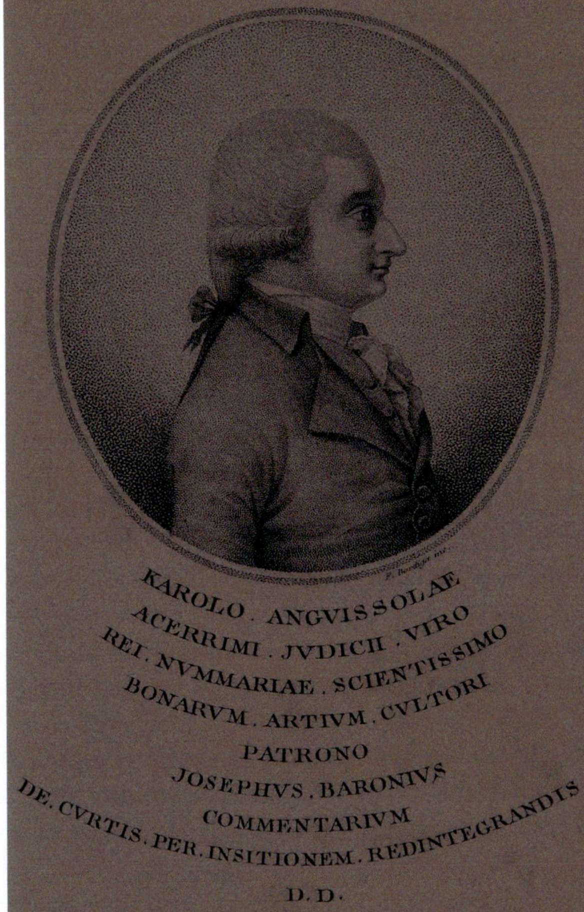

Contents

Compared to the flap the skin graft is a more recent invention. Why this should be is open to speculation. Perhaps surgeons were reluctant to remove skin totally from the body and its blood supply because of the difficulties they encountered with flaps [419]. More likely it was because they knew very little about the survival of tissue separated from the body and assumed that once removed it was dead [176]. At least some of the earliest attempts at grafting came about when amputated parts were replaced. These almost certainly met with failure and discouraged the use of purposeful free grafting [370].

The fourteenth century surgeon Guido Lanfranchi of Milan recounts in *Cyrurgia Parva* the story of a man who "came to me with his nose in his hand," and how he succeeded in re-implanting the amputated organ [520]. It is likely that this particular case involved only a portion of the nose which, when replaced, survived like any other free compound graft. A similar exploit was described by Leonardo Fioravanti who replanted the tip of a Spanish soldier's nose in 1570 [316].[1] These were isolated cases in which the surgeon was improvising on the spot in response to a medical emergency.

It was not until the seventeenth century that surgeons began to study the effects of removing and replacing pieces of skin in a systematic fashion. Since this was completely unexplored territory their first trials were conducted on animals. According to Thomas Birch [104], the earliest recorded attempt was undertaken by Walter Charleton (1620–1707),[2] in 1663. He removed a piece of skin from a dog and sutured it back into place. The fragment did not survive however and although the author had every intention of repeating his experiment, as he told the Royal Society, he was prevented from doing so when the dog escaped! The weekly report of the meeting of the *Royal Society* on 25 May 1664 says "The dog … foiled the Society by running away and, as far as can be determined, no further skin grafting was undertaken." Birch observes that in the same year another scientist (and later Fellow of the *Royal Society*), Robert Hooke, conducted a similar experiment, but due to various problems it failed and the results were never recorded [779]. We may observe that these sporadic attempts, whose exact scope was somewhat vague, very probably did not meet what we know today to be the indispensable requirements for a successful free graft.

Of quite a different calibre were the meticulous experiments on animals carried out over a period of 20 years by Giuseppe Baronio (1758–1814) (Fig. 4.1). He was probably inspired by John Hunter (1728–1793) [456][3] and Henry Louis Duhamel de Monceau (1700–1781) [261], whose works are cited in his book *Degli Innesti Animali* (*On Animal Grafts*) [54, 386], which was printed in Milan in 1804.[4] Baronio began his research on skin grafts in 1785, as he notes in a short work published in that year and dedicated to the Austrian nobleman Count Wilzeck. He pursued his studies with rigorous scientific method in a series of different animals and carefully recorded his findings.

Seeking to determine "whether grafting … would take place in larger animals", one of Baronio's earliest experiments was conducted on a ram (Fig. 4.2). He harvested two grafts about 9 cm long and 6 cm wide, one from either side of the animal's back, and used the graft from the left side to cover the defect on the right side and vice versa. Discovering that the margins of the graft tended to retract, he used adhesive tapes to fix them to the edges of the donor site, and carefully monitored the processes of healing and scar formation. As he triumphantly wrote: "Eight

1 The exploits of both Lanfranchi and Fioravanti will be described in detail in Chapter 6 which is devoted to nasal reconstructions.

2 Walter Charleton was an eclectic figure with numerous scientific interests, as is reflected in his monumental work *Natural History of Nutrition, Life and Voluntary Motion*, published in London by Henry Herringman in 1659. It is curious to note that the *Zeiss Index* cites the famous story of the escaping dog in its entry on Robert Hooke and not Walter Charleton (*The Zeiss Index. 900 B.C. to 1863 A.D.*, p 57, no. 245). Hooke was the curator of the Royal Society and although undoubtedly a great scientist his secretarial skills were limited. The records for this period were lost until 2006 when they were rediscovered in an attic in Dorset. Perhaps the controversy may now be solved.

3 Hunter's first book was on *The Natural History of Human Teeth* (1803). In it he describes inserting a tooth into a cock's comb. When he removed it sometime later he found that blood vessels had grown in from the surrounding tissue.

4 Giuseppe Baronio's book *Degli Innesti Animali* was translated into English and edited by Robert M. Goldwyn in 1985.

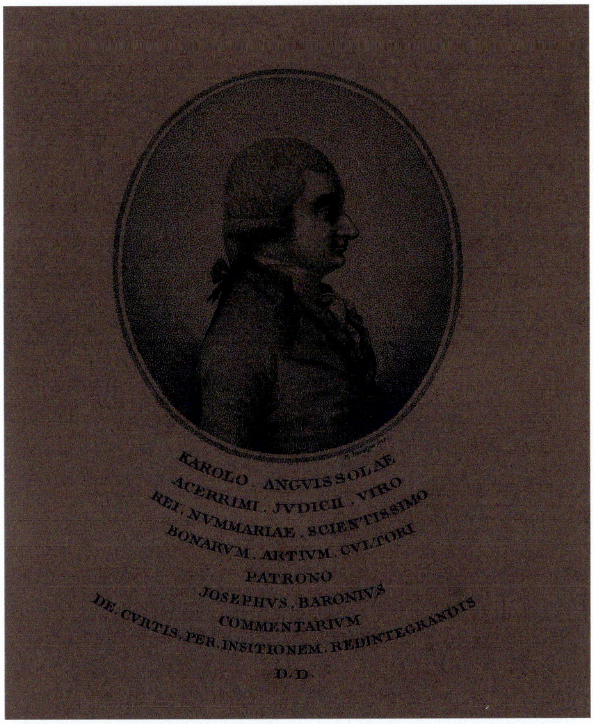
KAROLO . ANGVISSOLAE
ACERRIMI . JVDICII . VIRO
REI . NVMMARIAE . SCIENTISSIMO
BONARVM . ARTIVM . CVLTORI
PATRONO
JOSEPHVS . BARONIVS
COMMENTARIVM
DE . CVRTIS . PER . INSITIONEM . REDINTEGRANDIS
D.D.

Fig. 4.1 Portrait of Giuseppe Baronio (1758–1814). He was the first to carry out carefully planned experiments which showed that skin grafts were feasible. *Courtesy of Riccardo Mazzola, M.D., Milan*

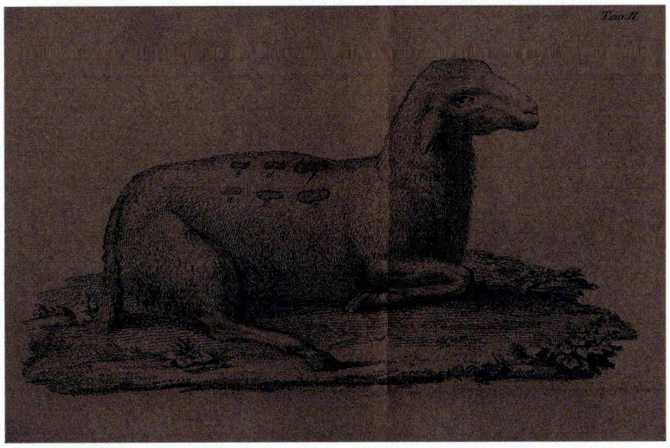

Fig. 4.2 Grafts on the back of a ram from Baronio's book. He did experiments on both autografts and homografts and the results were reported to the local scientific community in Pavia in the late eighteenth century. *Courtesy of Riccardo Mazzola, M.D., Milan*

days after the operation, when the grafts were uncovered, they were found to have healed over perfectly without the slightest suppuration. … eleven days in all after grafting, we made a cutaneous incision in the centre of the transplanted piece and were delighted to see blood issue forth, unequivocal proof of restored circulation." He followed the same procedure in a second experiment, this time waiting 18 minutes before re-implanting the crossed grafts. In this case a small amount of suppuration developed, but overall the grafts took as well as those in the first experiment and "blood issued forth and the circulation of blood had been restored even in these very areas of suppuration". We know now that a delay of 18 minutes will not compromise the vitality of skin graft tissue, even under less than ideal operating conditions. The suppuration reported by Baronio can probably be attributed to simple contamination, as animal experiments in his day were conducted in a non-sterile environment.

Baronio carried out trials on a total of 27 animals (rams, goats, dogs, and even a mare and a cow), always with the same positive results. These studies were of immense significance, serving first and foremost to demonstrate that grafts could be transferred and survive, a fact that up to then had not been scientifically proven. Indeed, this possibility was dismissed by leading surgeons including Alfred Armand Velpeau [1010, 1011] who, despite the fact that he himself had successfully re-implanted the skin torn away from a patient's finger, asserted that "this strange operation will never be practiced." Furthermore, by comparing the results of grafts carried out under different conditions and at different time intervals, Baronio succeeded in clarifying many of the biological aspects of the grafting and healing processes. The science of immunology still lay far in the future and with no knowledge of the rejection reaction, Baronio nevertheless noted that tissue transferred in the form of homografts, i.e. transplanted to another animal of the same species, regularly failed to survive.[5]

In a work that is otherwise a model of scientific objectivity, Baronio includes some curious digressions and observations. In Section V of *Degli Innesti Animali* he recounts a story that provides him with the occasion for "… some reflections on the method of healing wounds and of skin grafting as practiced by charlatans." Elsewhere he makes a few perplexing declarations, for example debridement of a wound tends to slow the healing process.

Baronio's book was the first in Europe after that of Tagliacozzi to deal with reconstructive surgery and represents a milestone in the history of medicine (Fig. 4.3). In his discussion of the biology of grafts, he refers to a "vital principle" that could unite two injured parts through the mediation of the "extra-vasated blood and coagulable lymph thrown out by the adhesive inflammation." Baronio believed firmly in the existence of an "organized vital substance" composed of blood entrapped by lymph (perhaps fibrin) that was instrumental in keeping the margins of a graft attached to those of the defect and furthermore stated that "a slight amount of inflammation" was conducive to healing. Unfortunately, the impact of his work, which was published in Italian in 1804 and translated into German in 1819, was limited. Reports of the skin flap operation used in India for nose reconstructions had just reached Europe, monopolizing the attention of surgeons and completely overshadowing the potential of the skin graft. Not only did they fail to integrate the technique into surgical practice, most surgeons never came to hear of it.

Among the medical achievements of Indian surgeons being discussed in Europe was a case involving a genuine graft rather than a flap. In 1817 Henry M. Dutrochet (1776–1847) [268] described an operation that his brother-in-law had witnessed in India: "A soldier in India, having had his nose cut off as a punishment, took himself to the Indians known for their operation to restore noses. They freshened the margins and chose an area of the buttock, which they beat vigorously with a slipper until there was considerable swelling. From this they cut a triangular piece of skin and subcutaneous tissue, which they placed on the nose and fixed with adhesive plaster." To the amazement of those Europeans present, this graft survived and its success was attributed to the preparation of the donor region by beating. As Henk J. Klasen [498] informs us, this unusual episode was cited by Leroux in the same year when he spoke before the *Societé d'Emulation de Paris*.

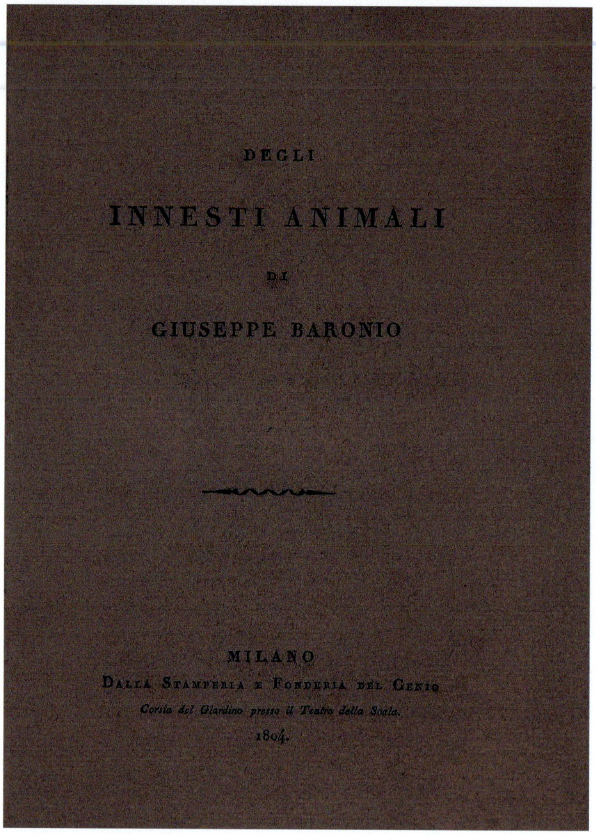
DEGLI

INNESTI ANIMALI

DI

GIUSEPPE BARONIO

MILANO

Dalla Stamperia e Fonderia del Genio

Corsia del Giardino presso il Teatro della Scala.

1804.

Fig. 4.3 Frontispiece of Baronio's book *Degli Innesti Animali* published in 1804. *Courtesy of Riccardo Mazzola, M.D., Milan*

The First Clinical Experiments

After these reports, the first attempts to graft skin in patients using the Indian method of beating were soon to follow in Europe. In 1823 Christian Heinrich Bünger

5 Baronio also observed that the defect left by the harvesting of the graft was larger in size than the graft itself. This phenomenon would later be described by Guillaume Dupuytren, although the explanation would have to await K. Langer, who in 1861 published his studies on the elasticity of skin and its lines of tension.

(1782–1842) of Marburg, reported the case of the repair of a nasal defect in a 33-year-old woman [142]. After beating the patient's thigh vigorously with a leather belt until it was red and swollen, a large piece of skin and subcutaneous adipose tissue was excised. This graft was trimmed and sutured to the defect, and on the third day, as Bünger wrote: "We doctors looked at each other in silence and we could not believe our eyes when we saw that the graft, which the day before had been chalk-white and had been deprived of the vital forces from the remainder of the body for at least 90 minutes, now had become a nose which for the most part had a pure scarlet colour and looked glossy and swollen." He continued: "[This] was a good demonstration that a fully separated skin graft that had been detached from the body itself for more than half an hour still maintained all the vital requirements necessary for its attachment to the parent." Legends about grafting were already commonplace but this is probably the first true case.[6, 7]

The unusual step of beating the donor region (which was also termed "flagellation") attracted the attention of Carl Thiersch (1822–1895), who would later develop the thin graft that bears his name [982]. In 1874 he wrote that this practice induced a beneficial inflammatory reaction: "Soft pounding causes the beginning of inflammatory self-proliferation … In the Indian rhinoplasty the surface of the stump was fresh and the piece of skin to be transplanted was prepared, while in our skin transplantation routine the opposite happens: the transplant is fresh and the base is inflammatorily prepared." As a result of these positive reports, flagellation of the skin became a common practice referred to as the ancient Indian method of skin grafting. In more recent times Gibson from Glasgow has investigated the effects of flagellation on grafts [368].

Another successful skin graft was reported by Sir Astley Cooper (1768–1841): "I amputated a thumb for a patient in Guy's Hospital and, finding that I had not preserved a sufficient quantity of skin to cover the stump, I cut out a piece from the thumb which I had removed, and applied it upon the stump, confining it by strips and adhesive plaster." He noted that after a few days the piece of skin "was firmly united and organized" [196, 197].

Despite these anecdotal reports of the successful grafting of skin, some of them by illustrious surgeons, the procedure was still not widely accepted at the beginning of the nineteenth century. The principles governing whether or not a graft would "take", i.e. attach itself to the recipient bed, remained for the most part a mystery. The guidelines that had been deduced on the basis of empirical observation were only half understood. In general, skin grafting was viewed as a difficult and unreliable procedure.

Even the renowned surgeon Johan Friedrich Dieffenbach (1794–1847) was forced to admit that his attempt to transplant skin from one arm to another in a neurological patient ended in total failure. The graft, which was fixed with an adhesive bandage, had undergone complete necrosis within one week. Aware that other colleagues had succeeded in this operation, he wrote: "It would be an interesting and well deserving work to unite in a small treatise on the transplantation of animal parts, all the observations disseminated in essays on physiology and surgery. We may still hope that at length, correct and repeated observations would probably enable us to penetrate this grand mystery of nature to understand the process, and thus to understand the boundaries, of this biological art." His reflections could not have been more apt; it was clear that grafts sometimes worked, but the pressing problem was to understand exactly why they so often failed (Fig. 4.4) [239, 244, 246].

Reports of experiments with skin grafts were also arriving from the United States. The first attempt was probably made by Jonathan Mason Warren (1811–1867), and involved a patient whose case has already been discussed in the chapter on flaps. A portion of the flap that War-

6 This story, if true, could be considered the first successful autograft carried out in Europe. As Baronio recounts, a charlatan vaunting what he claimed to be a balm with miraculous healing properties before a sceptical crowd, cut a piece of skin from his arm, replaced it in the same site and spread his ointment over it. The wound healed completely even though it was probably a compound graft containing adipose tissue as well as skin. This episode apparently inspired Baronio to take up the study of grafts.

7 A similar episode was recounted by Dionisio Andrea Sancassiani [886] in 1731. A female charlatan by the name of Gambacorta who made a living selling ointments in the squares of Florence cut a piece of skin from her leg and placed it on a plate which "she passed around so that the crowd of onlookers and the city authorities could witness" the truth of her claim. After replacing the skin and spreading her cream over it, the wound apparently healed "without leaving a trace".

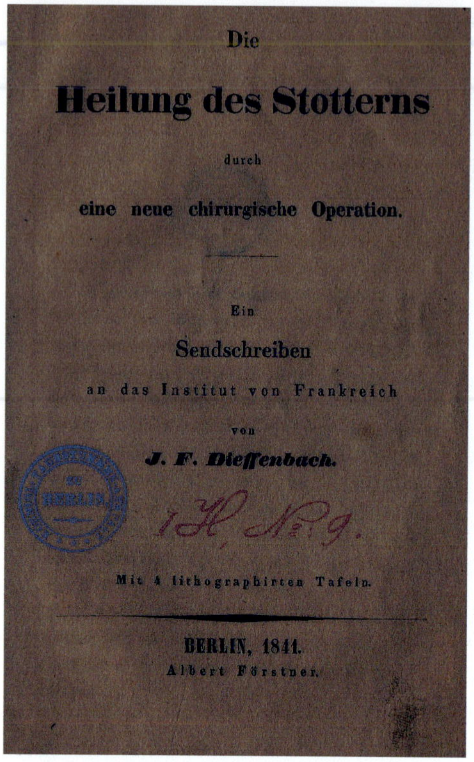
Die

Heilung des Stotterns

durch

eine neue chirurgische Operation.

Ein

Sendschreiben

an das Institut von Frankreich

von

J. F. Dieffenbach.

Mit 4 lithographirten Tafeln.

BERLIN, 1841.

Albert Förstner.

Fig. 4.4 Frontispiece of *Heilung des Stotterns* by Dieffenbach. Despite his early graft failures Dieffenbach encouraged the scientific community to investigate grafting. *Courtesy of Riccardo Mazzola, M.D., Milan*

ren had taken from the forearm of his patient for a nose reconstruction had failed. To repair this new defect, "the skin covering the ala was removed so as to leave no remaining appearance of redness", and a piece of skin from the arm was applied to the wound "by means of a lint moistened in blood which answered a much better purpose than the common adhesive plaster". Upon removal of the dressing, Warren could report with satisfaction that a complete union of the graft had taken place. This case, which was published in 1848, anticipated by many years the breakthroughs later made by European surgeons, but did not receive much recognition. Perhaps disappointment at the failure of his forearm flap distracted Warren from realizing the significance of his innovative repair, and led him to describe it with a certain nonchalance [1032].

Dieffenbach's suggestion that it would be useful to review in a single work the accumulated knowledge on skin grafts was taken up by Paul Bert (1833–1886). In a masterly doctoral thesis divided into four parts, Bert analysed the results of the disparate experiments and clinical cases published to date, and presented his own findings, which represented a continuation of Baronio's work. He made a clear distinction between grafts carried out on the same animal, between two animals of the same species, or in animals of two different species, coining the terms "autograft", "homograft" and "heterograft" [83, 85, 86]. Being unaware of the existence of the immune system, he was unable to explain the phenomenon of graft rejection, but did note, like Baronio, that autografts were almost always successful whereas both homografts and heterografts sooner or later were rejected by the recipient. Bert's description of the necessary conditions for the survival of the graft contributed significantly to future progress in tissue transplants. He underlined the importance of achieving good approximation of the graft, an atraumatic technique, careful immobilization of the graft, haemostasis and sterile operating conditions. In his work he noted the fact that "flagellation" served to improve the circulation to the donor region before the graft was taken.

In the first part of his thesis, Bert discusses *la greffe animale* and the different tissues that could be transplanted. In the second part he describes the results of his own experiments with different tissues (including teeth) implanted as autografts, homografts and heterografts crossed between various animals. In the third part he reviews the most important works by other authors, giving due credit to Baronio for his pioneering contributions. He then embarks on a general discussion of skin grafts, focusing special attention on the possible causes of failure. In the fourth part he analyses the requirements for a successful graft, considering in turn the donor area, the recipient site and factors external to the patient himself. Finally, the process of healing is subjected to close scrutiny; the resumption of blood circulation, secretions and innervation are accurately described [84].

Paul Bert's work represented an important contribution to plastic surgery, providing answers to many questions and guidelines on how to carry out a skin graft correctly. His observations were confirmed in another paper that, in retrospect, was of great significance and originality. In 1870 W. Hanff published a study on grafts that was corroborated by painstaking histological studies [411]. He demonstrated that grafts in frogs could take perfectly on the recipient area very soon after an operation, re-vascularizing within hours. Unfortunately, his studies were published when the surgical community was absorbed in discussing the clinical results obtained by J.L. Reverdin [837] just one year earlier. As so often happened, it was far easier for surgeons to assimilate clinical results than to interpret and apply the data from experimental studies, even though in the long term the genuine breakthroughs in plastic surgery would often be based on the latter.

Despite the undoubted if modest progress made by these laboratory studies and the sporadic reports of clinical successes, the outcome of grafting procedures during the nineteenth century remained unpredictable for a number of reasons. First of all, the process of rejection was not understood and many of the tissues used had no chance of succeeding since they were homografts. Others were full-thickness or even composite grafts containing a portion of subcutaneous tissue that we know are difficult. Finally, infection was almost inevitable in this period before the discovery of antiseptics, particularly in laboratory experiments.

Nonetheless, surgeons continued to experiment and progress was rapid during the second half of the nineteenth century, particularly following the invention of antisepsis by Lister in 1861 [567]. Equally important was the introduction of general anaesthesia by Morton in 1846 [714, 715]. This led to a greater willingness on the part of patients to undergo elective operations involving skin grafts. The groundwork was laid for the experiments of Reverdin. They marked the turning point that made the routine practice of skin and other tissue grafts possible [837].

Reverdin's Pinch Graft: The First Breakthrough

In 1866 Theodore Christian Albert Billroth (1829–1894) observed that in cases of severe burns, small islands of epithelium sometimes appeared in the granulation tissue. They then extended rapidly, contributing significantly to the epithelialization of the wound. In his opinion these represented surviving cells from the Malpighian layer and he hypothesized that they could play a crucial role in skin regeneration.

Inspired by this observation, Jacques Louis Reverdin (1842–1929), a young Swiss surgeon working in Paris, wondered what would happen if small pieces of skin were placed directly on granulating tissue. To find out he conducted a simple experiment. With a lancet and forceps he delicately lifted and cut small fragments of skin, laid them on the open wound of a patient, and waited (Fig. 4.5). To his amazement almost all of the fragments attached themselves to the recipient tissue, expanding rapidly and completing the epithelialization process. In a communication entitled *Greffes Epidermiques*, which he read before the *Societé de Chirurgie de Paris* a little more than one month after his operation, Reverdin described the results of his experiment in the most convincing terms [837]. His patient was a 53-year-old man who had suffered an avulsion injury to his forearm that refused to heal; several weeks had passed with only the formation of granulation tissue. On 24 November 1869 Reverdin removed a large number of tiny pieces of skin each about two square millimetres in size, from the patient's other arm "in an attempt to heal the wound with seeds of skin". Within one week these "seeds" began to grow and coalesce with one another, and in less than 5 weeks the wound was completely healed.

Reverdin reported his results immediately before an authoritative audience in a language that was current in the scientific world, and these circumstances helped convince the sceptical surgical community. The news that a simple procedure could resolve a case that in the past would have required amputation provided the confirmation that everyone had been waiting for. The *Societé de Chirurgie* warmly applauded Reverdin's work and immediately undertook to publish it. They also proposed that histological studies be undertaken, and as we have noted Hanff's experiments on frogs followed shortly after. The year 1869 marked the beginning of a new era in the history of the skin grafting which was no longer overshadowed by the constant threat of failure.

Reverdin was evidently an exceptional figure. Born in Geneva, he went to Paris to study at the Hôpital Necker under Jean Guyon.[8] After his brilliant debut working on grafts, he enrolled in the French army in 1870. The

8 Jean Casimir Félix Guyon (1831–1920) was the head of the Department of Surgery at the historic Hôpital Necker in Paris, and one of the founders of modern urology.

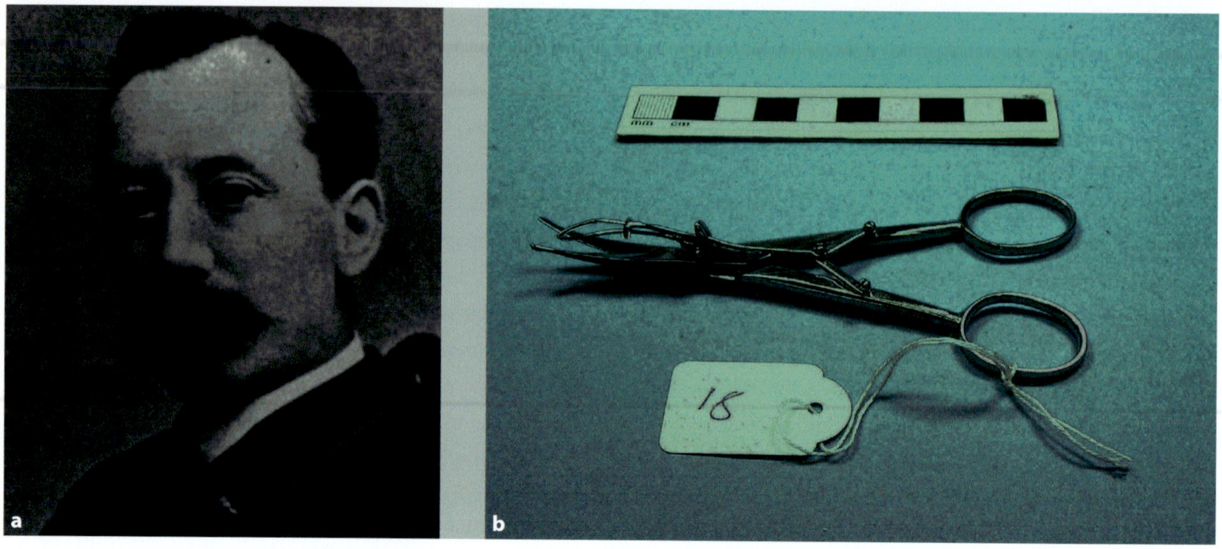

Fig. 4.5 **a** Jaques Louis Reverdin (1842–1929) devised pinch grafting. **b** Pinch graft scissors devised by Bryant. *From the Antony Wallace Archive, courtesy of the British Association of Plastic Reconstructive and Aesthetic Surgeons*

Franco-Prussian war at its height and this gave him, as it did so many other surgeons, ample experience treating wounds and amputations with skin grafts. Germany's isolation after the war perhaps explains why Reverdin's technique was first adopted in England. When George David Pollock (1817–1897), a surgeon at the Hospital for Sick Children in London, heard of the procedure he immediately went to Paris to learn how it was done [336]. After returning to England, he used it regularly and other surgeons followed suit; indeed, the technique that elsewhere was called the "pinch graft" was known in England as the "Pollock graft" [808–810].

The efficacy of Reverdin's seeding technique, combined with W. Hanff's demonstration that re-vascularization could take place quickly, convinced surgeons of the feasibility of the skin graft and they now sought to perfect the procedure and its results.

The next important contribution was made by George Lawson (1831–1903) who wondered whether larger grafts might not be just as successful. In 1870 he reported to a gathering of the *Clinical Society of London* the results of three experiments made using grafts containing both epidermis and dermis but no subcutaneous fat, in what may be considered the first full-thickness graft. Lawson called his innovation the "fourpenny graft" due to the size of the graft tissue, which was designed to cover the entire raw surface of the wound [536].

One of his patients was a 42-year-old woman suffering from a chronic ulcer that was so painful she wanted to have her leg amputated. She was instead persuaded by Lawson to undergo a graft procedure with skin taken from her arm, and after 3 weeks her ulcer had completely healed. It appears that Lawson was aware of Reverdin's work, because he sought to underline the advantages of his own graft: "[which] never became apparently lost amidst the surrounding granulations, as happened to many of the transplantations of minute portions of skin, but they maintained during the grafting period their own entity". He left the donor region to heal spontaneously by the second intention.[9]

Lawson confirmed the conditions for graft survival that Paul Bert had identified less than a decade earlier,

9 George Lawson became an ophthalmologist after serving in the army in the war against Russia. By the age of 39 had already written two books on his specialty. His single contribution to plastic surgery, *the fourpenny graft*, was of immense importance for it led to the acceptance and use of the full-thickness graft in reconstructive surgery. His biography appeared in 1968 [118].

stressing the importance of immobilizing the site with a bandage to protect it, "and thus to assist in retaining its vitality until established in its new taking". He observed re-vascularization and a return of sensitivity to the grafted tissue starting from the tenth day after the operation. The principal advantage of his graft was that it covered the entire raw surface whereas Reverdin's pinch grafts, although helping the healing of the defect, did not arrest the process of granulation, which led to the formation of larger quantity of scar tissue. Although Lawson's full-thickness graft represented a significant advance, his invention was largely overlooked and many decades would pass before its usefulness to reconstructive surgery was recognized.[10]

Two years later Louis E.L. Ollier (1830–1900), a brilliant surgeon who had studied under Claude Bernard at Montpellier, proposed certain modifications to Reverdin's technique. At the age of 30 he was appointed director of the department of surgery at Lyon,[11] and first suggested cutting larger pieces of graft tissue containing both epidermis and dermis. Another of his recommendations led to a significant improvement in the results. Neither Reverdin nor Lawson thought it necessary to prepare the surface of the wound before applying their grafts, even though the granulation tissue was sometimes so gelatious as to prevent the attachment of the seeded tissue. Ollier instead realized that "one must not cover the scarring tissue (the granulation being merely the stage preceding the healing of the defect), one must replace it". He insisted that it was not enough to "freshen" or debride the scar but it was necessary, as his mentor Claude Bernard had taught, to completely excise it and place the graft on healthy tissue after "a layer of new healthy granulation has formed". He still believed that granulations were necessary for the attachment, but that they should be fresh, well vascularized and presumably uninfected rather than old, exuberant and well on their way to becoming hypertrophic scar tissue.

The long-term results of Ollier's procedure were extremely encouraging. There was a considerable reduction in scar tissue and an improvement in the quality of the graft. The transferred tissue was supple, with normal colour and elasticity. He realized that his graft offered a promising alternative to the skin flap and declared that it "should be used whenever a flap was not possible".

The principles of the rejection reaction were still unknown and therefore Ollier did not hesitate to recommend the use of skin "from limbs amputated on account of accidents in healthy individuals"; regretfully, we do not know whether he ever attempted this procedure himself. Ollier was also a pioneer in the conservation of graft tissue and wrote that "an autograft stored in a refrigerating mixture for 25 days will maintain its normal colour". There is no record as to whether he used this tissue successfully as a graft. Ollier's contribution to our knowledge of grafts was fundamental and all the more impressive since his main interest was osteogenesis and the role of the periosteum. He was the author of more than one hundred papers on a wide range of subjects.

Thin Grafts

Another surgeon who made crucial contributions to graft surgery was Carl Thiersch (1822–1895). Born in the Bavarian city of Munich, he studied medicine at Ludwig-Maximillians University and then served as an army surgeon during the Franco-Prussian war (Fig. 4.6). This appears to have provided him with many opportunities to practise grafting operations, and his interest in this area continued throughout his long career.

Immediately after the war Thiersch conducted a simple yet elegantly designed experiment that helped to shed light on the anatomy and physiology of the graft. He carried out a series of autografts on the leg of a patient who was scheduled for amputation. These were performed at carefully spaced intervals, the last one 18 hours before the amputation. He conducted macroscopic and microscopic studies on the grafts concentrating in particular

10 Recognition of Lawson's contribution would not come until 1946, when L. Kock [502, 503] described his work and gave Lawson entire credit for the invention of the full-thickness graft, so often attributed to others.

11 Louis Ollier was born into a family with a long tradition of scientific interests that counted among its members a grand chancellor of the University of Toulouse, several magistrates and four generations of physicians, including his father, who practiced medicine in the city of Vans.

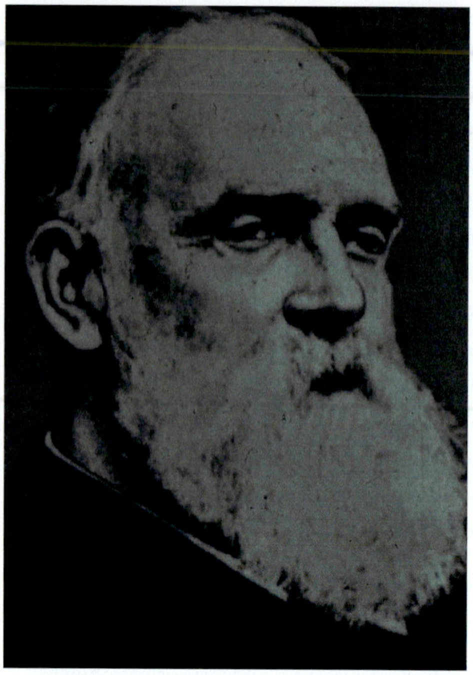

Fig. 4.6 Karl Thiersch (1822–1895) introduced the very thin graft

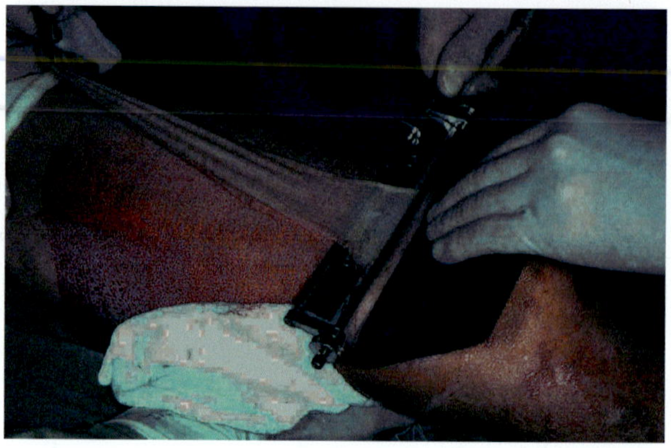

Fig. 4.7 Cutting a split skin graft with a Watson graft knife, one of several *guarded* instruments which followed the introduction of the adjustable dermatome designed by Humby. *PJS*

on the process of vascularization of the graft from the recipient bed. He succeeded in demonstrating the following:

- The process of healing begins with the deposition of a uniform layer of adhesive material (fibrin) between the graft and the recipient bed.
- Signs of re-vascularization between the graft and the recipient bed can be seen as early as 18 hours after the graft operation.
- The superficial layers of the graft, i.e. the epidermis, often fail to take whereas the deeper layer of the dermis, which contains surviving sebaceous and sweat glands, attaches more easily.

Thiersch published his findings in 1874 [983]. He concluded that the success of a graft depended not only on the characteristics of the granulations in the recipient area, but also on the thickness of the graft, for the superficial layers often seemed to create problems. His recommendation therefore was that the surgeon first remove the large granulations (as Ollier had suggested earlier), and then stretch the donor area flat before applying the thinnest, most uniform grafts possible, cut using his specially designed razor.

Thiersch's technique reflected an important shift in approach. Up to this time surgeons generally used full-thickness grafts, which were not only unreliable, but also created a new defect in the donor area that had either to be sutured or left to heal by the second intention. This posed serious limitations on the size of the graft that could be harvested. The thin graft instead left a sufficient amount of epithelium in situ, comprising at least all of the epithelium between the dermal papillae, the sebaceous and sweat glands and hair follicles (Fig. 4.7). This was enough to ensure a fairly rapid re-epithelialization and healing of the donor region. The surgeon could therefore take as much skin as was necessary to serve his purpose, an immense advantage that made a whole new range of clinical applications possible. He could now contemplate covering not only the raw portions of distant flaps, but also chronic ulcers, the stumps left after amputations, and above all deep extensive burns.

Although surgeons continued to prefer the full-thickness graft, Thiersch's technique was well received, particularly when it became clear that the attachment and survival of his thin grafts was easier to achieve than that of the full-thickness graft. According to McDowell [635, 636] the influence of Thiersch's work was so great that

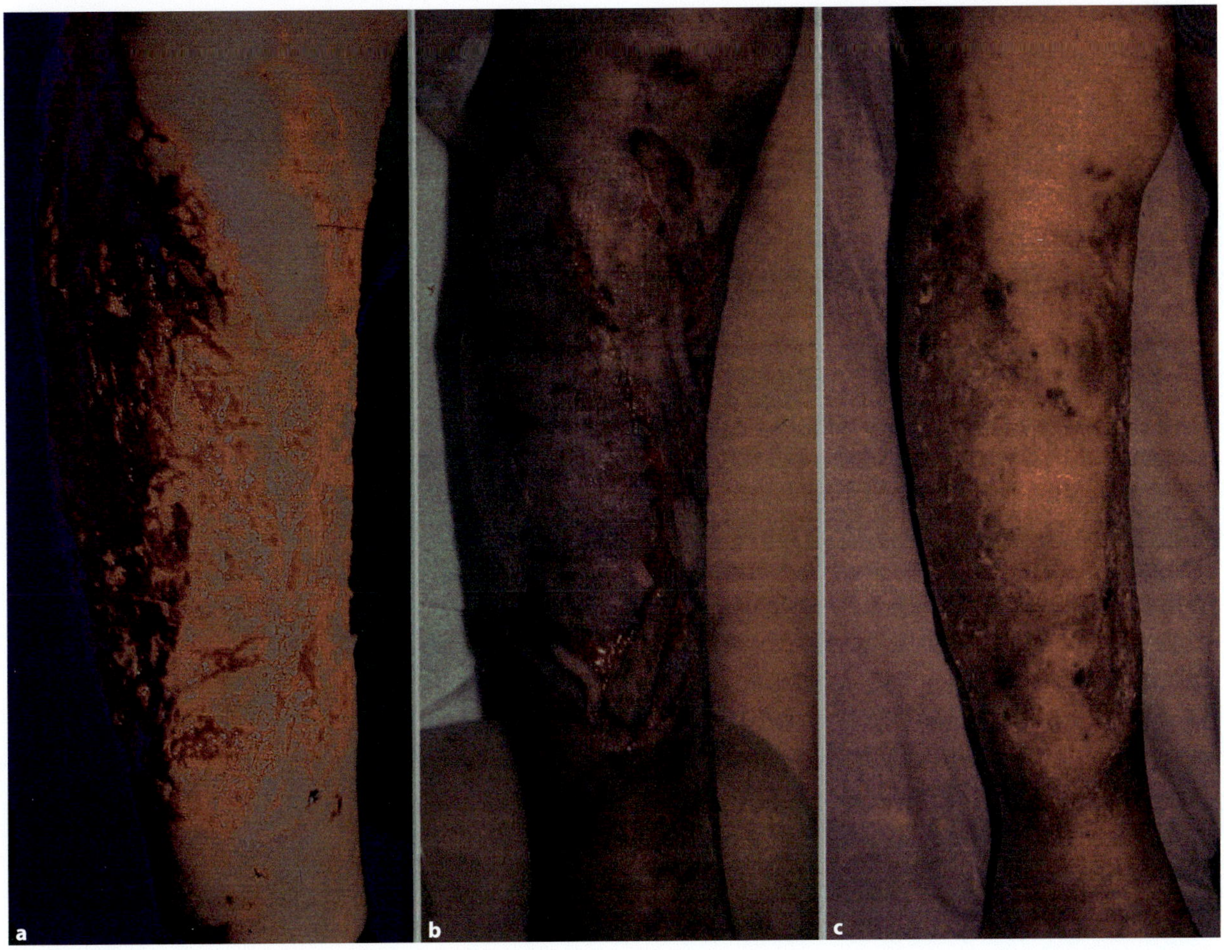

Fig. 4.8 Thin split skin grafts survive on recipient areas which are not ideal. The chronic granulations in this case (**a**) were scraped before application of the grafts (**b**) with good results (**c**). *PSR*

"he held back the development of split skin grafting for more than half a century". His most serious errors were to insist that the graft be as thin as possible, and that the best source was "the scar epithelium around the rim of the wound" (Fig. 4.8).

The Return of the Full-thickness Graft

While Carl Thiersch deserves credit for his work on the thin graft, the Scottish surgeon John Reissberg Wolfe (1824–1904) perfected the procedure of full-thickness grafting. Initially the two were viewed as rival techniques and both had their advocates, but in reality they were complementary, each one being appropriate for specific purposes. Both have earned a place in the armamentarium of reconstructive surgery.

Despite its advantages the fourpenny graft developed by Lawson in 1870 did not win broad acceptance and surgeons continued to use procedures based on Reverdin's seeding technique. Then, about two years after Thiersch published his work on thin grafts, Wolfe wrote a paper in 1875 contesting many of the accepted notions regarding graft surgery and describing a new method of his own [1047]. He took issue with Thiersch's recommendation that the graft should be taken from a site close to the defect. In his case he pointed out that the surgeon would have to: "cut skin off the face to repair the face, and in doing so … run a great risk of failure".

Furthermore, he questioned Tagliacozzi's insistence that a pedicle must be retained to guarantee the viability of his flap until it had acquired a sufficient blood supply from the surrounding area, a practice that imposed severe topographical limitations on the plastic surgeon. Thin free skin grafts demonstrated that a pedicle was not always necessary so they could be taken from any part of the body, to avoid conspicuous donor sites and prolonged immobilization. In reality, however, Wolfe's reasoning was only applicable to skin grafts and he neglected to take into account the fact that Tagliacozzi's thick flaps were intended for nasal reconstruction and required a thick flap containing fat.

Notwithstanding these conceptual errors, Wolfe's clinical work on full-thickness grafts represented a significant step forward. He introduced the notion that to ensure successful attachment, the graft had to be free of all subcutaneous areolar tissue and should be harvested in such a way as to include the dermis, but not the deeper layers. In an experiment on newly excised scars, he applied two grafts of different thicknesses to the same patient. One was cut as carefully as possible to include the dermis but none of the deeper layers (a full-thickness graft), and the other was taken leaving some subcutaneous areolar tissue and fat on the graft. While the first survived and quickly took on a normal colour and temperature, the second immediately became livid and by the fourth day had undergone extensive necrosis, leaving behind only a small portion of surviving tissue. Wolfe concluded: "If we want a skin graft to take by first intention we have to be sure that no areolar tissue is interposed between the flap and the defect."

With time Wolfe's recommendations achieved such a broad consensus that full-thickness free grafts came to be called *Wolfe grafts*. Indeed, if one followed his procedure the colour, elasticity and sensory responsiveness of the grafted tissue was quite similar, if not identical to that of normal skin, with minimal contracture. The Wolfe graft seemed to offer the ideal solution for every defect, although the problem of the closure of the donor site remained, limiting the size of the graft. Wolfe was an ophthalmologist and the problem of the donor area was not of great concerned him. Most of his grafts were to correct ectropion of the eyelids, which required only small grafts. He took these from the forearm but it is unclear how these were fixed in place. The quality of his full thickness grafts was close to normal skin and we now use them for bigger defects with excellent cosmetic results and minimal contracture (Fig. 4.9).

Wolfe was born in Breslau in 1824 and moved to Scotland when young. After studying in Glasgow and Paris he became an eye surgeon at the Aberdeen Royal Infirmary. Inspired by the nineteenth century ideals of liberty and patriotism, however, he abandoned his career for a life of adventure in the cause of nation-building, and eventually settled in Melbourne, Australia where he died in 1904.[12]

The full-thickness graft was introduced into the United States by O.F. Wadsworth in 1876 [1023]. When used on the face they can give good results even for large defects (Fig. 4.10a–c).

Further Progress in Skin Grafts

Up to this time, the skin flap had been the mainstay of reconstructive surgery, particularly in the case of facial defects, where large numbers of small flaps were used to replace missing tissue. For large defects in other parts of the body, pedicled flaps were employed but less frequently.

There were serious drawbacks to both of these procedures. Distant flaps often required long periods of immobilization as in the case of the cross leg flap devised by Hamilton, while repairs to the face invariably left disfiguring scars. Big flaps were difficult and the risk of infection ever present. The surgeon Fedor Krause (1856–1937)[13] perfected the use of the graft which he described

12 J.R. Wolfe was an active member of the fraternal organization of Freemasons. He became captivated by Giuseppe Garibaldi when the Italian hero and defender of liberty was invited to Scotland, which wanted independence from England. Indeed, he was so inspired by Garibaldi's cause that he gave up his position at the hospital to join the Italian leader's band of volunteers *I Mille*, which was preparing to set off for Sicily with the aim of uniting Italy. He became Chief Surgeon of Garibaldi's army in 1859, and later Inspector General of the Italian army's military hospitals.

13 Fedor Krause, who was born in 1856 and died at the venerable age of 91 in Halle in 1937. He was a professor of surgery who won fame for his work on bacteriology, osteomyelitis and tuberculous arthritis.

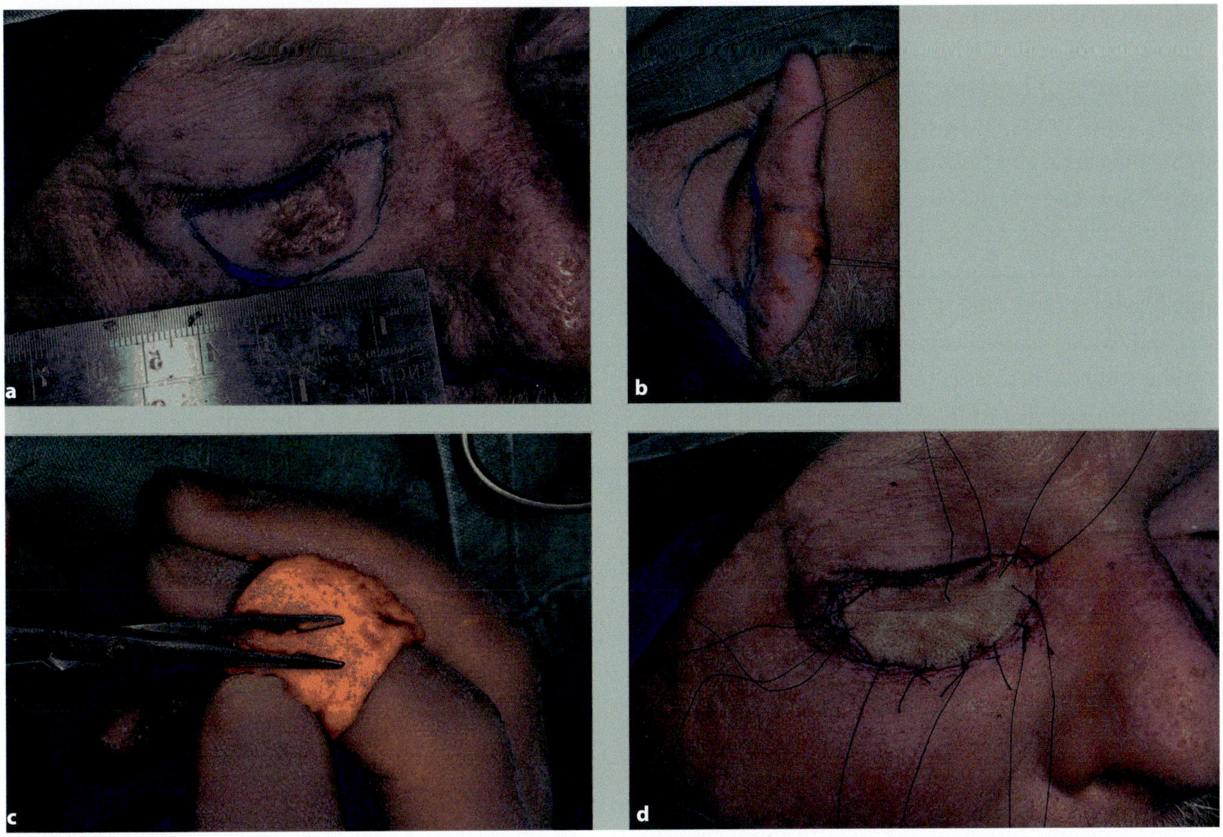

Fig. 4.9 **a** J.R. Wolfe (1824–1904) who was an ophthalmic surgeon in Glasgow devised his graft with the eyelid in mind to avoid ectropion. **b–d** In this case a post-auricular graft is used to fill a defect created by excising a basal cell carcinoma from the lower lid. *PJS*

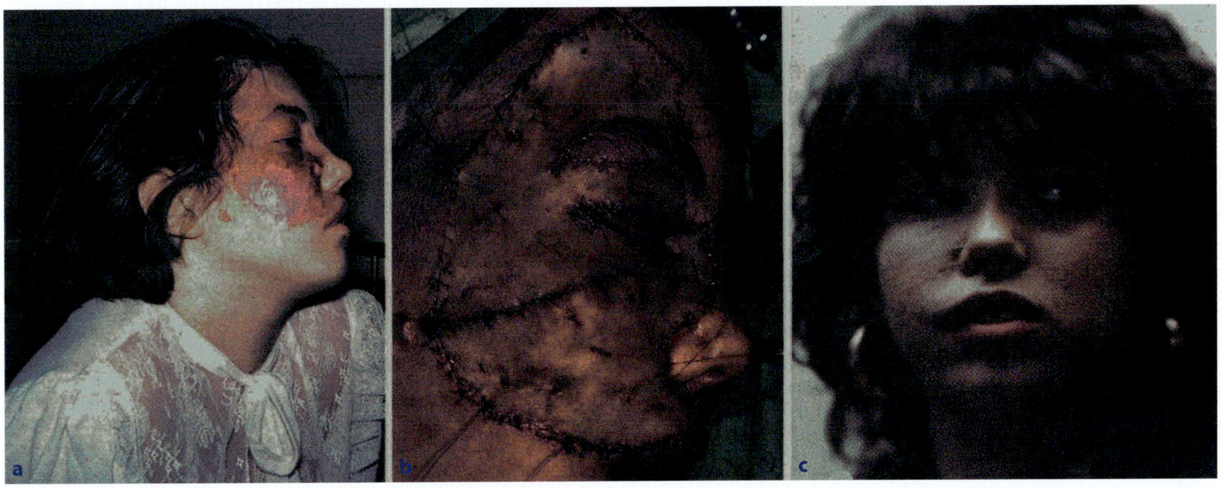

Fig. 4.10a–c Full thickness grafts give good results on the face even for large defects. This young patient had a capillary haemangioma excised and covered with two grafts from the groins. *PSR*

as a "non-pedicle flap that included the entire thickness of the cutis". In reality, Krause's graft shared many of the characteristics of Lawson's fourpenny graft and Wolfe's full-thickness graft, but he used it with success on large granulating areas and fresh defects following surgery for lupus[14] and cancer of the face.

In a study published in 1893, Krause described the results of over 100 grafts carried out on 21 patients with only 4 failures [508, 509]. Unlike his predecessors Lawson and Wolfe, he was not an ophthalmologist but a general surgeon and therefore thought in terms of large grafts. He noted that fresh wounds responded best, but he also treated chronic lesions after careful preparation of the surface by freshening to remove the granulations, and then washing with a mercury chloride and saline solution. The recipient area had to be perfectly clean and dry before the graft was applied and if there was any exposed bone it was chiselled until bleeding was induced. The graft was harvested with a scalpel and the areolar tissue removed, although Krause believed that the presence of a few lobes of fat would not compromise the success of the operation. Superficial bleeding was controlled by pressure rather than ligature whenever possible, because it was thought that the presence of a foreign body such as thread would interfere with the nourishment of the graft. In facial areas the graft was carefully sutured to the margins of healthy skin, but in other regions this was not always thought to be necessary. Krause introduced the use of non-adherent Vaseline dressings, to which he added a dilute solution of iodine. After 3 or 4 days the dressing was soaked off using a weak solution of boric acid.

Split Skin Grafts

As we have seen, Thiersch recommended the thinnest possible grafts whereas Lawson, Wolfe and Krause preferred the full-thickness graft. Neither of these techniques was without problems, however. Thin skin grafts were difficult to harvest and the tissue obtained—mostly viable epithelial cells interspersed with sebaceous glands and hair follicles—did not have the same characteristics as normal skin. Graft contraction was a problem not seen in full thickness grafts. The full-thickness graft, although it yielded superior results, could not exceed a certain size because of the defect that it left in the donor region.

These limitations would not be overcome until 1929 when Vilray P. Blair and James Barret-Brown developed the split-thickness skin graft, now universally known simply as the *split skin graft*. These were grafts of intermediate thickness which were harvested at the level of the stratum papillare and included some of the dermis while leaving an ample layer of epithelial cells in situ. Split skin grafts combined some of the advantages of both the thin and full-thickness grafts. They attached with relative ease, but since they included a portion of dermis, once healed their appearance and consistency were similar to that of normal skin [105].

The principal advantage of the split skin graft was that the donor region healed spontaneously. When necessary, fresh skin could be taken from the same area after about two weeks, which meant that an almost unlimited quantity of skin was obtainable. The exception was extensive burns.

Previously grafts had been cut using very sharp, unguarded knives similar to razors, and control of their thickness depended on the skill of the surgeon. Blair and Barret-Brown made a significant contribution to graft surgery with their invention of the electric dermatome, a special instrument that allowed the surgeon to regulate, within certain limits, the thickness and width of the harvested skin [72]. The drum dermatome which was used for cutting large symmetrical pieces of thick skin had its day but did not become popular (Fig. 4.11). Pneumatic dermatomes proved unreliable and cumbersome to use but the advent of electrical instruments made a big improvement (Fig. 4.12a–c).

In those cases where the size of the defect was large and split skin grafts cut with a dermatome were insufficient, surgeons could resort to a procedure devised by Otto Lanz (1865–1935). He was a Swiss surgeon who completed his training in Leipzig and was appointed professor of surgery in Amsterdam in 1906. McDowell [636] cited Lanz's discovery as an example of one of those "useful things invented for the wrong reasons". In reality Lanz's original intention was not to increase the potential size of the graft. He was concerned about the large open donor sites and devised an ingenious method to halve

14 Lupus is a term rarely used these days but refers to lupus vulgaris or tuberculosis of the skin, often the face.

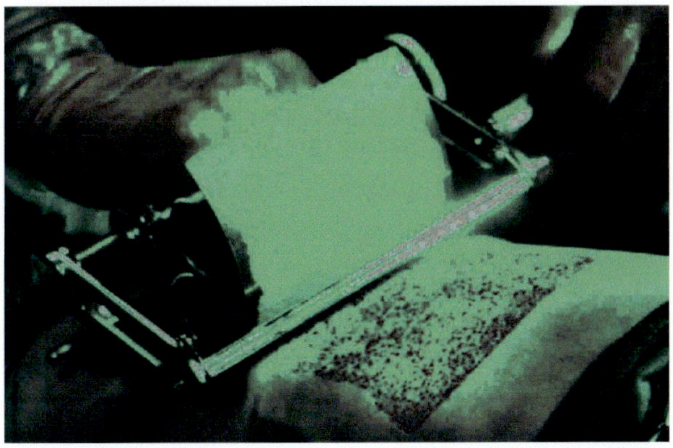

Fig. 4.11 The Padgett drum dermatome was used to cut large rectangles of thick skin graft but required experience and skill. *PJS*

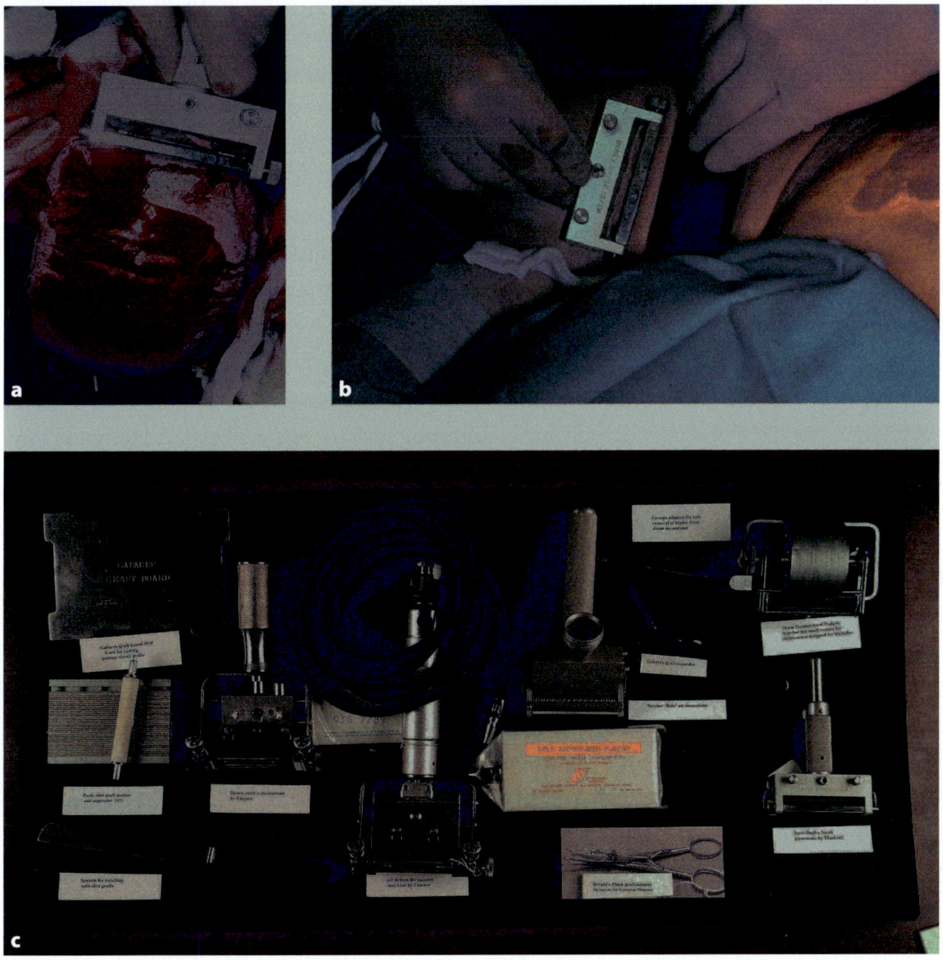

Fig. 4.12a–c Electrical dermatomes were more reliable and less cumbersome than the air driven model and their development allowed skin of a regular shape and thickness to be cut reliably even from awkward donor sites. They proved useful in burn patients. Here a graft is being taken from the scalp (**a**) and another from the more conventional area on the thigh (**b**). *PJS*. **c** A collection of mechanical dermatomes and other items: *left to right* Gabarro board above an early mesher, 1971 and graft spatula; dermatomes—Brown electric, Stryker 'Rolo'air, Zimmer air and Davis Duplex electric dermatomes; *upper right* a child's Padgett dermatome designed by McIndoe. *From the Antony Wallace Archive, courtesy of the British Association of Plastic Reconstructive and Aesthetic Surgeons*

the size of the donor site. He constructed an instrument furnished with a series of small knives that would make multiple cuts in the graft, which could then be stretched like an net to cover the defect. Indeed, one portion of the stretched graft might be used to cover the wound and the other to repair the defect in the donor region. His idea was the forerunner of modern mesh grafting (Fig. 4.13a–c) [530].

With the resolution of these various problems, grafting became a successful procedure and its practice spread rapidly. Over the years, as we have seen in Chapter 2, surgeons invented a variety of graft knives which simplified the procedure. Surgeons could now begin to concentrate on the biology of the graft with the aim of improving such aspects as re-vascularization and re-innervation of the grafted tissue. The latter was of crucial importance. As early as 1894, E.E. Goldman [385] published his observations on both processes and noted that nerve fibres initially formed in an irregular spotted pattern, which gradually extended to cover the entire graft. Some decades later Bengt Pontén [811] published an exhaustive review on the subject of the re-innervation of graft tissue.

Homografts and the Rejection Phenomenon

Today any student of medicine and most lay people know about the rejection phenomenon in organ transplantation. At the beginning of the twentieth century it was still a mystery. The failure of all but autografts puzzled the medical profession. Paul Bert in 1863 had noted that autografts were the only reliable tissues to survive but it was not understood why.

In 1903 C.O. Jensen [463] conducted a study which demonstrated that, while homografts initially attach themselves by the same process as autografts, after a period of time that could vary considerably, they were invariably rejected. This observation was confirmed by E. Lexer [560] and others explored the phenomenon (Schone 1912, Holman 1924, Bauer 1927). It is not certain who coined the term "rejection" but, as we will see, Medawar and Gibson used the term frequently.

During the first part of the twentieth century, surgeons, oncologists, geneticists and biologists had together arrived at some understanding of humoral immunity, but surgeons were still unable to resolve the problem of rejection. Indeed, it seemed that all attempts at skin homografts and organ transplants were doomed to failure. Then in 1943 a young Oxford zoologist, Peter Medawar [649–656] discovered the explanation for the phenomenon of rejection.

After conducting experimental work on animals, Peter Medawar was sent up to the Burns Unit at Glasgow Royal Infirmary in 1942. He set up a clinical study with Thomas Gibson,[15] a plastic surgeon who was treating a large number of burn victims from World War II. It became clear to them that the rejection of homografts arose out of an immune reaction—an antibody response of the host (*self*) that was triggered when antigenic (*non-self*) skin from a donor was introduced. Homografts were generally rejected during the second week after the graft operation, although in patients with serious burns the transplanted tissue sometimes lasted longer, probably due to a compromised immune system (Fig. 4.14a,b). E. Holman [446] had already noted in 1924 that the rejection reaction was donor-specific and that if skin from the same source was used a second time the rejection was immediate. Gibson observed the same phenomenon in what came to be referred to as "second set rejection" [369].

Nevertheless, much remained unclear and it was not until Medawar had returned to Oxford and completed his studies on homograft rejection—work which earned him the Nobel Prize, shared with MacFarlane Burnet, in 1960 and later a knighthood—that the process was completely explained. He demonstrated that it was an immunological phenomenon belonging to the category of actively acquired immunity: (1) once sensitivity to a foreign graft developed it became systemic, (2) a second set of allografts would be rejected immediately in an accelerated

15 After the studies on homografts, commissioned by the Medical Research Council, Tom Gibson's enquiring mind led him into further research and he eventually became Professor of Bioengineering at Strathclyde University, Glasgow. In 1970 he succeeded as Clinical Director of the Plastic Surgery Unit at Canniesburn Hospital, a unit he had helped establish with his colleague Jack Tough. He also served as second editor of the British Journal of Plastic Surgery for 10 years after succeeding A.B. Wallace another Scot from Edinburgh. Many know the name of Medawar but few realize Gibson's part in tissue transplantation [194].

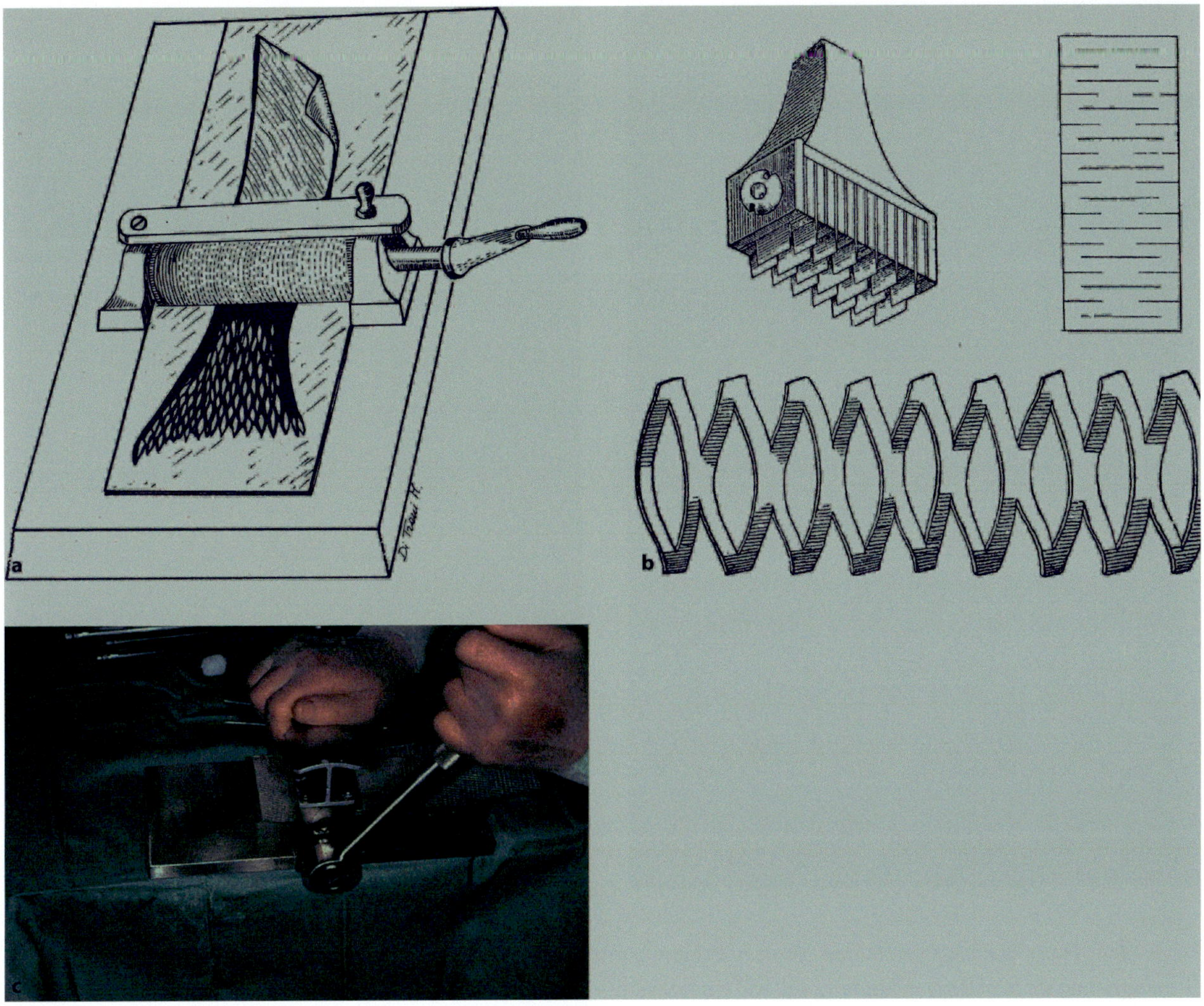

Fig. 4.13 **a** A diagram of the skin mesher. **b** The simple original instrument was conceived by the Dutch surgeon Otto Lanz (1865–1935) in 1908. **c** Several versions, with and without 'carriers', followed. *PJS*

process and (3) the entire process was donor-specific. Converse and Duchet [192] also showed, in 1947, that grafts between homozygote twins behaved like autografts and were accepted without problem by the host.

Thus, research on skin grafts led to the fundamental discoveries on which all modern organ transplant surgery and anti-rejection therapy are based.

Graft Viability and Preservation

As we have seen, ever since the first detailed studies on grafting were undertaken by Baronio and Thiersch, surgeons have been interested in the conservation of skin after it has been taken from the donor site until it is applied as a graft. Before the rejection reaction was understood and when homografts from cadavers or amputated limbs were being used, this appeared to be one of the key problems in graft surgery. In 1882 the American surgeon E.P. Brewer published a paper *On the limit of skin vitality* describing his experience with delayed grafting [130]. He took skin samples from cadavers and amputated limbs, wrapped them in damp gauze or paper, and stored them in a cool place (although it appears that he sometimes just kept them in his pocket) for 18–45 hours. He then grafted them to the host site. He reported that the grafts survived normally for a maximum of 36 hours,

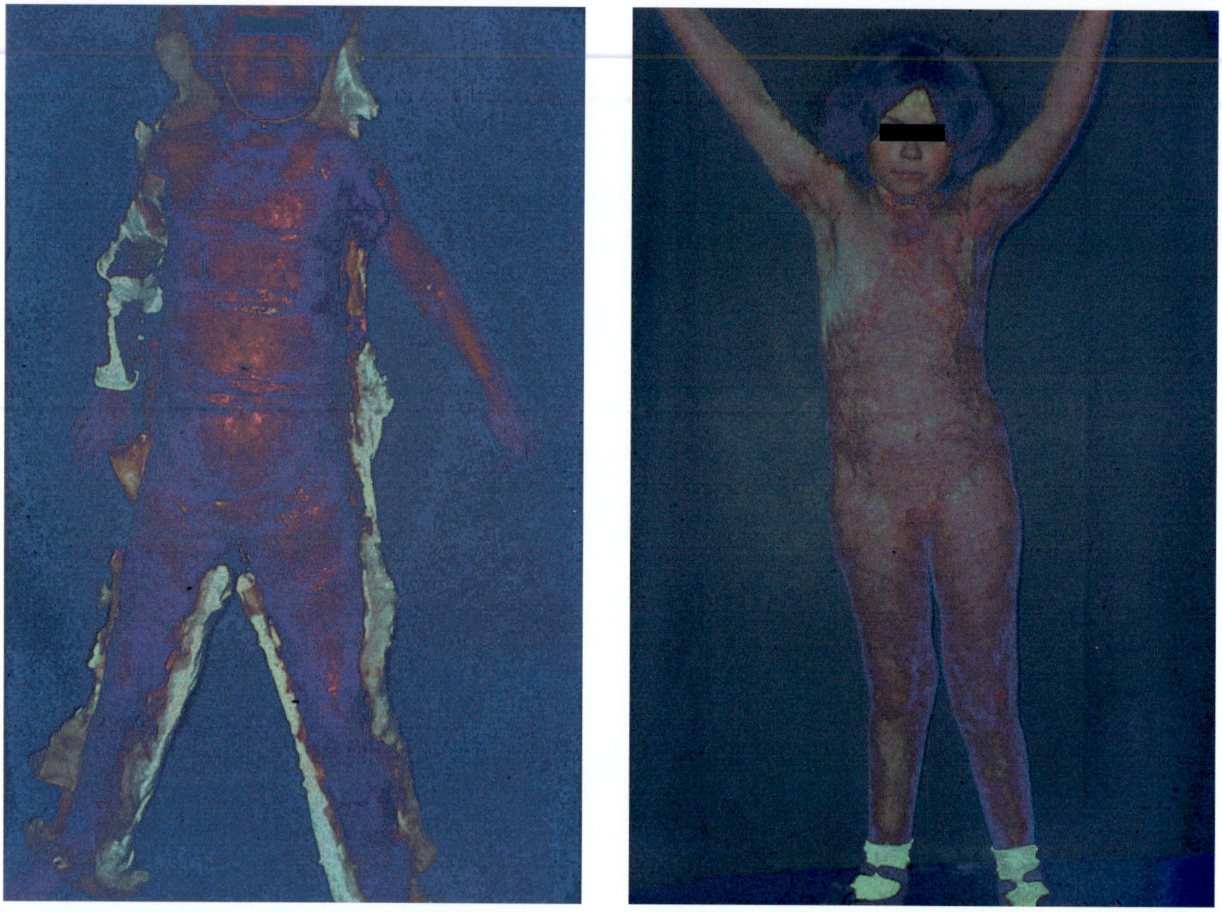

Fig. 4.14a,b Homografts are sometimes still used in large burns with limited donor sites particularly in developing countries. The alternating strips of large maternal grafts and narrow autografts give the longest edge from which the patient's 'self' tissue can epithelialize after the homografts are rejected. The patient's donor areas can then be cropped again. There was a successful outcome in this very large life-threatening burn in the 1960s. *PJS*

but sooner or later they failed. Given the lack of precise data on the conditions of preservation, his study merely demonstrated that graft tissue did not have to be implanted immediately.

The wars of the twentieth century saw a drastic increase in the number of serious burn victims, which made surgeons seek ways of preserving large amounts of viable tissue for use when needed.

Cooling, freeze-drying (lyophilization) or preservation in physiological solutions were compared. Early studies had been conducted by J. Wentscher [1042] who reported in 1898 that harvested tissue stored for 22 days at temperatures below 0 °C could still be successfully grafted. He demonstrated that freezing at temperatures as low as −50 °C did not compromise the vitality of the cells, whereas heating to +50 °C or soaking in chemical substances (antiseptics, etc.) was deleterious. Others investigated cooling in more recent times [182].

During World War II and the Korean War, surgeons had to treat large numbers of injured solders. Homografts were used as temporary, life-saving measures and the first skin banks were created, which were of vital importance in cases of mass casualties. Techniques for the conservation of both autografts and homografts by refrigeration, freezing and lyophilization were tested, and simple and effective procedures were developed to keep tissue viable and prolong survival before rejection.

It may be noted that much earlier, in 1912 Alexis Carrel [158] had studied the results of the freezing of tissue, and found that at low temperatures all biological processes appeared to be suspended. Jerome P. Webster [1038] and Tord Skoog [938] treated burns in the 1940s and 1950s with grafts of skin that had been frozen for storage and reported satisfactory results. In 1952 M. Allgower and T. Blocker [21] confirmed that frozen skin remains viable, as both Medawar [654] and Billingham and Medawar [102] had already observed. Unfortunately, freezing did not represent a very practical option under battlefield conditions.

The superiority of the lyophilized (freeze-dried) homografts to the fresh, refrigerated or frozen homograft was demonstrated by one of the authors of this book in 1960 [889, 890]. Such tissue can be stored for an indefinite length of time as long as it is kept in a vacuum. The question as to whether lyophilized tissue, once rehydrated can still be considered viable is not clear, if so their lowered viability is an advantage, for it means that any rejection is also slowed sometimes for months.

At present researchers are attempting to perfect methods of culturing new skin in vitro, a technique that could make significant improvements to the treatment of large burns.

Chapter 5

Grafts of Other Tissues

Contents

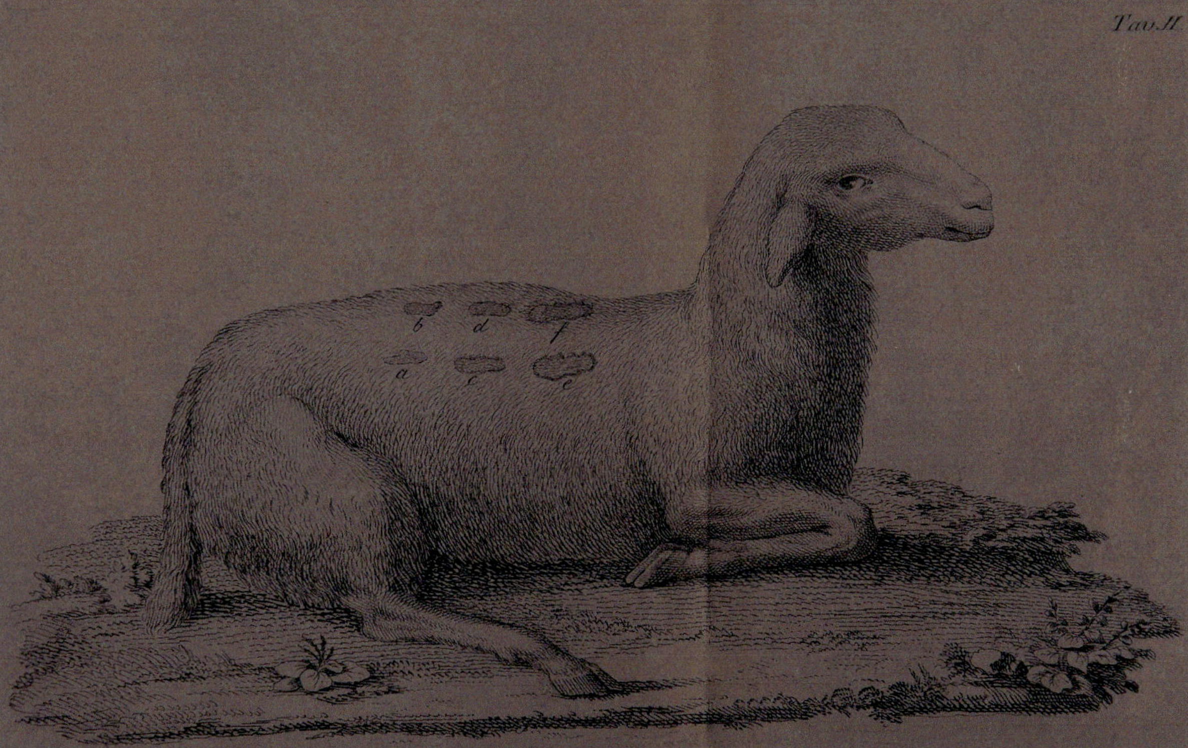

In addition to the skin, many other tissues such as bone, cartilage, tendons and even hair have been and still are grafted today. Like the skin graft the practice of tissue grafts is relatively recent. Before the introduction of antisepsis in the late nineteenth century, such operations were rarely successful and the only references to be found were in stories and legends such as that of Pelops' ivory shoulder, mentioned by Ovid in his Metamorphoses.[1]

Another more recent story is recounted by Job Janszoo van Meek'ren (1611–1666) in the opening chapter of his book on cranial fractures, which he claims was told to him by a missionary, Johannes Kraanvinkel [658]. It seems that a Russian aristocrat by the name of Butterljin had part of the top of his skull sliced off by a Tartar's sword. This segment was replaced in an operation that the Dutch author described as follows: "To fill up the space, the surgeon [whose name is not mentioned] took a piece from the skull of a dog that had been killed, corresponding in shape and size to the piece cut by the sword from the nobleman's head, and fitted it to the injured spot. In this way the nobleman was restored once again to health."

Perhaps the nobleman, elated by the success of his operation, spread the news too enthusiastically, for it reached the ears of the capital's Orthodox Russian priest who threatened to excommunicate poor Butterljin if the piece of dog's skull was not promptly removed from his head. It is a great pity that, due to this intransigence of the church, we have no follow-up on a case that might have proved extremely interesting! The only doubt that Edward Zeis [1060] seems to have expressed was: "How can we trust such a tale when it has been passed on so many times?"

There are isolated reports in the literature of the reimplantation of parts of the nose by bold surgeons such as Lanfranchi da Milano in the fourteenth century and Leonardo Fioravanti in the sixteenth century. These were probably composite grafts. However, it was not until the eighteenth century that grafting and the problems connected with the procedure would attract the serious attention of the surgical community.

The first surgeon to carry out a composite graft was Henry Louis Duhamel du Monceau (1700–1746). His work on animals attracted considerable attention, in particular a series of autograft experiments in which he transplanted the spurs from roosters to the well vascularized tissue of their crests [262]. It appears that these grafts were at least partially successful and in some cases the skin, muscle, bone or the entire spur attached to the new site. This experiment was repeated in 1767 by John Hunter who noted that for a graft to attach successfully it had to be implanted in a well vascularized site [456, 457].[2]

Others during the course of the eighteenth century experimented on animals without paying much heed to the question of where the grafts came from, i.e. a different individual or a different species. For example, in 1807 Antelme Baltasar Richerand sought somewhat audaciously to transplant part of the muzzle of a dog to a rabbit [839] and in 1815 Pierre Francois Percy attempted a heterograft of bone [791].

In 1922 Pierre Mauclaire published a text on grafts, Les Greffes Chirurgicales [618, 619], in which he listed the attempts made by various surgeons (Piedeguel, Espagnol, Bossu, Hunter, Flemant, Buffon and Wiesmann) to re-attach amputated digits. He also mentions the reimplantation of an ear by Hange and Wiessman, and a muscle transplant carried out in 1877 by Zahn and Zieklenko. While his review was both timely and useful, the reported success of some of the operations leaves us somewhat sceptical. Furthermore, in his entire book Mauclaire dedicates only three lines to Giuseppe Baronio (1758–1814) and it is doubtful that he was really acquainted with the work of this scrupulous researcher, for he went no further than to observe that he was "the Italian who grafted the tail of a cat to a rooster". We have already described the importance of Baronio's work in the last chapter. In our discussion of the skin graft, we have also seen how Johan Friedrich Dieffenbach (1794–1847), perplexed by the failure of his attempts where others had succeeded, called upon scientists to review the accumulated experience in grafts and seek to understand their mechanism (Fig. 5.1) [245, 246].

---

1 As recounted by Ovid, Pelops, the brother of Niobe, was cut into pieces and served to the gods at a banquet by his father, Tantalus, to test their divinity. Demeter, mourning for Persephone, did not perceive the wicked act and ate a piece of the shoulder. The gods gave Pelops life again and an ivory shoulder!

2 John Hunter was probably the first surgeon to propose the transplantation of teeth.

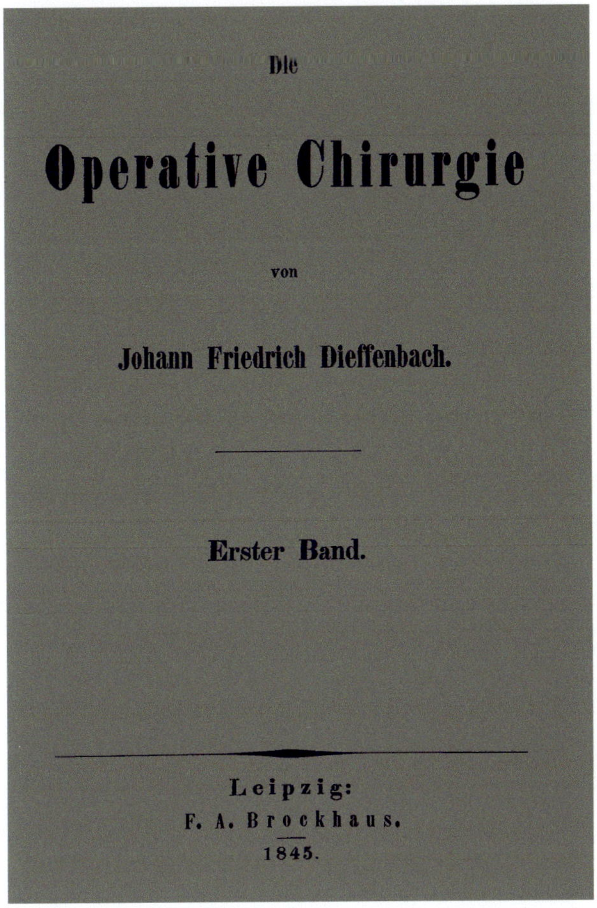

Die

Operative Chirurgie

von

Johann Friedrich Dieffenbach.

Erster Band.

Leipzig:
F. A. Brockhaus.
1845.

Fig. 5.1 Frontispiece of Dieffenbach's most important work Die Operative Chirurgie published in 1845. Unlike others who were successful, Dieffenbach encountered problems with his grafts and this made him investigate their use scientifically. Baronio had answered many of the questions some years before. Courtesy of Riccardo Mazzola M.D., Milan

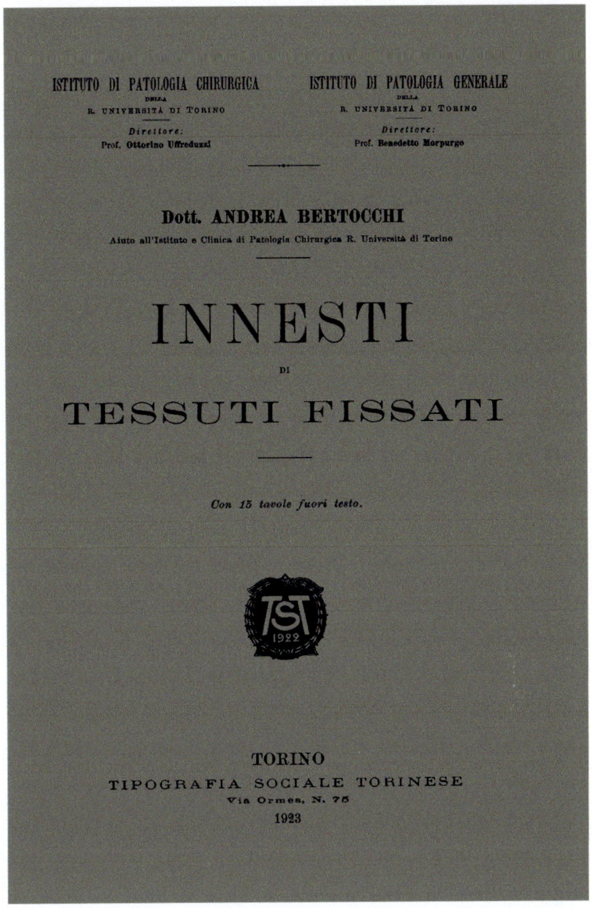

ISTITUTO DI PATOLOGIA CHIRURGICA
DELLA
R. UNIVERSITÀ DI TORINO
Direttore:
Prof. Ottorino Uffreduzzi

ISTITUTO DI PATOLOGIA GENERALE
DELLA
R. UNIVERSITÀ DI TORINO
Direttore:
Prof. Benedetto Morpurgo

Dott. ANDREA BERTOCCHI
Aiuto all'Istituto e Clinica di Patologia Chirurgica R. Università di Torino

INNESTI
DI
TESSUTI FISSATI

Con 15 tavole fuori testo.

TORINO
TIPOGRAFIA SOCIALE TORINESE
Via Ormea, N. 75
1923

Fig. 5.2 Frontispiece of Bertocchi's book Innesti di Tessuti Fissati (1823). Bertocchi suggested the use of grafts which had been "fissati" (fixed) either in alcohol of formalin. Courtesy of Riccardo Mazzola M.D., Milan

Indeed, no one had very clear ideas on the subject and we should not be surprised that Andrea Bertocchi [87] stimulated by the somewhat speculative paper on the nature of biological tissues published by Jean Nageotte [722] attempted a series of grafts of "tessuti fissati", i.e. harvested tissue preserved in 70° or 80° alcohol and/or 10% formalin. These grafts obviously failed, but Bertocchi succeeded in getting some useful data from his work. He demonstrated, for example, that a range of tissues such as vessels, bone, cartilage, tendons, connective tissue, nerves and fat treated in this way "... were able to create a connective substrate in which the living cells of the surrounding tissues could regenerate". Even if many of his conclusions are debatable, Bertocchi correctly observed that the reaction of the host tissues stimulated by these grafts was less marked than their response to fresh homografts. His discussion of cartilage is interesting. He observed that it was not reabsorbed and therefore could still provide mechanical support for the surrounding host tissue (Fig. 5.2).

Bone Grafts

It had not escaped the attention of surgeons that pieces of bone that became detached during the course of surgical procedures or as a result of traumata often survived if left in their original site. In 1809 Daniel Merrem (1790–1859) described this phenomenon in intracranial operations, noting that pieces of skull removed during surgery re-attached when they were put back in place [661]. Around this time surgeons began to study bone grafts using animals. Paul Bert was one and he wrote his Doctoral Thesis on animal grafts (Fig. 5.3). Louis Xavier Édouard Léopold Ollier (1830–1900) also did extensive research on tissue grafts in animals and described the case of a patient whose femur had been so badly broken that one condyle remained connected by only a few strands of tissue. They were certainly insufficient to nourish it. However, when immobilized it united to the shaft in several weeks [747–750]. Finally, Richard von Volkmann (1830–1899) reported, at a meeting in Berlin in 1872, the case of a compound gunshot wound in which the bone was shattered very badly. However the fragments healed successfully after being replaced in situ [1021]. This report received wide publicity and was instrumental in convincing surgeons of the feasibility of bone transplants. In 1915 Fred Houdlett Albee (1876–1945) took the next logical step and investigated whether fragments of bone might survive if used as grafts in other sites. His observations convinced him that they did and he published his results in 1916 [9].

Once the idea had been accepted the vexed question regarding the source of osteogenesis, which had never been answered, was re-opened. Many physicians of antiquity, most prominently Hippocrates, Celsus and Galen, had speculated on the biology of bone. Hippocrates did not believe that this tissue could regenerate, whereas Galen postulated the existence of a vital sap in the bone that stimulated the mending of fractures. Later Delamotte, Havers and others established, on the basis of their experiments and from empirical observation, that bone was a living tissue and therefore should be able to reproduce like any other. The question remained by what mechanism?

By contrast to those studying skin grafts whose efforts were concentrated on perfecting the grafting technique and making it safe and reliable, doctors studying bone grafts where consumed with theoretical questions as to the exact nature of bone regeneration. This was very pertinent to fracture healing but distracted them from the possibilities of bone grafting. In the end, however, much of this academic speculation would lead to significant practical advances.

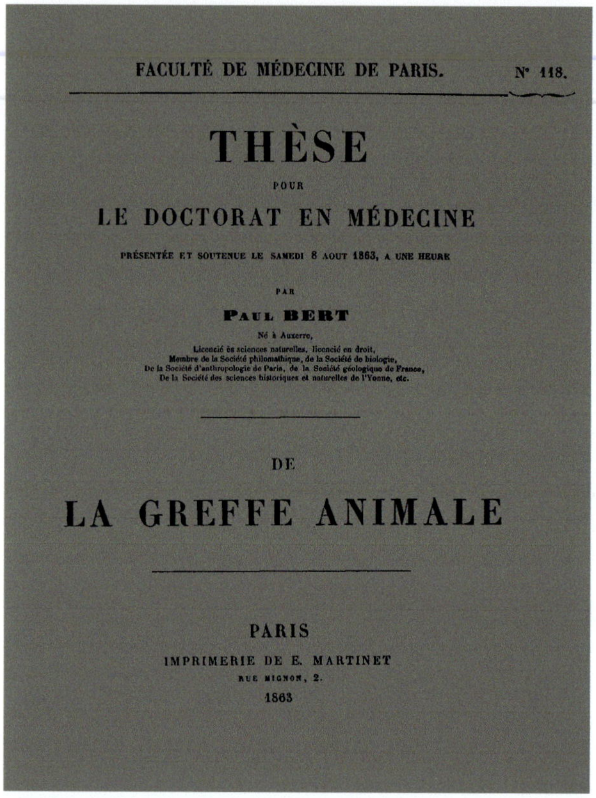
FACULTÉ DE MÉDECINE DE PARIS. N° 118.

THÈSE

POUR

LE DOCTORAT EN MÉDECINE

PRÉSENTÉE ET SOUTENUE LE SAMEDI 8 AOUT 1863, A UNE HEURE

PAR

PAUL BERT

Né à Auxerre,
Licencié ès sciences naturelles, licencié en droit,
Membre de la Société philomathique, de la Société de biologie,
De la Société d'anthropologie de Paris, de la Société géologique de France,
De la Société des sciences historiques et naturelles de l'Yonne, etc.

DE

LA GREFFE ANIMALE

PARIS

IMPRIMERIE DE E. MARTINET
RUE MIGNON, 2.
1863

Fig. 5.3 Frontispiece of Paul Bert's thesis La Greffe Animale which was relatively short. In the same year (1863), he published his book with the same title (Fig. 5.7) and this covered the subject in much greater depth. Courtesy of Riccardo Mazzola M.D., Milan

For example, interest soon focused on the periosteum. As early as 1684, Antoine de Heyde[3] observed the production of new bone in the haematoma that formed between the two broken ends of a fracture. He later demonstrated that the periosteum in frogs was capable of generating new bone. However, one of the most pivotal discoveries was made in 1739 by Duhamel du Monceau. He conducted systematic studies on the reproduction of bone in young animals. He noted the formation of a gelatinous

3 De Heyde's work Anatomia Mytuli, Subjecta Centuria Observationum in 1684 appeared at a very early stage and predates most others.

substance beneath the periosteum that he hypothesized was the source of osteogenesis, and succeeded in demonstrating that “le perioste fait l’os”; i.e. that the periosteum was involved in the generation of bone and was therefore a key factor in the healing of fractures [24].

Just a few years later, Michele Troja (1747–1827) carried out an important series of experiments. He had come to Paris on a fellowship to complete his surgical training under Lieutaud and Desault, and while there undertook a study of the process of bone regeneration in animals [997, 998]. He analysed the healing of fractures under varied conditions in frogs, birds and dogs. After removing pieces of bone from the tibia, the excised area of bone healed completely. He believed that this was due to the cellular activity of the periosteum.[4] It would seem that the small fragments of bone were removed subperiosteally. He did not appear to believe that the bone marrow played any significant role. Troja’s contribution to our understanding of the complex process of bone regeneration was acknowledged by Francesco Frusci in his painstaking and well documented book on the subject, published in 1851 [342].

One hundred years after Troja, the central role of the periosteum was again emphasized by the British surgeon James Syme (1799–1870) [966, 967], who wrote: “The evidence is now sufficient for putting beyond all question the power of the periosteum to form new bone, independently of any assistance from the old bone.” This notion gained adherents in Germany and Russia as well as England, but it was in France that further corroboration for the theory was published by Joseph Francois Malgaigne (1805–1865) in 1834 [598], Alfred Armand Velpeau (1795–1867) in 1839 [1010, 1011] and above all by Marie Jean-Pierre Flourens (1794–1867) in 1842 [322, 323].[5]

In 1842 Flourens published the first results of his experiments on the periosteum. He repeated Troja’s experiments, after giving his predecessor due credit.[5] “It was the experiments by Troja that gave me the idea, experiments recognized to be most excellent and great.” Flourens in turn showed while new bone was formed by the periosteum existing bone was absorbed by the marrow. Another crucial piece had been added to the puzzle. He continued and broadened his studies, producing further supporting data that were published in an exhaustively detailed book in 1847.[6]

After Flourens, more work on osteogenesis was conducted by Ollier beginning in 1858 [747–750]. He succeeded in shedding light on aspects regarding graft compatibility, in particular the importance of the donor. He concluded that, as with skin grafts, only autografts of bone had a good chance of surviving. Although nothing was known of immunology at the time, he perceptively observed: “Based on our experience, we must renounce the notion of a graft of periosteum from animal to a human subject. We have almost always observed extrusion of the grafts practiced between different animals … Therefore, it should only be from a man that we take the periosteal graft or, better still, from another region of the same individual … There is nothing to suggest that it would be useful to repeat Percy’s work and repair a human tibial defect with a bone segment taken from the tibia of a cow.”

Ollier’s experiments were comprehensive and, after publishing his first results in 1862, he produced a one thousand page treatise in 1867 that covered the entire subject of grafts. He analysed every aspect, including survival, vascularization, reabsorption, and the differences between the bone graft and the periosteal graft. Aware of the clinical implications of his work, he also studied the conservation and refrigeration of bone tissue and attempted to test his conclusions in the operating room. In 1861 he used a flap containing a segment of frontal bone—and therefore not a true free bone graft—

4 Michele Troja reported the results of his experiments to The Societé Royale de Medécine and published them in the Mémoires de l’Académie des Sciences (Paris) in 1775. A more exhaustive review followed in the form of a book, published first in French and then in a Latin edition that was dedicated to Joseph Lieutau. This book was republished in Naples, where Troja had been appointed to the chair in urology in 1779. He was an outstanding anatomist and surgeon and in addition to his work on grafts, published important papers in the areas of urology and ophthalmology.

5 See Recherches sur le Dévelopment des Os et des Dents (Research on the Development of Bone and Teeth).

6 Marie Jean-Pierre Flourens was professor of comparative anatomy at the University of Paris as well as secretary of the Académie des Sciences. He made contributions to our understanding of embryology, the blood circulation and the nervous system.

to reconstruct a nose. Four years later he attempted to treat the necrotic elbow of a young osteomyelitis patient by inserting four autografts of bone into a recipient bed consisting of scar tissue. Most disappointingly the operation failed, probably due to the poor vascularity of the tissues. As he was forced to report, despite the absence of infection, 9 months later nothing remained of the grafted bone tissue.

There is no doubt that the work conducted by Ollier at Montpellier under Claude Bernard did much to stimulate interest in bone grafts and laid the groundwork for future progress, as did his research on skin grafts discussed in an earlier chapter. Although there had been previous attempts to graft bone, no one before Ollier had undertaken a study of the subject in such a thorough and systematic manner. Oddly enough, despite the mass of supporting data that he had gathered, Ollier remained pessimistic about the feasibility of bone grafts. Perhaps discouraged by the failure of his elbow graft, he went so far as to declare that bone grafts are "not only undesirable but even dangerous in human patients".

Nevertheless, many of the conclusions drawn by Ollier were entirely correct. He demonstrated that for a graft to survive the tissue must be still viable, it should be at least partially covered by periosteum and autografts were always preferable to allografts.

Early Bone Grafting

Not only researchers, but many surgeons supported the hypothesis that the periosteum played a central role in bone regeneration. Bernard Rudolph Konrad von Langenbeck (1776–1851) was persuaded of this and well before many of his colleagues, he used the periosteum successfully to recreate bone. His clinical work focused on the head and he was able to demonstrate, as Ollier had done for other parts of the body, that osteogenesis in the facial bones and skull was predominantly periosteal in origin [524, 526].

In 1859 von Langenbeck resected the maxilla of a patient, leaving the periosteum in situ. When he examined the involved area some time later, he discovered that the missing section of the maxillary bone had completely regenerated. For this reason he always included periosteum in the flaps that he raised for his cleft palate repairs. Such was his faith in the regenerative capacity of this tissue that he included periosteum from the frontal bone in his flaps for nose reconstructions.

Notwithstanding the convincing evidence published by Ollier, another hypothesis was emerging that ascribed the regenerative capacity of bone exclusively to the osteoblasts. The eminent Scottish surgeon Sir William MacEwen (1848–1924) questioned all previous notions regarding osteogenesis with a paper that he presented to the Royal Society in London in 1880. He described the successful reconstruction of a missing 10-cm section of a boy's humerus using several pieces of bone from other patients who had been operated on for tibial curvature. Although each graft included periosteal tissue, he proposed that the osteoblasts were responsible for bone formation and that the periosteum served merely the sustaining function of a "living membrane" [637–639].

Other colleagues continued to support Ollier's thesis. G. Axhausen declared in 1908 that bone was replaced through the osteogenic activity of its "living periosteum" [43, 44]. Others, without actually contradicting Ollier, suggested that the osteogenic function of the periosteum was not absolutely essential. Among these were Ernst Ziegler (1849–1905) [1058], Jakimowitsch [462] who conducted his own experiments in 1881 and Ambrogio Ferrari [309] who carried out a careful series of bone grafts and managed to demonstrate that the periosteum was not indispensable to bone regeneration, although he noted that the new procedure of antisepsis was crucial to the success of the operation. Ferrari also studied grafts in dogs, rabbits and chickens. In one experiment he implanted autografts that had been treated with a 3% solution of phenol and checked the survival of the tissue from the 10th to the 19th day of the study. He reported that out of a total of 15 grafts, 2 failed due to infection whereas 9 showed clear signs of re-vascularization which he demonstrated by injecting a carmine solution into the blood vessels.

The role of the periosteum in the survival of bone grafts was superseded by a new theory at the end of the nineteenth century. The Viennese surgeon Michael Barth published a series of studies between 1893 and 1908 [56–59] confirming the dissertation thesis of a Russian medical student, Radzimowski of Kiev [824]. They argued that whether or not the transplanted bone tissue included periosteum was irrelevant, because the contribution of the graft itself was only transitory; afterwards it would "degenerate in its entirety and become replaced by new bone". The graft in reality served as a platform upon which new bone could be deposited and it did not matter whether the tissue was vital or not, because it was the surrounding tissues and not the graft that were responsible for new bone formation. This also provided an explanation for the scattered reports of the supposed success with bone tissue that had been boiled, ground or chemically fixed.

Barth soon found supporters for his theory, among them N.J. Baschkirzew and N.N. Petrow [62]. They reported in 1912 that neither periosteum nor cancellous marrow were essential to the survival of a graft because the transplanted tissue was destined to be reabsorbed. During this process, they postulated that "physiochemical stimulants" were released that induced metaplastic bone formation by the neighbouring tissues. The cells of the grafted bone tissue all died sooner or later, depending upon how far they were located from the vascularized tissue needed for their survival. According to these authors, the role of the periosteum was at best uncertain; it probably facilitated the adherence of the graft tissue to the recipient bed, slowing the reabsorption process and allowing consolidation of the new vascular network and in addition furnished a mechanical stimulus to the formation of new bone.

Two years later, in 1914, Dallas B. Phemister (1882–1951) published his landmark paper on The Fate of Transplanted Bone, demonstrating that both the periosteum and endosteum were necessary to the regeneration of bone and suggesting that the haversian intratrabecular spaces played a role as well. Most importantly, he proved that a graft consisting of many small pieces of bone without periosteum survived better and produced more bony callus than a single large graft with periosteum, probably due to better vascularization [797].

The so-called Phemister graft quickly won almost universal acceptance among surgeons and its advantages were confirmed shortly afterwards by William Edward Gallie (1882–1952) and D.E. Robertson [355]. In 1915 Albee reported the first case of Pott's syndrome treated with a bone graft applied as an internal splint [9].

By the end of the 1920s the bone graft had become a routine procedure in orthopaedic surgery, and was soon employed regularly in plastic surgery (Fig. 5.4a–d). Before this it had been used sporadically, for example, in 1896 James Israel (1848–1909) used bone tissue taken from the tibia to reconstruct a nose [461]. Despite the fact that the graft was inserted through an external, longitudinal incision, the cosmetic result was quite good. Charles Nélaton (1851–1911) and Louis Ombrédanne (1871–1956) carried out similar operations with equally satisfactory results [727].

Cartilage Grafts

At the same time as research was being done on bone and its biology, investigations were carried out on cartilage during the nineteenth century although its use in the operating room would not become a reality until some decades later.

Albrecht Teodore Middeldorpf (1824–1869) attempted to implant pieces of cartilage in the peritoneum, but reported that these were completely reabsorbed [665]. This experiment, notwithstanding its disappointing results, is described in Mauclaire's comprehensive review of grafts. Ollier's interest in grafts extended to cartilage although he was convinced that, as with bone tissue, for a cartilage graft to survive it needed to be transplanted with its perichondrium. In 1872 F.W. Zahn experimented with grafts of foetal cartilage but without success [1056, 1057].

Many of the disputes over the biology of bone also cropped up in discussions of cartilage. Mauclaire believed that the superficial layer of the cartilage rather than the perichondrium was responsible for chondrogenesis, and a variety of other theories proliferated.[7]

Although initial results were not encouraging, surgeons began to use cartilage grafts at the end of the nineteenth century. The first to publish his findings was Friedrich Mangold (1859–1909), who used ink injection studies to show that cartilage implanted with its perichondrium could survive for 9 months in rabbits. Encouraged by these results, he decided to use a cartilage graft to close a laryngeal defect. He began by implanting a piece of rib cartilage 3 × 5 cm in size beneath the skin of the patient's neck. After 8 months he raised a composite flap from the neck to close the gap in the larynx. This was in 1900 and was probably the first clinical case of a cartilage graft.

7 Mangold, 1887; Salty Kow, 1900; Giani, 1911; and J.S. Davis (1917) [224].

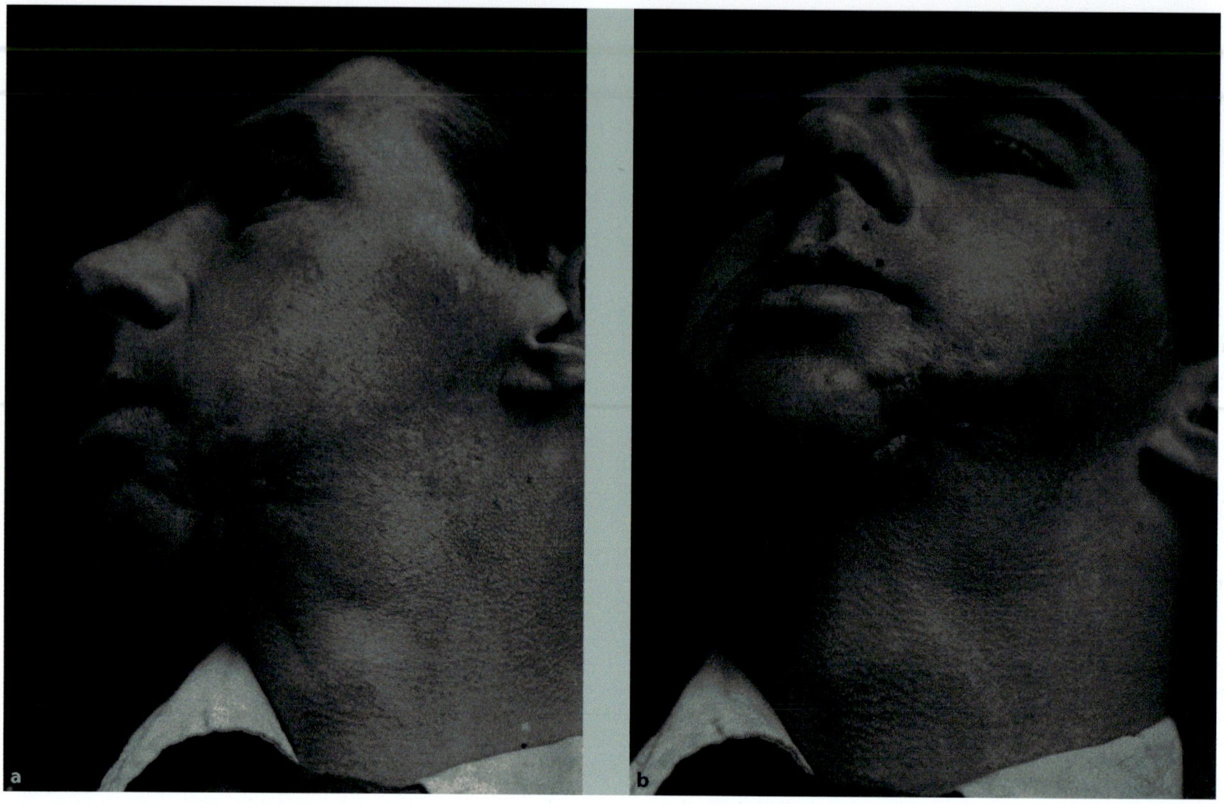

Fig. 5.4a,b A case of loss of the central portion of the mandible, bone grafted by Thomas P. Kilner at Sidcup during World War I. He became Nuffield Professor of Plastic Surgery in Oxford. Reproduced by permission of the Gillies Archives, Queen Mary's Hospital, Sidcup, UK

Mangold then applied the procedure to correct a saddle nose in two different patients in 1900. The first was a 15-year-old girl whose nose had been destroyed by lupus, while the second was a boy whose nostrils "flapped in the wind like veils". Mangold repaired the deformity by inserting a piece of cartilage 4.5 cm long, 1 cm wide and 1.5 cm thick harvested from the costal cartilage of the seventh rib. He described the operation as follows: "A small incision was made across the glabella, the skin was undermined with a small Kocker's forceps down to the tip of the nose and the graft was inserted so that it would hold the tip up … The side of the graft that was not covered by perichondrium was placed under the skin … two small tongues of cartilage were placed in the wings of the nostrils." In a second step, the surgeon carried out a V-Y plasty to correct the tip of the nose.

Mangold was a genuine pioneer in the area of cartilage grafts and a figure of some stature in the scientific community, but regretfully little or nothing is known about the man himself. Both W. Bethmann of Leipzig and the plastic surgeon Leo Clodius of Zurich have attempted to research his biography, as Frank McDowell notes [636], but without success. It seems that Friedrich Mangold practised at Karola Children's Hospital in Dresden-Almstad, but the hospital was completely destroyed by bombs in 1945 and all of its records were lost. Mangold died at the age of 49 from an infection caught during the dissection of a cadaver.

Paul Bert, who we have already encountered in the chapter on skin grafts, also carried out experiments on cartilage grafts and concluded that they could survive and even lead to the formation of bone [83–86]. He also confirmed, after comparing autografts with heterografts, that the recipient bed was crucial to the success or failure of a graft. These studies were followed by investigations into the survival of chondrocytes and the cartilaginous

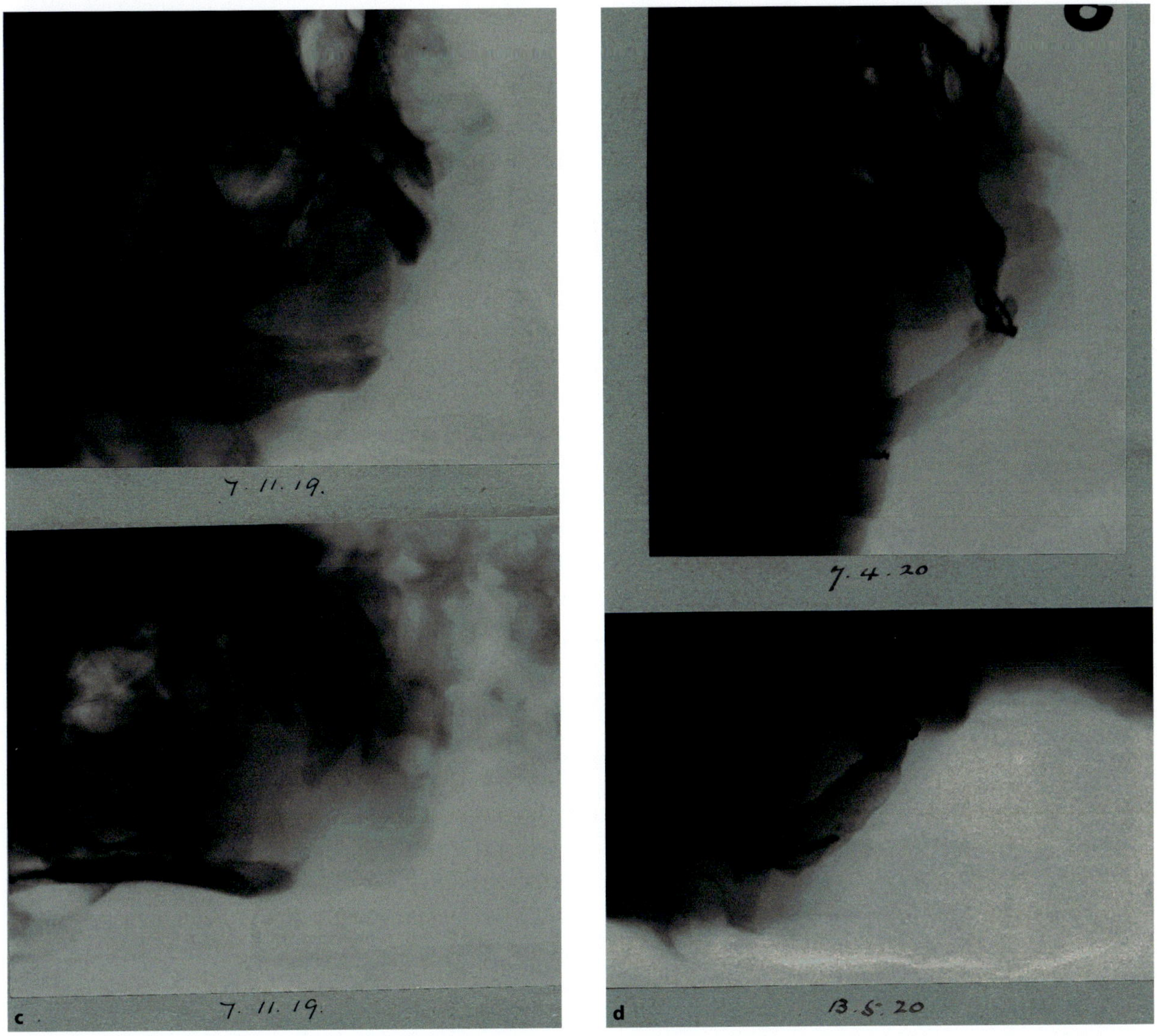

Fig. 5.4c,d *(continued)* A case of loss of the central portion of the mandible, bone grafted. Reproduced by permission of the Gillies Archives, Queen Mary's Hospital, Sidcup, UK

matrix in graft tissue, including homografts and preserved tissue. But here, as with bone grafts, disagreements arose. For example, F.W. Zahn [1056, 1057] contested Bert's conclusions, declaring that adult cartilage was almost always reabsorbed, whereas foetal cartilage often survived and even produced bone.

Fisher transplanted costal cartilage with and without perichondrium to reconstruct the ear and the nose and concluded that perichondrial tissue was not essential to the survival of the graft [318]. Hippolyte Morestin (1868–1919) successfully used cartilage to reconstruct defects of the orbital, malar and mandibular bone [701]. Heinrich Hellferich (1851–1945) also transplanted epiphyseal cartilage and discovered through histological studies that the closer the cells were located to the perichondrium, the better their chances of survival [425, 426].

In this period, the development of a saddle nose due to lupus was common and cartilage was often used to correct the defect. A paper published in 1902 by the French surgeon Charles Nélaton (1851–1911) reported his success with this operation [725, 726], while Mauclaire cites the excellent results obtained by Morestin, Koenig,

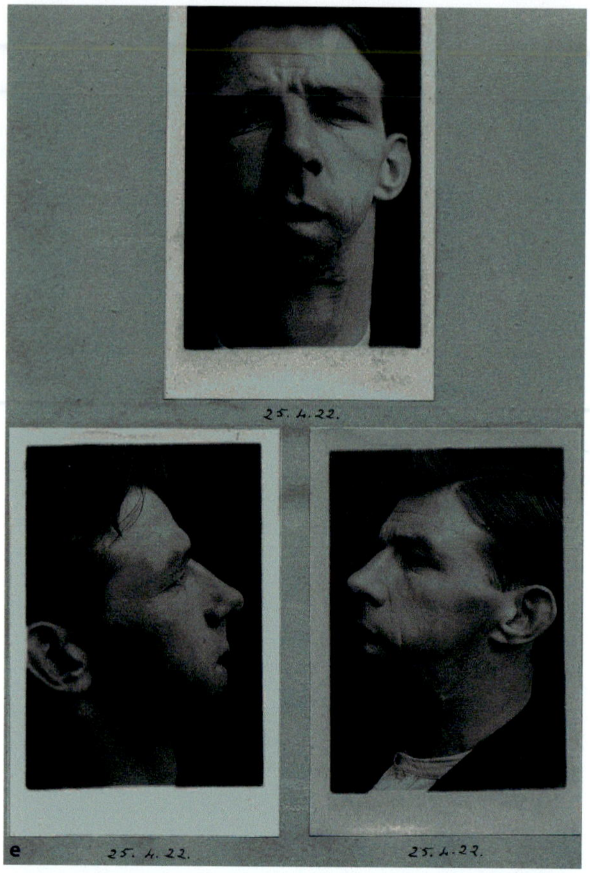

Fig. 5.4e *(continued)* A case of loss of the central portion of the mandible (post-operative view). Reproduced by permission of the Gillies Archives, Queen Mary's Hospital, Sidcup, UK

Henly, Johnson and Carte, sometimes with grafts placed directly under the skin of the nose and in other cases by implanting the cartilage under the flap destined for the nasal reconstruction (Figs. 5.5, 5.6) [618, 619].

Morestin used a piece of costal cartilage to reconstruct the tarsal plate of a patient's lower eyelid, and reported after one year that this tissue was still present and intact. According to Mauclaire [618, 619], Lotheinsen used costal cartilage to close a cranial defect in 1902, and in orthopaedic patients to fill osteomyelitic cavities with cartilage.

While most reports of nasal reconstruction describe the use of cartilage to rebuild the dorsum, Dubrueil [255] applied cartilage with great skill to recreate the alar of the nose. Others adopted cartilage grafts to reconstruct ears or, like Buddinger in 1900, to repair the tarsus of an eyelid. Mauclaire mentions all of these achievements, but nevertheless remained sceptical about the survival of cartilage grafts, although he did concede that the reabsorption of the graft was compensated for by its gradual replacement with fibrous tissue.

Heterografts with cartilage taken from animals were also attempted, but it seems that these invariably failed, although Morestin claimed that he successfully repaired a skull defect with such a graft. Then in 1923 Harold Neuhof [729] reported the results of detailed histological studies on the outcome of animal grafts in human recipients. He determined that over time the cartilage was absorbed and replaced with fibrous tissue, but that even so it could be used to repair the nose and ear with good permanent results. Apart from provoking a slight reaction in the host tissues, it provided supporting fibrotic tissue and the nose was still flexible. Like his colleagues, Neuhof used costal cartilage for his nasal reconstructions, inserting the graft into a subcutaneous pocket in the flap that was destined to be transferred to the nose.

In contrast, the results of his skull reconstructions were not as satisfactory and his experiments with homografting portions of joints were a total failure. He made his first attempt in 1907. After excising the upper third of the tibia in a sarcoma patient, he attempted to replace it with a partial joint taken from the amputated limb of another patient. This graft failed, but he mentions the names of a series of colleagues including Wolf and Muetter whom, he claims, carried out the same operation successfully.

In the period just before World War II, Lyndon A. Peer conducted a series of studies on cartilage grafts, publishing his results in the 1950s [783, 785, 786]. He demonstrated that the nasal septum, costal cartilage and ears were excellent sources of graft tissue both with and without perichondrium. He also challenged Neuhof's theory of bone regeneration, for he found neither resorption of the graft tissue nor invasion of the site by the surrounding tissues. His conclusions were convincing since he managed to follow-up some of his patients for 14 years.

Cartilage is still used for grafts today, because it is easy to harvest and carve and will maintain its form and volume for a long period of time, properties that make it invaluable for the reconstruction of the nose and the ear.

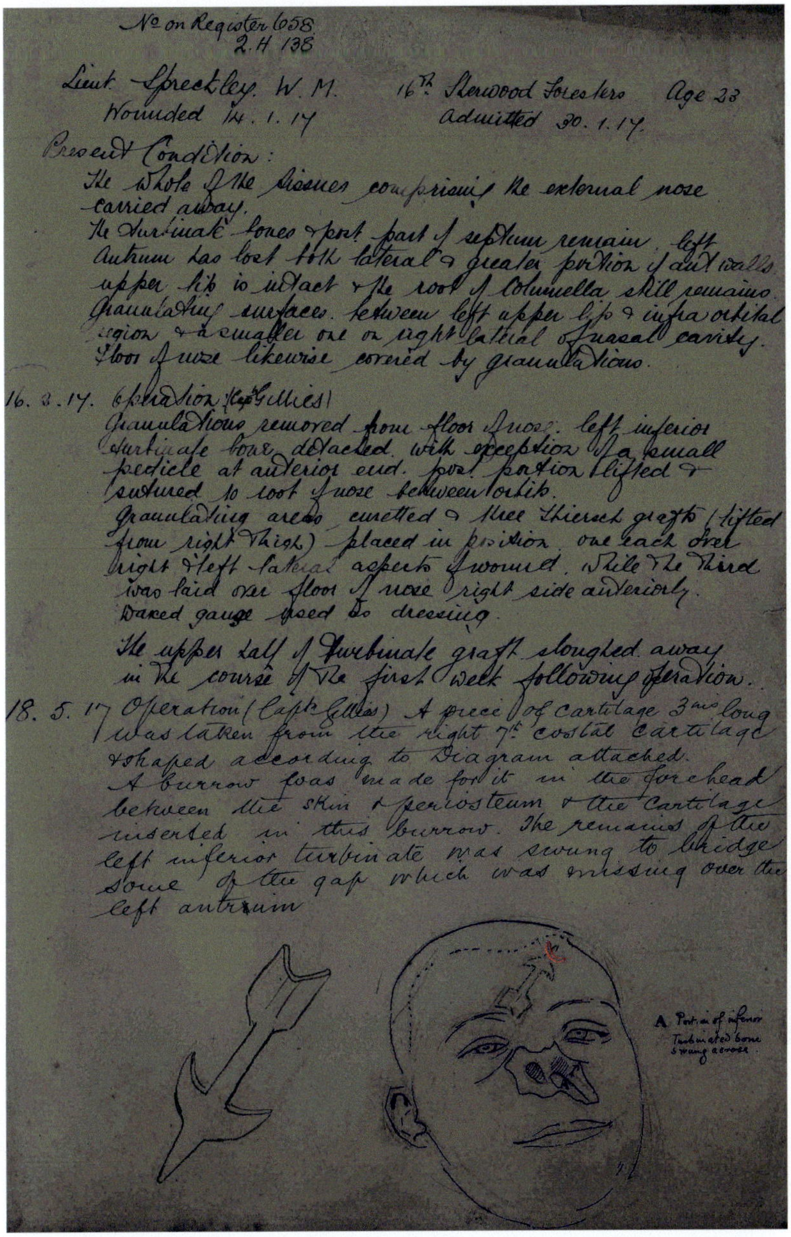

No on Register 658
2.H 138

Lieut. Spreckley. W. M. 16th Sherwood Foresters Age 23
Wounded 14.1.17 admitted 30.1.17.

Present Condition:
The whole of the tissues comprising the external nose carried away.
The turbinate bones & post. part of septum remain. left antrum has lost both lateral & greater portion of ant. walls
upper lip is intact & the root of columella still remains.
Granulating surfaces between left upper lip & infra orbital region & a smaller one on right lateral of nasal cavity.
Floor of nose likewise covered by granulations.

16.3.17. Operation (Capt Gillies)
Granulations removed from floor of nose. left inferior turbinate bone detached with exception of a small pedicle at anterior end. post. portion lifted & sutured to root of nose between orbits.
Granulating areas curetted & three Thiersch grafts (lifted from right thigh) placed in position, one each over right & left lateral aspects of wound, while the third was laid over floor of nose right side anteriorly.
Waxed gauze used as dressing.
The upper half of turbinate graft sloughed away in the course of the first week following operation.

18.5.17 Operation (Capt Gillies) A piece of cartilage 3ins long was taken from the right 7th costal cartilage & shaped according to Diagram attached.
A burrow was made for it in the forehead between the skin & periosteum & the cartilage inserted in this burrow. The remains of the left inferior turbinate was swung to bridge some of the gap which was missing over the left antrum

A. Portion of inferior Turbinated bone swung across.

Fig. 5.5 A sketch and operation notes made by Gillies following the insertion of a cartilage graft under the skin of the forehead which was subsequently used in a flap for nasal reconstruction (see Fig. 5.6). Reproduced by permission of the Gillies Archives, Queen Mary's Hospital, Sidcup, UK

Fat Grafting

While free grafts of fat tissue have been used since the nineteenth century, the procedure has never won the complete acceptance amongst surgeons. The technique has always been limited due to the high failure rate and the associated risk of infection.

The first surgeon to attempt the fat graft seems to have been Gustav Adolf Neuber (1850–1932) in 1893 [728]. He transferred fat tissue to correct an unsightly depressed scar in the periorbital region and the operation was a complete success, as Morton and Norman recorded [716], describing the surgeon's elation at the absence of complications. Neuber reported his results to

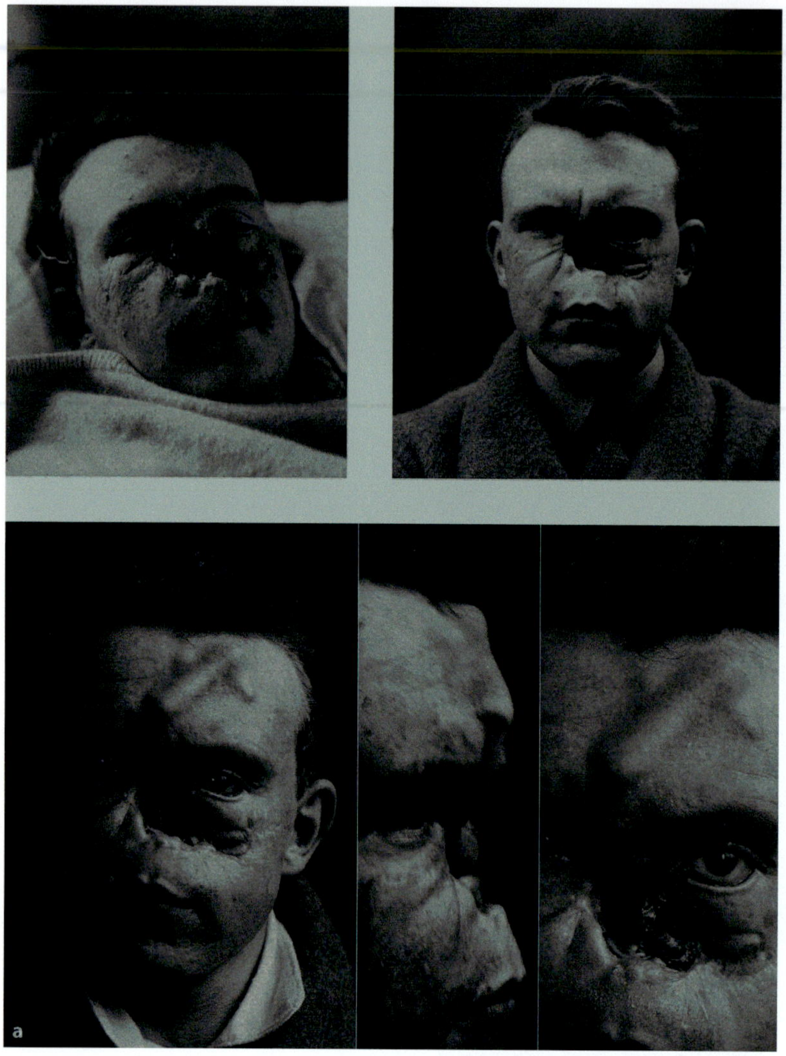

Fig. 5.6a,b Pre-operative views of the patient in Fig. 5.5 showing the cartilage beneath the forehead skin. Reproduced by permission of the Gillies Archives, Queen Mary's Hospital, Sidcup, UK

the German Surgical Society, recommending that surgeons who adopted this procedure employ many small grafts of fat tissue because these had a greater chance of surviving. "Pieces larger than a walnut"—at least in his experience—showed a high failure rate. Neuber furthermore reported that his attempts to use fat tissue to fill bone cavities were not successful due to the nearly complete lack of blood vessels in their walls.

When other surgeons heard of Neuber's exploit they quickly followed suit. Just three years later in 1896, P. Silex reported the use of fat grafting to correct depressed scars around the eyes, noting that the technique not only served to fill the defect but also prevented the skin from re-attaching to the orbital bone beneath the scar [927]. In the same year F. Verderame correctly noted a certain drawback to the procedure—the tendency of the graft to contract due to scarring or resorption and therefore recommended over-correcting for the defect [1012]. More than ten years later Erich Lexer (1867–1937) published a paper entitled Cosmetic Fat Transplants in which he described the use of fat grafting to correct the saddle nose defect, large defects in the breast, and even a case of facial hemiatrophy [559, 560].

From these disparate results one may deduce that there was some unpredictability in the results of fat grafting. Morestin however firmly believed in its utility and in 1912 reported his experience with the repair of depressions in various regions of the face using the technique [698, 699].

An unusual graft was carried out in 1910 by A. Bier. He utilized a lipoma to correct a case of facial hemiatrophy [94]. Earlier Vincenz Czerny (1842–1916) had ex-

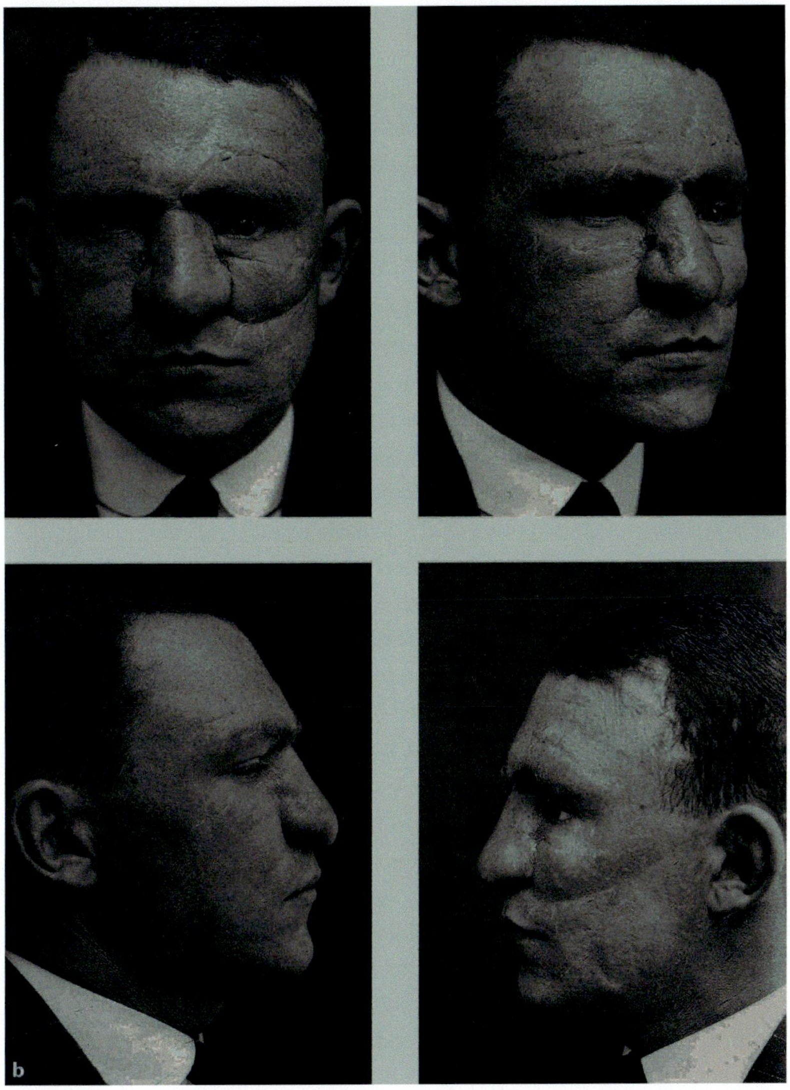

Fig. 5.6a,b *(continued)* Post-operative views of the patient in Fig. 5.5 showing the cartilage beneath the forehead skin. Reproduced by permission of the Gillies Archives, Queen Mary's Hospital, Sidcup, UK

cised an entire lipoma and transferred it to fill the defect in a breast that had been treated for fibrocystic mastitis [211].[8] It appears that this operation was successful and the lipoma was not reabsorbed. Lipomas were used by other surgeons, some of whom observed that the tumour stopped growing once it was grafted, but they did not speculate on the possible reasons for this. Breast reconstructions with fat were also attempted in 1911 by Stieda [960] and one year later by Klap [497] and Goebel [382], but unfortunately we do not know the long-term outcome of these operations. In 1959 John Watson published a review on the application of free fat grafts in mammoplasty [1036]. The results of all these efforts were dependent on the amount of resorption that took place and it seems that the various techniques advocated to minimize this problem were never completely successful [228]. The arrival of silicone implants largely superseded the use of free fat grafts for breast augmentation.

The interpositioning of fat was used to prevent recurrence after the treatment of ankylosis of the temporomandibular joint by Bier, Neuhof and Lexer in the

8 In 1913 Rigollot-Simonnot [841] used a homograft of lipoma to correct a depressed scar, but did not report the results of his operation. We do have the report of an autograft lipoma carried out by Péraire and Bonamy in 1914—Tumeur des deux seins cher une femme et transplantation lipomateuse. Bull Mem Soc Chir Paris 2:60.

reports already mentioned. Fat grafts have also been employed on occasions by neurosurgeons; for example, by Bonnet in 1915 [618, 619], Rehn [832, 833] and Eden [272]. In more or less the same period, Rehn and Eden conducted experiments with fat grafts in rabbits [273].

Again it was who conducted histological studies that shed crucial light on the behaviour of the fat graft. In 1923 he reported the results of detailed studies on a series of fat grafts that he had followed for a period of several months. He demonstrated that after 6 months one could see fat escaping from the many dead cells of the graft, only to be formed into cysts. In addition, he noted extensive fibrosis and the formation of enlarged adipose cells. The graft seemed to be stable at this point, but as the author prudently observed: “Its final destiny was more than a little unpredictable.” These studies ought to have laid to rest the dispute over the outcome of fat grafts, but the argument continued between supporters of the cell replacement theory, who claimed that the histiocytes eventually absorbed the fat freed from the dead adipose cells, and the advocates of the cell survival theory, who insisted that the fat was actually maintained in surviving hypertrophic adipose cells.

Independently of these opposing theories, there was general agreement that fat grafts tend to shrink over time. Lyndon Peer demonstrated that large grafts (exceeding 250 g) undergo a reduction in size of around 45%, while smaller grafts did better and could maintain up to 75% of their original size.. At this point, since it was clear that the only reason why small grafts survived best was because they became vascularized more readily, efforts were directed at this process.

This point had already been explored by Bert in 1865 (Fig. 5.7) and his conclusions were confirmed by Carl Thiersch (1822–1895) [1036] and later by Davis and Traut in 1925 [226]. If vascularization could be improved, particularly in the initial stages, it was assumed that the quantity of surviving tissue would increase. In 1929 O. Loewe had the insight to suggest that skin dermis might be included with the fat tissue, not only to add support and density to a graft that otherwise was often almost liquid in consistency, but also to facilitate vascularization [573]. In 1936–1937 Peer [784] and then Peer and Paddock in 1937 [787] studied the outcome of the dermo-fat autografts and showed that 45% of the tissue would survive if it exceeded 250 g. It appeared that the vascularization of fat grafts was improved when dermis was included and today when seeking to correct a small defect such as a depressed scar on the face, the surgeon is much more likely to use a dermal graft than a fat graft.

The use of these free grafts developed over many years beginning with early experiments, progressing to tentative clinical applications and then finding an accepted place in reconstructive surgery. Some of them have failed or been abandoned because of complications. Skin grafts are a mainstay of plastic surgery. Bone grafts are used in plastic surgery but have mainly become the province of the orthopaedic surgeon. Cartilage is occasionally used and free grafts of dermis and fat are a rarity. When free grafting techniques were added to the flaps which were already established, reconstructive options became much wider. At this stage in our history we should conclude by mentioning the advent of microvascular techniques. They have added another dimension to the story and when large compound defects following trauma or cancer resection need to be reconstructed, other tissues such as bone as well as skin can be transplanted reliably at one operation (Fig. 5.8a–c) [973, 974].

The fibula alone or with skin has also been transfered microsurgically to treat long bone defects.

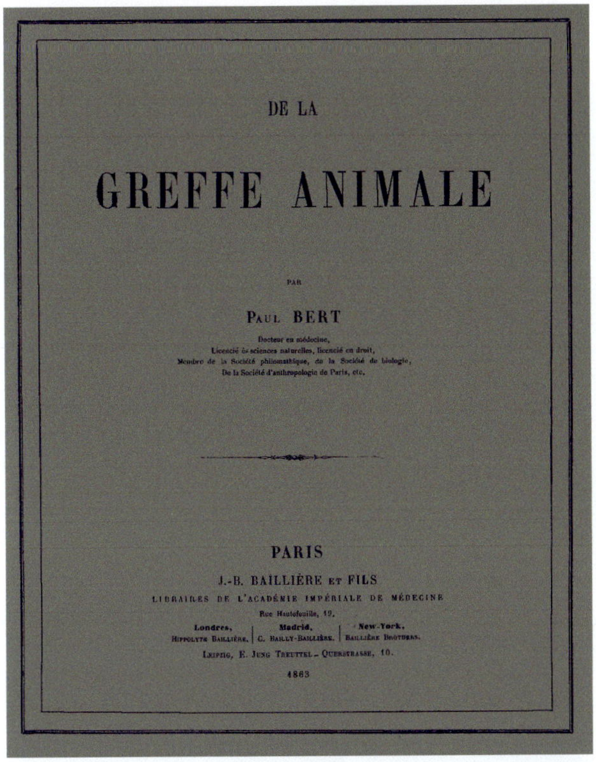

DE LA

GREFFE ANIMALE

PAR

PAUL BERT

Docteur en médecine,
Licencié ès sciences naturelles, licencié en droit,
Membre de la Société philomathique, de la Société de biologie,
De la Société d'anthropologie de Paris, etc.

PARIS

J.-B. BAILLIÈRE ET FILS

LIBRAIRES DE L'ACADÉMIE IMPÉRIALE DE MÉDECINE

Rue Hautefeuille, 19.

Londres, Hippolyte Baillière. | Madrid, C. Bailly-Baillière. | New-York, Baillière Brothers.

Leipzig, E. Jung Treuttel – Querstrasse, 10.

1863

Fig. 5.7 Frontispiece of Paul Bert's most important work La Greffe Animale (1863). He continued where Baronio left off and was probably the first to suggest the terms autograft, homograft and heterograft. His contribution to the understanding of the behaviour of cartilage grafts was very important. Courtesy of Riccardo Mazzola M.D., Milan

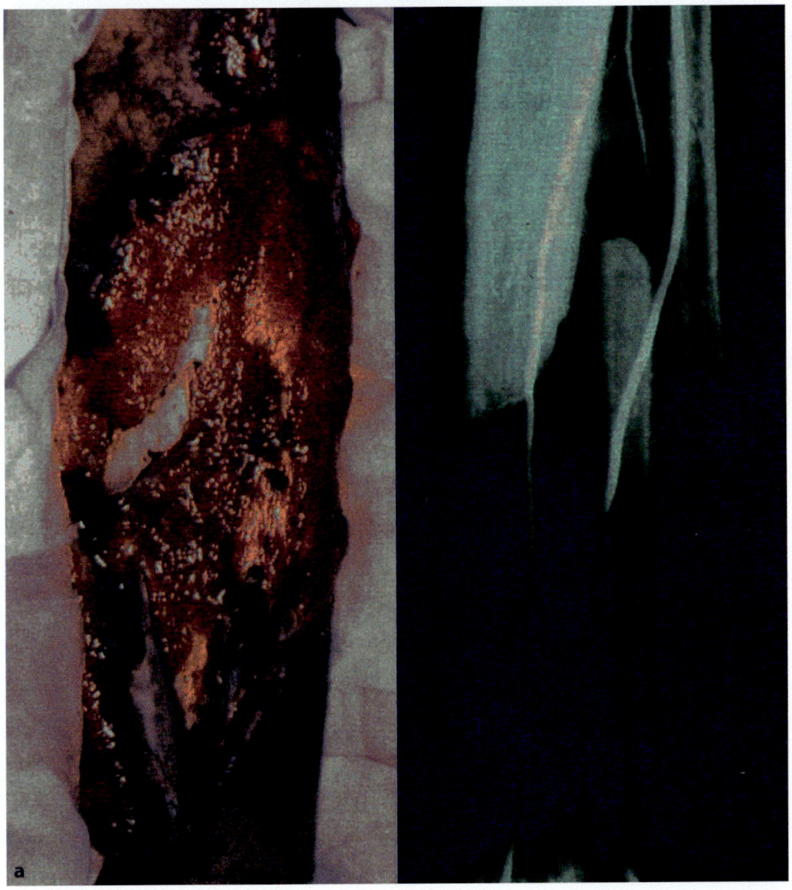

Fig. 5.8 A road accident victim from 1975. **a** A compound fracture of the tibia with segmental bone and skin loss. **b, c** *see next page*

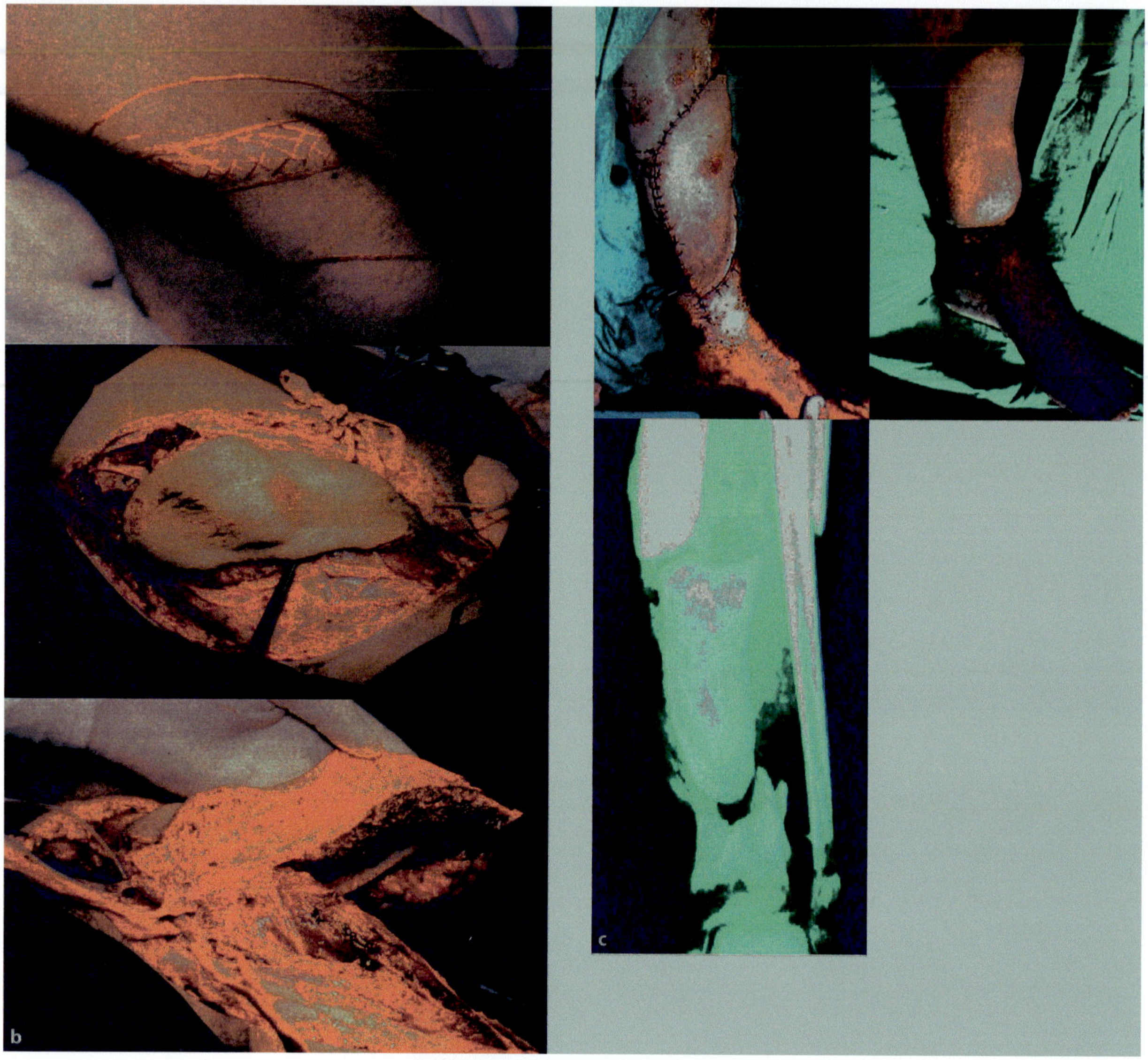

Fig. 5.8 *(continued)* A road accident victim from 1975. **b, c** Microsurgical transfer of iliac crest bone and skin using the deep circumflex iliac vessels. The flap was bulky and further orthopaedic surgery was required to treat bony non-union. PSR

Chapter 6

Some Notes on Anaesthesia

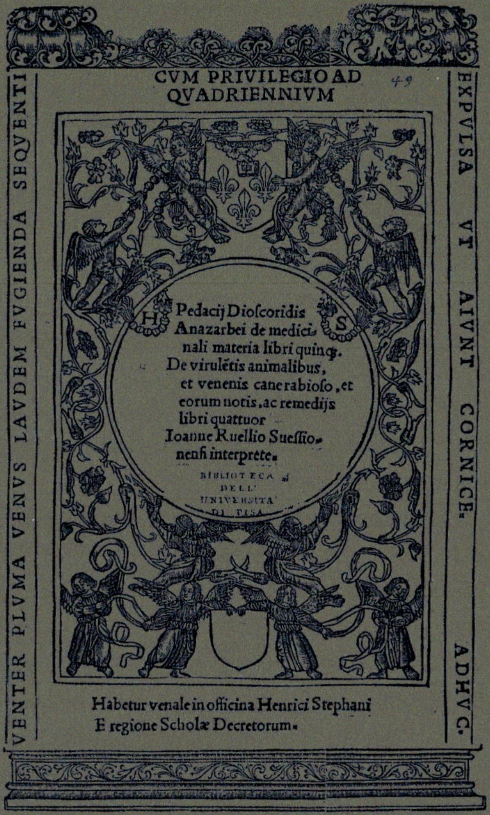
CVM PRIVILEGIO AD QVADRIENNIVM

Pedacij Dioſcoridis Anazarbei de medicinali materia libri quinq.
De viruletis animalibus, et venenis cane rabioſo, et eorum notis, ac remedijs libri quattuor
Ioanne Ruellio Sueſſionenſi interprete.

Habetur venale in officina Henrici Stephani E regione Scholæ Decretorum.

VENTER PLVMA VENVS LAVDEM FVGIENDA SEQVENTI EXPVLSA VT AIVNT CORNICE ADHVC.

Contents

And the Lord God caused a deep sleep to fall upon Adam and he slept and he took one of his ribs and closed up the flesh instead thereof … *Genesis 2, 21*

In the work *Triumph Over Pain* (1938), René Fulop-Miller [345] observed that primitive man considered pain to be the work of the devil or malign spirits. They could be overcome if one had the will and courage to fight them. Healers, priests and magicians were called upon to assist in the battle by inducing a state of hypnosis in the patient possessed by the evil spirits. With the advent of Christianity, magic was replaced by the power of prayer—no doubt often reinforced by alcohol. Indeed, some have maliciously suggested that this was the one of the reasons why so many monasteries engaged in the production of beer, wine and spirits. Although there is no proof for this theory, it is a fact that up to and beyond the year 1000 A.D. it was primarily among the religious orders that those who practised the medical arts were to be found. They dispensed medicines but did no surgery which involved shedding blood.

Surprisingly, sophisticated surgical techniques were first developed in those areas of the world where plants extracts with powerful sedative effects were available for example opium in India (where nasal reconstructions were being carried out in 1500 B.C.) and coca in Mesoamerica. *Datura stramonium*, a plant with strong analgesic properties, was known in both Asia and pre-Columbian America. Other narcotics that were traditionally used in rituals or for recreational purposes, for example mescaline, also have analgesic properties.

In the ancient civilizations of the West a variety of botanical preparations were employed as painkillers (Fig. 6.1). The Egyptians, followed by the Arabs, were well acquainted with the analgesic properties of the poppy (*Papaver somniferum*) and hemp (*Cannabis indica*). A clay tablet dating from 2500 B.C. found among the ruins of the Palace of Nineveh in Mesopotamia tells us that a mixture of henbane seeds (*hyoscyamus*) and gum was chewed by the Babylonians to sooth toothache. Hemlock (*Conium maculatum*), lettuce-opium (*Lactucarium*), and the mandrake (*Atropa mandragora*) were used by the Egyptians, Babylonians and Hebrews. They also seem to have been familiar to the ancient Greeks and Romans. Celsus, Pliny the elder and the seventh century surgeon Paolus Aegineta of Alexandria used them. One of the first to describe the mandrake and its properties was Dioscorides Pedacius around 60 B.C. in his book *De Medicina Materia* (Fig. 6.2)

The medical text of Susruta, a work of immense antiquity, mentions henbane and hemp and the surgeons of ancient India no doubt knew of and used other plants capable of relieving pain. T.E. Keys [492]. The *Pandit* or Hindu scholar Vallala (925 B.C.) employed two drugs during cranial operations, one to induce an unconscious state (*sammohini*) and another to reawaken the patient (*sanyibani*), but disappointingly the exact nature of the drugs is not recorded.[1]

References to simple analgesics can be found in many classical texts. In Greece a potion called *nepenthe*[2] attributed to the god of healing Aesculapius was used to anaesthetize patients (c.400 B.C.). Greek and Roman physicians also wrote of a remarkable mineral which they found had analgesic properties, the "stone of Menphis". As Marcus Kleiman [499] explains, this stone probably contained carbonates that produced carbon dioxide, a gas that could have a mild sedative effect, when exposed to vinegar. The mandrake root was cited by the Romans as an effective anodyne (Fig. 6.3); Pliny (79 A.D.) administered it in wine, while the military surgeon Dioscorides Pedacius (54 A.D.) wrote that "the mixture of mandrake and wine" could be taken orally, administered as an enema or inhaled as a vapour (Fig. 6.4).[3] Chauncey D. Laeke recently suggested that the plant they knew may have contained an alkaloid with an effect on the nervous

1 This information can be found in Pandit Vallala's work, *Bohja Prabandha*.

2 Nepenthe is first known to have been used in Egypt, and is the drug that Helen slipped into Ulysses' wine in the *Odyssey*. Mention of its use as an anaesthetic is not rare in the literature; we can find nepenthe cited in the Talmud (Samme de Shinta), in *The Arabian Nights* (*bhang*) and finally by Shakespeare in *Othello* ("drowsy syrup").

3 Pedacius Dioscorides was a Greek surgeon who served in the army of the emperor Nero from 54 to 68 A.D. He described about 600 plants and plant essences in what is probably the first work on botanical medicine as an applied science. The principles of Dioscorides were followed unquestioningly by physicians and botanists for many centuries in Europe. See Figs. 6.2–6.4.

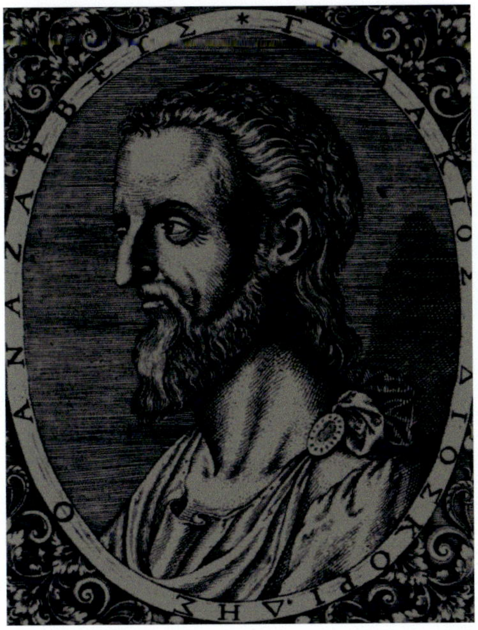

Fig. 6.1 Portrait of Dioscorides Pedacius (c.50 A.D.). Among his extensive studies on the properties of herbs he described the mandrake and its analgesic effects. *Courtesy of the Library of the University of Pisa*

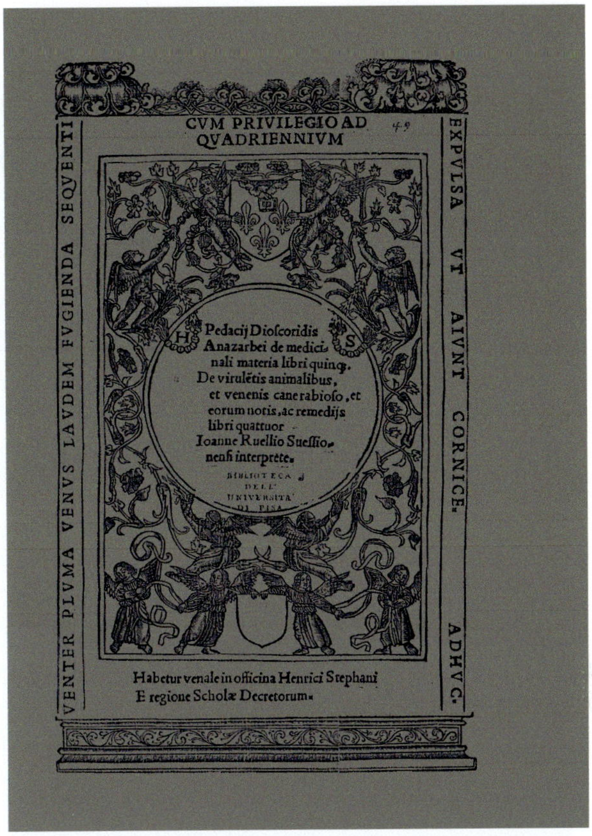

Fig. 6.2 Frontispiece of the first edition of Dioscorides Pedacius' work *Anazarbeo de Materia Medica*. *Courtesy of the Library of the University of Pisa*

system similar to that of atropine. The mandrake was also known in ancient China; documents record its use by the physician Pien Ch'iao around 225 B.C. and by Hua T'o in 220 A.D.

The *Scuola Salernitana* perfected what they called the *confetio soporis* (sleeping potion). Apart from henbane and hemp, which in India were burned so that their smoke could be inhaled, this combination probably represents the first inhalation anaesthetic in the history of medicine. In reality the ingredients, opium, hyoscyamine, mulberry juice, lettuce-opium, hemlock and ivy, were already well known. They were cited by Dioscorides,[4] again in the *Pharmacopoeia of Bamberg* [732] and also in the *Montecassino Codex* [492]. The "sleeping potion" was quite simple to prepare and use: a sponge was soaked in a solution containing all the ingredients, allowed to dry, and then stored until needed. Just before the operation, the sponge could be dampened and placed over the mouth of the patient, who would then inhale its volatile substances.

Ugo Borgognoni and his son Theodorico, Bishop of Cervia (1205–1298) [122, 981] modified the recipe contained in the *Pharmacopoeia of Nicola*, and their *spongia soporifera* proved so effective that it was adopted all over Italy. Foreign physicians such as Henry de Mondeville who came to study at Bologna University took their

4 See *Dyascorides de Herbis Feminini* where the first description of the *spongia soporiphera* may be found. This was first produced in Latin and later translated into the Florentine dialect in 1597.

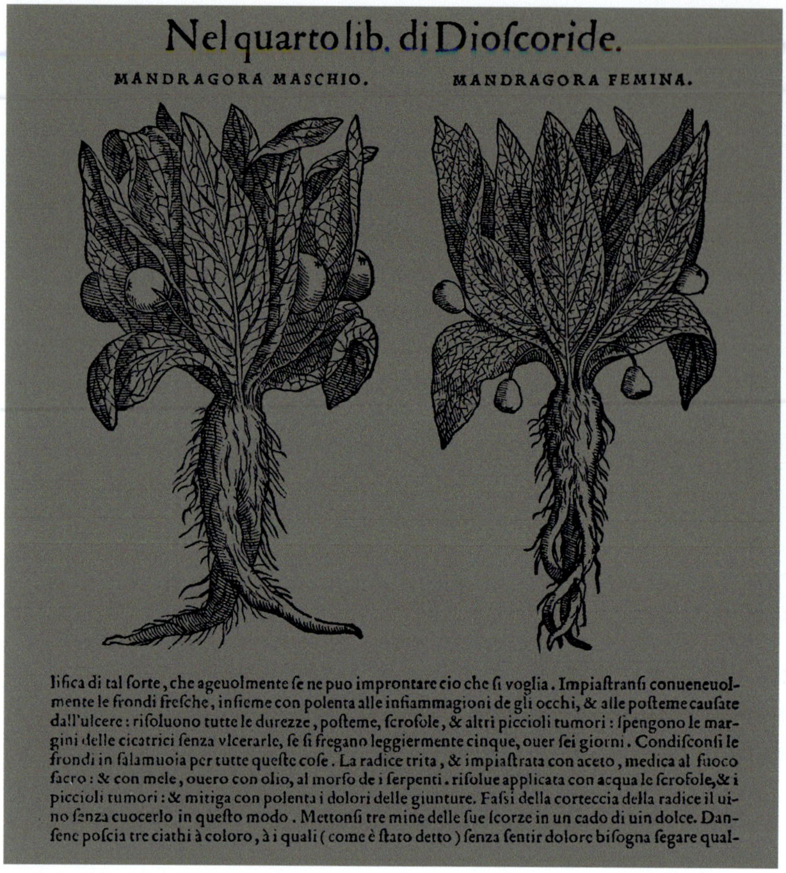

Nel quarto lib. di Dioſcoride.

MANDRAGORA MASCHIO. MANDRAGORA FEMINA.

lifica di tal ſorte, che ageuolmente ſe ne puo improntare cio che ſi voglia. Impiaſtranſi conueneuolmente le frondi freſche, inſieme con polenta alle infiammagioni de gli occhi, & alle poſteme cauſate dall'ulcere: riſoluono tutte le durezze, poſteme, ſcrofole, & altri piccioli tumori: ſpengono le margini delle cicatrici ſenza vlcerarle, ſe ſi fregano leggiermente cinque, ouer ſei giorni. Condiſconſi le frondi in ſalamuoia per tutte queſte coſe. La radice trita, & impiaſtrata con aceto, medica al fuoco ſacro: & con mele, ouero con olio, al morſo de i ſerpenti. riſolue applicata con acqua le ſcrofole, & i piccioli tumori: & mitiga con polenta i dolori delle giunture. Faſsi della corteccia della radice il uino ſenza cuocerlo in queſto modo. Mettonſi tre mine delle ſue ſcorze in un cado di uin dolce. Danſene poſcia tre ciathi à coloro, à i quali (come è ſtato detto) ſenza ſentir dolore biſogna ſegare qual-

Fig. 6.3 A page from the fourth book of Dioscorides *Anazarbei de Medicali Materia* translated by Ioanne Ruello where the mandrake and its effects are described in detail. *Courtesy of the Library of the University of Pisa*

knowledge of this innovative technique back to their own countries. Theodorico provides a detailed description of the sponge in his surgical text *Cyrurgia*, concluding with the following instructions: "to reawaken the patient, apply repeatedly to his nostrils a sponge soaked in vinegar". At the *Scuola Salernitana* a sponge soaked in fennel juice was preferred for this purpose!

During the sixteenth century, the philosopher Giambattista della Porta claims to have introduced improvements to Theodorico's *spongia soporifera* that made it even more effective in inducing a profound state of sleep. From the same period, references can be found suggesting that a certain Valerio Cordus managed to synthesize a gas similar to ether, but he does not appear to have employed this as an anaesthetic.

Various techniques not involving drugs were used to relieve the pain of operations including cold, concussion, hypnosis and blood letting. Carotid compression is said to have been tried and Parė in the sixteenth century used nerve compression.

Inhalation Anaesthesia

Joseph Priestley [346, 816] swimming somewhat against the tide, emigrated from America to England in 1791. He promulgated the thesis that inhaling oxygen could be beneficial to patients suffering from lung diseases. Soon physicians on both sides of the Atlantic were using oxygen and nitrogen to treat asthma, catarrh and consumption. In 1795 another American, the chemist Latham S. Mitchell, declared that nitrous oxide was poisonous and indeed a "principle of contagion" that could serve as a vector for the spread of infection. Undeterred by this alarming hypothesis, a medical student and chemist Humphrey Davy [227] tried inhaling the gas himself and discovered that instead of having a noxious effect it induced rather pleasant sensations, including the irresistible impulse to laugh. In 1800 the young man, who was a surgeon's assistant at the time, suggested that the substance (which came to be known as *laughing gas*) might be used as an anaesthetic, and its effectiveness was later

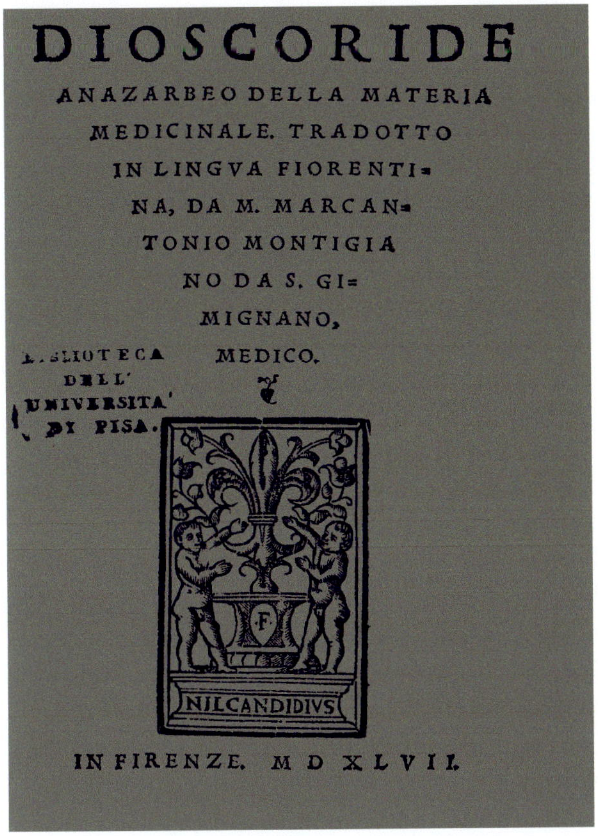

DIOSCORIDE
ANAZARBEO DELLA MATERIA
MEDICINALE. TRADOTTO
IN LINGVA FIORENTI-
NA, DA M. MARCAN-
TONIO MONTIGIA
NO DA S. GI-
MIGNANO,
MEDICO.

IN FIRENZE. M D XLVII.

Fig. 6.4 Frontispiece of the translation into Italian (Florentine at that time) of Dioscorides' book by Marcantonio Montigi of San Giminiano, Tuscany in 1547. *Courtesy of the Library of the University of Pisa*

demonstrated by William Allen during an operation carried out in the presence of Sir Astley Cooper at Guy's Hospital in London. In 1844 Horace Wells of Boston gave a public demonstration of the gas which was unsuccessful and met with cries of "humbug" [179].

Michael Faraday [302], who had studied under Davy, conducted his own experiments in 1818 using various agents and it did not escape him that ether had a marked soporific effect. Henry Hill Hickman [430], a member of the *Royal College of Surgeons* in both London and Edinburgh, tested the effects of CO_2 on animals but his attempts to demonstrate his findings before his colleagues in London, and then in Paris where he had been invited by Baron Larrey, a military surgeon in Napoleon's army, failed ignominiously.

In the meantime, clandestine *laughing gas parties* and *ether frolics*—the nineteenth century equivalent of today's pot and cocaine parties, where mixtures of nitrous oxide and ether were inhaled—had become quite the rage in America. William E. Clarke, a young chemistry student from Rochester, New York, who had attended a few such parties and noted the analgesic effect of the gas, had the brilliant notion of testing its efficacy as a dental anaesthetic. On a cold January day in the year 1842 he administered ether to a certain Miss Hobbie, impregnating a towel with the fluid and asking her to inhale the fumes while being operated on by her dentist, Dr. Elijah Pope.

Learning about the effects of laughing gas and ether the surgeon Crawford W. Long (1815–1878) [574] in the town of Jefferson, Georgia, persuaded a friend, Mr. James M. Vanble, to undergo anaesthesia with ether before he began surgery to remove two benign tumours from his neck. The courage of the surgeon, and above all of the patient, was amply rewarded for the experiment proved a resounding success. The patient declared that he had felt no pain whatsoever and remembered little or nothing of the operation. Long continued to use this technique, but only published an account of it in 1849 [516].

In September 1846, a dental surgeon by the name of William T. Morton unaware of Long's work but knowing that ether was being used as a topic local anaesthetic, consulted his former professor, the physician and chemist Carl Thomas Jackson (1805–1880), regarding how ether inhalation might be used during surgery. After testing the effects on himself and an assistant he began using the gas in his orthodontic operations, following Jackson's instructions. Unlike Long, Morton published his findings immediately, in the form of a letter to the *American Journal of Dental Science* [713]. As G. Hayward [420] recounts, he also tried without success to have his gas patented under the name of *Letheon*.

Of much greater consequence to the history of surgery, Morton offered his services to John C. Warren, chief surgeon at Massachusetts General Hospital.[5] Much interested in his discovery, Warren not only agreed to

5 John Collins Warren was the son of John Warren (1753–1815), founder of the renowned Harvard Medical School, and in his turn the father of Jonathan Mason Warren (1811–1867), the first surgeon in the United States to carry out a nasal reconstruction.

attempt an operation with Morton there to administer his remarkable gas, but invited a number of his colleagues to observe the procedure, which took place on the morning of 14 October 1846. Morton never looked back from that momentous day; he abandoned the profession of dentistry and transformed himself into an anaesthetist administering ether during operations using an apparatus of his own design [714–716]. Here is Warren's description of the procedure carried out during an operation to remove an angioma: "The apparatus was applied to the mouth of the patient by Dr Morton for about 3 minutes, at the end of which time he fell into a state of insensibility. I immediately made an incision about 3 inches long through the skin of his neck, and began to dissect the major nerves and blood vessels without any expression of pain on the part of the patient. After a short time he began to speak incoherently and seemed to be in a state of agitation for the remainder of the operation. Immediately afterwards, when asked whether he had suffered greatly, he affirmed that he had felt as if his neck had been scratched, but later when interrogated by me, his declaration was that he did not feel any pain at the time, even if he was aware that the operation was in course."

Following Morton's triumph however, Jackson, who seems to have had an extremely contentious nature, denounced him as a swindler and claimed priority for the discovery of the properties of ether in 1840. Years of litigation followed. Jackson even wrote two letters to Elia de Beaumont, dated 13 November and 1 December 1846, defending his claim, and requested that the French scientist read the letters before the *Académie des Sciences* of Paris. De Beaumont obliged in January 1847. Nevertheless, due to the renown of Massachusetts General Hospital and the prestige of John C. Warren, who was the son of the founder of Harvard Medical School, the operation carried out on 14 October received universal attention and the date has been recognized ever since in the medical world as Ether Day.

The term *anaesthesia* was coined by the poet and physician Oliver Wendell Holmes in a letter which he wrote to Morton on 21 November 1846, explaining how "this signifies insensibility—more particularly [as used by Linnaeus and Cullen] the absence of tactile sensibility". It is perhaps appropriate to recall here that the sense of touch and the sense of pain are closely related as they involve the same neuron pathways.

On 7 November 1846, John C. Warren's son, Jonathan Mason Warren (1811–1867), undertook the first cleft lip repair carried out under general anaesthesia with ether, on a six-hour-old infant (*sic*!).

In the following year Morton published a complete account of his use of ether for surgical anaesthesia but unfortunately another surgeon who had been present as an observer on that historic day, Henry Jacob Bigelow (1818–1890), with an enthusiasm and rapidity perhaps worthy of the inventor himself, presented a communication on the procedure to the *American Academy of Arts* and Sciences on 3 November 1846, followed by an article in the *Boston Medical and Surgical Journal*, and by another communication delivered on 9 November 1846 before the Boston Society for Medical Improvement [98–100].

The news of this remarkable breakthrough, which would revolutionize the practice of surgery, spread like wildfire around the world; in December 1846—just two months after the operation carried out by Warren in Boston–the procedure was already being used in London, with surgeons in the rest of Europe soon following suit [320].

The success of ether as an anaesthesia stimulated research on other agents and in March 1847 the French physiologist M.J.P. Flourens (1794–1867), whose important contributions we have discussed in our chapter on grafts, reported on the effects of chloroform in animals [322, 324]. His paper does not seem to have been read by many surgeons, but one who did immediately grasp its implications was Sir James Young Simpson [929] who already had some experience with ether. He reported that chloroform appeared to be a less irritating substance and began using it on all of his patients, including Queen Victoria during the delivery of her eighth child.

In 1848 Thomas Nunnerly tried to combine ether with other agents with mixed success. Ethylene, which according to Priestley had been discovered in 1779 by Becker and Ingenhouss, was first used as an inhalation anaesthetic by Ludimar Hermann [428]in 1864.

Cyclopropane was first described in 1882 by August von Freund (1835–1892), but was considered too toxic for use as an anaesthetic agent [337, 1035]. Only much later did studies at the University of Wisconsin in the 1930s and then the University of Maryland in 1939 lead to the development of a mixture of ether and cyclopropane that was demonstrated to be effective and less toxic.

Intravenous Anaesthesia

It appears that Sir Christopher Wren, the Royal Architect who built St Paul's Cathedral in London but began his career as an astronomer and physiologist, was the first to conceive the idea of injecting substances into the veins. He carried out his first experiment on a dog in 1656, studying the intoxicating properties of wine and ale by injecting them via a goose quill attached to a pig's bladder directly into one of the animal's veins. He also investigated the effects of a solution of opium, and must have reported good results for within in a short time this solution was being administered to patients.

In this same period, experiments on the transfusion of blood and the intravenous administration of physiological solutions had begun. In 1662 Johann Daniel Major (1634–1693) injected patients with medicinal agents [597], but attempts to administer anaesthetics by this means were not made until the nineteenth century. One of the pioneers of intravenous anaesthesia, according to Keys [492] was N.P. Krawkoiw. Working in Saint Petersburg with a group of close collaborators he introduced the use of methylpropylcarbinol while his Russian colleagues were routinely giving Hedonal (methylpropylcarbinol urethane) to hundreds of patients intravenously. By the outbreak of the First World War a whole battery of anaesthetic drugs was available, not only ether and chloroform, but also agents containing for example procaine hydrochloride, paraldehyde and morphine.

The discovery of barbiturates further increased the armamentarium. Perhaps the first was Pernoston which was introduced by R. Bumm in Germany in 1927. Experiments with other preparations culminated in the discovery of the immensely successful drug Nembutal in 1930 by Fitch, Waters and Tatum [319]. Other reports of thiobarbiturates soon followed [583].

In 1935 Harold Kind identified the active ingredient in curare as *d-tubocurarine* [493]. Claude Bernard had already described the muscle paralysis which this substance induced, after conducting experiments on the neuromuscular end plates in animals [80]. The fascinating history of curare is recounted in two books, one by Kenneth Bryn Thomas (1916–1978) [985] and the other by J. Vellard [1009] and the history of its use in anaesthesia is told in a paper by Harold Randall Griffith and Enid G. Johnson in 1942 [395].

Local Anaesthesia, Regional Anaesthesia and Other Breakthroughs

In 1555 a Spanish explorer, Augustin de Zarate, travelling through Peru observed the peculiar properties of the coca plant. The Indios, who still chew the leaves today, were familiar with the effects in deadening the sense of cold and hunger, but the active principle, cocaine, was only isolated in 1860 by Albert Niemann (1834–1861) [733].

Cocaine was probably first used in the operating theatre in October 1884, when Carl Koller administered the agent intra-nasally and found that it caused the complete anaesthesia of the nasal mucosa. Soon cocaine was being used as a local anaesthetic, by direct application in ophthalmology and intra-nasally in otorhinolaryngology. Otis and Knapp, as Keys writes [492], also recommended cocaine as a local anaesthetic for urethra operations. In an important series of experiments, in 1885 James Leonard Corning (1855–1923) injected cocaine as a spinal anaesthesia first into dogs and then into humans [200]. He noted that when injected subcutaneously it could reduce bleeding for prolonged periods of time in the anaesthetized region [199]. In 1886 he published the first treatise on local anaesthesia [201]. Others were developing similar techniques in Scandinavia around this time [885].

The effect of the juice extracted from the opium poppy was well known in Antiquity and this substance was one of the key ingredients in Theodorico's *spongia soporifera*. The Westphalian surgeon Friedrick Wilhelm Serteurner [918] isolated the active principle in 1806, calling it *morphine*. Laudanum, an alcohol solution containing morphine, became an extremely popular narcotic painkiller in the nineteenth century. In Italy morphine was first used as a local anaesthetic by Spessa during the excision of a fistula in 1871.

The addition of epinephrine (adrenaline) to cocaine (and later other local anaesthetic agents) represented a significant development. Adrenaline's vasoconstrictive effect slowed the resorption of the local anaesthetic, thereby diminishing its toxicity and making it possible to administer larger doses. It also prolonged the anaesthetic effect itself and reduced bleeding.

In Scotland, Alexander Wood (1817–1884) invented the metal needle in 1853 [1048], while in France Charles Pravaz devised a similar needle in the same year. This simple instrument greatly facilitated the administration of drugs, and in 1887 the first local anaesthetic plexus block was successfully carried out.

Further Developments

The administration of inhalation anaesthetics via a mask was very limiting in surgery of the face. This procedure was improved by the invention of various types of masks, the first of which were designed by Warren and Schimmelbusch. Naturally such masks could not be used when the surgeon had to work in or around the mouth and in 1869 Friedrick Trendelenburg (1844–1924) proposed an alternative route for the delivery of the anaesthetic—a tracheostomy [996]. This offered a safe and secure method of anaesthetizing patients who had to undergo long operations on the face or upper airways.

Vesalius in 1543 [1017] and Robert Hooke in 1667 demonstrated that it was possible to insert tubes into the trachea orally and intubation was later used in attempts to resuscitate people who had drowned or been executed by hanging.

It was not until 1858 that John Snow anaesthetized a rabbit using chloroform by inserting a tube into its trachea. In 1878 MacEwen introduced a flexible endotracheal tube which was only 3/8 inches in diameter. It was Franz Kuhn in Germany in 1911 who used a thin-walled tube made of metal, passed through the nose to administer anaesthesia in a patient.

During World War I the great number of facial injuries treated at the Queen Mary Hospital, Sidcup in England, stimulated the search for different ways of giving anaesthesia avoiding a mask (Fig. 6.5). Among those who worked at this task were R. Eade followed by Ivan Magill (Fig. 6.6). and his colleague E.S. Rowbotham [873]. They introduced the routine use of endotracheal anaesthesia with the obvious lasting benefits for surgery. Rowbotham was also successful at blind nasal intubation with a wide-bore tube in 1920.

One problem in those early days was the expiration which originally required another tube inserted in the trachea. Magill conceived what was later called the *Magill attachment*. This allowed the discharge of the gases without the need of a second tube and endotracheal anaesthesia became safer and eventually routine.

In the years that followed, Magill and others devised and refined many new techniques and pieces of apparatus which made difficult anaesthesia possible (Fig. 6.7) [590–594]. New drugs and anaesthetic agents were invented and the advent of the ventilator introduced the era of modern anaesthesia (Fig. 6.8).

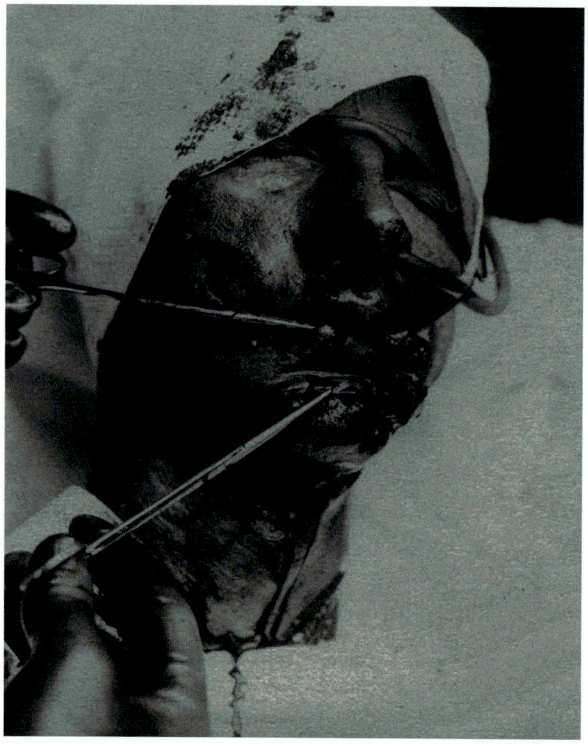

Fig. 6.5 **a** Surgery on the face posed difficulties in maintaining the airway while not interfering with the operation. This soldier is having surgery to repair a lower lip wound with an intranasal tube in September 1917 before Magill arrived at Sidcup. **b** see next page

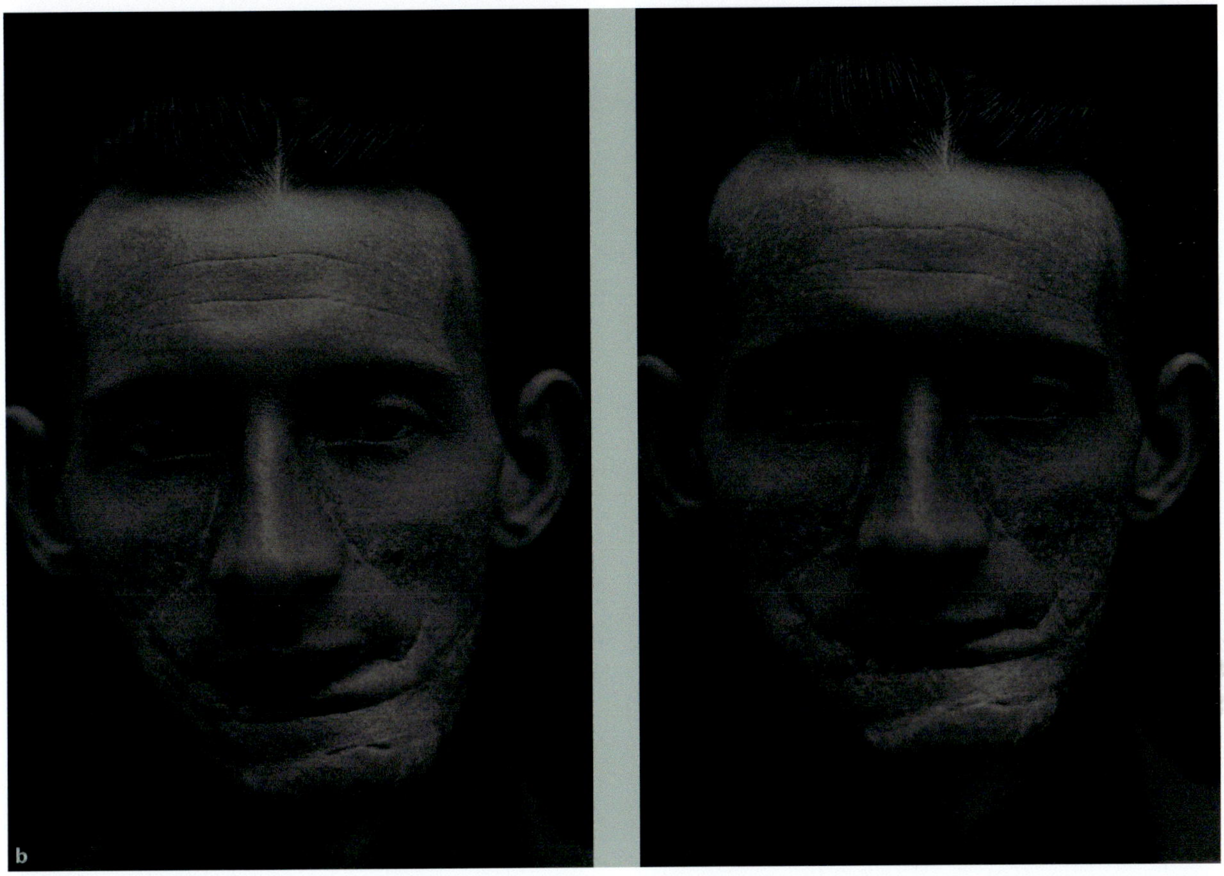

Fig. 6.5 *(continued)* **b** The final result after 11 operations. He later died of tuberculosis. *Reproduced by permission of the Gillies Archives, Queen Mary's Hospital, Sidcup, UK*

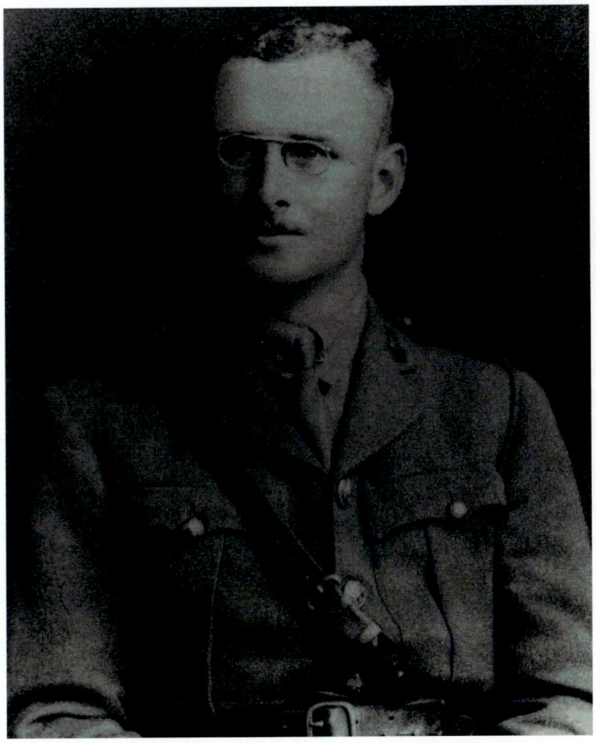

Fig. 6.6 Ivan Magill (later to become Sir Ivan) at Sidcup during World War I. *Reproduced by permission of the Gillies Archives, Queen Mary's Hospital, Sidcup, UK*

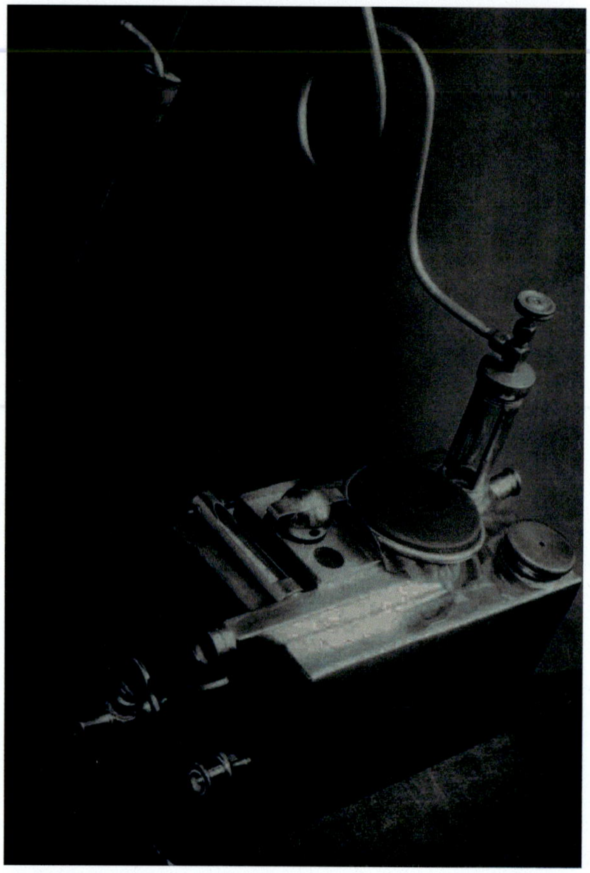

Fig. 6.7 Many pieces of apparatus were devised to permit effective, safe anaesthesia on soldiers with severe injuries who underwent facial reconstruction at the Military Hospital in Sidcup. One example is this apparatus, used for warming ether, made by Archibald Lane. *Reproduced by permission of the Gillies Archives, Queen Mary's Hospital, Sidcup, UK*

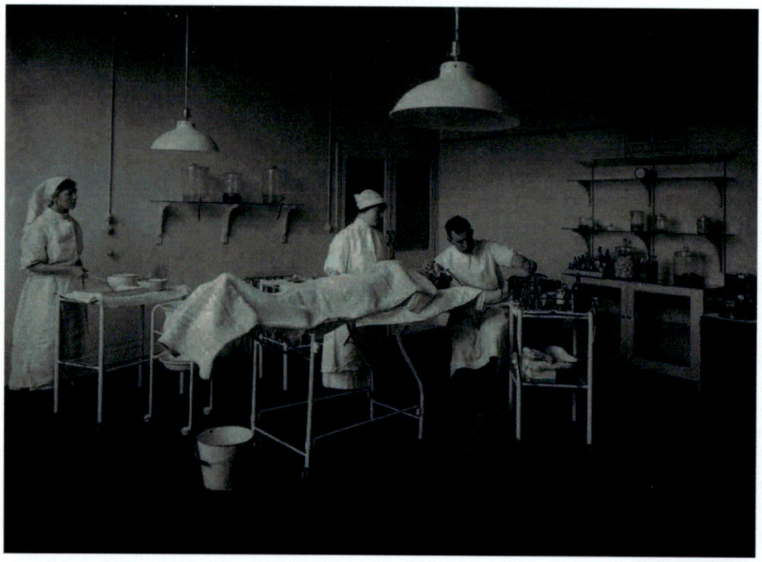

Fig. 6.8 By comparison to present the day, anaesthetic equipment was very basic. *Reproduced by permission of the Gillies Archives, Queen Mary's Hospital, Sidcup, UK*

Chapter 7

Nasal Reconstruction

ICON OCTAVA.

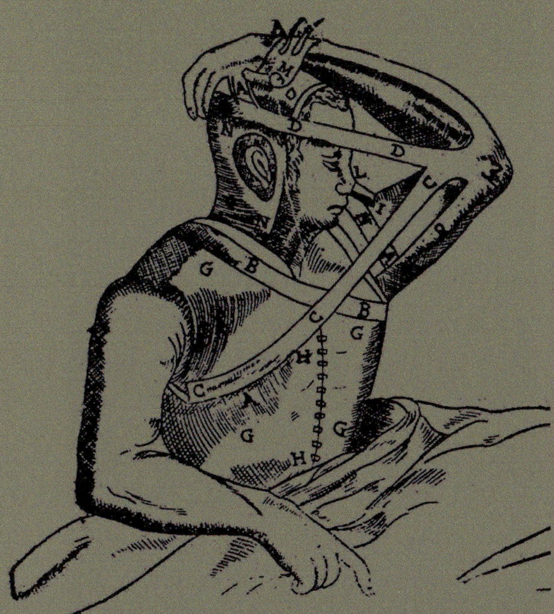

Contents

For more than twenty-five centuries plastic surgery focused almost exclusively on the reconstruction of the face, and it was the nose that received the greatest amount of attention from earliest times. Over the years the techniques that were used for nasal reconstructions evolved and were applied to other parts of the body, but many of the original principles have remained almost unchanged.

The history of the surgical reconstruction of the nose can be divided into four distinct periods:

- Antiquity (Prehistory to the Middle Ages)
- The Renaissance (from the fourteenth to the sixteenth centuries)
- Decline (from the sixteenth to the eighteenth centuries)
- Rebirth (after 1793)

Antiquity

Fractures of the nose were one of the first problems to be treated by surgery and the methods were not so very different from those used today.

The Edwin Smith papyrus [128, 537] which dates according to its translator J.H. Breasted to the Early Dynastic Period (c.3000–2500 B.C.), sheds fascinating light on the practice of surgery on the nose in ancient Egypt. It presents three separate cases describing their symptoms in sufficient detail to allow us to make a diagnosis: swelling, pain, bleeding and crepitation of the bony fragments. The text then provides a description of the treatment to be administered: "Thou shouldst force it [the broken nose] to fall, so that it is lying in its place and clean out the interior of both his nostrils with two swabs of linen until every worm of blood which coagulates in the inside of his two nostrils comes forth. … insert two plugs of linen saturated with grease in the inside of his two nostrils. Thou shouldst put [him] at his mooring stakes until the swelling is drawn out, thou shouldst apply stiff rolls of linen by which his nose is held fast, thou shouldst treat him afterward [with] grease, honey [and] lint every day until he recovers" (Fig. 7.1).[1]

Similarly in Greece, Hippocrates (460–375 B.C.) [434–437] recommended: "When the bones of the nose are depressed, they should be raised into their normal position by means of an instrument called a Shalak; a hollow wooden tube is then kept in the nostrils so as to retain the bones in their natural position."[2] It is interest-

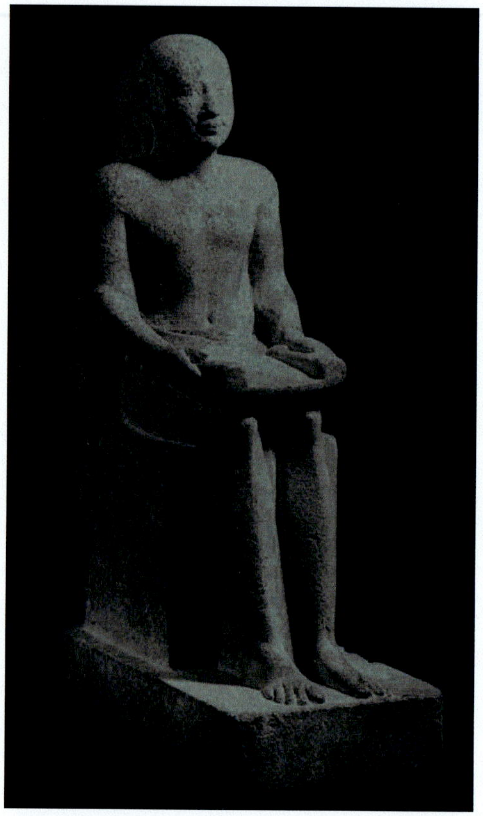

Fig. 7.1 Statue of Imhòtep (c.2900 B.C.) possibly the earliest image of a doctor from antiquity. He was the physician to King Zoser (2980–2900 B.C.) and became so famous that he was elevated to the status of a God until superseded by Asclepios in Greece (Aesculapius to the Romans). *Courtesy of FMR Art.spa Bologna*

1 According to the translator of the Edwin papyrus, James Henry Breasted of the Oriental Institute of Chicago, the ancient Egyptians accredited this treatment to Imhotep, a physician and master sculptor (his name is linked to the Step Pyramid) who lived during the third dynasty (c.2650 to c.2575). Considered a semi-deity, some centuries later he was elevated in rank to a god of healing. He was described by Sir William Osler as "the first figure of a physician to stand out clearly from the mist of antiquity."

2 See *Chirurgia ex Greco in Latinum Conversa* by Vivo Vidi, in the chapter *De Luxatorum Fracturumque Assium Coaptatione Mochlicove Sermo Septuagesimus.*

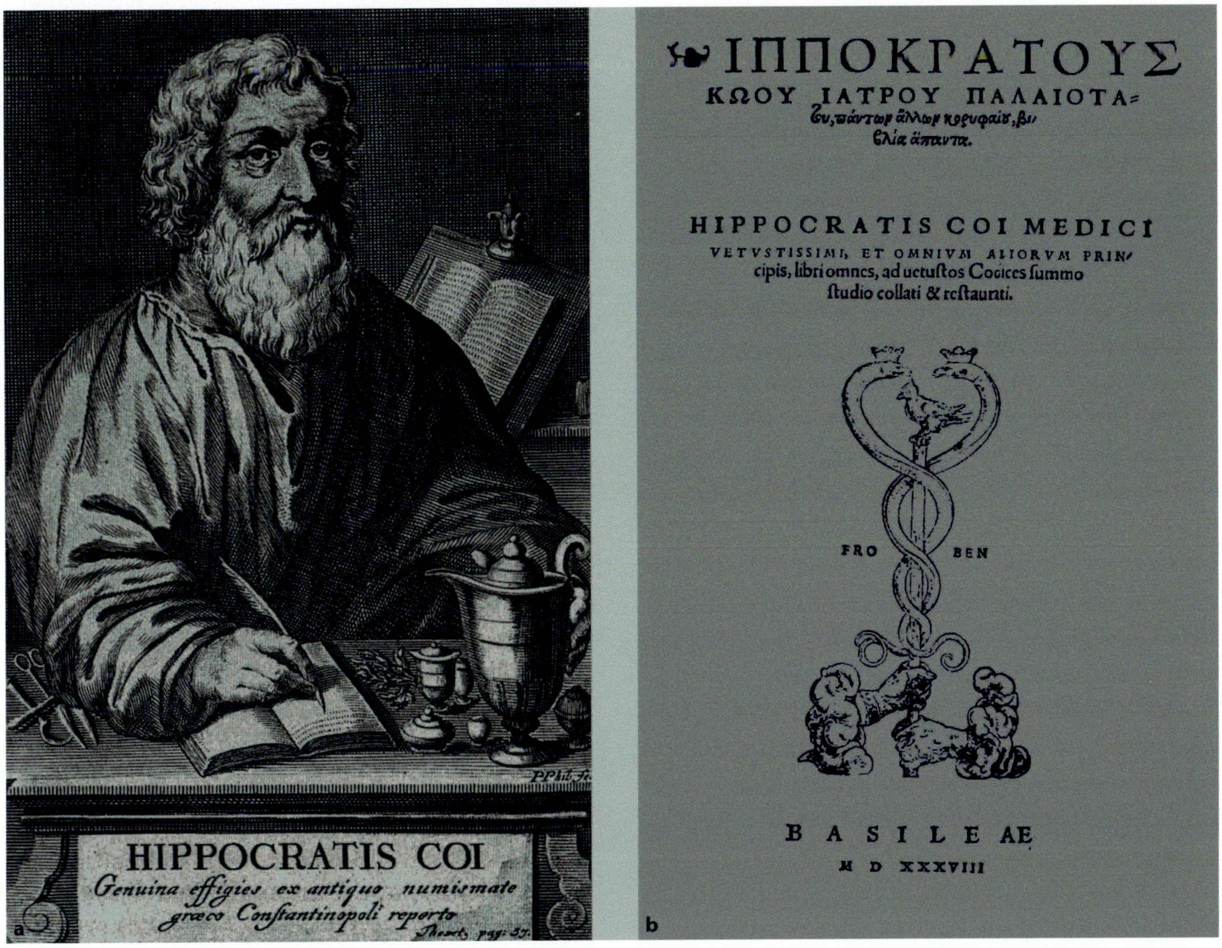

Fig. 7.2 **a** Portrait of Hippocrates. There was a belief that he was descended from Asclepios. His works are collected with those of his pupils in *Corpus Hippocraticum*. *Courtesy of FMR Art.spa Bologna*. **b** Frontispiece of *Corpus Hippocraticum* (Greek version, Basle 1538). *Reprinted from* Surgery an Illustrated History *by Ira M Rutko, (1993) with permission of Elsevier*

ing to note that Hippocrates had already observed and made the distinction between the saddle nose which was the result of trauma and that due to a congenital abnormality. In fact, his description of children with a depressed nose bridge accompanied by the loss of teeth and ulceration of the palate is highly suggestive of a form of syphilis, one that was unknown in Europe at the time (Fig. 7.2a,b) [389].

The principle of raising the depressed bone fragments and holding them in the correct position after a trauma was reiterated by Anthyllus (second century B.C.). In the translation of one of his works by Bussmaker and Daremberg [149] we read: "In fractures of the nose, it is well to fill the nostrils completely with cotton or silk and not to extract it until the nose has taken its shape."

Centuries later Paulus Aegineta (625–690) once again underlined the importance of repositioning the nasal bones, adding that: "When the fracture is of the inner parts, this is to be done with the head of a probe immediately, during the course of the first day, or not long afterwards, because the bones of the nose will become consolidated by about the tenth day … But they are to be placed in the proper position with the index finger and thumb externally." To fix the fragments and keep them from moving "… two wedge-like tents formed of a twisted linen rag are to be applied, one to each nostril" [3, 4].

Nasal Reconstruction in Ancient India

While in ancient Egypt and Greece physicians limited themselves to treating simple fractures, in India by 1500 B.C. they were already carrying out reconstruction of amputated noses. The frequency with which these operations were conducted can be explained by the fact that since earliest times, perhaps as far back as 3000 B.C., amputation of the nose was a traditional punishment for sexual misdemeanours. A demand for rhinoplasty existed, as explained by Shah Tribowandas (1850–1904)[3]: "The mutilation of the nose is a practice for avenging a wrong that is peculiar, I believe, to this country ... Here cutting off the nose is a special way of manifesting vengeance. Of all the organs of the body, the nose is considered to be the organ of respect and reputation. The usual saying—when a person is told that he has no nose—means that he has forfeited delicate feelings of honor ... A noseless person thus is not only humbled, but is held to be an unfortunate being. Thus the people in India who are deprived of their noses feel the greatest humiliation; they try to shun society and are even ready to sacrifice their lives." [920]

D.J. Brian [131] confirms that cutting off the nose was often carried out as a punishment. He observes that in the province of Gujerat the Council of Brahmins was charged with enforcing these sentences. The executioner, after shaving the head of the condemned person, cut off the nose with a pair of sharp shears. This procedure was often accompanied by further mutilation of the face with acid.

There is confirmation that this punishment was fairly widespread in the epic poem Ramayana [34] which recounts the story of the virtuous Prince Rama. Among his many trials and tribulations he was seduced as part of a nefarious plot by Surpunakha, the beautiful sister of his adversary King Ravana.[4] However, Rama's brother Laksham[5] managed to unmask Surpunakha and as a punishment cut off her nose, in this way dishonouring her.[6] The poem recounts that King Ravana charged a surgeon with the reconstruction of his sister's nose but disappointingly for us does not say how it was done. This poem, which dates from around 1500 B.C., clearly demonstrates that the amputation and subsequent reconstruction of the nose were well known in India three and a half millennia ago (Fig. 7.3a,b).

There is another example of the application of this punishment en masse in relatively recent times. When King Gurkha Prithvi Narayan conquered the Nepalese city of Kitipoor in 1767 A.D. he inflicted this punishment on its inhabitants. They had courageously resisted his siege and inflicted grave losses on his troops. The King's brother had lost an eye in the battle. He ordered the amputation of the nose and upper lip of the 865 males who had been taken prisoner, with the sole exception of unweaned babies and the players of wind instruments. The king also changed the name of the city to Naskatapoor which means "the city without noses" [29, 329].

The practice continued in India during colonial times, as we know from the case of the cart driver Cowasjee. In 1792 he was condemned by the Sultan Tipu to have his nose and right hand cut off. Even today the custom does not seem to have completely disappeared. A report in the British literature relates the incident of an Indian husband who cut of his wife's nose for committing adultery in 1983 [131].

It is not known whether this practice spread from India to other countries at the time. We do have evidence that in the time of Diodorus Siculus in the first century A.D. there was a penal colony in Egypt, where all the prisoners had to undergo amputation of their noses. The colony was called Rhinocolura, from the Greek ρηινο = nose and κολουροσ = to cut [1025].

Regardless of this sociological background the historians Brian [131] and Almast [23] agree that this operation was being practised routinely around 1500 B.C. and perhaps even before. It probably started during the earliest period of Hindu medicine when its principles

3 Trivobandas himself carried out more than 300 nose reconstructions.

4 The name Surpunakha probably derives from *shoorp*, a bamboo basket used to separate grain from bran and therefore, symbolically, good from evil and *nakka* which means "fingernail". Thus the name signifies an exotic woman with long nails who separates good from evil.

5 The word Laksham derives from *laksha* (sign) and *man* (mind), meaning a person of sharp intelligence.

6 The story is depicted in a large bas relief around the inner courtyard of the temple of Angkor Wat, Cambodia.

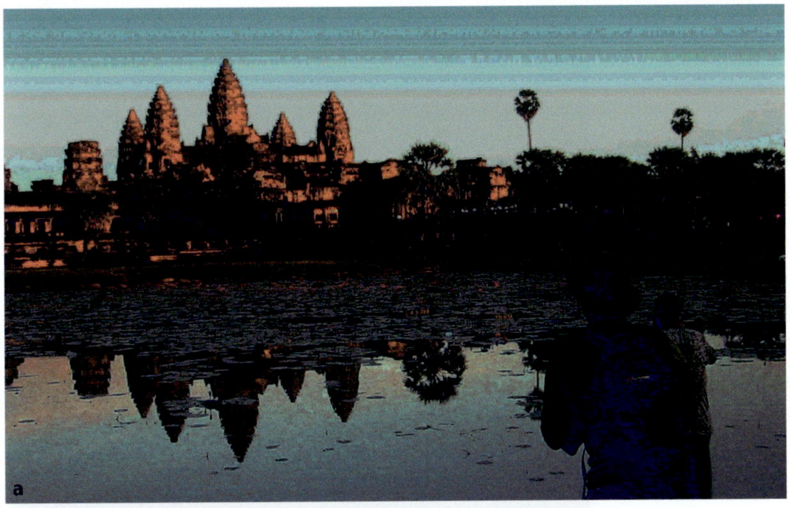

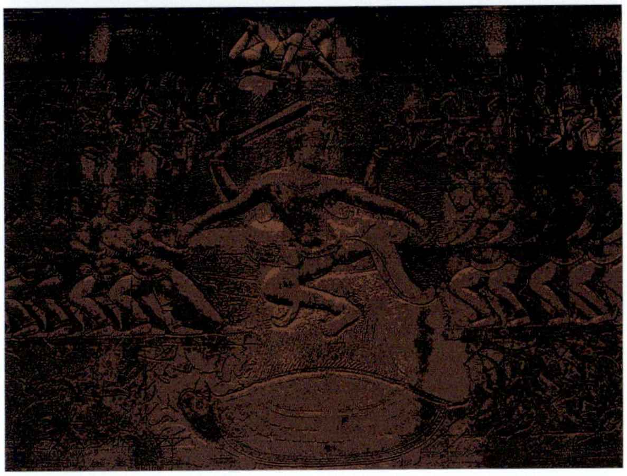

Fig. 7.3 **a** The temple of Angkor Wat, near Siem Reph in Cambodia, is considered to be the largest religious building in the world and dates from the ninth century A.D. **b** The galleries of three floors are decorated with bas-reliefs, one of which depicts the epic poem Ramayana dating from c.1500 B.C. Part of the legend recounts the practice of nasal reconstruction. *PSR*

were set down in the sacred writings known as the Vedas. The first record comes from the Susruta-Samhita[7], in which the surgeon Susruta[8] gives a description of the technique of nasal reconstruction. He claims to have learned the method from the great master Dhanvantari. The Susruta-Samhita is the text that records the Ayurvedic system of medicine, which by tradition was received by Dhanvantari from Brahma. It is composed of 12 books divided into 186 chapters, the first 27 being of direct interest to the surgeon. It forms the fundamental

7 There exists some doubt as to the true identity of Susruta. G. Muhopadhyaya (1872–1935) [717] wrote that "nothing certain is known, even taking into account that he was the son of Viskvamitra, because we are not sure when these personages lived". It has also been suggested that the Susruta-Samhita could represent a compilation of works written over a period of several centuries by different authors. Recently, V.K. Baskaradoss [63] accepts that Susruta was probably the son of the sage Viskvamitra and his wife Divodasa Kasi Raja, (herself a pupil of Dhanvantari) and points out that Viskvamitra is mentioned repeatedly in the Indian epic Ramayana which is placed sometime around 1800 B.C. Another reason to think that Susruta lived earlier than is usually accepted is the fact that he mentions in the Samita the name of Lord Krishna who is clearly described in another epic, the Mahabhrata, which is dated around 1300 B.C. Therefore there are good reasons to believe that the date of birth of Susruta was much earlier than 600 B.C.

8 Muhopadhyaya also assembled considerable information on the surgical instruments used by the Hindus. He describes 125 tools, which were generally made of iron but for special purposes might also be of copper, lead, tin, silver or gold, with handles beautifully molded in the form of animals or birds. The author compares these to the instruments used by the ancient Greeks and Romans and in some cases to their modern equivalents.

text of medicine and surgery upon which all later Indian works are based. Rhinoplasty is described in chapter 16,[9] where Susruta begins by proposing "Wine should be used before the operation to produce sleepiness and even insensibility to pain. The patient who has been fed does not faint, and the one who is rendered intoxicated does not feel the pain of the operation." We then learn how Susruta carried out his procedure: "First the leaf of a creeper, long and broad enough to fully cover the whole of the severed or clipped off part, should be gathered, and a patch of living flesh, equal in dimension to the leaf should be sliced off from down upward, from the region of the cheek and after scarifying [the margins] with a knife, swiftly adhered to the severed nose. Then the cool-headed physician should steadily tie it up with a bandage decent to look at and perfectly suited to the end for which it has been employed. The physician should make sure that the adhesion of the severed parts has been fully effected and then insert two small pipes into the nostrils to facilitate respiration and prevent the flesh from hanging down." (Fig. 7.4) [90]

There follow recommendations on bandaging to ensure that the flap remains adherent to the nose. Susruta had probably learnt from experience that early attempts at remodelling were dangerous and advises against early secondary surgery.[10]

It is probable that the method described by Susruta continued to be practised without substantial variation for centuries. In fact we have no evidence of any changes until the innovations introduced by Vagbat [1000] in the fourth century. In his work *Ashtanga Hridyans*[11] Vagbat described in detail the usual procedure of cutting a flap from the patient's cheek and demonstrated his awareness that its survival depended upon leaving an adequate pedicle for its nourishment. His most original contribution was a bold step. It predates, by more than 15 centuries, the solution to the problem of recreating the nasal lining. He achieved this by folding the end of flap on itself. He also described a novel technique for suturing the flap using cotton thread and sharp needles. Haemostasis was achieved by compression and respira-

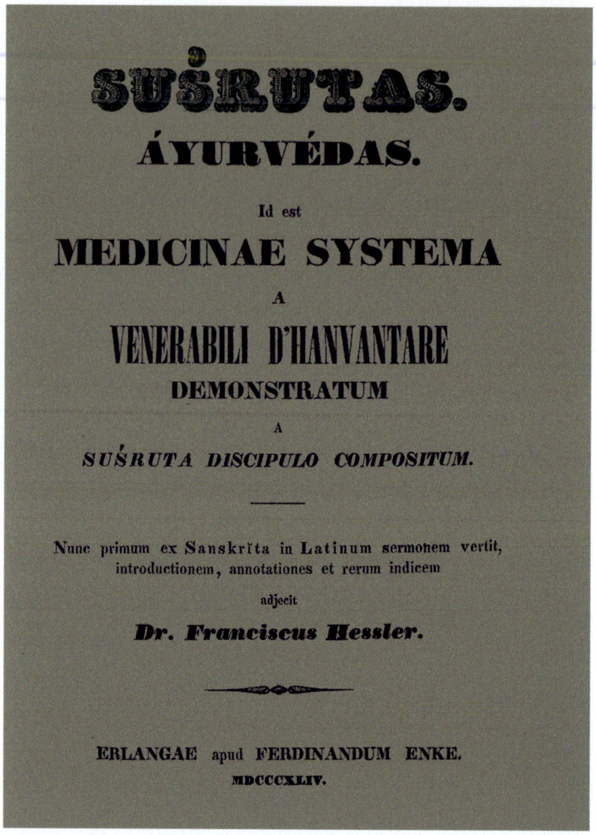

SUŚRUTAS.
ÁYURVÉDAS.
Id est
MEDICINAE SYSTEMA
A
VENERABILI D'HANVANTARE
DEMONSTRATUM
A
SUŚRUTA DISCIPULO COMPOSITUM.

Nunc primum ex Sanskrīta in Latinum sermonem vertit, introductionem, annotationes et rerum indicem adjecit

Dr. Franciscus Hessler.

ERLANGAE apud FERDINANDUM ENKE.
MDCCCXLIV.

Fig. 7.4 Frontispiece of Susruta's *Ayurvedas* translation into Latin in 1846. It covered all aspects of known medicine. *Courtesy of Riccardo Mazzola, M.D., Milan*

9 Dhanvantari was the physician of the gods. He was born with a cup of nectar in one of his many hands and held in another is a leech, the traditional cure for swelling.

10 The Susruta-Samhita was first translated by Hessler into Latin in 1844, and then by Vellurs into German, but both of these versions were only partial. Probably the English edition by Bhishagratna published in 1907 represents the first complete translation of the original Sanskrit text. For a more complete discussion of the Susruta-Samhita and on Indian medicine in general, readers may consult *Fundamental and Plastic Surgery Considerations in Ancient Indian Surgery* by G.D. Singhal, Vaiyda Kirti et al., Banaras Hindu University Press, 1981.

11 A commentary on *Ashtanga Hridyans* was recently published by K.S. Goleria [387] and the text was translated from Sanskrit into English by Kaviraj Atridev Gupta in 1950.

tion ensured, as in Hippocrates' time, by inserting tubes into the nostrils.

Descriptions of the sophisticated nasal reconstructions being carried out in India did not reach Europe until the end of the eighteenth century, by which time the method had been modified from the procedure described by Susruta and Vagbat. The flap was now cut from the forehead rather than the cheek. Antia and Daver [29] record that there were at least three families of healers who were renowned for practising the frontal flap long before it was exported to Europe. The were the Maharattas of Kumar, near Puné in the northwest part of India, the Kangahaira family, originally from the northern Punjab city of Kanga and finally a Nepalese family whose name is not known.

Despite exhaustive research carried out by S.C. Almast [22] on the surgical practice of the Kangahaira family, it is not clear when the technique of the frontal flap was developed. He discovered that their methods were carefully transmitted from father to son and never to outsiders. Married daughters might participate in the operation but only if they and their husbands lived with the family. Unmarried daughters were not allowed to be present for fear that when they married and left home, the secrets might spread outside the family circle. It has been established that the Kangahaira were active near Delhi during the war of Krushhetra, i.e. around the year 1000 B.C. However, there are many clues that they were practising in Kanga long before, perhaps as early as 1400 B.C. when Raj Sausar Chaud I controlled the region. So great was their fame that patients came from every part of northwestern India including present-day Pakistan, drawn not only by their reputation but perhaps also by faith in the benevolent power of the patron goddess of Kanga. Almast [22] reports fascinating details about the family's practice, such as the fees they demanded, the existence of a register of patients, and the fact that they were required to sign a consent form absolving the surgeon of all responsibility should the outcome be unsuccessful.

Little is known about the Maharatta family except that for centuries they practised nasal reconstructions using the frontal flap. The only evidence we have shows that they were still active in the eighteenth century, when medical officers of the East India Company witnessed their operations.[12]

We have no information on the practice of rhinoplasty outside India during antiquity, apart from a single, somewhat improbable, instance. In 1979 J.P. Remensnyder and colleagues [834] published a paper suggesting that the Emperor Justinian, son of Constantine IV, may have undergone reconstructive surgery for an amputated nose. Justinian was deposed by a military insurrection in 695 and during his imprisonment had his nose cut off. He wore a golden prosthesis for some time but then, according to Remensnyder, possibly underwent a surgical reconstruction around the year 700 in an unknown city in eastern Europe. This hypothesis is based on the documented facts of the Emperor's overthrow, imprisonment and mutilation, to which the authors have linked a statue depicting the emperor with a normal nose and a scar on his forehead—extremely slender grounds on which to build such a significant claim!

The Renaissance

The reconstructions that were being carried out as a matter of course by Indian surgeons were completely unknown in Europe. Ammon and Baumgarten [24, 25] and Manna [608] claim that Celsus (25 B.C. to 50 A.D.) carried out nasal reconstruction on the basis of the fact that he used flaps on the face, especially to repair lips [167, 168]. There is however no evidence that he reconstructed noses. In fact Celsus made his way onto the list of the pioneers of nasal reconstruction, in the absence of sufficient proof that he had ever conducted such an operation.

The single case described by Lanfranchi da Milano in Chapter II of his *Cyrurgia Parva* [520] might be considered another exception to the general rule that nasal reconstructions were unknown in the West. He speaks of

12 Some of the Eastern practitioners were credited with such a degree of skill that tales were told of the freshly severed nose being thrown into a fire to prevent it being sewn back. No confirmation of such fantastic tales can be found in historical documents or the medical literature.

"a completely detached nose, in an individual who came to me with his nose in one hand", which he claims to have successfully reimplanted.[13] However, this episode does not represent a true reconstruction but rather a reimplantation or, more exactly, a compound free graft (Fig. 7.5).

Theodoric of Cervia (1205–1298), son of the eminent professor of surgery Ugo Borgognoni, whose book *Cyrurgia* [979, 980] was included by Guy de Chauliac in his collection of the works of the ten most famous surgeons of the century, has been credited with performing nasal reconstructions with flaps. In reality it appears that in his discussions on the repair of nasal injuries, he simply recommended replacing traumatic flaps "with delicacy and care",[14] which is quite different from a genuine reconstruction.[15]

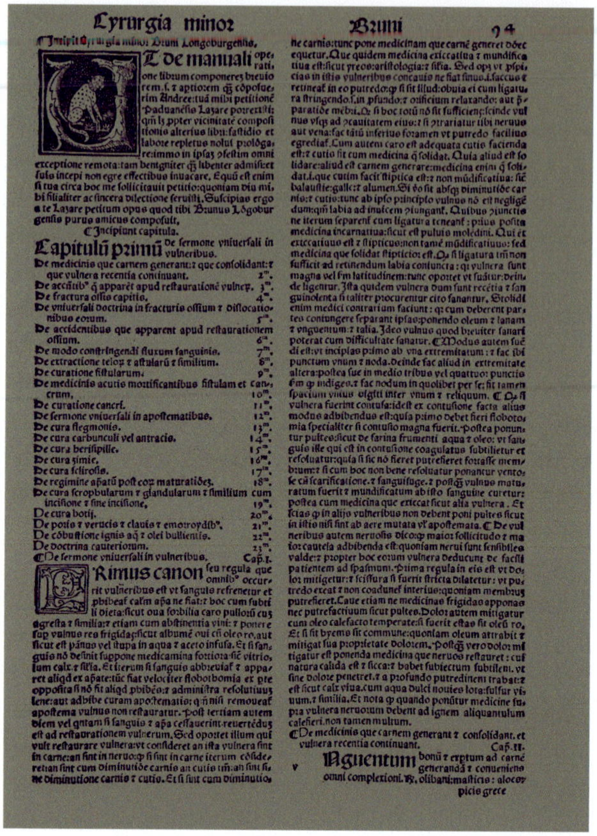
Cyrurgia minor
Bruni
94

Fig. 7.5 First page of Lanfranchi's *Cyrurgia Parva*, compiled in 1298 and included by Guy de Chauliac in his *Cyrurgia Magna* published in 1468 in Lyon. *Courtesy of Riccardo Mazzola, M.D., Milan*

The Branca Family

In the fifteenth century nasal reconstructions were being carried out for the first time in Europe by a gifted Sicilian surgeon, Gustavo Branca, and his equally brilliant son Antonio. Just where they learned the technique remains a mystery. If we accept the claims of various authors including Wright[16], who are supported by historical sources such as Carl Ferdinand von Graefe (1787–1840) [391] "… there is reason to believe that the Saracens introduced the Art into Sicily, even though it is not clear just where and when the Arabs might have practised the technique of rhinoplasty in order to be able to export it…". More solidly grounded is the claim of Almast [23] that the Sus-

13 Lanfranchi wrote *Cyrurgia Parva* in 1298 but it did not appear in print until 1478 when Guy de Chauliac published his collection *Cyrurgia Magna* in Lyon. Oddly enough, although he included Lanfranchi's contribution in his book, de Chauliac did not believe in the feasibility of nose reimplantations. In Tract II, Lib. II, p 31 he declares that "Si nasus ex toto exciderit amplius non potest reuniri, unitio enim in organicis est impossibili" (If the nose is totally excised it is impossible to reunite it, to reconstruct the organic unit is impossible).

14 See *Cyrurgia*, Book IV, Chapter VIII.

15 Federico da Montefeltro (1420–1482), Duke of Urbino and a professional soldier was said to have undergone a rhinoplasty when young. At the age of nineteen he was struck in the face by a lance while jousting in the lists and lost his right eye. A myth arose that he had his large nasal bridge removed surgically so that he could see the right side of the battlefield through his one good eye and spot attempts to poison his food while banqueting. This legend was accepted and supported in more recent times by Harold Gillies and Ralph Millard. The true story is recorded by one of the authors [892].

16 A copy of the book by J. Wright, with no cover and therefore no indication of the publisher or year of publication, may be found in the Biblioteca della Fondazione Sanvenero Rosselli in Milan.

ruta-Samhita was known to the Arabs because, as he has demonstrated, the Hindu text was translated into Arabic by a certain Mauke during the reign of King As-Massur in 775. The work is also cited by Ibn Abi, who lived during the first half of the thirteenth century

There is mention that Gustavo Branca was originally from Provence and visited Persia before finally settling in the Sicilian city of Catania. If this is true, he would perhaps have had the opportunity to learn of the methods being used in India, but unfortunately there is no way for us to confirm or disprove this hypothesis.

The suggestion that the Branca family may have been inspired by the works of Celsus seems equally implausible, for the text *De Medicina* by the Roman author was not rediscovered and published until 1478 in Florence. Therefore it remains uncertain where and how the Branca family learnt the technique. Furthermore, as Gnudi and Webster [379–381] point out, the flaps that Celsus described "were without transposition and without separation from the underlying base of the part to be transplanted" and therefore in reality constituted advancement flaps.

What is known for certain is that on 11 February 1412 Gustavo Branca and his descendents were granted a license to practise surgery by the Aragon king of Sicily, Ferdinand I [202].[17] This does not necessarily mean that Gustavo was equipped with any medical training because, as we have seen, such preparation was not required of surgeons in that period.

Medicine was still an esoteric art and in accordance with widespread custom the Branca family kept the technical details of their operations a jealously guarded secret. Since they did not write a single line about themselves, we would be hard-pressed to know anything of their methods were it not for the fact that historians and other authors took an interest in their remarkable feats of reconstructive surgery. The first to mention the Brancas in this context was Pietro Ranzano (1441–1492) the Bishop of Lucera, who wrote in the eighth volume of his *Annales Mundi* [828]: "Very famous in those days was Branca the Sicilian. Among all the barber-surgeons of the world he was the most brilliant. He discovered in this art many things worthy of admiration and almost incredible, since he conceived how to shape and restore mutilated noses. His son Antonio added not a few things to the wonderful invention of the father. He created not only the nostrils but somehow was able to repair lips and mutilated ears. Moreover he made ulcers heal that appeared incurable [even] with the help of the medical art." (Fig. 7.6a,b)[18]

It seems therefore that the Branca family, like Celsus before them, also used flaps to reconstruct lips and ears.

Another author who wrote about the Branca family's activities was Bartolomeo Fazio (1400–1457) the historian of King Alphonse I of Naples. In *De Viris Illustribus* [304][19], after describing in the same admiring terms as the bishop the miraculous reconstructions they were capable of, he goes on to provide a fairly detailed account of one of these operations: "In speaking of this century I have thought both Branca and his son especially worthy to be remembered because Branca, the elder, was the originator of an admirable and almost incredible procedure. He conceived how to repair and replace noses that had been mutilated or cut off and developed his ideas into a marvelous art. And the son Antonius added to his father's wonderful discovery. For he conceived how mutilated lips, ears and noses might be restored. Whereas his father had taken the flesh for the repair from the mutilated man's face, Antonius took it from the muscles of his arm, so that no distortion of the face should be caused. On the arm that was cut open and into the wound itself, he bound the [site of the] mutilated nose so tightly that the patient might not move his head at all. After fifteen days or sometimes twenty, little by little with a sharp knife he cut away the flap which had become attached to the nose; finally he severed it entirely from the arm and shaped it into a nose with so much in-

17 The licence that was granted to Gustavo Branca is conserved among the Lettere della Segrezia of Palermo, Ad 1406-10, Nr. 38, Fol. 76.

18 Pietro Ranzano was born in Palermo in 1442. He became Bishop of Lucera in the Kingdom of Naples in 1476. The several volumes comprising his *Annales Mundi* were conserved in the Library of the Franciscan Fathers of Palermo, but around the end of the eighteenth century it was decided to transfer them to the Municipal Library. During this move volume 8 was lost, but fortunately Vincenzo Auria [38] had included the passage reproduced here in his book *Sicilia Inventrice* (1704).

19 *De Viribus Illustribus* was printed two centuries later, in Florence in 1745.

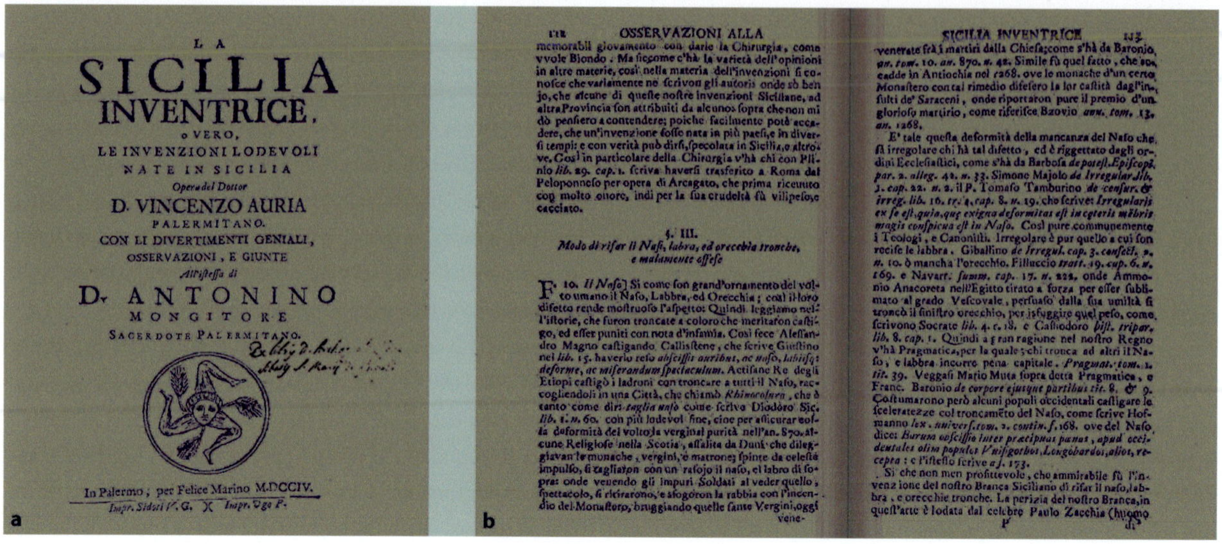

Fig. 7.6 **a** Frontispiece of *La Sicilia Inventrice* (1704) by Vincenzo Auria which includes **b** an account of the Branca family's activity in the field of nasal reconstruction reported in the fifteenth century by Pietro Ranzano, Bishop of Lucera, in his *Annales Mundi*. *Courtesy of Riccardo Mazzola, M.D., Milan*

genuity that it was scarcely possible with the eye to detect the flap that had been added, since the deformity of the face had been entirely removed."

The Branca family are also cited in glowing terms in a letter written in 1503 by an Apulian poet at the court of Frederick II of Naples, Elisio Calenzio [151] who advises his friend Orpiano, who had lost his nose, to consult them without delay: "Orpianus, should you want to have your nose restored come to me. Truly, the thing is most wonderful! Branca, a Sicilian and a man of great ability, has learned the art of restoring a nose, either by supplying it from the arm of the patient or by affixing upon the part the nose of a slave. Having seen this I was determined to write to you, to whom no news could be more interesting. Be assured that, if you come, you may go home again with as much nose as you please."[20]

Calenzio was obviously labouring under a misapprehension when he wrote of the possibility of attaching the nose of one person to another. This is the first time this notion is mentioned and, as we shall see, it not only took root but in the following century became the source of an important obstacle to the spread of the correct method of nasal reconstruction.

The technique of the arm flap was also adopted by Heinrich von Pfolsprundt [796], an aristocrat, Bruder des Deutschen Ordens (Brother of the German Order) and a surgeon with the Prussian army. In 1460 he wrote a book describing the technique in great detail.[21] In fact, the account which he gives corresponds to the method used by Antonio Branca half a continent away and we may ask ourselves how he could have learned of the technique if the Branca family was so secretive about their work. Von Pfolsprundt gives us a hint when he writes "Ein Wall hatch mich gelernht"; in other words, he learned the procedure from "ein Wall", this being an old German word for "ein Welshe" or someone who speaks a Romance language, a term that is still used today in southern Germany and Austria to refer to a person originally from the south, i.e. an Italian. One may suppose therefore that von Pfolsprundt had the occasion to meet an Italian surgeon who was travelling through Germany.

20 Calenzio's letter was published by Stephen Gourmelin [389] in *Chirurgie Artis*.

21 The book by Heinrich von Pfolsprundt was finally published four centuries after his death, in 1868, in *Buch der Bündth-Ertznei* by H. Haeser and A. Middeldorpf (Berlin).

The description furnished by von Pfolsprundt was so accurate and detailed that any skilled surgeon would have been able to repeat the operation simply by following his instructions. Thus, the author appears to be contradicting himself when he urges the reader not to share the knowledge contained in his book: “Should someone come to you because his nose has been cut off and he desires to have a new one, you must abstain from showing [the operation] to anyone else if you do not wish him to learn the art by imitating you.” Evidently keeping the details of their procedure secret remained an obsession with all the surgeons of the period (Fig. 7.7).

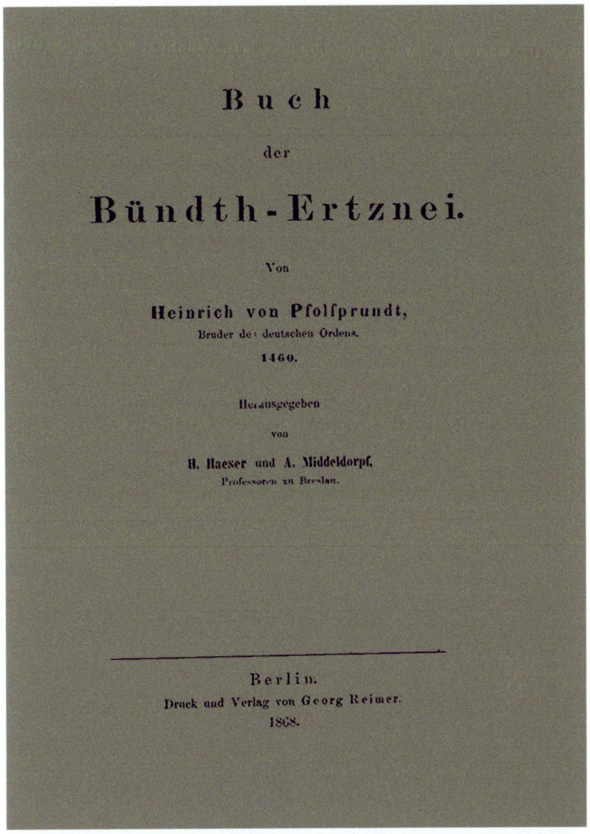

Buch

der

Bündth-Ertznei.

Von

Heinrich von Pfolfprundt,

Bruder des deutschen Ordens.

1460.

Herausgegeben

von

H. Haeser und A. Middeldorpf.

Professoren zu Breslau.

Berlin.

Druck und Verlag von Georg Reimer.

1868.

Fig. 7.7 Frontispiece of Haeser and Middeldorpf's *Buch der Bündth-Ertznei* which includes the work of Pfolsprundt compiled around 1460. The book was printed in Germany in 1808. *Courtesy of Riccardo Mazzola, M.D., Milan*

An Italian who was able to describe Antonio Branca's method even if he had never seen him work, probably because he had the opportunity to meet some of Branca's former patients, was Alessandro Benedetti (1450–1512) [347]. In *Anatomiae sive Historia Corporis Humani* published in 1502 in Venice and Paris [70, 71], he explains[22]: “Their method consists in cutting a small piece of flesh from the patient's arm in the shape of a nose and applying it to the stump. For this they cut the top layer of skin on the arm with a scalpel. After this they bind the arm to the head if the nose has been recently cut off; otherwise, if need be they scarify the nose so that it will adhere to the raw surface. When the wounds have healed together they take from the arm with a scalpel [vulneris cohereat, conglutinatis vulneribu, e brachio tanto cultello demunt, quantu instaurari conueniat] as much flesh as is needed for the restoration. Blood vessels from the nose supply nourishment to the flap and finally a covering is obtained. … And so with great dexterity they shape a new nose. They construct nasal passages with great skill. … During the beginning of the treatment [however] I recommend that you not handle the nose lest it come away in your hand!” (Fig. 7.8) [70]

Benedetti's description is interesting because for the very first time the problem of the blood supply to the flap from the recipient bed is specifically mentioned.

The question has been raised as to whether Benedetti, who describes the rhinoplasty procedure with such confidence, had actually ever carried out such an operation himself. We are inclined to believe that he did, because he mentions various details that no surgeon could have known except from direct experience. For example, he observes that “sometimes on the skin [of the flap] hair may grow”, a phenomenon that all surgeons are well acquainted with, especially in the case of poorly vascularized flaps. He furthermore writes of the reconstructed nose: “this appendage does not tolerate severe winters”, a phenomenon which he would have had ample opportunity to observe in the relatively northern city of Padua, unlike the Brancas in the hotter climate of Sicily. It may be noted that Benedetti never cites the illustrious Sicilian surgeons directly in his book.

When Antonio Branca died at the end of the fifteenth century the art of nose reconstruction was immediately taken up and continued by the Vianeo family in Calabria.

22 See *Anatomiae sive Historia Corporis Humani*, Book V, Chapter XXXIX, *De naso*.

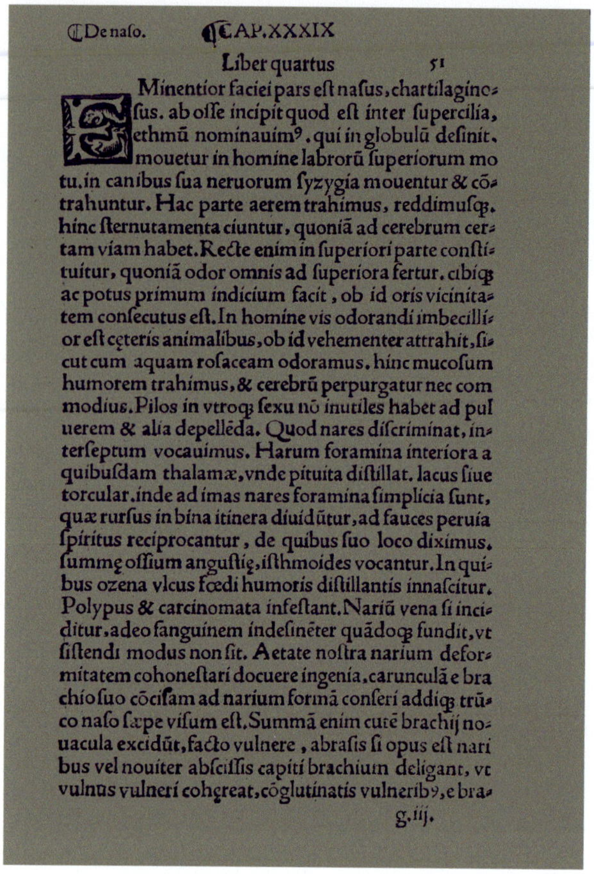
¶De naſo. ¶CAP.XXXIX
Liber quartus 51
EMinentior faciei pars eſt naſus, chartilagino-
ſus. ab oſſe incipit quod eſt inter ſupercilia,
ethmũ nominauim9. qui in globulũ deſinit.
mouetur in homine labrorũ ſuperiorum mo
tu. in canibus ſua neruorum ſyzygia mouentur & cõ-
trahuntur. Hac parte aerem trahimus, reddimuſq;.
hinc ſternutamenta ciuntur, quoniã ad cerebrum cer-
tam viam habet. Recte enim in ſuperiori parte conſti-
tuitur, quoniã odor omnis ad ſuperiora fertur. cibiq;
ac potus primum indicium facit, ob id oris vicinita-
tem conſecutus eſt. In homine vis odorandi imbecilli-
or eſt cęteris animalibus, ob id vehementer attrahit, ſi-
cut cum aquam roſaceam odoramus. hinc mucoſum
humorem trahimus, & cerebrũ perpurgatur nec com
modius. Pilos in vtroq; ſexu nõ inutiles habet ad pul
uerem & alia depellẽda. Quod nares diſcriminat, in-
terſeptum vocauimus. Harum foramina interiora a
quibuſdam thalamæ, vnde pituita diſtillat. lacus ſiue
torcular. inde ad imas nares foramina ſimplicia ſunt,
quæ rurſus in bina itinera diuidũtur, ad fauces peruia
ſpiritus reciprocantur, de quibus ſuo loco diximus.
ſummę oſſium anguſtię, iſthmoides vocantur. In qui-
bus ozena vlcus fœdi humoris diſtillantis innaſcitur.
Polypus & carcinomata infeſtant. Nariũ vena ſi inci-
ditur, adeo ſanguinem indeſinẽter quãdoq; fundit, vt
ſiſtendi modus non ſit. Aetate noſtra narium defor-
mitatem cohoneſtari docuere ingenia, carunculã e bra
chio ſuo cõciſam ad narium formã conſeri addiq; trũ-
co naſo ſæpe viſum eſt. Summã enim cutẽ brachij no-
uacula excidũt, facto vulnere, abraſis ſi opus eſt nari
bus vel nouiter abſciſſis capiti brachium deligant, vt
vulnus vulneri cohęreat, cõglutinatis vulnerib9, e bra-
g.iij.

Fig. 7.8 Description of the *Italian Method* by Alessandro Benedetti (1450–1512) in *Anatomiae sive Historia Corporis Humani* published in 1502 (Venice and Paris) which predates Gaspare Tagliacozzi's book by about 50 years. *Courtesy of Riccardo Mazzola, M.D., Milan*

The Vianeo Family

The Vianeo family became quite as celebrated for their skill as the Brancas although where they learnt the technique remains a mystery. According to one sixteenth century author, Gilberto Nazareno Cognatus (1506–1567), a young surgeon by the name of Pavone who had studied with the Branca family left Sicily and settled in Calabria [186]. The surgeon Edward Zeis (1807–1868) [1059, 1060], who found support for his opinion in a manuscript by Garmannus (1640–1708) [358], suggested that "Vianeo" might be a corruption of the name Pavone, and on this basis concluded that the first Vianeo was a student of the Brancas. However, there are insufficient data to support this hypothesis, and furthermore the name "Vianeo" can be found spelled in many different ways, including "Bojano", "Vojano" and "Fojaneo". The most convincing argument for a link between the two medical families is the sheer geographical proximity of Catania and Calabria.

What is certain is that Vincenzo Vianeo, the founder of this family of surgeons, lived in a small town in Calabria called Maida at the beginning of the sixteenth century and carried out operations following the method of Antonio Branca. We also know that one of his grandsons, Bernardino, moved from Maida to Tropea along the coast, no doubt because of the obvious advantages offered by the larger, "Royal City" to someone of his profession (Fig. 7.9).[23] Working alongside Bernadino in Tropea were his sons Paolo and Pietro, the latter of whom would remain active for another fifteen years. Recent research by Franco Rambollà [826] suggests that the wife of Pietro, Laura Guarna, continued to practise after the death of her husband until at least 1588. A chronicle of the period mentions that she treated a French patient, whose name was not recorded, in that year (Fig. 7.10a,b).[24]

In keeping with the tradition of their profession, the Vianeos left no written record of their work, and any information that we have must be gleaned from scattered testimony such as the story of a patient by the name of Camillo Porzio (1530–1580). Porzio was teaching philosophy and law in Naples having studied at the University of Pisa [813, 814].[25] At the age of 35, it seems that a jealous husband cut off his nose. The unfortunate profes-

23 The title of Città Reale (Royal City), bestowed by the king, was much sought after by the larger commercial centres in the kingdom, for it brought with it various tax concessions.

24 Rambollà discovered many interesting facts concerning the Vianeo family. It was he who demonstrated that they moved from Maida to Tropea and that Vincenzo had been born between 1410 and 1420. It appears that Bernardino died at the age of 74 in 1538, while Paolo died in 1555 and Pietro in 1571.

25 On the story of Camillo Porzio's misadventure and how he came to lose his nose, see also the introductory notes by Agostino Gervasio to Porzio's book *L'Historia d'Italia e la Descrizione del Regno d Napoli* [813].

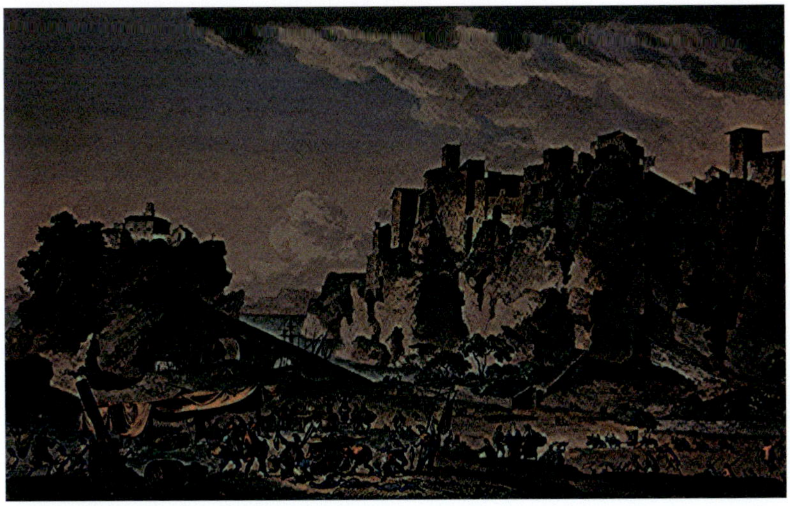

Fig. 7.9 A view of Tropea from an engraving of the seventeenth century *Courtesy of Riccardo Mazzola, M.D., Milan*

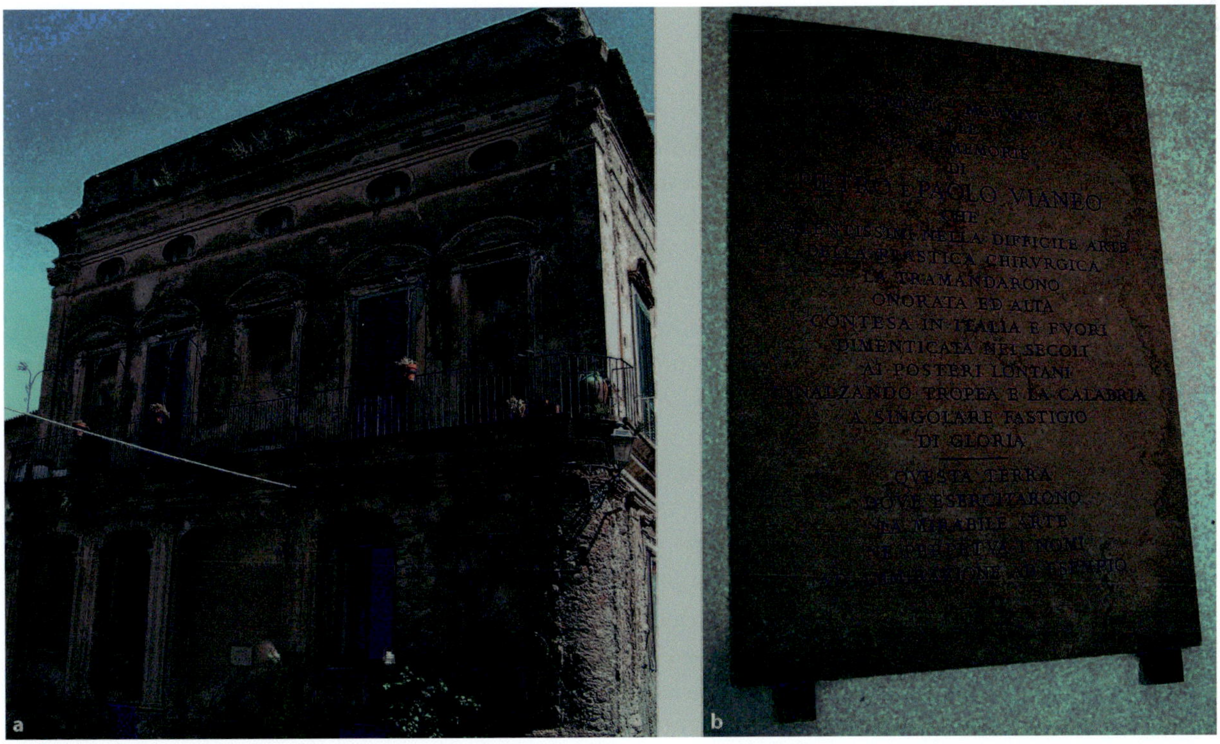

Fig. 7.10 **a** The façade of the Borgognoni Palace in Tropea where the Vianeos worked in the fifteenth century and where they were visited by Leonardo Fioravanti. **b** The plaque commemorating the Vianeos. *Courtesy of Mrs Rosanna Prato, Pisa*

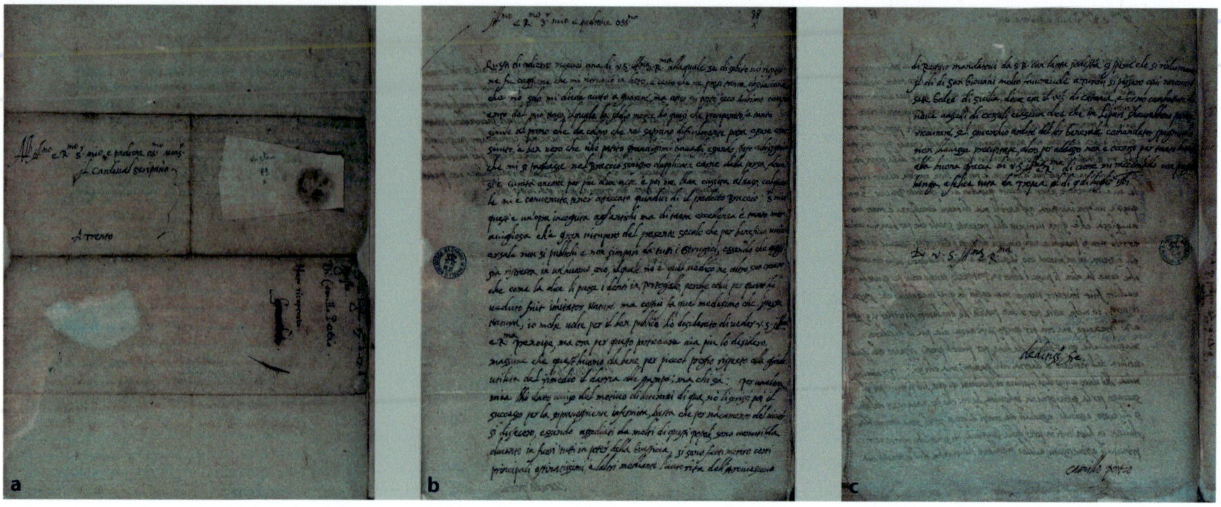

Fig. 7.11a–c The original letter written on 9 July 1561 by Camillo Porzio to his friend, Cardinal Gerolamo Siriprando. The address shows that the Cardinal was attending the Council of Trent which lasted from 1545 to 1563. Porzio outlines the nasal reconstruction he was undergoing in Tropea. *By permission of the Biblioteca Nazionale di Napoli*

sor took himself to Tropea in order to have a new one made and from there wrote a letter on 9 July 1561 to his friend the cardinal Girolamo Siriprando[26] of Lucca, describing his experience (Fig. 7.11a–c). He concluded with satisfaction: "[my new nose] will be difficult to detect by anyone who does not know about it". That the result was more than acceptable may also be deduced from the fact that he later wedded the lady—by this time providentially widowed—who was the cause of his medical adventure (Fig. 7.12a,b).

Further news of the Vianeo family can be obtained from a book published in 1600 by Gabriele Barri [55]. He evidently had limited knowledge of the subject for he wrote: "Vincenzo, a famous surgeon, is the physician who first conceived the art [although we know that in reality he was not the first] of reconstructing mutilated lips and noses. His nephew Bernardino, the son of his brother, inherited this art … " Barri does not mention Paolo Vianeo, although he does write that "a citizen called Pietro Vianeo is still living in the city [of Tropea], he as well being a surgeon who, among other things, restores lips and noses".

Perhaps the most illustrious witness to the bravura of the Vianeo family was the surgeon Ambroise Paré (1510–1590) who wrote: "the young cadet of the family of Saint-Thoan, tired of the burden of wearing a silver nose for so many years, set off for Italy and thanks to his remarkable courage recovered his nose, to the great amazement of all who had known him before."[27] Despite apparently being impressed with the result, Paré was against nasal reconstruction because he thought the procedure was excessively painful for the patient and the immobilization added lengthy discomfort (Fig. 7.13) [768, 770].

Before Paolo and Pietro Vianeo died they had another visitor who deserves credit. This was Leonardo Fioravanti (1518–1588) [314, 317]. According to many at the time, he transformed rhinoplasty from a secret practice performed by artisans to its rightful domain within scientific surgical endeavour [893, 894]. He was a physician with untraditional ideas who generated so much controversy that he was accused of being a charlatan by many of his peers.[28] Fioravanti had studied medicine at the University of Bologna but devoted himself primarily to surgery, thus incurring the disdain of his colleagues

26 The letter to Cardinal Siriprando is conserved in the Biblioteca Nazionale of Naples (codex XIII, A, 52).

27 See *Opera Chirurgica*, Book XXII, Chapter 2, "Qua arte exacta naris portio reparari".

28 For example, Fioravanti was strongly opposed to the practice of blood letting, which was still extremely widespread in his day.

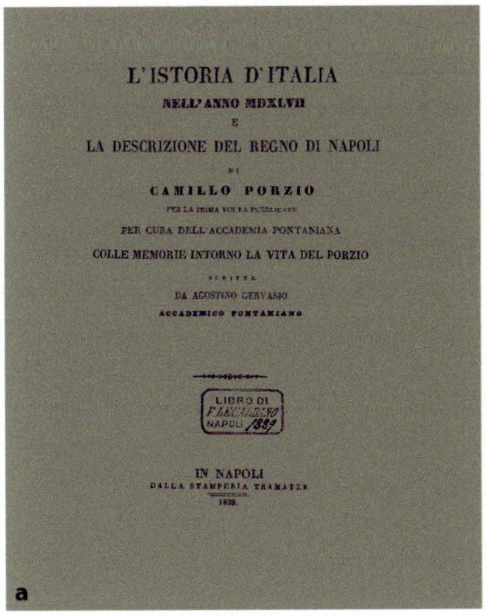
L'ISTORIA D'ITALIA
NELL'ANNO MDXLVII
E
LA DESCRIZIONE DEL REGNO DI NAPOLI
DI
CAMILLO PORZIO
PER LA PRIMA VOLTA PUBBLICATE
PER CURA DELL'ACCADEMIA PONTANIANA
COLLE MEMORIE INTORNO LA VITA DEL PORZIO
SCRITTE
DA AGOSTINO GERVASIO
ACCADEMICO PONTANIANO

IN NAPOLI
DALLA STAMPERIA TRAMATER
1839.

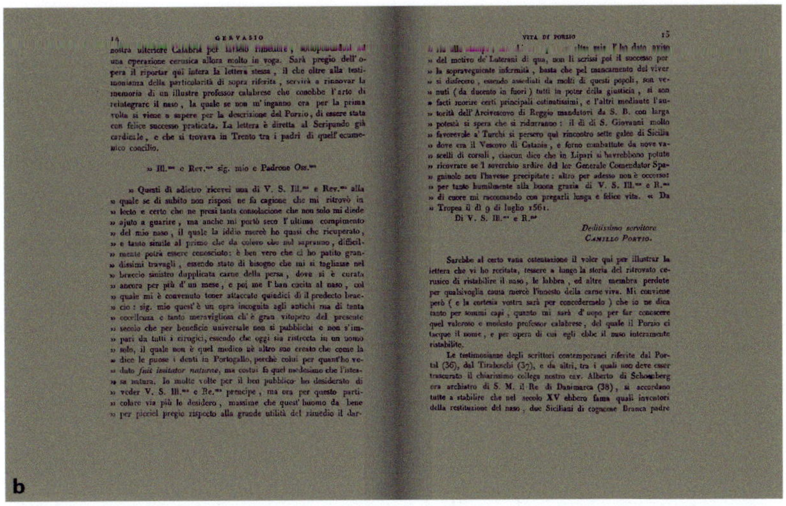

Fig. 7.12 **a** Frontispiece of Camillo Porzio's book *L'Historia d'Italia*, finally published in 1839, where the activities of the Vianeo brothers are reported. **b** The printed version of his letter to the Cardinal. *Courtesy of Riccardo Mazzola, M.D., Milan*

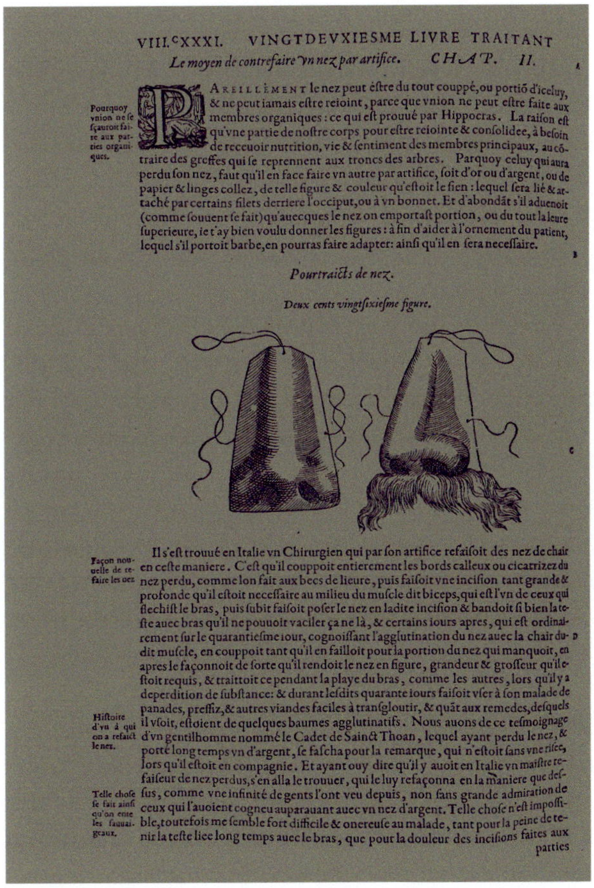
VIII.cXXXI. VINGTDEVXIESME LIVRE TRAITANT

Le moyen de contrefaire vn nez par artifice. CHAP. II.

Pourquoy vnion ne se sçauroit faire aux parties organiques.

PAREILLEMENT le nez peut estre du tout couppé, ou portiō d'iceluy, & ne peut iamais estre reioint, parce que vnion ne peut estre faite aux membres organiques : ce qui est prouué par Hippocras. La raison est qu'vne partie de nostre corps pour estre reiointe & consolidee, à besoin de receuoir nutrition, vie & sentiment des membres principaux, au cōtraire des greffes qui se reprennent aux troncs des arbres. Parquoy celuy qui aura perdu son nez, faut qu'il en face faire vn autre par artifice, soit d'or ou d'argent, ou de papier & linges collez, de telle figure & couleur qu'estoit le sien : lequel sera lié & attaché par certains filets derriere l'occiput, ou à vn bonnet. Et d'abondāt s'il aduenoit (comme souuent se fait) qu'auecques le nez on emportast portion, ou du tout la leure superieure, ie t'ay bien voulu donner les figures : à fin d'aider à l'ornement du patient, lequel s'il portoit barbe, en pourras faire adapter: ainsi qu'il en sera necessaire.

Pourtraicts de nez.

Deux cents vingtsixiesme figure.

Façon nouuelle de refaire les nez

Il s'est trouué en Italie vn Chirurgien qui par son artifice refaisoit des nez de chair en ceste maniere. C'est qu'il couppoit entierement les bords calleux ou cicatrizez du nez perdu, comme lon fait aux becs de lieure, puis faisoit vne incision tant grande & profonde qu'il estoit necessaire au milieu du muscle dit biceps, qui est l'vn de ceux qui flechist le bras, puis subit faisoit poser le nez en ladite incision & bandoit si bien la teste auec bras qu'il ne pouuoit vaciler ça ne là, & certains iours apres, qui est ordinairement sur le quarantiesme iour, cognoissant l'agglutination du nez auec la chair dudit muscle, en couppoit tant qu'il en failloit pour la portion du nez qui manquoit, en apres le façonnoit de sorte qu'il rendoit le nez en figure, grandeur & grosseur qu'il estoit requis, & traittoit ce pendant la playe du bras, comme les autres, lors qu'il y a deperdition de substance: & durant lesdits quarante iours faisoit vser à son malade de panades, pressiz, & autres viandes faciles à transgloutir, & quāt aux remedes, desquels il vsoit, estoient de quelques baumes agglutinatifs. Nous auons de ce tesmoignage d'vn gentilhomme nommé le Cadet de Sainct Thoan, lequel ayant perdu le nez, & porté long temps vn d'argent, se fascha pour la remarque, qui n'estoit sans vne risee, lors qu'il estoit en compagnie. Et ayant ouy dire qu'il y auoit en Italie vn maistre refaiseur de nez perdus, s'en alla le trouuer, qui le luy refaçonna en la maniere que dessus, comme vne infinité de gents l'ont veu depuis, non sans grande admiration de ceux qui l'auoient cogneu auparauant auec vn nez d'argent. Telle chose n'est impossible, toutefois me semble fort difficile & onereuse au malade, tant pour la peine de tenir la teste liee long temps auec le bras, que pour la douleur des incisions faites aux parties

Histoire d'vn à qui on a refaict le nez.

Telle chose se fait ainsi qu'on ente les sauuageaux.

Fig. 7.13 Paré's nasal prostheses from *Les Oeuvres*. The French surgeon preferred prostheses to nasal reconstruction. *Courtesy of Riccardo Mazzola, M.D., Milan*

who continued to believe that medicine was a noble art and surgery a lowly, manual profession (Fig. 7.14). They may also have been envious of his successful business set up for the production and sale of unguents and balms [313].[29]

Fioravanti left Bologna at the age of 31 [315][30] and travelled extensively throughout Italy and Sicily, eventually enrolling as a surgeon with the Spanish army which was sent by the viceroy of Naples to North Africa. While in Africa he had his first experience of reconstructive surgery, which he recounts in his book *Il Tesoro della Vita Humana* (Fig. 7.15) [316]. Like Lanfranchi da Milano, he was called upon to treat a 29-year-old soldier by the name of Andres Gutierrez whose nose had been cut off during a brawl. Fioravanti says "The nose fell into the sand. The quarrel ended and the poor man remained without his nose. And I, who happened to be standing there, took it up and after peeing upon it to wash away

29 His unguents and balms were popular in England at the time.

30 See Fioravanti, *Il Reggimento della Peste* [315].

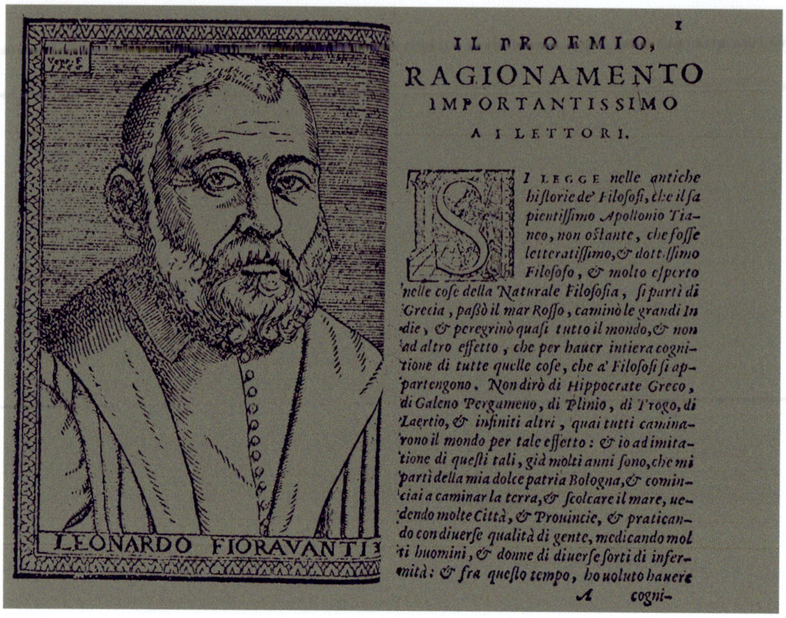
IL PROEMIO,
RAGIONAMENTO
IMPORTANTISSIMO
A I LETTORI.

SI LEGGE nelle antiche hiſtorie de' Filoſofi, che il ſapientiſſimo Apollonio Tianeo, non oſtante, che foſſe letteratiſſimo, & dottiſſimo Filoſofo, & molto eſperto nelle coſe della Naturale Filoſofia, ſi partì di Grecia, paſſò il mar Roſſo, caminò le grandi Indie, & peregrinò quaſi tutto il mondo, & non ad altro effetto, che per hauer intiera cognitione di tutte quelle coſe, che a' Filoſofi ſi appartengono. Non dirò di Hippocrate Greco, di Galeno Pergameno, di Plinio, di Trogo, di Laertio, & infiniti altri, quai tutti caminarono il mondo per tale effetto: & io ad imitatione di queſti tali, già molti anni ſono, che mi parti della mia dolce patria Bologna, & cominciai a caminar la terra, & ſolcare il mare, uedendo molte Città, & Prouincie, & praticando con diuerſe qualità di gente, medicando molti huomini, & donne di diuerſe ſorti di infermità: & fra queſto tempo, ho uoluto hauere

A cogni-

Fig. 7.14 Portrait of Leonardo Fioravanti (1518–1588) with the first page of his book. He studied at the University of Bologna and was one of the rare surgeons to graduate in Medicine. *Courtesy of Riccardo Mazzola, M.D., Milan*

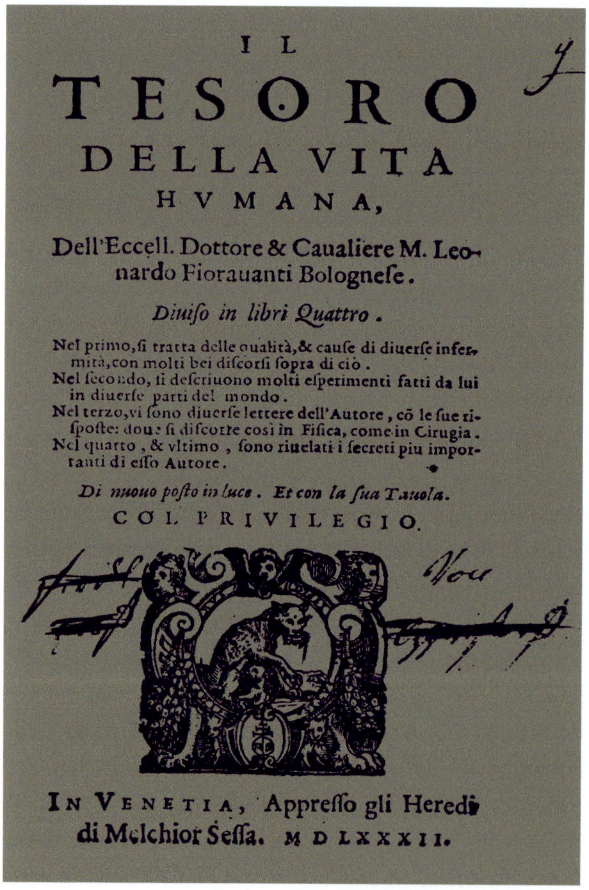
IL
TESORO
DELLA VITA
HVMANA,

Dell'Eccell. Dottore & Caualiere M. Leonardo Fiorauanti Bologneſe.

Diuiſo in libri Quattro.

Nel primo, ſi tratta delle qualità, & cauſe di diuerſe infermità, con molti bei diſcorſi ſopra di ciò.
Nel ſecondo, ſi deſcriuono molti eſperimenti fatti da lui in diuerſe parti del mondo.
Nel terzo, vi ſono diuerſe lettere dell'Autore, cō le ſue riſpoſte: doue ſi diſcorre così in Fiſica, come in Cirugia.
Nel quarto, & vltimo, ſono riuelati i ſecreti piu importanti di eſſo Autore.

Di nuouo poſto in luce. Et con la ſua Tauola.

COL PRIVILEGIO.

IN VENETIA, Appreſſo gli Heredi di Melchior Seſſa. M D LXXXII.

Fig. 7.15 Frontispiece of *Il Tesoro della Vita Humana* by Fioravanti. *Courtesy of Riccardo Mazzola, M.D., Milan*

the sand, I stitched it into place once again very firmly, and dressed it with a balsam of our own making, and let the bandage remain for eight days, thinking that in any case it would have served for naught. Instead when I unbound it, the nose had stuck so well that all Naples came to hear of this marvel, and this is well known for the said Andreas doth live yet and can testify to the same." (Fig. 7.16)

Fioravanti had great faith in the benefits of urine, as can be read in the surgical text by Pietro and Ludovico Rostinio [864] published in 1564. They wrote that with regard to "long, penetrating wounds, where a mere ligature is not enough for closing … In such cases Leonardo from Bologna would recommend that the wounds be washed with urine which has just been discharged and still is warm. The reason is that warm urine attracts the blood and cleanses the fresh wound. It is wonderful to see how such washing is very beneficial to new wounds."

Another example of the use of urine may be found in Fioravanti's own account of what may have been the very first splenectomy done in Italy, from his book *Il Reggimento della Peste*. The patient was a Greek woman suffering from splenomegaly and the outcome of the operation, which he carried out in Palermo with the help of the unskilled surgeon Adriano Zaccarello, was so successful that she was seen attending mass at the Church of Madonna dei Miracoli just twenty-one days later! Encouraged by

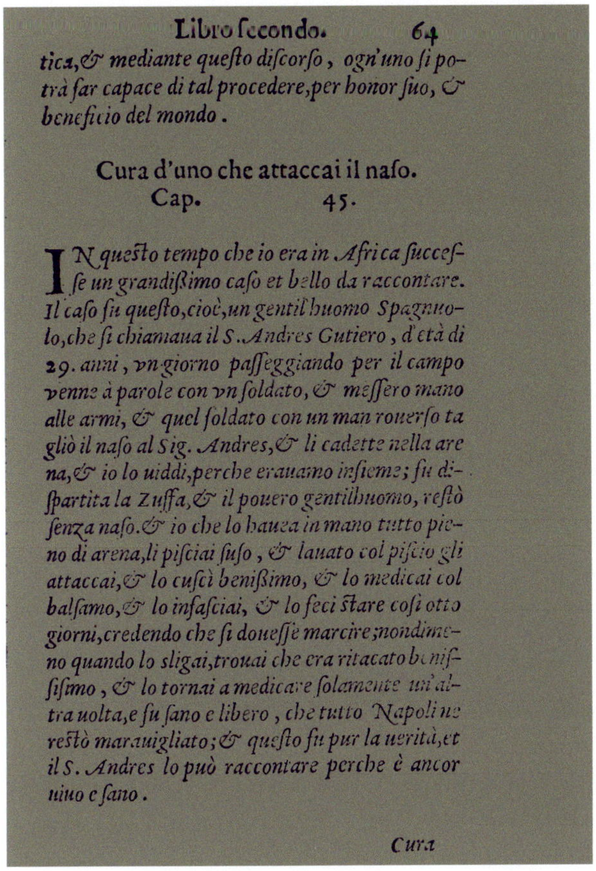

Libro ſecondo. 64

tica, & mediante queſto diſcorſo, ogn'uno ſi potrà far capace di tal procedere, per honor ſuo, & beneficio del mondo.

Cura d'uno che attaccai il naſo. Cap. 45.

IN queſto tempo che io era in Africa ſucceſſe un grandiſsimo caſo et bello da raccontare. Il caſo fu queſto, cioè, un gentil'huomo Spagnuolo, che ſi chiamaua il S. Andres Gutiero, d'età di 29. anni, vn giorno paſſeggiando per il campo venne à parole con vn ſoldato, & meſſero mano alle armi, & quel ſoldato con un man rouerſo tagliò il naſo al Sig. Andres, & li cadette nella arena, & io lo uiddi, perche erauamo inſieme; fu diſpartita la Zuffa, & il pouero gentilhuomo, reſtò ſenza naſo. & io che lo haueа in mano tutto pieno di arena, li piſciai ſuſo, & lauato col piſcio gli attaccai, & lo cuſcì beniſsimo, & lo medicai col balſamo, & lo infaſciai, & lo feci ſtare coſi otto giorni, credendo che ſi doueſſe marcire; nondimeno quando lo sligai, trouai che era ritacato beniſſimo, & lo tornai a medicare ſolamente un'altra uolta, e fu ſano e libero, che tutto Napoli ne reſtò marauigliato; & queſto fu pur la uerità, et il S. Andres lo può raccontare perche è ancor uiuo e ſano.

Cura

Fig. 7.16 In this page from *Il Tesoro della Vita Humana*, Fioravanti describes how he replanted the nose of a Spanish soldier in Africa. *Courtesy of Riccardo Mazzola, M.D., Milan*

this success, Fioravanti sought to repeat the operation a short time later in Naples when a patient with an injured spleen was brought to him. In this case, after removing the organ it was necessary to clean the blood clot from the abdominal cavity. Fioravanti asked everyone around the operating table to urinate (sic!) on the unfortunate patient, certainly a more antiseptic procedure than washing out the abdominal cavity with a pail of water, and the patient recovered without complications.

Returning to Fioravanti's contribution to rhinoplasty, after his tour of duty in Africa Fioravanti went to Catania, only to discover that the Branca family, whose technique he hoped to learn, were no longer practising. He therefore continued to Calabria, determined to witness the operation carried out by the Vianeo family, before returning to Naples:"And thus I embarked for Calabria to go to Naples; but first I went to a city called Turpia, where at that time lived two brothers, one called Pietro and the other Paulo, noble and influential men in the city, and most worthy surgeons who could make a nose for anyone who had lost his own by some accident. In this city I made a halt, with a mind to see if I could somehow get to know how they proceeded when carrying out such an operation."

Despite fact that they usually guarded their secret from all strangers and other surgeons in particular, the Vianeo brothers appear to have accepted their visitor without much hesitation, probably because Fioravanti did not present himself as a surgeon. He writes: "I went to the house of those two physicians pretending that I was a gentleman from Bologna, and had come to see them because I had a relative whose nose had been cut off at Serravalle in Lombardia while fighting against the enemy, and I wished to know whether it would be opportune for him to come to them or not. Furthermore, I told them that in Bologna there was a Senator by the name of Cornelio Albergati, whose nose had been cut off by a street thief, and that he had learned of the fame of these surgeons from letters. These were the reasons for which I wished to observe." No doubt happy at the prospect of acquiring two wealthy new patients, the brothers gave Fioravanti permission… "to go every day to their house where they had five noses in the course of reconstruction and I, … pretending that I had not the courage to look, turned my face elsewhere but my eyes saw very well and thus I succeeded in discovering the entire secret operation from beginning to end, and learned it".

Here, after describing the preliminaries, which included the administration of a pre-operative purgative, Fioravanti proceeds to the technique itself: "In the left arm, between the shoulder and the elbow, they took hold of the skin with pincers and, lifting it, they passed a large knife between the pincers and the flesh of the muscle, then inserting from one end to the other a piece of wool or linen; and they medicated the wound until the skin had thickened, after which they scarified [the stump of] the nose, then they detached the skin from the arm by cutting it at one extremity and they sutured it to the nose and bound it with such artifice and skill that there was no possibility of moving the arm from the face until the skin had grown into the nose; and when it had grown, they cut the other end still attached to the arm and, after having scarified the lip of the mouth, they sewed to it

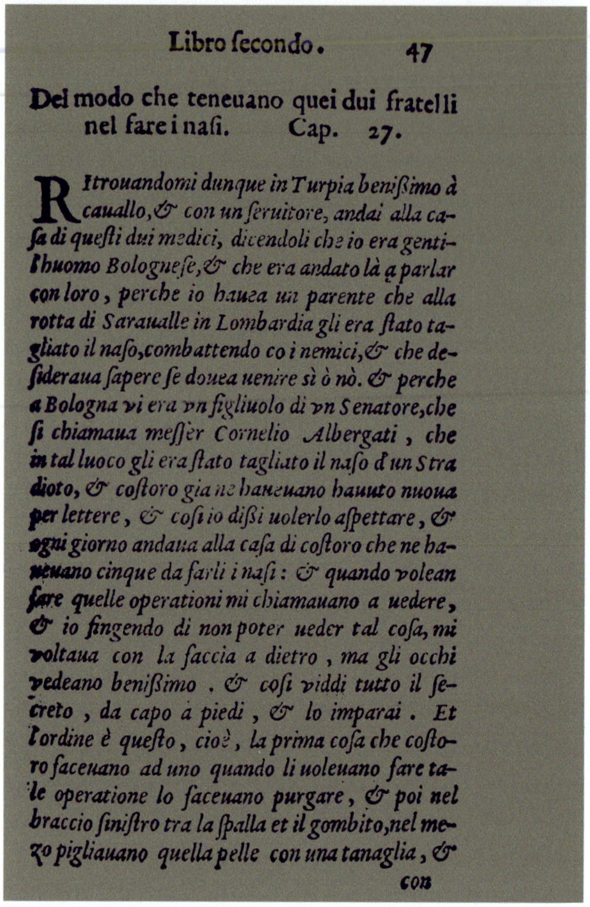

Libro ſecondo. 47

Del modo che teneuano quei dui fratelli nel fare i naſi. Cap. 27.

Ritrouandomi dunque in Turpia beniſſimo à cauallo, & con un ſeruitore, andai alla caſa di queſti dui medici, dicendoli che io era gentilhuomo Bologneſe, & che era andato là à parlar con loro, perche io hauea un parente che alla rotta di Saraualle in Lombardia gli era ſtato tagliato il naſo, combattendo co i nemici, & che deſideraua ſapere ſe douea uenire sì ò nò. & perche a Bologna vi era vn figliuolo di vn Senatore, che ſi chiamaua meſſèr Cornelio Albergati, che in tal luoco gli era ſtato tagliato il naſo d'un Stradioto, & coſtoro gia ne haueuano hauuto nuoua per lettere, & coſi io diſſi uolerlo aſpettare, & ogni giorno andaua alla caſa di coſtoro che ne haueuano cinque da farli i naſi: & quando volean fare quelle operationi mi chiamauano a uedere, & io fingendo di non poter ueder tal coſa, mi voltaua con la faccia a dietro, ma gli occhi vedeano beniſſimo. & coſi viddi tutto il ſecreto, da capo à piedi, & lo imparai. Et l'ordine è queſto, cioè, la prima coſa che coſtoro faceuano ad uno quando li uoleuano fare tale operatione lo faceuano purgare, & poi nel braccio ſiniſtro tra la ſpalla et il gombito, nel mezo pigliauano quella pelle con una tanaglia, &

con

Fig. 7.17 The page from *Il Tesoro della Vita Humana* which describes Fiorovanti's visit to the Vianeo brothers in Tropea. The book was published by the *Collegio dei Dottori* in Bologna when Gaspare Tagliacozzi was a medical student and it possibly stimulated his interest in nasal reconstruction. *Courtesy of Riccardo Mazzola, M.D., Milan*

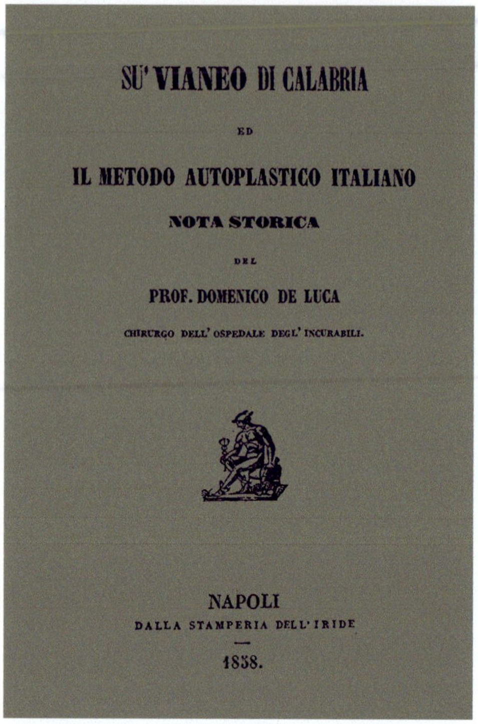

Fig. 7.18 Frontispiece of de Luca's book about the Vaineo family from 1858. *Courtesy of Riccardo Mazzola, M.D., Milan*

the skin of the arm, and tended it until it had fused with the lip and then they applied [to the site] a metal form in which the new nose could grow to the right size and form, even if it remained somewhat more white than the face. Such is the method that these men used in re-making the nose." (Fig. 7.17)

A full account of the operation is provided in *Il Tesoro della Vita Humana*, which was printed around 1570.[31] The book was a notable success, and was recommended to the members of the University of Bologna's Collegio dei Dottori, to which Fioravanti himself belonged [378].

Before leaving the Vianeo family it is interesting to note that they were not completely forgotten and reappeared in the nineteenth century in *Su Vianeo di Calabria, Il Methodo Autoplastico Italiano* by Domenico de Luca published in Naples in 1858 (Fig. 7.18).

31 According to Gnudi and Webster, the book was first published in Venice in 1570, but this does not mean that his work was not familiar to the faculty in Bologna beforehand. The work formed his thesis and we know that he graduated in 1568.

Gaspare Tagliacozzi

There was another outstanding surgeon working in Bologna at the time. This was Gaspare Tagliacozzi (1545–1599), whose name is familiar to many plastic surgeons. He was so gifted that while still a student he was assigned the post of lettore (lecturer) under the supervision of the professor anatomy and surgery Giulio Cesare Aranzio (1530–1599) (Fig. 7.19). It is probable that Tagliacozzi read Fioravanti's account of the Vianeo's technique and this awakened his interest in the subject. We may even be allowed to suspect that if he had not come across *Il Tesoro della Vita Humana*, Tagliacozzi would have become an anatomist rather than immersing himself in this miraculous new form of surgery.

Tagliacozzi was born in Bologna on 2 March 1545 and died there in 1599, although for centuries these dates remained uncertain.[32] There was also confusion about his birthplace which was sometimes said to be the town of Tagliacozzo in the Abruzzi [362, 623].[33] These details have formed the object of debate and inaccurate citations. It was only when the detailed study of M. Gnudi and J. Webster [379–381] was published in 1935 that these questions were settled beyond doubt. The two historians found the name "Gaspar filius Joannisandreae Tagliacossa" dated 2 March 1545, written in the baptismal registry of the Church of San Pietro in Bologna. In that time it was the custom to baptize babies within two days of their birth and it seems highly unlikely that the child would have been brought all the way from the mountainous town in the Abruzzi to Bologna in March. Furthermore Gnudi and Webster were able to show from documents in the archives of the archbishop that the wealthy and influential Tagliacozzi family had lived in the city for at least two centuries. They failed to find any link with the Abruzzi town of Tagliacozzo.

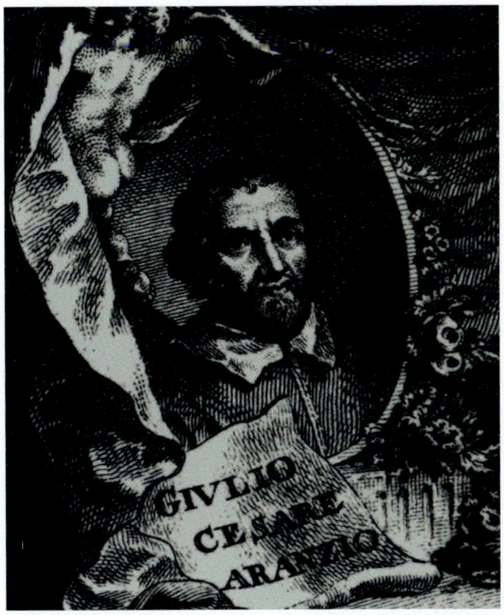

Fig. 7.19 Portrait of Giulio Cesare Aranzio (1530–1589) who taught Tagliacozzi in Bologna. He made a study of blood circulation and published a book, *De Humano Foetu Libellus*, describing the physiology of pregnancy. *Courtesy of FMR Art. spa Bologna*

Tagliacozzi enrolled as a medical student at the University of Bologna in 1565, and began teaching anatomy at the Ospedale della Vita e della Morte even before he completed his studies in 1570 [623]. According to the historian G.G. Forni [330], the hospital was probably the most important of the sixteen found in the province of Bologna at that time and provided cadavers for the university's anatomical dissections. After Tagliacozzi graduated, Aranzio got him the position of lecturer in surgery

32 G.A. Mercklinus [659] wrote incorrectly in a short biography in 1658 that Tagliacozzi was born in 1553. P.A. Orlandi [758] stated in 1714 that Tagliacozzi died in 1553 and this erroneous information was repeated by J.J. Mauget [620] in 1731 and by N.F.T. Eloy [277] in 1755, whereas G. Fantuzzi [301] in 1790 and Michele Medici [657] in 1857 stated the year of his birth to be 1546.

33 Giuseppe Baronio (1758–1814) [54] believed that Tagliacozzi was born in Tuscany, while Giuseppe Gattinari [362] claimed that he was from the region of Abruzzi where there is a town by the name of Tagliacozzo. To add to the confusion, in this town is a square dedicated to "Gaspare Trigambe, famoso chirurgo dei miracoli, professore di Chirurgia a Bologna, del quale un busto ed una statua sono esibiti nell'Archiginnasio" [Gaspare Trigambe, famous surgeon of miracles, professor of surgery at Bologna, of whom a bust and a statue are on display in the Archiginnasio]. The historian G. Marini [611] wrote an article on "questo chirurgo dei miracoli, Gaspare Triganbe, nato a Tagliacozzo" [this surgeon of miracles, Gaspare Triganbe, born in Tagliacozzo]. It is probable however that Trigambe was a legendary figure, and in any case there is no evidence that he was the same person as Gaspare Tagliacozzi.

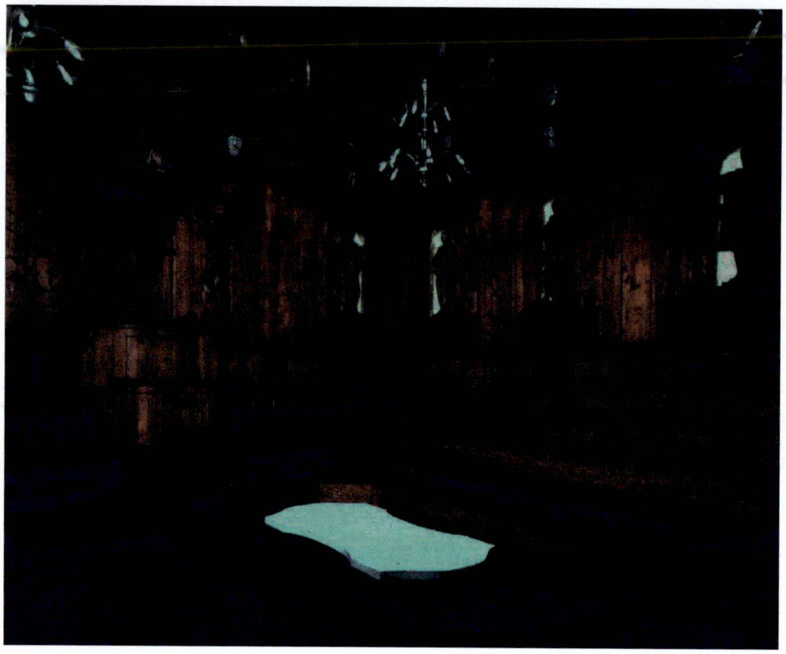

Fig. 7.20 The restored Anatomical Theatre in Bologna where Tagliacozzi lectured. *PJS*

at the university (Fig. 7.20). In the meantime, this exceptional young man enrolled in the faculty of philosophy and after completing his studies in 1576, became a full member of the *Collegio di Arti e Medicina*, better known as the Collegio dei Dottori (Fig. 7.21).

The Letter of Tagliacozzi to Mercurialis

Aranzio[34] played an important role in Tagliacozzi's professional career. He not only secured the post of lecturer in both anatomy and surgery for him but then designated him as the successor to his chair. As well as these well-deserved favours he apparently gave him operating experience, as Gnudi and Webster report: "Tagliacozzi was directly indebted to Giulio Cesare Aranzio for his first practical lessons on the Art." Does this mean that Aranzio also taught his student the technique of rhinoplasty? This would be plausible because he himself had mastered the procedure, as we learn from a work discovered by Gnudi and Webster. It appears that the Polish physician, Wojciech Oczko visited Italy from 1565 to 1569, remaining for a considerable time in Bologna. In his book Przymiot he wrote admiringly "what Aranzio, professor of surgery, used regularly to do [facere solebat] during my days in Bologna, employing the skin of the arm and without touching the muscle … and there resulted a beautiful nose". However little is known about Tagliacozzi's activities as a surgeon before 1568, the year he wrote his famous letter to Mercurialis.

During the sixteenth century Gerolamo Mercurialis (1530 to c.1604) was one of the most influential figures in Italian medicine. He studied in Bologna and taught at the University of Pisa before becoming professor of medicine at Padua. He was the author of a systematic treatise on skin diseases in 1572 and a well-known illustrated compendium on medical gymnastics in 1573.[35] As a cultivated intellectual with a broad range of interests, he was appointed Superintendent of the Vatican Monuments by the Pope.

34 Giulio Ceseare Aranzio made several significant contributions to the development of anatomy during the sixteenth century. He published *Observationes Anatomicas* and *De Humano Faeto Opusculum* and initiated construction of the university's famous anatomical theatre which was completed in 1637, 48 years after his death.

35 This probably represents the first published text on physiotherapy.

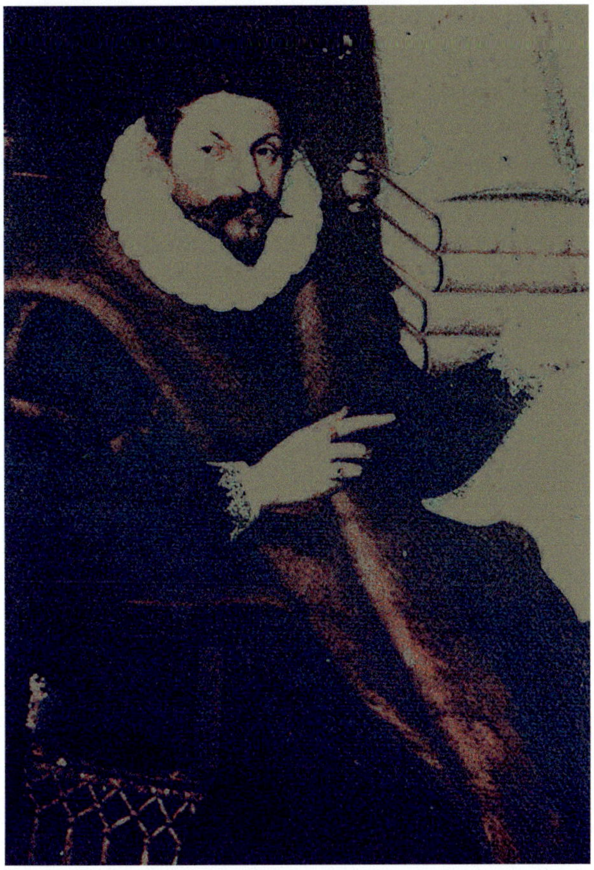

Fig. 7.21 Portrait of Gaspare Tagliacozzi (1545–1599). *Courtesy of Riccardo Mazzola, M.D., Milan*

In 1585 Mercurialis published the first edition of *De Decoratione Liber* in which he mentions the nasal reconstructions that were being carried out in Italy: "In our time applause has been accorded for the discoveries of those who restored noses, certainly in Calabria," and adds, "There is also the excellent Tagliacotius in Bologna, who recently showed me, when I was there visiting, two patients whose noses had been reconstructed."[36]

Tagliacozzi was fully aware of Mercurialis' influence in academic circles and "In Bologna on the 22nd day of February in the year of our Lord 1586" wrote him a letter to inform him that since his visit he had successfully completed another two nasal reconstructions. This letter was reproduced in its entirety by Mercurialis in the second edition of *De Decoratione Liber* (Fig. 7.22), which was published in Frankfurt in 1587 [660].[37] For twelve years, until Tagliacozzi finally published his book, this four-page letter constituted the only source of information available on the rhinoplasty technique as it was practised in Bologna (Fig. 7.23). In his letter Tagliacozzi provided a concise and lucid description of the operation, although he expressed concern that its brevity might induce the inexpert surgeon: "… like a sailor who has learned [to navigate] from books, to attempt the operation without success, to the detriment both of the patient and the very reputation of the Art."

Tagliacozzi had good reason to be worried because he had already seen how his method could be misinterpreted or completely misunderstood. As he wrote: "Vesalius, Paré, Gourmelin and others have written that a small hole or cavity is prepared on the arm, in which the mutilated nose is buried until the flesh grows into it, and that this flesh is moulded into a shape of a nose."[38] This of course was a wholly incorrect interpretation of the technique, which was to raise a flap on the arm and stitch it to the nose before separating it at a later operation. The nose was not "buried" beneath the skin of the arm.

Tagliacozzi furnished instructions on the preparation of the patient for the operation. For example, "Briefly, any cacochymia [he probably meant any general illness] must be removed … [Patients suffering from] a venereal disease must be ruled out absolutely … The bowels should be moved daily or be stimulated appropriately." However, most of his letter covered the technical details of the operation itself. "An incision is made in the skin of one of the arms, right or left, down to the flesh, right down to

36 See *De Decoratione Liber*, Chapter XVIII (De scissuris cutis), p 23.

37 See also the *Observationes Medicarum* … by Johannes Aschenk von Grafenberg, in 1594, p 200.

38 Vesalius obviously did not fully grasp the nature of the operation for he wrote: "… the principle is to lift the muscle at its thickest and most fleshy point and to separate it completely from the underlying parts. Once this is done one must very carefully separate the epidermis and dermis from the muscle … We unite the flap of muscle to the face in such a manner as to prevent any movement of the head or arm for a period of forty days." Paré also believed that 40 days of immobilization were necessary and concluded that this period was too long for most patients to tolerate.

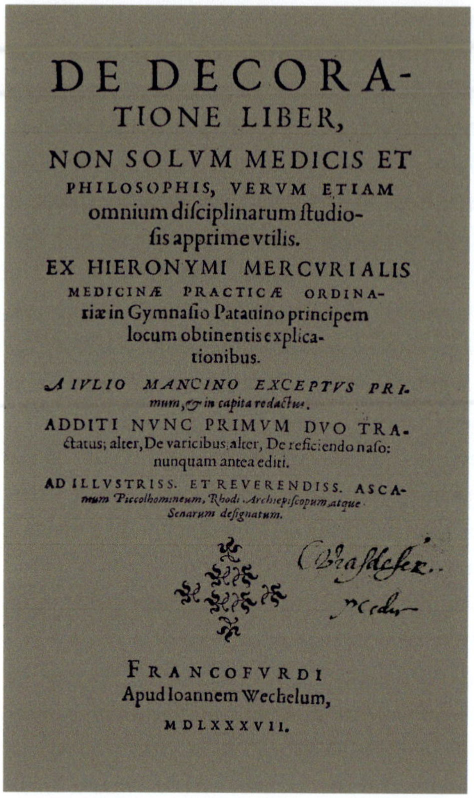

DE DECORA-
TIONE LIBER,
NON SOLVM MEDICIS ET
PHILOSOPHIS, VERVM ETIAM
omnium diſciplinarum ſtudio-
ſis apprime vtilis.
EX HIERONYMI MERCVRIALIS
MEDICINÆ PRACTICÆ ORDINA-
riæ in Gymnaſio Patauino principem
locum obtinentis explica-
tionibus.
*A IVLIO MANCINO EXCEPTVS PRI-
mum, & in capita redactus.*
ADDITI NVNC PRIMVM DVO TRA-
ctatus; alter, De varicibus; alter, De reficiendo naſo:
nunquam antea editi.
AD ILLVSTRISS. ET REVERENDISS. ASCA-
*nium Piccolhomineum, Rhodi Archiepiſcopum atque
Senarum deſignatum.*

FRANCOFVRDI
Apud Ioannem Wechelum,
MDLXXXVII.

Fig. 7.22 Frontispiece of the second edition of *De Decoratione Libere* by Gerolamo Mercurialis (1530–1604) from 1587 which includes Tagliacozzi's letter describing his method. Tagliacozzi's own book appeared one year later. Mercurialis had already written about the nasal reconstructions carried out by the Vianeos and Tagliacozzi in the first edition of 1585. *Courtesy of Riccardo Mazzola, M.D., Milan*

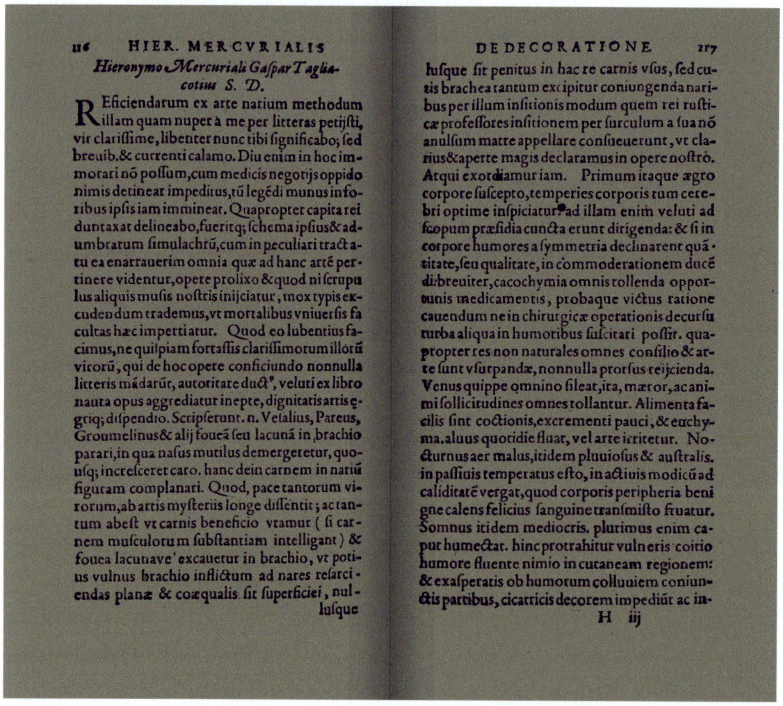

116 HIER. MERCVRIALIS

*Hieronymo Mercuriali Gaſpar Taglia-
cotius S. D.*

REficiendarum ex arte narium methodum
illam quam nuper à me per litteras petijſti,
vir clariſſime, libenter nunc tibi ſignificabo; ſed
breuib. & currenti calamo. Diu enim in hoc im-
morari nō poſſum, cum medicis negotijs oppido
nimis detinear impeditus, tū legēdi munus in fo-
ribus ipſis iam immineat. Quapropter capita rei
duntaxat delineabo, fueritq; ſchema ipſius & ad-
umbratum ſimulachrū, cum in peculiari tracta-
tu ea enarrauerim omnia quæ ad hanc artē per-
tinere videntur, opere prolixo & quod ni ſcrupu
lus aliquis muſis noſtris inijciatur, mox typis ex-
cudendum trademus, vt mortalibus vniuerſis fa
cultas hæc imperti atur. Quod eo lubentius fa-
cimus, ne quiſpiam fortaſſis clariſſimorum illorū
virorū, qui de hoc opere conficiundo nonnulla
litteris mādarūt, autoritate duct⁹, veluti ex libro
nauta opus aggrediatur inepte, dignitatis artis ę-
griq; diſpendio. Scripſerunt. n. Veſalius, Pareus,
Groumelinus & alij foueā ſeu lacunā in brachio
parari, in qua naſus mutilus demergeretur, quo-
uſq; increſceret caro. hanc dein carnem in nariū
figuram complanari. Quod, pace tantorum vi-
rorum, ab artis myſteriis longe diſſentit; ac tan-
tum abeſt vt carnis beneficio vtamur (ſi car-
nem muſculorum ſubſtantiam intelligant) &
fouea lacunave excauetur in brachio, vt poti-
us vulnus brachio inflictum ad nares reſarci-
endas planæ & coæqualis ſit ſuperficiei, nul-
luſque

DE DECORATIONE 117

luſque ſit penitus in hac re carnis vſus, ſed cu-
tis brachea tantum excipitur coniungenda nari-
bus per illum inſitionis modum quem rei ruſti-
cæ profeſſores inſitionem per ſurculum a ſua nō
anulſum matre appellare conſueuerunt, vt cla-
rius & aperte magis declaramus in opere noſtro.
Atqui exordiamur iam. Primum itaque ægro
corpore ſuſcepto, temperies corporis tum cere-
bri optime inſpiciatur: ad illam enim veluti ad
ſcopum præſidia cuncta erunt dirigenda: & ſi in
corpore humores a ſymmetria declinarent quā-
titate, ſeu qualitate, in commoderationem ducē
di: breuiter, cacochymia omnis tollenda oppor-
tunis medicamentis, probaque victus ratione
cauendum ne in chirurgicæ operationis decurſu
turba aliqua in humoribus ſuſcitari poſſit. qua-
propter res non naturales omnes conſilio & ar-
te ſunt vſurpandæ, nonnulla prorſus reijcienda.
Venus quippe omnino ſileat, ita, mæror, ac ani-
mi ſollicitudines omnes tollantur. Alimenta fa-
cilis ſint coctionis, excrementi pauci, & euchy-
ma. aluus quotidie fluat, vel arte irritetur. No-
cturnus aer malus, itidem pluuioſus & auſtralis.
in paſſiuis temperatus eſto, in actiuis modicū ad
caliditatē vergat, quod corporis peripheria beni
gne calens felicius ſanguine tranſmiſto fruatur.
Somnus itidem mediocris. plurimus enim ca-
put humectat. hinc protrahitur vulneris coitio
humore fluente nimio in cutaneam regionem:
& exaſperatis ob humorum colluuiem coniun-
ctis partibus, cicatricis decorem impediūt ac in-

H iij

Fig. 7.23 Tagliacozzi's letter to Mercurialis in the second edition of *De Decoratione Libere*. *Courtesy of Riccardo Mazzola, M.D., Milan* the surface of the muscle; in other words, simple and solid skin is taken from the anterior brachial region."

One of his next points was destined to be either misinterpreted or completely ignored and remained a controversial issue for 150 years. Tagliacozzi wrote: "The removal of the bandage should be decided on the basis of the union and on a satisfactory nourishment of the skin and this will vary considerably according to the varying temperament of the patient. But when one observes a good union of the wound and a good nourishment of the skin, then one may cut the arm from the face." Tagliacozzi did not specify exactly how much time should elapse before dividing the flap, leaving it instead to the judgement of the surgeon. But he did conclude that "a period of about fourteen days is in general necessary for the process of thickening and solidification to become complete." We will see that these straightforward recommendations were often ignored by Tagliacozzi's detractors, who claimed that the patient must remain for no less than forty days in a very uncomfortable position with his arm attached to his face. This they believed made the operation unendurable. Tagliacozzi, no doubt having already had to persuade worried patients, took care to explain in his letter that "on the contrary the procedure is so well tolerated that, even leaving aside the outcome, [this procedure] has won universal admiration".[39]

Tagliacozzi's instructions concluded with an explanation of how to splint and bandage the flap, a complex but necessary manoeuvre to ensure the proper shape of the new nose. Finally, he listed with pride the aristocratic patients, three Italians and a Belgian, whom he had successfully treated and announced to his illustrious colleague in Padua that he was writing a treatise in which every aspect of the operation would be thoroughly discussed.[40]

Tagliacozzi's Nasal Reconstruction

In 1598, twelve years after his letter to Mercurialis, Tagliacozzi published *De Curtorum Chirurgia per Insitionem* (Fig. 7.24) [969] under the auspices of the University of Bologna and with the financial support of Vincenzo Gonzaga, Duke of Mantua.[41] The result was a unique work—the first text on plastic surgery in the history of medicine. In over 700 pages the author analyses the principles of the operation, discusses the indications and contraindications, explains the healing process (*cohalescere*) as the flap becomes attached to the recipient site, and describes the surgical instruments (often of his own design) that were required. The problems of postoperative care and the prevention of complications are not neglected. All of the difficulties that a surgeon might encounter in the creation of a new nose are raised and discussed in detail. Finally he explains how the flap could be used to repair other parts of the face.

Twenty-one woodcut engravings (*icones*) illustrate the various stages of the procedure. The author expresses himself pleased to be able to, as he put it: "at last bring this area of surgery to the true level of an Art, so that it can be transmitted in writing and any man may confidently and successfully operate in accordance with the rules that he finds here before him" (Figs. 7.25a,b, 7.26a,b).

Tagliacozzi did not claim to have been the inventor of the technique; indeed he generously cites the contributions of his predecessors, the flaps of Celsus, Galen and Paulus Aegineta, and the descriptions by Vesalius and Alessandro Benedetti. He refers to Benedetti as "a truly eloquent man, Veronese by birth"[42] and reports in full his description of the operation. Gustavo Branca is also mentioned and Tagliacozzi strongly criticizes *il Maestro siciliano* for never having described his operation, but states that in his judgement it was probably quite different from his own.

Tagliacozzi's academic position and social connections undoubtedly contributed to the success of his book.

39 Thomas and Goldwyn translated Tagliacozzi's writings in their book of 1996 [984] and we have used them in this section.

40 Gnudi and Webster succeeded in tracking down the names of another eleven patients who were treated by Tagliacozzi after 1580, including the Duke of Piacenza, the Duke of Mantova, and a member of the family of Grand Duke Ferdinando of Tuscany (Tagliacozzi happening to be in Florence on a visit to the Grand Duke).

41 The dedication on the front page of the book is to Principe Vincenzo Gonzaga, not simply Duke of Mantova.

42 Alessandro Benedetti was born in Legnago, a town close to Verona.

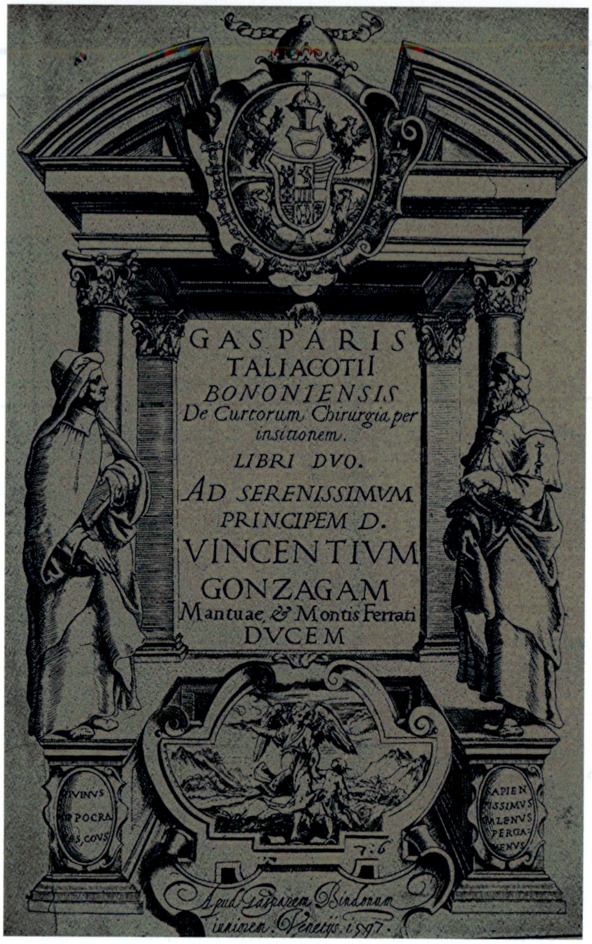

Fig. 7.24 The frontispiece of *De Curtorum Chirurgia per Insitionem* with the dedication to *Principem D. Vincentium Gonzagam* who supported Gaspare Tagliacozzi. *Courtesy of Riccardo Mazzola, M.D., Milan*

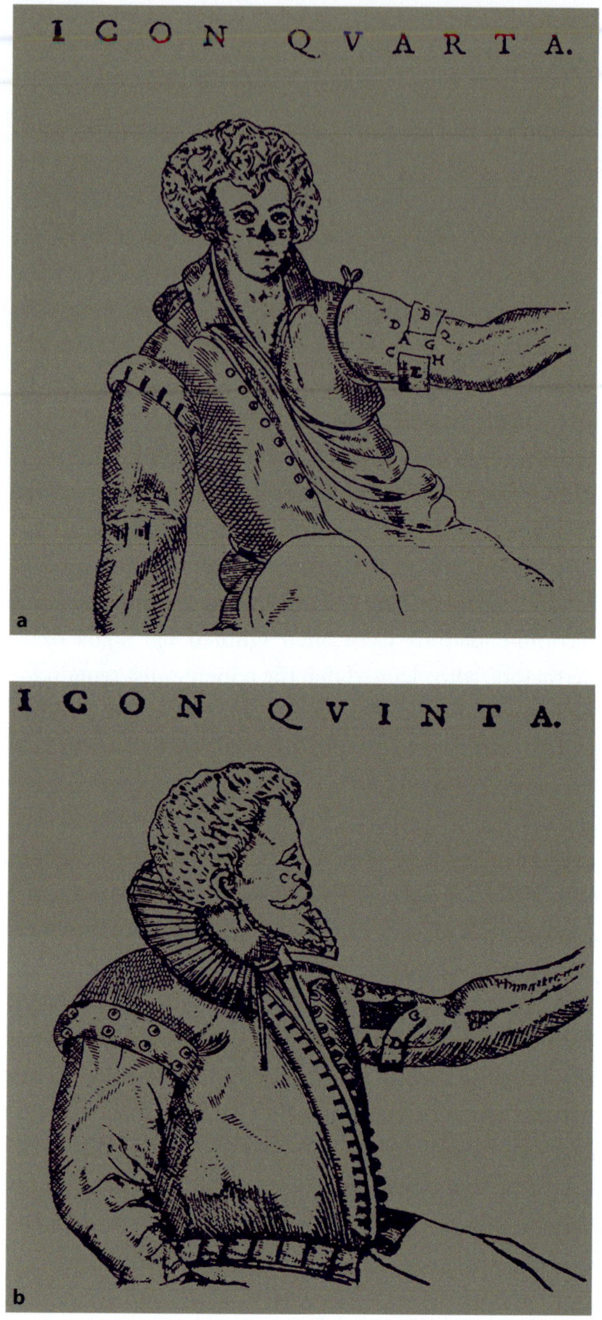

Fig. 7.25a,b Two iconae (numbers 4 and 5) from the book by Tagliacozzi showing the early stages of the reconstruction. *Courtesy of Riccardo Mazzola, M.D., Milan*

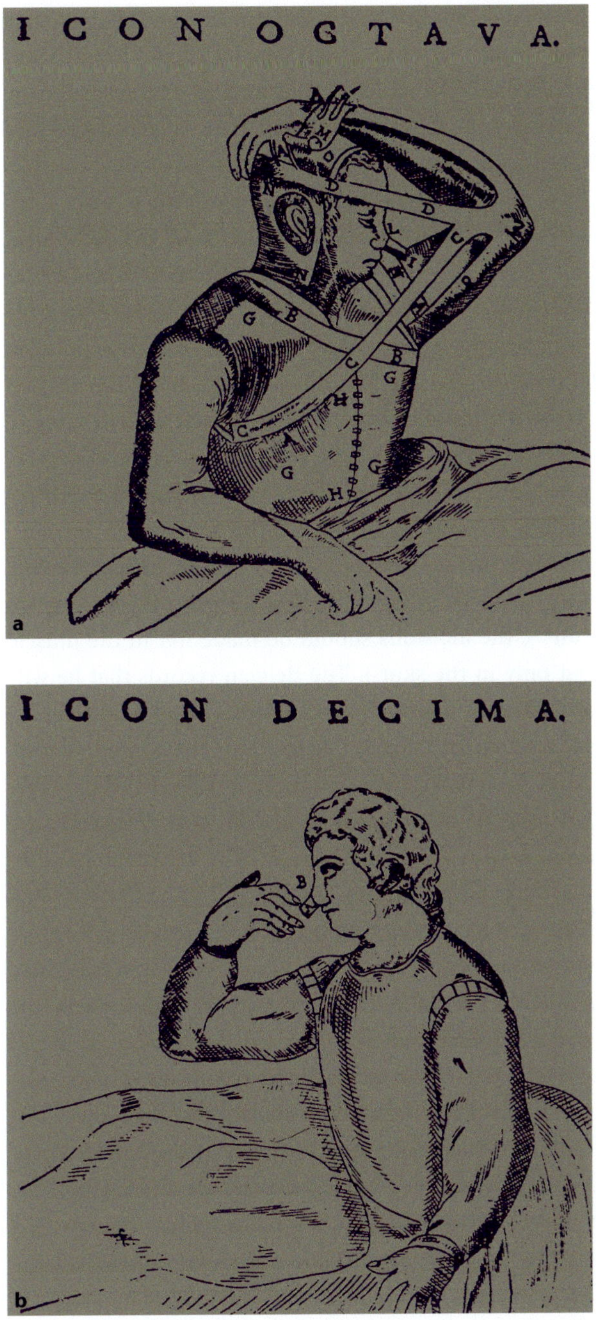

Fig. 7.26a,b Iconae 8 and 10 showing the flap fixed to the nose and after separation from the arm. *Courtesy of Riccardo Mazzola, M.D., Milan*

His friendship with the powerful Gonzaga family[43] and the patronage of the Duke enabled him to have the best artists of the period prepare his illustrations. The first edition was published in Venice, where some of the most prestigious printing houses in Europe were established. The volume is a fine example of the printer's art. It opens with a page bearing the title and the author's dedication to the Duke printed in black against a red background, followed by a title page decorated with a fine engraving, and also contains sixteen pages of *laudi* including one by the son of the author, Giovanni Andrea Tagliacozzi.

The official edition was printed in folio by Bindoni in Venice in 1587 and bore the necessary imprimatur issued by the Venetian *Consiglio dei Dieci*, (Council of the Ten) the body empowered by the Church to grant the necessary authorization and *certificato di registrazione* for the publication of any work. *De Curtorum Chirurgia* was so well received that further editions were published in rapid succession. Another indication of its success was the fact that as soon as the first edition appeared, a pirated version was published by Roberto Mejetti. This was decidedly inferior to the original, being printed in a smaller and less elegant format with illustrations of much poorer quality. Furthermore, contrary to what is stated on the first page—"Cum Indici quadruplici"—the fourth index is missing. The dedication to Prince Gonzaga was left out and of the twelve Laudi only the one written by Tagliacozzi's son was included. It is not known whether Bindoni, who possessed the copyright to the work, attempted to prosecute Mejetti for infringement but even if he did, his rival continued his activity of publishing pirated editions undeterred.[44]

Tagliacozzi's Students and Supporters

Despite the success of his book, Tagliacozzi's method did not win a large following among the cognoscenti, for in this period innovative and technically difficult operations were often rejected out of hand by their authors'

43 The Gonzaga family governed the city of Mantua; both powerful and enlightened, they sponsored many artists, musicians and writers including Anthony Van Dyck, Peter Paul Rubens, Torquato Tasso and Claudio Monteverdi.

44 In Frankfurt in 1598 *De Curtorum Chirurgia per Insitionem* was reprinted in ottavo format by Johan Saur; two centuries later it was still being widely read for there was a German edition prepared in 1831 by Dr. Maximilian Troschel and printed in Berlin by G. Reimer. Finally, Jean Manget included the complete text (but without any illustrations) in his *Biblioteca Chirurgica*, an encyclopedia of surgery printed in Geneva in 1721 by two different publishers, Gabriel de Tournes and Cramer and Parachon.

less enterprising colleagues. Nevertheless, some surgeons adopted the method and testified to its efficacy.

In 1614 William Fabricius Hildanus (1560–1634) published the story of a Swiss girl who "fell into the hands of soldiers [belonging to the Duke of Savoy, who was engaged in a war against Geneva in 1590] and they, after seeking in vain to violate her chastity, cut off her nose ..." Two years later the virtuous maiden went to Lausanne to consult a surgeon by the name of Griffon who had learned the technique of nasal reconstruction "from an Italian travelling through Lausanne who had known the famous Tagliacotius, the original inventor of this operation and of this procedure". It is credible that Griffon had the procedure explained to him by a colleague since Tagliacozzi's book was not published until five years later and it seems improbable, although theoretically not impossible, that the Swiss surgeon might have come across a copy of the second edition of Mercurialis' *De Decoratione Liber* containing Tagliacozzi's famous letter, which had been published just one year earlier [433].

Among Tagliacozzi's students the most well-known is Giovanni Battista Cortesi (1554–1636) (Fig. 7.27). Despite being born into a poor family he aspired to become a surgeon. He was taken on as an assistant at the Ospedale della Vita e della Morte in Bologna where Tagliacozzi was teaching and with admirable perseverance managed to complete the course of study in medicine and earn his degree. Tagliacozzi recognized the gifts of this unusually motivated student and sought to teach him as much as possible and assisted him in his career. In 1598 Cortesi was appointed professor of surgery at the University of Messina in Sicily, where in 1625 he published his own work, *Miscellaneorum Medicinalium* (Fig. 7.28) [203]. In it he reproduces some of the text and illustrations from *De Curtorum Chirurgia* and declared that while he was studying under Tagliacozzi he "had managed to learn so much of [his maestro's] Art that he himself had succeeded in reconstructing not a few noses" (Fig. 7.29a,b). Cortesi also visited the nearby city of Tropea, where he learned that "Pietro Vianeo and his family had by this time died out, but one could see the forceps that they used to carry out their operations."[45] Another account of Tagliacozzi's method appeared in 1625; written by A. Molinetti (d.1675), it described a reconstruction that was carried out by his father with excellent results ("qui refacitus elegantissime nares viderim") [681]. Outside Italy we find various advocates of the technique, one of the most important being Thomas Feyen, better known as Fienus (1567–1631). He was a native of Antwerp whom we know was studying medicine in Bologna around the year 1590. In 1602 he published *De Principuis Artis Chirurgicae Controversiis*, a surgical text in twelve volumes which included a compendium of Tagliacozzi's work [311]. Fienus underlines various crucial points regarding the method. For example, in Chapter 2 he emphasizes that no muscle tissue should be included in the flap: "Non fit scission in musculi brachii, sed tantum cute" ("the incisions should be made not in the muscle but only in the skin"). The Belgian records that he witnessed many operations conducted by Tagliacozzi during his sojourn in Bologna: "I can testify that Gaspar Tagliacozzi, professor of anatomy at the University of Bologna, has restored many noses by his cut, noses I myself have seen, both while in the process of restoration and after they have been restored", although reading his work one cannot help wondering how often he was actually present for he wrote "Ex carne brachii alterius hominis posse instaurari nasum" ("the new nose may be taken from the arm of another man").

A curious work on Tagliacozzi and his method was published in Sweden by Nicolai Rosén (1706–1773) [862]. He was professor of surgery at the University of Uppsala where he became passionately interested in the subject of rhinoplasty after serving as the "opponent"[46] during the presentation of his thesis by a student, Isaac Fritz, on *Chirurgia Curtorum*, i.e. "transplant surgery". The thesis is interesting because it probably represents the only work published in the eighteenth century that discusses not only rhinoplasty but the entire literature on reconstructive surgery to date. In it Fritz cites the Vianeo family and three of Tagliacozzi's engravings are

45 Cortesi died in Calabria but not, as has been suggested, during this journey in search of traces of the Vianeo family, but rather during a later trip undertaken to visit a patient of high lineage.

46 The title of *Opponent* is still used in Sweden today to refer to the professor who has been assigned to discuss the candidate's doctoral thesis with him.

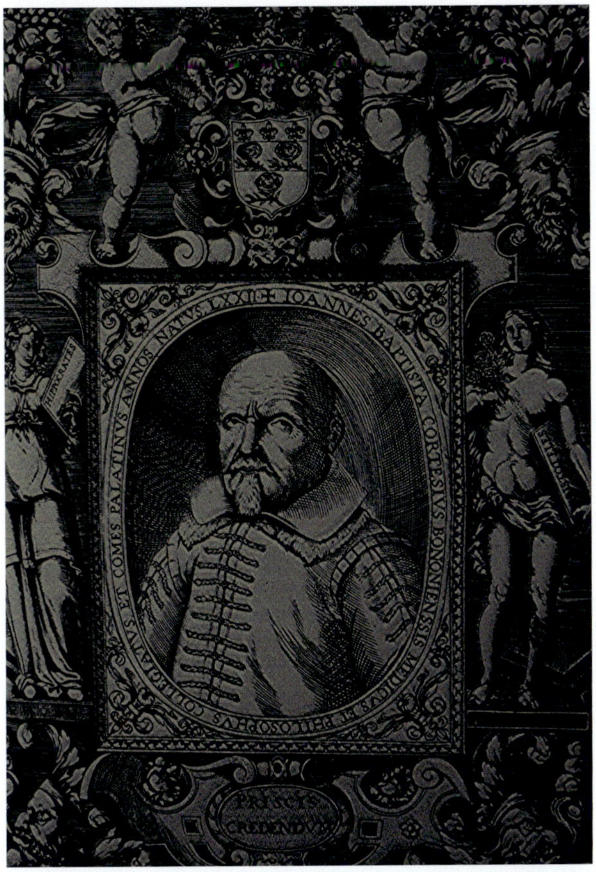

Fig. 7.27 Portrait of Giovanni Battista Cortesi (1554–1636) who was a devoted pupil of Tagliacozzi in Bologna before obtaining the Chair of Surgery in Messina. *Courtesy of Riccardo Mazzola, M.D., Milan*

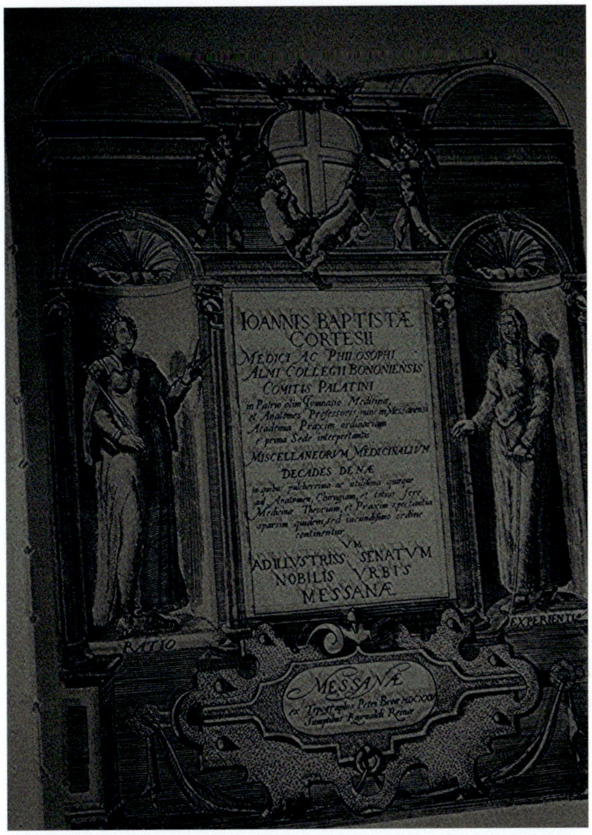

Fig. 7.28 Frontspiece of *Miscellaneorum Medicinalium* by Cortesi which contains a description of Tagliacozzi's method. *Courtesy of Riccardo Mazzola, M.D., Milan*

reproduced. The thesis was included in von Rosén's book (Fig. 7.30) [862].

The Death of Tagliacozzi

On 26 November 1598 all the activities of the University of Bologna were interrupted in order that the faculty might pay homage to Professor Gaspare Tagliacozzi, who had passed away on November 7th. All lessons were suspended and the entire *Collegio dei Dottori* gathered to listen to the *Oratio Funebre* delivered by Muzio Piacentini [798].

In accordance with his wishes, the surgeon was buried at the Monastery of the Sisters of San Giovanni in Bologna. There are various versions of the events that followed and some doubt remains as to the veracity of the facts. Giordano [378] says that Tagliacozzi's body was shortly afterwards exhumed and buried in unconsecrated ground, a story that is supported by Fielding H. Garrison [360, 361] but refuted by V. Rinieri [842]. It does appear that there was an attempt to have the Bolognese surgeon denied a Christian resting place, but in the face of this attempt, his family and colleagues from the *Collegio dei Dottori* protested. They managed to have the life and work of the illustrious professor presented before the Tribunal of the Inquisition. The religious judges, despite the unspoken prejudice against surgery and its practitioners which still prevailed in many conservative circles, concluded that the conduct of Gaspare Tagliacozzi during

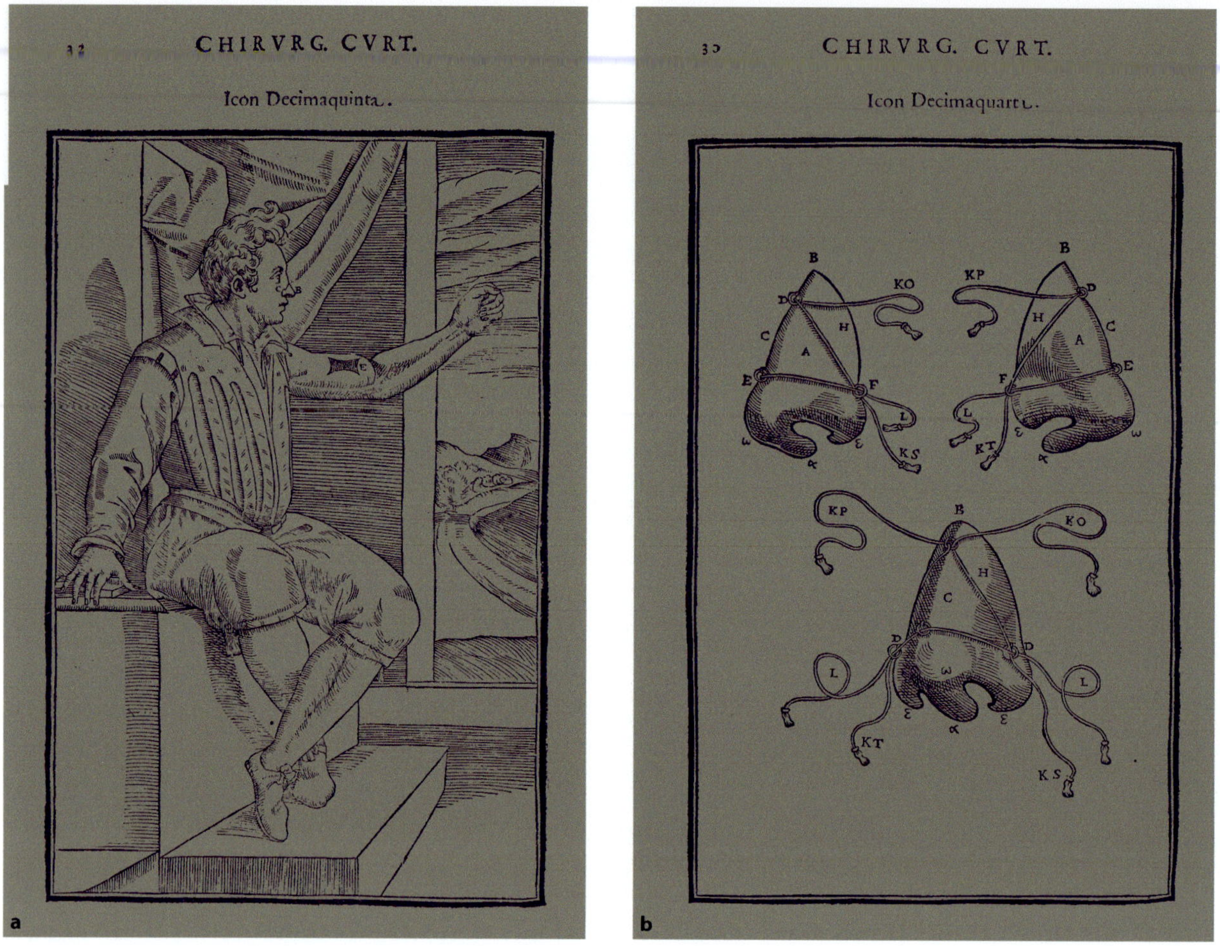

Fig. 7.29a,b Copies of iconae from Tagliacozzi's book in the *Miscellaneorum Medicinalium* by Cortesi. The splint was used to shape the reconstructed nose. *Courtesy of Riccardo Mazzola, M.D., Milan*

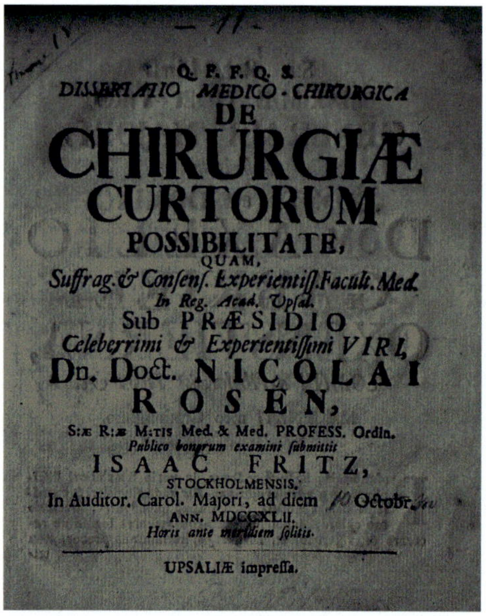

Q. F. F. Q. S.
DISSERTATIO MEDICO-CHIRURGICA
DE
CHIRURGIÆ
CURTORUM
POSSIBILITATE,
QUAM,
Suffrag. & Consens. Experientiss. Facult. Med.
In Reg. Acad. Upsal.
Sub PRÆSIDIO
Celeberrimi & Experientissimi VIRI,
Dn. Doct. NICOLAI
ROSEN,
S:æ R:æ M:tis Med. & Med. PROFESS. Ordin.
Publico bonorum examini submittit
ISAAC FRITZ,
STOCKHOLMENSIS.
In Auditor. Carol. Majori, ad diem Octobr.
ANN. MDCCXLII.
Horis ante meridiem solitis.

UPSALIÆ impressa.

Fig. 7.30 Frontispiece of the book *De Chirurgie Curtorum Possibilitate* by Nicolai Rosen which contains the work of Fritz. It was printed in Sweden in 1742 with a complete description of Tagliacozzi's method. This book was probably the first dedicated entirely to Plastic Surgery after Tagliacozzi. *Courtesy of Riccardo Mazzola, M.D., Milan* his lifetime had always been marked by sincere religious faith and that the accusations against him were based on "malignant fabrications by envious persons". Just who these *invidiosi* were can be easily guessed [155].

Gnudi and Webster [381] report that during their examination of the copy of the *Curtorum Chiurugie per Insitionem* conserved in the Archiginnasio of Bologna, they found a note stating that Tagliacozzi's "reputation was restored with full honor, as was his innocence". They also discovered the following annotation in the registry of the Church of San Paolo dated 25 November 1603, four years after the surgeon's death: "The remains of the Most Excellent Dr. Togliacozzi were once again carried into the Church of San Giovanni Battista" (where they had been buried on 26 November 1598 and then exhumed).[47] P. Capparoni [155] explains that four years passed before the bones of Tagliacozzi were brought to their final resting place, because the family decided to erect a chapel in his memory and three years were required for its construction.[48]

The Decline of Rhinoplasty

Many factors contributed to limit the spread of Tagliacozzi's technique of nasal reconstruction. The first edition of *De Curtorum Chirurgia* was printed in a limited number of copies and its author died just two years later at the age of 53. If Tagliacozzi had lived longer, his continued surgical and teaching activities would surely have contributed to the spread of his method.[49]

However, the end of the sixteenth century witnessed a decline in the art of surgery all over Europe and Italy was no exception, despite the significant discoveries that were being made in other fields of medicine by such figures as Vesalius, Redi and Bellini. J.G. McCarthy [628] has written that "ironically the Age of Enlightenment was not the Age of Enlightenment for plastic surgery". This period of obscurantism continued well into the seventeenth century and certainly did nothing to encourage the spread of Tagliacozzi's teachings.

The attitude of the Church, even if its past interdictions were no longer formally observed, continued to pose an obstacle to the acceptance of modern surgical methods. In 1163 the Council of Tours had condemned all cruel procedures including the practice of anatomy and surgery and this decision had never been formally revoked, although it was often ignored with impunity during the last decades of the sixteenth century.[50] There is no question that in ecclesiastical circles there was opposition to surgery and this existed even in the relatively enlightened University of Bologna. In the Tagliacozzi's case the specific accusation that he had acted against the will of God led to his exclusion, however briefly, from burial in consecrated ground.

The fact was that the opposition of his colleagues played a primary role in preventing the spread of Tagliacozzi's innovative procedures. This bias was in many cases inspired by pure envy rather than a scientifically objective appraisal of the feasibility of reconstructive surgery. Furthermore, this resistance was difficult to overcome because his critics often possessed limited knowledge of his methods.

Consider for example the antagonism of Andrea Vesalius (1514–1564) to Tagliacozzi's surgical procedure [1013–1017]. This was probably based on the misunderstanding that the pedicle had to remain attached for forty days. Instead, Tagliacozzi left the decision up to the surgeon although he recommended a period of approximately fifteen days.[51]

The same misconception appears to have influenced the positions of Dionise Chacon as well as Ambroise Paré [767] who declared that the required period of forty days was "extremely difficult and burdensome for the patient". Furthermore, Paré declared that "the form of the nostrils

47 The Church of Saint John the Baptist is situated in the parish of Saint Paul in Bologna.

48 Antonio, the son of Gaspare Tagliacozzi, is also buried in this chapel.

49 Marc Antonio Ulmi wrote that he did the Tagliacozzian rhinoplasty in Montechiaro near Brescia [999] in his book published in 1602, so he was one of very few Italians who still practised the method after the master.

50 Vesalius for instance was only condemned to a pilgrimage to the Holy Land and only 20 years after he had left his anatomical activities.

51 See *De Curtorum Chirurgia per Insitionem*, Chapter VII, par. XXIX.

could not be that which it was before" despite the fact that he had seen the remarkable results in a patient whom he had sent to the Vianeos. The French surgeon continued to advocate the use of the artificial nose. Paré designed many prostheses, including obturators for the palate and lips with or without moustaches! (Fig. 7.13). Given the technical difficulties of reconstructive surgery and the relative scarcity of surgeons who were practised in the art, it is not surprising that many patients preferred this solution. Among these was the Danish astronomer and philosopher Tycho Brahé, who had lost his nose in a duel. He was dissuaded by Fallopius from undergoing rhinoplasty and opted for an artificial replacement, becoming known in his town as "the man with the golden nose".

The physician Gabriele Fallopius from Padua (1523–1564) was in fact strongly opposed to the idea of reconstructive surgery. This appears to be based on even less understanding of the method than the other opponents. He wrote that the time required for the operation was "in generally three months, in some cases even six and sometimes more than an entire year" (Fig. 7.31) [297, 298]. In his lectures on the subject he never failed to mention the case of an unfortunate goldsmith whom he passed in the streets of Padua every day, who had gone to Bologna to obtain a new nose and returned, according to Fallopius, with a "quid carnis", a mere lump of flesh passing for a nose.[52] By citing such examples, it was easy to convince his students that the prosthesis was a preferable solution to "potiusquam isthaec subire tormenta" ("supporting such tortures instead") (Fig. 7.32).[53] Even after many surgical advances over subsequent centuries some surgeons and their patients preferred a prosthesis to nasal reconstruction [577] and this remains so to this day.

Perhaps Vesalius and Fallopius were among the *invidiosi* who petitioned to have the professor's coffin moved? It is certainly a fact that Tagliacozzi's opponents consistently and mistakenly cited the *caro* (flesh) or *muscul*i (muscle) as the main component of the flap, just as philosopher Tommaso Campanella (1568–1639) used the term *caro brachii* (flesh of the arm) when describing a reconstruction carried out by the Vianeo family [153]. Fioravanti was one of the rare authors to refer correctly to the skin in discussing the procedure.

Another fanciful misconception associated with Tagliacozzi's procedure remained for a long time. As Zeis [1060] observed, it seemed incomprehensible that someone like Girolamo Sbaraglia (1641–1710), a professor at the same university, could have been so misinformed as to claim in his description that a patient had received the nose of a porter and "the story finished badly in that the nose fell off when the donor died".[54] Perhaps the case described by Johan Baptiste von Helmont (1577–1644) [427][55] derives from the same legend. He tells the story of a Belgian soldier who: "having lost his nose in a battle, went to the surgeon Tagliacozzus in Bologna to be provided with a new one. Since he was afraid of having a cut made in his own arm, he hired a porter for the purpose and after paying him a fee a nose was carved out of the arm of this person." Unfortunately, any description of how the flesh was transferred from the arm of the donor to the face of the recipient is omitted. We are therefore left wondering whether these two individuals remained attached to each other for the required period of several weeks! "Then about thirteen months after his return home, his implanted nose grew stiff and some days later decayed and fell off. On investigation of this strange and unexpected happening it was discovered that at about the same moment that the nose grew stiff the porter had died: witnesses to this are still alive in Brussels."

A story recounted by Nicolaus de Blegny (1653–1722) [117] echoes these tales: "… a man whose nose had been completely severed a number of days earlier, had the wound scraped open and to the remainder of his nose, the freshly cut-off nose of his own servant was applied, with the ensuing success of the two joining and growing together. But upon the death of that servant the nose putrefied at the same time as the body from which it had been taken." There being no limit to human invention, it

52 See *De Decoratione*, chapter XI.

53 Another quotation said to be used by Fallopius was that patients went to Bologna to get a new nose and returned with a "nasello". This refers to a well-known ugly fish.

54 See *Oculorum et Mentis Vigiliae …* , *Bononiae Studior* by Sbaraglia published in 1704. Sbaraglia strongly opposed Tagliacozzi and became and enemy of Malpighi who was his supporter.

55 See *Opera Omnia*, published posthumously in 1682.

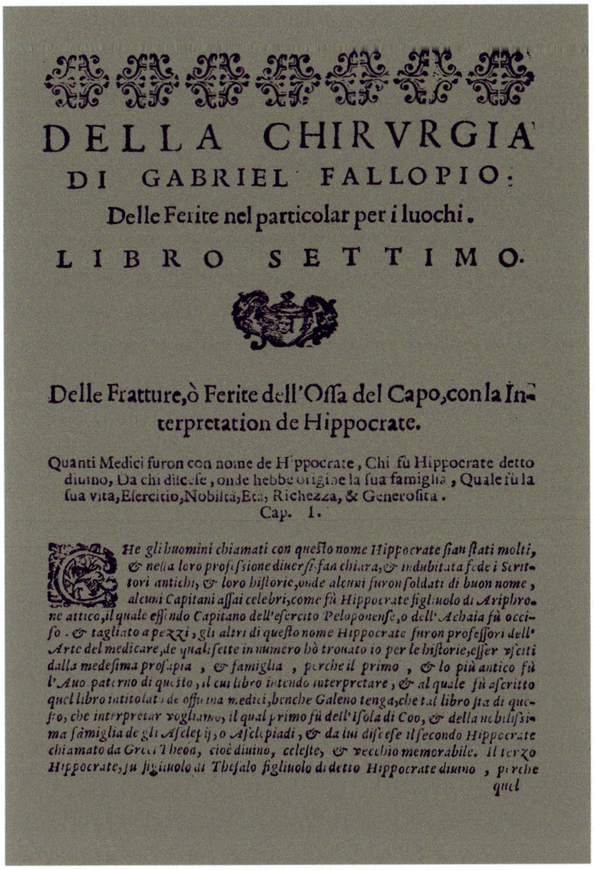

DELLA CHIRVRGIA DI GABRIEL FALLOPIO: Delle Ferite nel particolar per i luochi. LIBRO SETTIMO.

Delle Fratture, ò Ferite dell'Ossa del Capo, con la Interpretation de Hippocrate.

Quanti Medici furon con nome de Hippocrate, Chi fù Hippocrate detto diuino, Da chi discese, onde hebbe origine la sua famiglia, Quale fù la sua vita, Esercitio, Nobiltà, Età, Richezza, & Generosità. Cap. I.

Fig. 7.31 Frontispiece of *Della Chirurgia* by Gabriele Fallopius (1523–1564), Professor of Anatomy and Surgery at the University of Padua. He was opposed to nasal reconstruction. *Courtesy of Riccardo Mazzola, M.D., Milan*

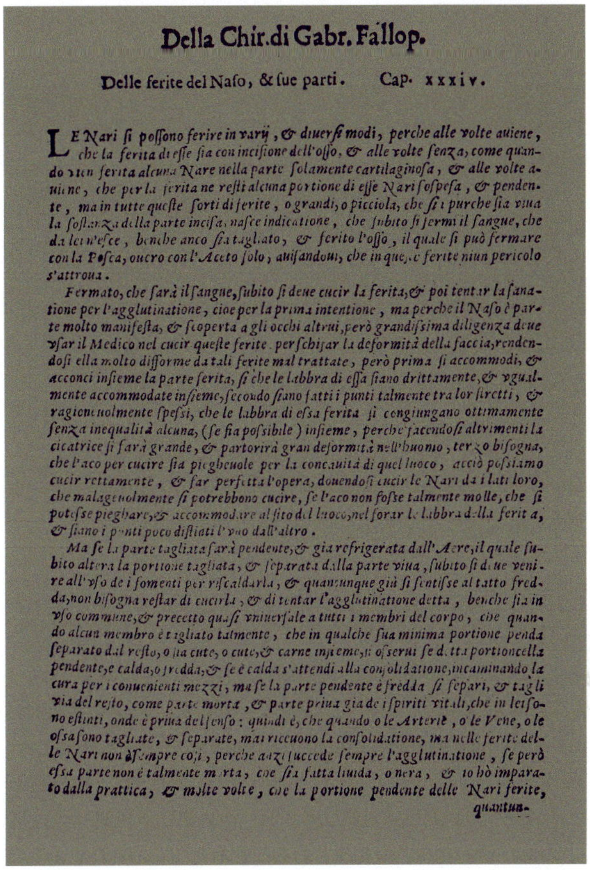

Della Chir. di Gabr. Fallop.

Delle ferite del Naso, & sue parti. Cap. xxxiv.

Fig. 7.32 Fallopius criticizes Tagliacozzi's method on this page of Chapter 34 of *De Chururgia Lib 7. Courtesy of Riccardo Mazzola, M.D., Milan*

should not surprise us to come across other stories such as the one recounted by the Jesuit Athanasius Kircher (1602–1680) of two individuals who had exchanged skin and were afterwards able to communicate with one another by telepathic means over a distance of thousands of miles [495, 496].

On the rare occasions when the surgical texts of the period discussed rhinoplasty, they contained highly inaccurate information. For example, in 1684 in an article reporting on his experience with the arm flap, Mattheus Gottfried Purmann (1648–1721) [819] cites Tagliacozzi as working in the fifteenth century. Even in the eighteenth century Magatus advised against reconstruction: "if the nose be cut off it can only be replaced by grafting" [589].

In an era when magic commanded greater respect than medicine it is not surprising that these false, sometimes fanciful stories did not help the acceptance of the procedure.

Critics of Tagliacozzi could even be found in non-scientific circles. Samuel Butler (1612–1680) ridiculed the surgeon's work in his long satirical poem *Sir Hudibras*

Learned Tagliacotius from
the brawny part of Porter's Bum
cut supplemental noses, which
would last as long as parent-breech;
but when the date of Nock was out
off dropt the sympathetic snout.

Voltaire was even more caustic when in 1785 he wrote of Tagliacozzi: "Thus the great Aesculapius of Etruria repaired all the lost noses with a new business: he took a piece from the arse of the poor man and applied it directly to his nose …"

The general climate was so hostile to Tagliacozzi's method that the Faculty of Medicine of Paris in 1742 rejected the thesis presented by two candidates, Dubois and Vandenesse, entitled "A curta nares ex brachio reficienda" ("How to remake a nose from an arm") on the grounds that such an operation was impossible.

The Revival of Reconstructive Surgery

Against the chorus of voices raised in criticism of Tagliacozzi, Reneaume de la Garanne [357] in the year 1723 suggested a modification which represented a genuine improvement and perhaps marked a turning point in the history of rhinoplasty. He claimed that it was not necessary to wait for the suppuration and granulation beneath the bipedicle arm flap, and that one of its edges could be sutured directly to the face during the first stage of the operation. He also proposed shortening the period during which the face and arm had to remain united to 16 days–in other words, the length of time recommended by Tagliacozzi.

At the end of the eighteenth century the practice of rhinoplasty began to spread across Europe once again, albeit by means of side-roads since the spark that ignited this rebirth did not come, as one might have expected, from articles published in journals, but from reports appearing in popular press.

The first sign of a revival—one which did not, however, have immediate repercussions in Europe—appeared in India where an English-language newspaper, the *Madras Gazette*, published an article in 1793 with the headline "A Singular Operation". Written by two physicians attached to the East India Company, it described a nose reconstruction which they had witnessed, carried out by a member of the Maharatti family of healers. The following year in England a letter to the editor signed "B.L." appeared in the *Gentlemen's Magazine*—a somewhat more elite, but certainly not a scientific publication (Fig. 7.33) [46]. The impact that this letter eventually had on the development of rhinoplasty in Europe was so prodigious that it deserves to be reproduced here in its entirety.

Mr. Urban,

A friend has transmitted to me, from the East Indies, the following very curious and in Europe, I believe, unknown chirurgical operation, which has long been practised in India with success, namely affixing a new nose on a man's face. The person represented in Plate I is now in Bombay.

Cowasjee, a Maharatta of the caste of husbandmen, was a bullock-driver with the English Army in the war of 1792 and was made a prisoner of the Tipu who cut off his nose and one of his hands. … For about 12 months he had remained without a nose, when he had a new one put on by a man of the brickmaker caste, near Pauna (Fig. 7.34). *This operation … has been practiced from time immemorial. Two medical gentlemen, Mr. Thomas Caruso and Mr. James Trindelay*[56] *of the Bombay Presidency, have seen it performed as follows:*

A thin plate of wax is fitted to the stump of the nose, so as to make it a nose of good appearance. It is then flattened and laid on the forehead. A line is drawn around the wax, and the operator then dissects off as much skin as it covered, leaving undivided a small slit between the eyes. This slit preserves the circulation until a union has taken place between the new and the old parts. The cicatrix of the stump of the nose is next pared off, and immediately behind this part an incision is made through the skin, which passes about both alae, and goes along the upper lip. Skin is now brought down from the forehead and, being twisted half round, its edge is inserted into this incision, so that a nose is formed with a double fold above, and with the alae and septum below fixed in the incision. A little Terra Japanica is softened with water, and being spread on a slip of cloth, five or six of these are placed over each other, to secure the joining. No other dressing but this cement is used for four days. It is then renewed, and cloth dipped in ghee [a kind of butter] *is applied. The connecting slips of skin are divided about the twenty-fifth day, when a little more dissection is necessary to improve the appearance of the new nose. For five or six days after the operation the*

56 By long-established custom in Britain surgeons are referred to not by the title of Doctor (Dr) but rather Mister.

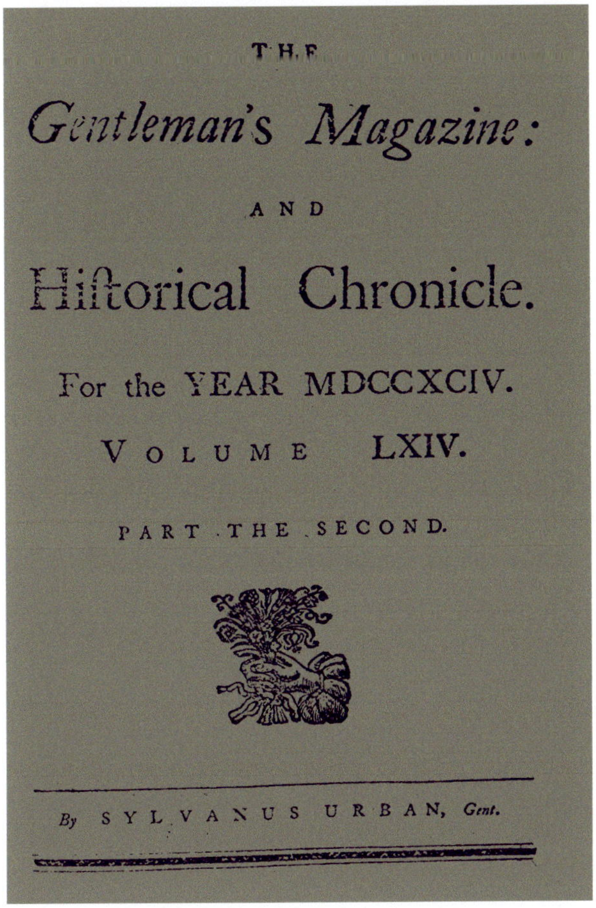

THE

Gentleman's Magazine:

AND

Hiſtorical Chronicle.

For the YEAR MDCCXCIV.

VOLUME LXIV.

PART THE SECOND.

By SYLVANUS URBAN, Gent.

Fig. 7.33 Frontispiece of the *Gentleman's Magazine* published in October 1794. *Courtesy of Riccardo Mazzola, M.D., Milan*

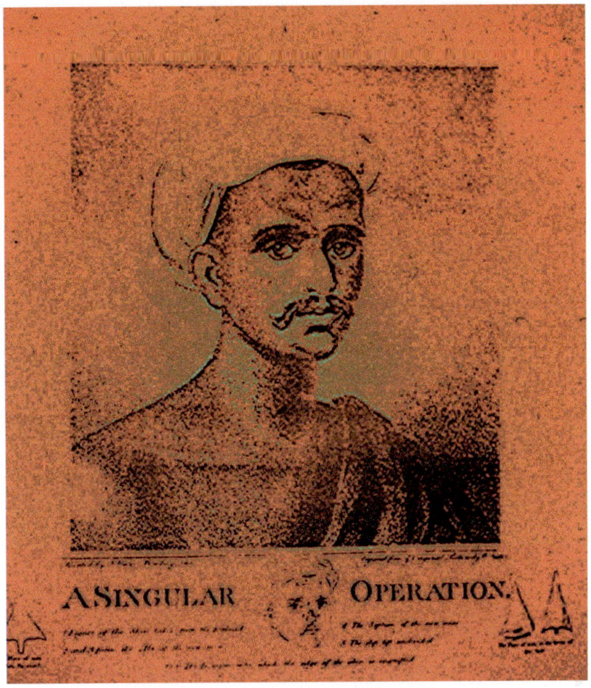

Fig. 7.34 Portrait of Cowasjee with small drawings of the operation, from the *Gentleman's Magazine. Courtesy of Riccardo Mazzola, M.D., Milan*

patient is made to lie on his back; and on the tenth day bits of soft cloth are put into the nostrils to keep them sufficiently open. The artificial nose is secure and looks nearly as well as the natural one; nor is the scar on the forehead very observable after a length of time. The picture from which this engraving was made was printed in January, ten months after the operation.

Yours &c. B.L. (Fig. 7.35a,b).

Even though it did not appear in a medical publication, the letter raised considerable interest among English surgeons. Later Zeis [1059, 1060] criticized the English for having occupied India for so long before discovering the technique and sharing it with the rest of the world.

The identity of the author, B.L., long remained a mystery. One year after the letter in *Gentlemen's Magazine*, an article in the Bombay Gazette attributed it to a certain "Mr Lucas, skilled surgeon of Madras" and many repeated this information as accurate, including the author of an article published in the *Philadelphia Medical Museum Magazine* in 1806 and J.C. Carpue who affirmed in his famous text on rhinoplasty [157] "Mr Lucas, an English surgeon, with this operation was successful in many cases." Finally, in 1971, T.J.S. Patterson [780, 781] after thorough research established that the author was a certain Colly Lyon Lucas, chief surgeon and member of the Medical Board of Madras. It is not known whether C.L. Lucas ever carried out a rhinoplasty operation himself. Others have made contributions to this fascinating tale [335, 633].

Mr. URBAN, Oct. 9.

A FRIEND has tranſmitted to me, from the Eaſt Indies, the following very curious, and, in Europe, I believe, unknown chirurgical operation, which has long been practiſed in India with ſucceſs; namely, affixing a new noſe on a man's face. The perſon repreſented in *plate I.* is now in Bombay.

Cowasjee, a Mahratta of the caſt of huſbandman, was a bullock-driver with the Engliſh army in the war of 1792, and was made a priſoner by Tippoo, who cut off his noſe and one of his hands. In this ſtate he joined the Bombay army near Seringapatam, and is now a penſioner of the Honourable Eaſt India Company. For above 12 months he remained without a noſe, when he had a new one put on by a man of the Brickmaker caſt, near Poonah. This operation is not uncommon in India, and has been practiſed from time immemorial. Two of the medical gentlemen, Mr. Thomas Cruſo and Mr. James Trindlay, of the Bombay preſidency, have ſeen it performed, as follows: A thin plate of wax is fitted to the ſtump of the noſe, ſo as to make a noſe of a good appearance. It is then flattened, and laid on the forehead. A line is drawn round the wax, and the operator then diſſects off as much ſkin as it covered, leaving undivided a ſmall ſlip between the eyes. This ſlip preſerves the circulation till an union has taken place between the new and old parts. The cicatrix of the ſtump of the noſe is next pared off, and immediately behind this raw part an inciſion is made through the ſkin, which paſſes around both *alæ*, and goes along the upper lip. The ſkin is now brought down from the forehead, and, being twiſted half round, its edge is inſerted into this inciſion, ſo that a noſe is formed with a double hold above, and with its *alæ* and *ſeptum* below fixed in the inciſion. A little *Terra Japonica* is ſoftened with water, and being ſpread on ſlips of cloth, five or ſix of theſe are placed over each other, to ſecure the joining. No other dreſſing but this cement is uſed for four days. It is then removed, and cloths dipped in ghee (a kind of butter) are applied. The connecting ſlips of ſkin are divided about the 25th day, when a little more diſſection is neceſſary to improve the appearance of the new noſe. For five or ſix days after the operation, the patient is made to lie on his back; and, on the tenth day, bits of ſoft cloth are put into the noſtrils, to keep them ſufficiently open. This operation is very generally ſucceſsful. The artificial noſe is ſecure, and looks nearly as well as the natural one; nor is the ſcar on the forehead very obſervable after a length of time. The picture from which this engraving is made was painted in January, 1794, ten months after the operation.

Fig. 1. the plate of wax when flattened.

Fig. 2. and 3. the plate of wax in the form of the noſe.

Fig. 4. 1. figure of the ſkin taken from the forehead; 2. and 3. form of the *alæ* of the new noſe; 4. *ſeptum* of the new noſe; 5. the ſlip left undivided; 6. 6. 6. the inciſion into which the edge of the ſkin is ingrafted.

Yours, &c. B. L.

Fig. 7.35 The "B.L." letter to the Editor of the *Gentlemen's Magazine*, October 1794. This was the first time that news of the rhinoplasties performed in India reached Europe and caused great interest in the medical circles of England and Germany. *Courtesy of Riccardo Mazzola, M.D., Milan*

The Nineteenth Century

Despite the curiosity generated by the news from India, no one seemed to showed interest except a young surgeon in London by the name of Joseph Constantine Carpue. He began to collect as much information as he could, seeking out and interviewing members of the army and civil servants who had spent time in India. Sir Charles Mallet assured him that rhinoplasty was quite commonplace and had been performed there "since time immemorial". A certain Mr Barry employed by the East India Company told him that nasal reconstructions were carried out by the Koomas with a razor, and that the operation lasted an average of thirty minutes.[57] Fired with enthusiasm by these accounts, Carpue sought to learn more about the procedure. He managed to ascertain that "the patient lay on his back on a table with his head resting on a cushion", but could not discover any information on the administration of analgesics. Determined to attempt the operation himself, he first practised on eleven cadavers.

This period of preparation lasted almost twenty years. Then in 1814 an army officer came to Carpue seeking advice having lost his nose following, he claimed, a course of treatment with mercury for a liver disorder. Carpue suspected that the cause of the necrosis was syphilis and before proceeding, tested the healing capacity of the patient by making a series of small incisions around his nose. These healed without complications and Carpue decided to operate on 23 October 1814.

He following the procedure described in the letter by B. L. scrupulously. First he made a model in wax, then raised a frontal flap and sutured it to the region of the nose inserting gauze into the new nostrils. He attempted to suture the defect in the forehead as best he could. The entire operation lasted thirty-seven minutes. Carpue attributed the past failures to reproduce Tagliacozzi's method to the cold northern climate which prevented adequate circulation to the new nose[58] and therefore kept his patient in a heated room to simulate the Indian climate. When after three days he removed the bandages he was unable to contain his delight at what he saw, exclaiming, "My God, there's a nose!"

He did not have to wait for long before another patient came to see him. He was another soldier who had lost the left side of his nose during the Peninsular campaign against Napoleon. So, before the end of 1816 he was able to publish his celebrated book, *An Account of Two Successful Operations for Restoring a Lost Nose, Including Descriptions of the Indian and Italian Methods* [157]. He hoped that this would restore the reputation of nasal reconstruction and the use of flaps (Fig. 7.36).

Carpue's book contained both a detailed description of his two cases and a comparison of the traditional Hindu and Italian methods. The publication of his account revived interest in the letter that had appeared twenty years before in the *Gentleman's Magazine* and stimulated general interest among surgeons. Among them was the illustrious German C.F. von Graefe [391, 393]. He grasped the potential of Carpue's work and realized that the flap could be used for other types of reconstruction. He promptly translated Carpue's book into German and began experimenting with the techniques himself.

Von Graefe was born in Warsaw on 8 March 1787, and lived near Poznan until 1805 when his family moved to Dresden. A precocious student, after studying the classics he completed his medical studies at the age of 20 and moved to Halle where the university was, as he wrote: "in a state of profound deterioration. The students were cast into their profession still ignorant not only of anatomy and medicine, but even of the most ordinary operations of the Art. The harelip was never even treated."[59]

Von Graefe deserves some credit for rescuing surgery from this state of affairs. In 1810 at the age of 24 he was offered the chair of surgery at the universities of Halle and Königsberg, but turned down these positions to join the more prestigious faculty in the University of Berlin in 1811. This was the period of the Napoleonic Wars and after the outbreak of the War of Liberation (1813–1815) he was asked to leave the university and serve as Surgeon

57 Koomas was the name of a caste of bricklayers in Hindustan.

58 According to Carpue: "The climate of North Europe is less favourable to the success of the operation than that in the South" and attributed this factor to "the little demand and frequent failure in execution" that discouraged surgeons from attempting nose reconstructions.

59 See the *Lancet Gallery of Medical Portraits*, published in London in 1834.

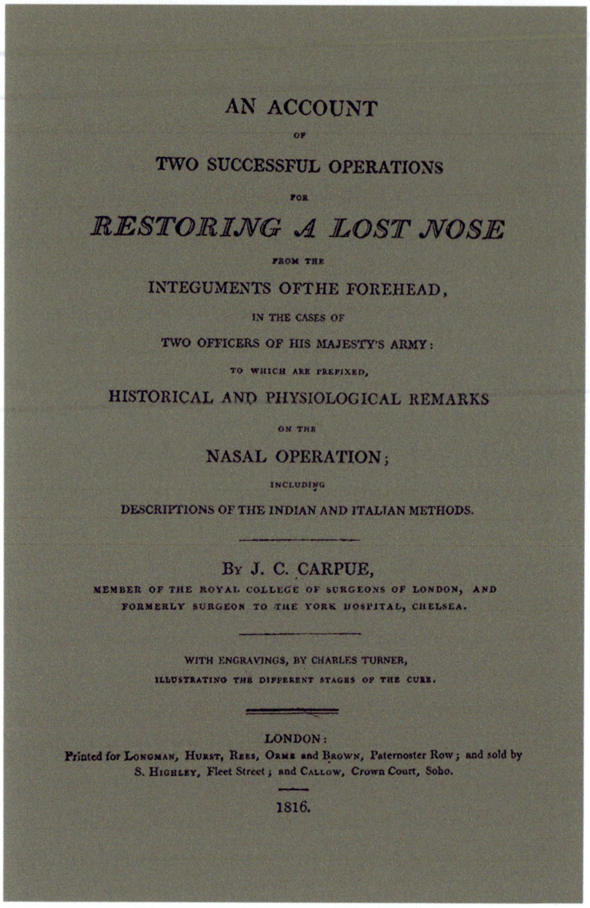

AN ACCOUNT
OF
TWO SUCCESSFUL OPERATIONS
FOR
RESTORING A LOST NOSE
FROM THE
INTEGUMENTS OFTHE FOREHEAD,
IN THE CASES OF
TWO OFFICERS OF HIS MAJESTY'S ARMY:
TO WHICH ARE PREFIXED,
HISTORICAL AND PHYSIOLOGICAL REMARKS
ON THE
NASAL OPERATION;
INCLUDING
DESCRIPTIONS OF THE INDIAN AND ITALIAN METHODS.

BY J. C. CARPUE,
MEMBER OF THE ROYAL COLLEGE OF SURGEONS OF LONDON, AND FORMERLY SURGEON TO THE YORK HOSPITAL, CHELSEA.

WITH ENGRAVINGS, BY CHARLES TURNER,
ILLUSTRATING THE DIFFERENT STAGES OF THE CURE.

LONDON:
Printed for LONGMAN, HURST, REES, ORME and BROWN, Paternoster Row; and sold by S. HIGHLEY, Fleet Street; and CALLOW, Crown Court, Soho.

1816.

Fig. 7.36 Frontispiece of Carpue's book (1816) which contains his account of two successful nasal reconstructions and descriptions of the Indian and Italian methods. *Courtesy of Riccardo Mazzola, M.D., Milan*

General to the German Army.[60] Von Graefe died in 1840 at the age of 53 in Hannover, where he had been summoned to operate on the heir apparent, Prince George for cataracts. Memorial services were held all over the country in tribute to this exceptional man, who had made fundamental contributions to the modernization of the entire field of surgery.

As early as 1818 von Graefe expressed his preference for the Italian method of nasal reconstruction so as to avoid the unsightly scarring on the forehead and the risk of meningitis, which at that time was believed to be associated with the Indian method. Before adopting the arm flap he had also experimented with local advancement flaps of the type described by Celsus and revived in France in the nineteenth century as the *procedée du tiroir*. After these studies he concluded that "it had been a profound error to abandon and even worse, ridicule the art of Tagliacozzi".

Von Graefe based his procedure on Tagliacozzi's technique, but divided the operation into a series of phases spread out over a period of many months. After raising the flap on the arm (phase 1), he waited three months before sectioning one extremity (phase 2), and then another four months before attaching this to the nasal stump (phase 3). He may appear to have been over cautious, but we must remember that he was conducting an operation that had not been attempted for two centuries. The possible complications were not at all clear and past descriptions of the operation was contradictory and often unreliable. In the fourth phase the flap was detached from the arm, while the fifth was reserved for any necessary remodelling. This approach was referred to as *von Graefe's modification of the Italian method* (Fig. 7.37).

However, von Graefe soon realized that this procedure could be modified without any risk and reduced the time between each of the first three stages. Indeed he noted that waiting too long before attaching the flap to the nose was counterproductive because, having reached an optimal stage of vascularization (what Tagliacozzi called *aetas virilis*), it began to become fibrotic. In von Graefe's book *Rhinoplastice* published in 1818 we can see an illustration of a flap with its proximal end divided. Compared to the defect on the arm, the flap has shrunk to half its original size (Fig. 7.38).

In his constant search for ways to improve the technique, von Graefe abandoned the forceps designed by

60 Von Graefe was awarded numerous decorations for his war service. With great efficiency he set up surgical field units in the area lying between the Rhine and the Weser Rivers, where more than 100,000 wounded soldiers were treated. In this period surgeons were still using the amputation procedure described by Ambrose Paré two centuries earlier; Von Graefe modernized and improved the technique so that, as he observed, in a series of 13 operations, all of the patients not only survived, but their convalescence lasted a mere 13 days. He was also a pioneer in the technique of blood transfusion [163].

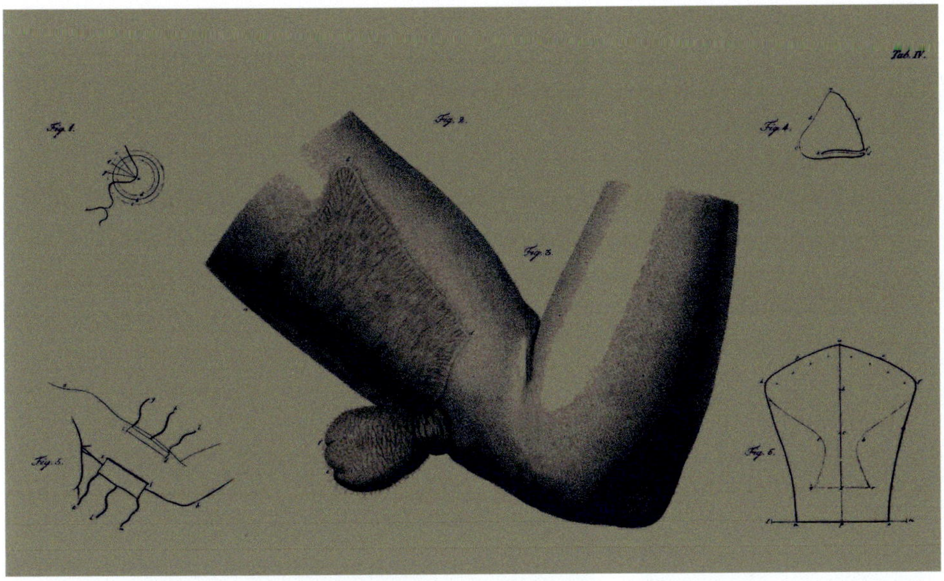

Fig. 7.37 A picture from *Rhinoplastice* by Von Graefe. He originally divided the proximal end of the flap after 4 months and left it hanging for many weeks. The open flap probably became stiff and fibrotic so consequently the new nose did not need skeletal support. *Courtesy of Riccardo Mazzola, M.D., Milan*

Tagliacozzi to hold the skin while cutting the flap. Instead, he made a bipedicle flap 15 cm long and 6 cm wide down to muscle with a knife. He then divided one end after four weeks rather than the three months originally proposed, and after another two or three weeks attached it to the nose. The separation of the flap from the arm was made 6–12 days later, when the blood supply from the face appeared adequate. He still continued to wait for some time before attempting any remodelling of the new nose. His shortening of the process seems to have been influenced by the claim made by de la Garanne almost a century earlier, that 16 days was sufficient for the flap to take [357]. He shortened his time periods even further, combining phases 2 and 3 so that the flap was attached to the nose immediately after the sectioning of the first pedicle. This approach came to be known as *the German method* (Fig. 7.39a,b).

Other surgeons experimented unsuccessfully to circumvent the most awkward step of the Tagliacozzi procedure, the fixing of the arm to the face. For example Heinrich Christian Bünger (1782–1842), professor of anatomy at Marburg, tried to attach a graft composed of skin and muscle taken from the anterior surface of the thigh to the raw stump of the nose [142]. An assistant[61] pressed the free graft against the recipient site until the bleeding had stopped and then it was sutured. Not surprisingly, this experiment ended with the necrosis of the compound graft.

Jacques Mathieu Delpech (1792–1832) played a similar, if more limited, role in France to that of von Graefe in German. He conducted research on the comparative advantages of frontal and brachial flaps and wrote what may be considered the first important work on plastic surgery to be published in France [234]. In June 1832 he carried out his first successful nasal reconstruction by the Indian method. Shortly afterwards a similar attempt using the Italian method ended in failure, probably because he detached the flap from the arm prematurely. In other experiments he followed a procedure that corresponded exactly to the modified German method, although he claimed to have learned of von Graefe's work much later through a German student who was visiting

61 The assistant was Dr. Ulman, who later became professor of surgery at Marburg before E. Zeis.

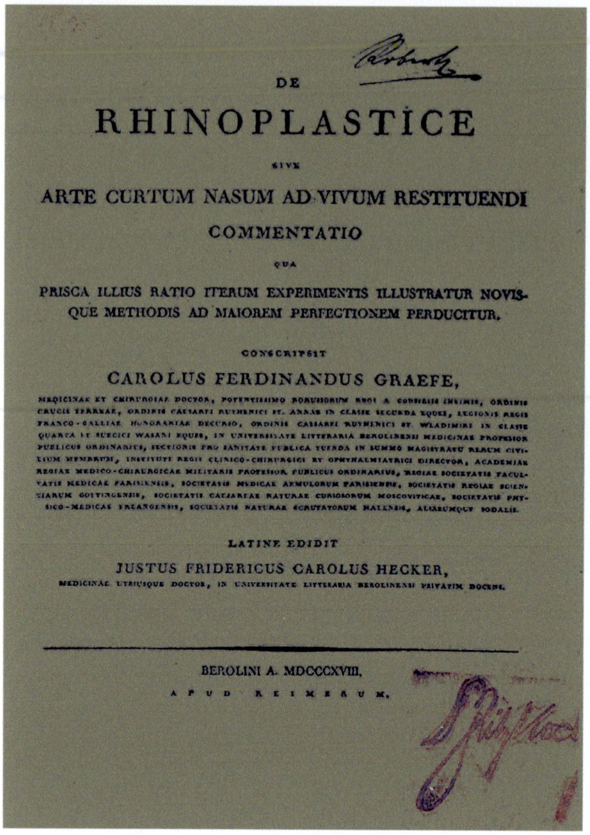

DE

RHINOPLASTICE

SIVE

ARTE CURTUM NASUM AD VIVUM RESTITUENDI

COMMENTATIO

QUA

PRISCA ILLIUS RATIO ITERUM EXPERIMENTIS ILLUSTRATUR NOVISQUE METHODIS AD MAIOREM PERFECTIONEM PERDUCITUR.

CONSCRIPSIT

CAROLUS FERDINANDUS GRAEFE,

MEDICINAE ET CHIRURGIAE DOCTOR, POTENTISSIMO BORUSSORUM REGI A CONSILIIS INTIMIS, ORDINIS CRUCIS FERREAE, ORDINIS CAESAREI RUTHENICI ST. ANNAE IN CLASSE SECUNDA EQUES, LEGIONIS REGIS FRANCO-GALLIAE HONORARIAE DECURIO, ORDINIS CAESAREI RUTHENICI ST. WLADIMIRI IN CLASSE QUARTA ET SUECICI WASANI EQUES, IN UNIVERSITATE LITTERARIA BEROLINENSI MEDICINAE PROFESSOR PUBLICUS ORDINARIUS, SECTIONIS PRO SANITATE PUBLICA TUENDA IN SUMMO MAGISTRATU RERUM CIVILIUM MEMBRUM, INSTITUTI REGII CLINICO-CHIRURGICI ET OPHTHALMIATRICI DIRECTOR, ACADEMIAE REGIAE MEDICO-CHIRURGICAE MILITARIS PROFESSOR PUBLICUS ORDINARIUS, REGIAE SOCIETATIS FACULTATIS MEDICAE PARISIENSIS, SOCIETATIS MEDICAE AEMULORUM PARISIENSIS, SOCIETATIS REGIAE SCIENTIARUM GOTTINGENSIS, SOCIETATIS CAESAREAE NATURAE CURIOSORUM MOSCOVITICAE, SOCIETATIS PHYSICO-MEDICAE ERLANGENSIS, SOCIETATIS NATURAE SCRUTATORUM HALENSIS, ALIARUMQUE SODALIS.

LATINE EDIDIT

JUSTUS FRIDERICUS CAROLUS HECKER,

MEDICINAE UTRIUSQUE DOCTOR, IN UNIVERSITATE LITTERARIA BEROLINENSI PRIVATIM DOCENS.

BEROLINI A. MDCCCXVIII.

APUD REIMERUM.

Fig. 7.38 Frontispiece of the book *Rhinoplastice* in which Von Graefe (1787–1840) gives details of his experience. He favoured the Italian method and made several modifications to the technique over the years. *Courtesy of Riccardo Mazzola, M.D., Milan*

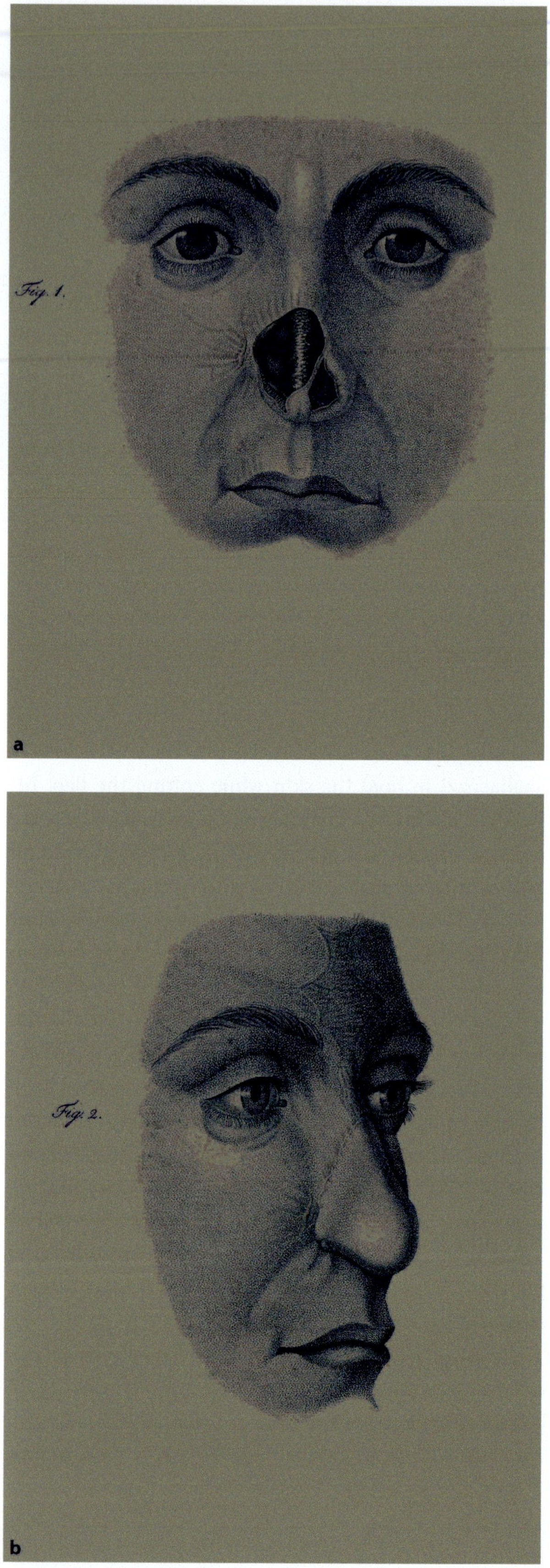

Fig. 7.39a,b A case from Von Graefe's book. *Courtesy of Riccardo Mazzola, M.D., Milan*

Montpellier.[62] Delpech's unstinting praise for his German colleague, whom he referred to as "a most distinguished surgeon", would seem to indicate that he was acting in good faith.

Delpech advocated the Indian method because it allowed him to apply the flap to the recipient site immediately, avoiding some of the problems of the brachial flap, such as suppuration, hypertrophic scarring, and contraction of the thickened edges of the flap. The French surgeon came across his first patient while walking through the streets of Montpellier with his colleague Louis Labat. He gives an unusually circumstantial description of the encounter and of the patient's defect, which continues for three pages: "In the month of April 1820 we met … a young beggar 12 years of age showing a very peculiar congenital deformity which stimulated our interest. We invited him to come and be examined. He did as we requested and here are our observations. The whole right side of the face was very regular and even pleasant, but the left side was horribly disfigured by an abnormal opening of this side of the nose. A large fissure which exposed the inner part of the fossa nasalis from the lower part of the nose went up to the medial corner of the left eye."

In his work *Chirurgie Clinique de Montpellier* [233] published between 1823 and 1828, Delpech described a total of five reconstructions carried out using the Indian method. Sometimes partial necrosis of the flap occurred, but it was never so serious as to compromise the final outcome, which he found with the Italian flap. In his discussion of the rhinoplasty technique he appears to be claiming a position of priority for the school of Montpellier, at least in France, assuring his readers that: "this operation which we have been carrying out for the last ten years[63] and which many of our pupils have repeated in accordance with our teachings in the cities of France, seems to have been ignored or despised up to the present time in the rest of the kingdom. It was necessary that travellers from India bring us the news of a procedure practised successfully for many years by a half-civilized people, in order to make us believe in the possibility of such a reconstruction, which seems since then to have remained almost exclusively in the hands of the English and the Germans."

On the day that Delpech began his attempt to reconstruct the nose of the 12-year-old boy the operating theatre must have been thronged with observers, because we have the eyewitness accounts of no fewer than three surgeons: Philibert Joseph Roux (1780–1854) [871], Louis Labat (1803–1847) [513] and finally Philippe Frederich Blandin (1789–1849) [108, 113].

Rhinoplasties were also being performed in Italy. Bartolomeo Signoroni [926] wrote about his experience with both the modified von Graefe method in1833 and the Indian method in 1836. In 1838 Pietro Sabattini (1810–1864) published a paper describing a nose reconstruction carried out using the Indian method, to which he added a genuine innovation—an arterial flap cut from the lower lip to refashion the upper lip [875] (see Chapter 4).

It appears that the French surgeons, who were undoubtedly skilful and inventive were somewhat reluctant to accept of the achievements of colleagues from other countries. Delpech's comments on his English and German rivals are an example. In their eagerness to compete they occasionally announced the discovery of already well-established concepts. This seems to have been the case with Michel Serre [917] who reported in 1842 *la Méthode Français pour Deplacement*, which is very similar to the advancement flap described by Celsus [167, 168] eighteen centuries earlier. Zeis criticizes him severely for this, declaring: "it appears quite evident that 'the French method' is based essentially on French vanity".

By now however, rhinoplasty was being practised almost everywhere in Europe and had spread to the other side of the Atlantic. Jonathan Mason Warren (1811–1867) undertook the long voyage to Europe in order to learn the technique and in 1837 published an account of the first nasal reconstruction carried out in the United States [1033, 1034]. Many others[64] followed suit and, in 1900,

62 See *Chirurgie Clinique de Montpellier*, vol 2, p 548 (1828).

63 In this work, published in 1823, Delpech declares that he first began doing nasal reconstructions ten years before, that is in 1813 or three years before the publication by Carpue, a claim which appears somewhat improbable.

64 Among the most well known authors who wrote about nasal reconstructions in this period were Robert Liston (1794–1847) [569, 570]; Joseph Francois Malgaigne (1806–1865) [599, 600]; Alfred Armand Marie Velpeau (1795–1867) [1010, 1011]; Friedrick August von Ammon (1799–1861) and Moritz Baumgarten [24, 25]; and Antoine Joseph Jobert de Lamballe (1799–1867) [464].

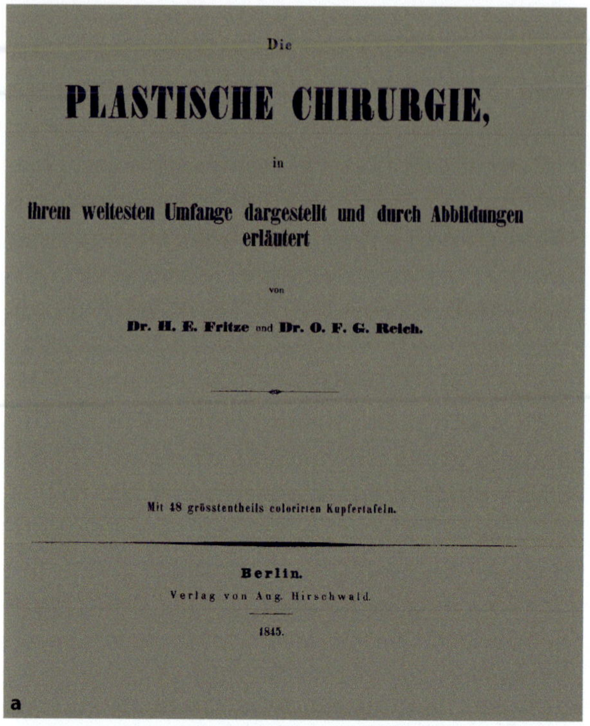
Die

PLASTISCHE CHIRURGIE,

in

ihrem weitesten Umfange dargestellt und durch Abbildungen erläutert

von

Dr. H. E. Fritze und **Dr. O. F. G. Reich.**

Mit 48 grösstentheils colorirten Kupfertafeln.

Berlin.
Verlag von Aug. Hirschwald.

1845.

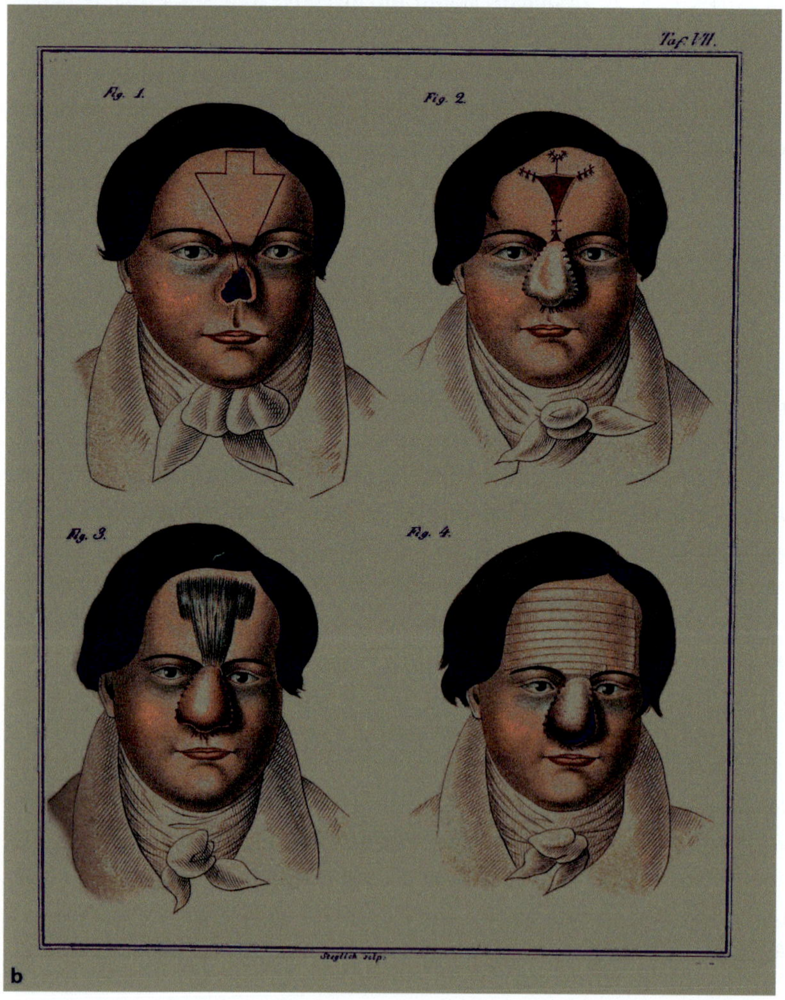

Fig. 7.40a,b The frontispiece and page from the book by Fritze and Reich *Die Plastische Chirurgie* which shows the vertical position of the flap which led to congestion and a dog ear. *Courtesy of Riccardo Mazzola, M.D., Milan*

Keegan [490] compiled a review on the subject and found no less than 152 cases in the literature during the course of the nineteenth century. To this he added his own hundred reconstructions carried out during his five years of service in India using the frontal flap procedure.

Initially the flap for nasal reconstruction was drawn vertically in the mid frontal region, but the resulting twist of the pedicle tended to jeopardize the blood supply to the flap (Fig. 7.40a,b). Surgeons began experimenting with ways to avoid this problem. Johan Frederick Dieffenbach (1794–1847) proposed creating a very narrow frontal pedicle, but this led to congestion and swelling, a problem which he suggested treating by the application of leeches or alternatively by tying off some arterial branches (Fig. 7.41) [245, 246]. The latter measure was criticized by Blandin, Serre and Bernard Rudolph Conrad von Langenbeck (1810–1887) [522]. Von Langenbeck pointed out that the problem of congestion was caused by poor venous outflow rather than the arterial supply.

Torsion of the pedicle often resulted in a fold with thickening of the tissue at the base of the flap—the future root of the nose—and as well as being aesthetically unpleasing, this jeopardized the circulation. Obviously surgeons were reluctant to trim this *dog ear* at the first operation as this would compromise the blood supply. Once again Dieffenbach offered a solution, which in this case was more readily accepted by his colleagues, that of extending one of the two vertical incisions down to the side of the nose so that, after rotating the flap, this portion of the pedicle could be inserted into the longer nasal incision (Fig. 7.42a,b).[65] The rotation could be carried out more easily, the twist causing pressure on the veins was lessened, and the exposed surface was reduced to a minimum. Later Dieffenbach modified the procedure again, suggesting that the frontal flap be incised at an oblique angle (Fig. 7.43a,b) in order to reduce the rotation, a solution that was strongly seconded by the Finnish surgeon Julius von Szimanosky (1829–1868) [782]. Further refinements were introduced by Jacques Lisfranc (1790–1847) [565] and Louis Labat [513].

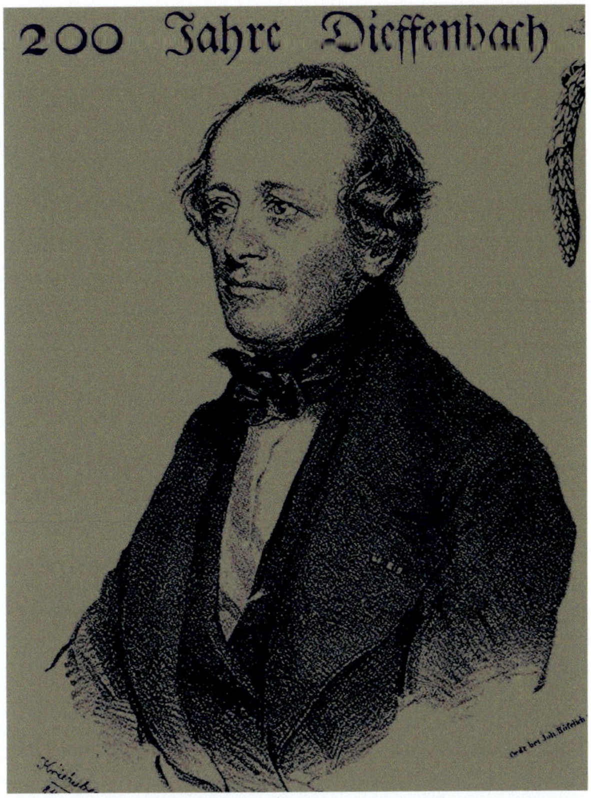

Fig. 7.41 Portrait of Dieffenbach who made modifications to the flap incisions to try to avoid circulatory problems and the dog ear. He eventually placed it obliquely. *Courtesy of Riccardo Mazzola, M.D., Milan*

Although an advocate of the frontal flap, Dieffenbach suggested an improvement to von Graefe's modified brachial flap procedure in 1845. When making the bipedicle flap on the arm at the first stage, he designed it so that the distal end was wider to allow later reconstruction of the nasal alae. This was already being done in the direct forehead method.

Although most surgeons seemed to prefer the technique of the frontal flap, improvements to the brachial flap continued to be introduced. One modification was proposed by Paolo Fabrizi (1806–1859) in 1841. He sug-

65 The attribution of the *inset pedicle* technique to Dieffenbach was not universally accepted. For example, the French claim that Lallemand [519] had already used this approach in 1824 to correct a lower lip defect by rotating a flap, cut from the neck of the patient, through approximately 180°. Zeis [1060], who had little patience with the claims of the French school of surgery, refuted this, affirming that the defect in Lallemand's case was actually a continuation of the donor site and that the pedicle was much wider. Hence the flap was entirely different from the long, thin frontal pedicle proposed by Dieffenbach (see Zeis Index pp 204–205).

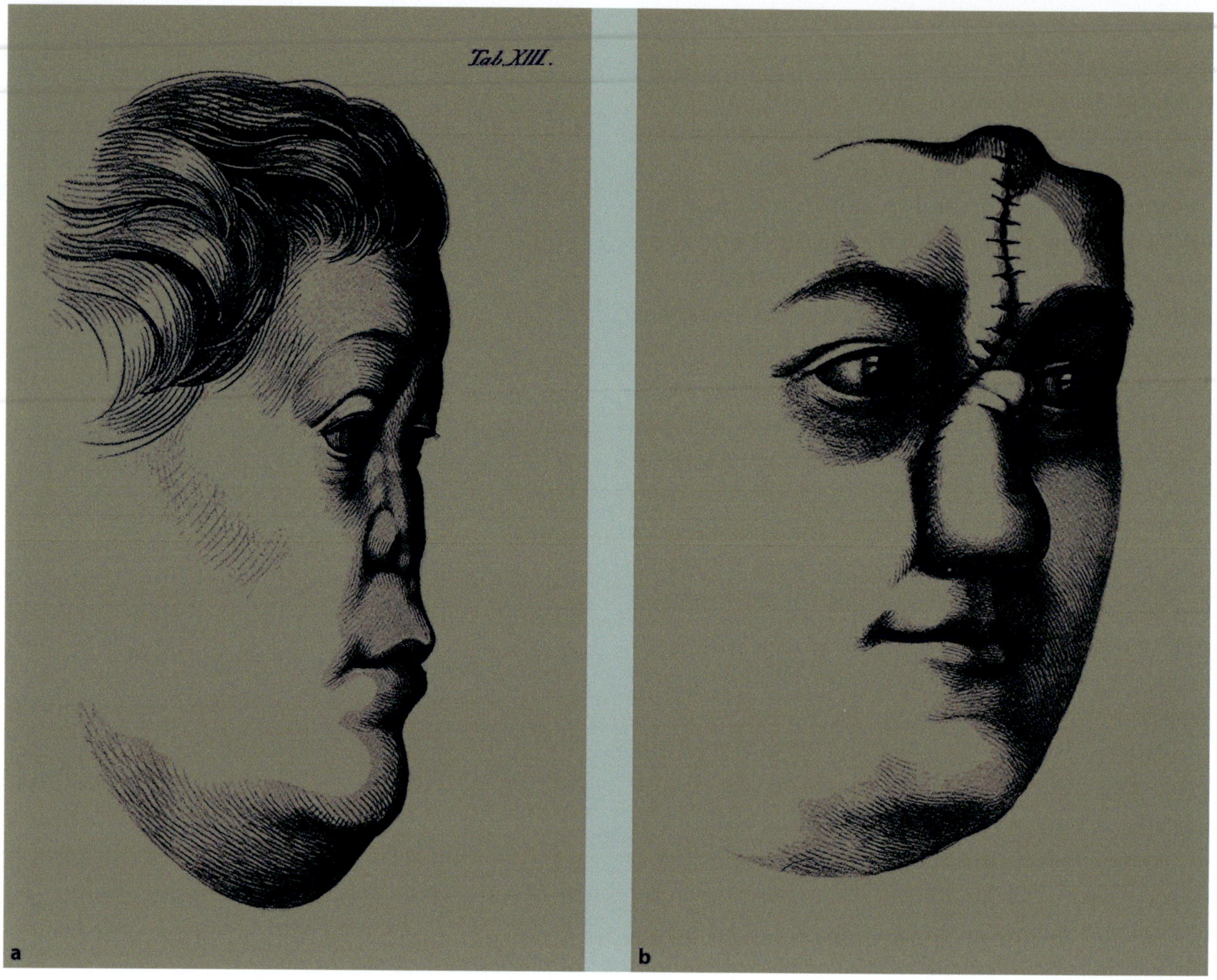

Fig. 7.42a,b Drawings from Dieffenbach showing how he extended the flap incision to the side of the nose. *Courtesy of Riccardo Mazzola, M.D., Milan*

gested moving the position of the brachial flap distally to the forearm, with its proximal end located about one inch from the elbow [294]. This made the position of immobilization much more bearable for the patient. It is interesting to note that James Israel, who trained with Langenbeck, reported his experience to the *Society of Surgeons of Berlin* in 1896. He had already published on saddle nose deformity in 1887 and on this occasion used free autogenous bone from the tibia to reconstruct the saddle nose deformity in two men with syphilis (see Chapter 13). His third case was a woman suffering from lupus which had destroyed her nose. Like Fabrizi, he used a flap from her forearm but in addition, incorporated a piece of ulnar bone as a compound flap [461]. He gets credit as the first to use bone grafts in nasal reconstruction but as McDowell reports the history of bone grafting is chequered and difficult to clarify [634, 636] (see Chapter 13—saddle nose). During the same period, surgeons in the United States were experimenting with different rhinoplasty techniques; among them were Pancoast and Mutter in Philadelphia, and Mott, Post and Buch in New York. The work of Aristide Auguste Verneuil (1823–1895) in this area also deserves mention [1013].

Perhaps the largest series of nasal reconstructions carried out by a single surgeon in the nineteenth century was that of Tribowandas, who operated on over three hundred patients during his career. Born in 1850 to a poor family in Junagadadh, he completed his medical studies in Bombay and then returned home to begin his practice. He was perhaps aided in his career by the presence in the region of a famous bandit, Kadu Makrani,[66] whose principal activity was cutting off noses on commission.[67]

Reconstruction of the nasal lining was always a problem which nineteenth century surgeons attempted to resolve. In fourth century India, Vagbat [1000, 1001] had recognized the need for nasal lining but his folded flap was not the complete solution. It helped form the inner surface of only the very end of the nose but left a raw area elsewhere. The final result was less than optimal both aesthetically and functionally because of fibrosis as many experienced surgeons particularly in France who had adopted the folded frontal flap admitted [233, 234, 513]. Dénonvilliers [236] observed that all surgery had managed to accomplish thus far was to "substitute a disgusting deformity with a ridiculous one."

The suggestion of Nicola Petrali was an improvement. He proposed the incision of a small central tongue at the end of the flap to form the columella, and folding its two lateral portions to create the lining for the nostrils [794]. A similar approach was suggested by Ernest Blasius (1802–1875) [116], Dieffenbach [245] and Serre [917].[68]

All of these methods required a longer flap for sufficient skin to fold round the inside of the nostrils. This led surgeons, mostly in France and Germany, to experiment first with different types of frontal oblique flaps based on the supraorbital vessels and then with flaps based on the temporal vessels. Other flaps were proposed, such as the ones based on the scalp to move forehead skin. Various surgeons reviewed the available methods and added their own modifications [925].

By the end of the century another technique for lining the nose had developed using free skin grafts. One of these used skin from the post-auricular area. The advent of cartilage and bone grafts made it possible to achieve even more satisfactory results [702] (see Chapters 4 and 5).

The chapter would be incomplete without, at least mentioning tissue expansion. The advent of this technique has been discussed briefly already and its use as a preliminary in forehead rhinoplasty has allowed easier direct closure of the secondary defect with the production of a thinner, more malleable flap for nasal reconstruction.

---

66 Tribowandas became so famous in India that even today the popular expression "Kadu cuts off noses but Tribowandas remakes them" is used to describe a problem that can be resolved. There are also songs celebrating his remarkable skill.

67 Due to the large number of patients demanding his services, Tribowandas often worked at two operating tables simultaneously. After sectioning and preparing the flap of the first patient, an assistant was assigned to watch over him while the surgeon began operating on the second patient. Tribowandas noted that this waiting period allowed the flap, which was initially pale and cold, to regain its normal colour and temperature.

68 The debate regarding who first developed the procedure of the trilobed flap to reconstruct the columella and the lining of the nostrils was finally settled when it was demonstrated that, although Petrali published the first description in 1842, Blasius had been using the method since 1838, publishing his results in 1848.

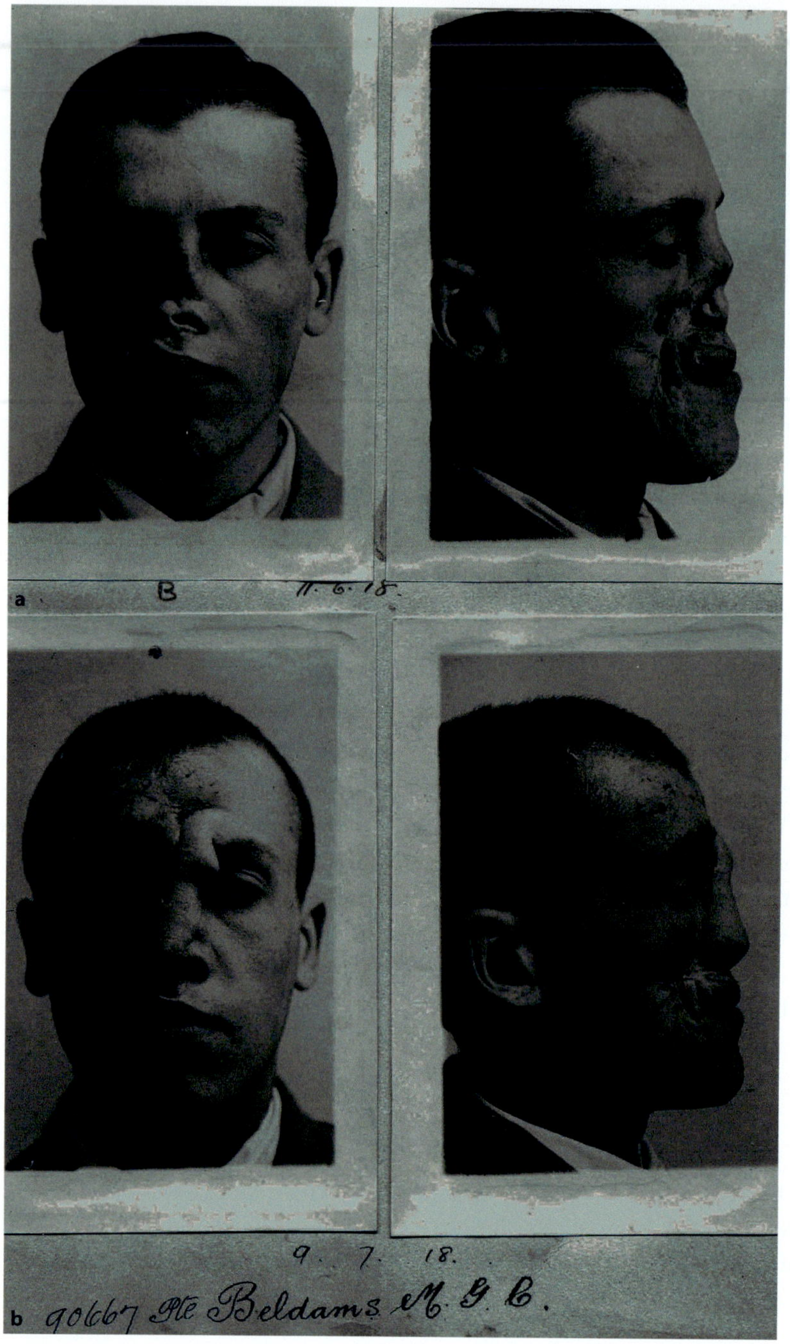

Fig. 7.43a,b A nasal reconstruction using an oblique forehead flap performed by Gillies during the First World War at Queen Mary's Hospital, Sidcup. *Reproduced by permission of the Gillies Archives, Queen Mary's Hospital, Sidcup UK*

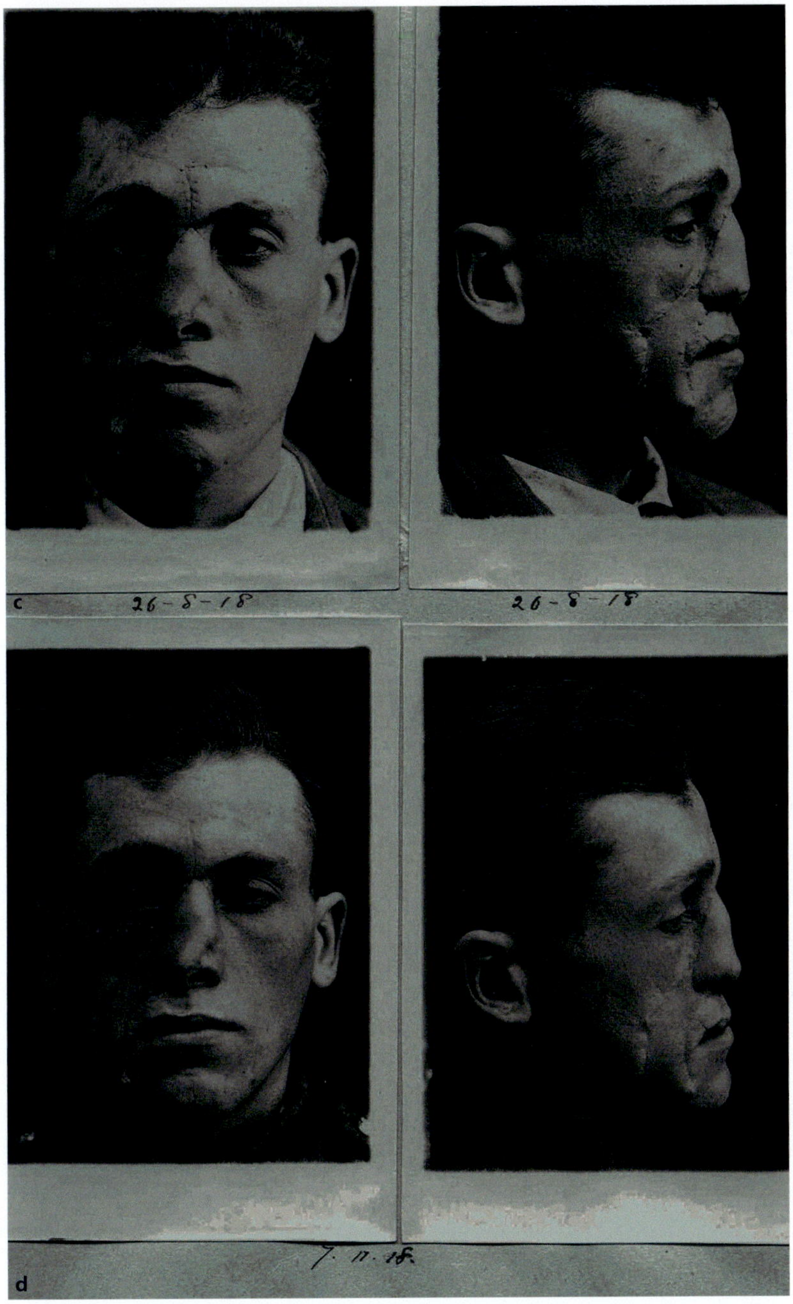

Fig. 7.43c,d *(continued)* A nasal reconstruction using an oblique forehead flap performed by Gillies during the First World War at Queen Mary's Hospital, Sidcup. *Reproduced by permission of the Gillies Archives, Queen Mary's Hospital, Sidcup UK*

Chapter 8

Cleft Lip and Palate

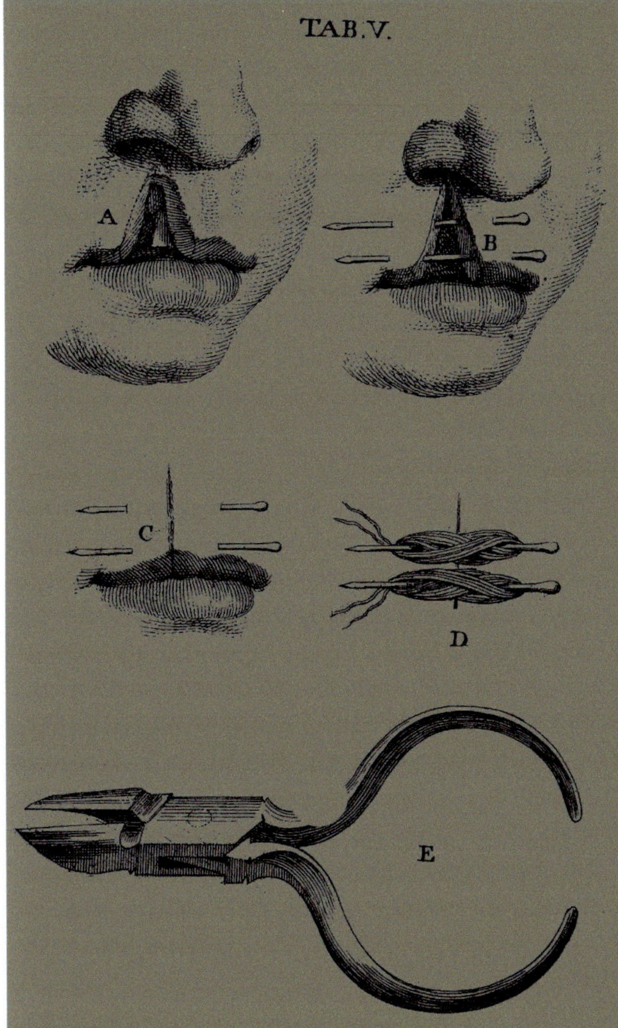

Contents

Cleft lip (harelip) and cleft palate are the most common congenital malformations of the face and affect approximately 1 in 1,000 newborn infants, although their frequency has diminished considerably in developed countries where pre-natal examinations allow an early diagnosis and the mother can interrupt her pregnancy if a defect in the foetus is found.

The reaction to the birth of a deformed child has varied widely from culture to culture. John Marquis Converse [191] noted that: "... in ancient times many congenital deformities, including the cleft lip and palate, were considered to be evidence of the presence of an evil spirit in the affected child". This was particularly true in the case of facial deformities and the infant was "removed from the tribe or cultural unit and left to die in the surrounding wilderness", a practice that was common in Antiquity and still happens today in certain African tribes. In Sparta the unfortunate newborns were abandoned on Mount Tagete, while in Rome they was drowned in the Tiber River or thrown off the Tarpeian rock. Rather than condemning this practice, the philosopher Plato justified it in one of his dialogues in the *Republic*, explaining that it was a means of removing evil omens and preserving the soundness of the race.

The fact that there are very few records of clefts from this early period is probably due to this practice and it seems likely that even if a child survived the early weeks their chances of thriving were poor.

The Cleft Lip

Cleft Lip in Antiquity

No report appears in the medical literature of the Egyptians, Greeks, Etruscans or Romans, even though the healing arts were well developed in ancient Egypt. In the medical papyrus discovered by George Ebers (1837–1898) there is an entire section devoted to mouth diseases, but no mention is made of clefts of the lip or palate [271].[1] Similarly, while 48 cases of trauma, many involving the face, are described in the treatise on surgery known as the papyrus of Edwin Smith (1822–1906) [128, 710],[2] the authors do not seem to have been aware of the existence of facial clefts [537].

In a monograph on the subject, George Dorrance (1874–1949) discussed the case of a mummy that had been reported in 1929 by Smith and Dawson in their work *Egyptian Mummies* published in London [250]. The skull clearly showed the signs of a cleft hard palate. W.G. Holdsworth [441] interpreted this as evidence that the Egyptians knew of the condition, but in fact it represents an isolated and perhaps unique archaeological finding and there is no reason to believe that the body had been preserved simply because it possessed this deformity. As Dorrance comments, given the sheer mass of archaeological and anatomical material that has survived, it is remarkable that "only a single case of a cleft palate has come to light" from the civilization of ancient Egypt.

Facial clefts were apparently unknown in Greece. The fact that no reference to the condition can be found in the *Corpus Hippocraticus*, which represented a compendium of the medical knowledge of the period, might lead one to suspect that this congenital deformity did not exist in the region. Tord Skoog (1915–1977)[3], however, has demonstrated that such was not the case [936]. He describes a terracotta statuette found in 1969 in the Potters' Quarter of Corinth. Dating from 700–300 B.C., the figurine portrays a clown with a complete cleft lip modelled in meticulous detail, so that the secondary defects of the premaxilla and the alae of the nose are clearly visible. No attempt had been made to repair even these minor defects, and the ancient Greek jester evidently sought to make the best of his handicap by employing it in the service of his art (Fig. 8.1).

1 The Ebers papyrus was discovered in 1862 and acquired by George Ebers in 1873. He published a German translation in 1875. Today the manuscript is conserved at the University of Leipzig.

2 The Edwin Smith papyrus was purchased by Edwin Smith in 1873, translated into English by James H. Breasted [128] and published in Chicago in 1930. It appears that this papyrus was compiled around 2600–2200 B.C., although the *Encyclopedia Britannica* suggests that it actually represents a copy made around 1600 B.C. of a work dating as far back as 3000 B.C.

3 Tord Skoog (1915–1977). After training in Finland with Soivio and England with McKindoe and Gillies he became Professor of Plastic Surgery in Uppsala from 1959 until his death. He organized the first post-war International Congress of Plastic Surgery in Sweden in 1955. See obituary by P. Santoni-Rugiu (1977) *Chir Plast* 3:1.

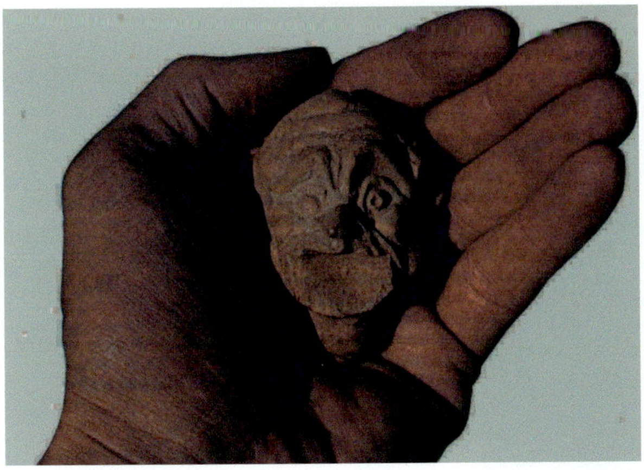

Fig. 8.1 A statuette from the potters' quarter of Corinth c.700–300 B.C. showing a clown with a harelip. This appears to be the only representation of a cleft in ancient Greece. *Courtesy of the Skoog family, Uppsala*

The silence of the Etruscans on the subject is even less accountable since it is known that they practised advanced dentistry and produced sophisticated prostheses, some of them made of gold.[4] One example was found in Corneto near Tarquinia. It had eight loops, five of which were attached to healthy teeth while three surrounded the artificial teeth (Fig. 8.2a,b). This predates by about 3,000 years the first modern prostheses made in the United States in the nineteenth century. It is certainly extraordinary that no evidence of lip or facial clefts has come down to us from a civilization that was so familiar with intra-oral pathologies (Fig. 8.3a,b) [956].

How was this defect treated in ancient Rome? As we have already seen in the chapter on the flaps, Aulus Cornelius Celsus (25 B.C. to 50 A.D.) used local flaps to treat cases of full thickness lip loss while smaller defects were repaired by abrading the margins and suturing them together [167, 168]. On the basis of these descriptions Aristide Auguste Verneuil [1013] and Alfred Louis Velpeau [1010] claimed that Celsus might have tried the use of the skin flap to repair congenital clefts in the first half of the nineteenth century. However, Dorrance [250] refuted their suggestion and since we have not been able to find any mention of lip clefts in *De Medicina*, it may be presumed that the defects so skilfully repaired by Celsus were not congenital.

Pliny the Elder (23–79 A.D.) wrote that a healthy palate was necessary for normal speech, but did not give an example of deformity affecting speech [804]. Claudius Galen (131–201 A.D.) also mentioned the palate, having studied its role in speech. However, his descriptions concern speech abnormalities and there are no specific references to congenital defects [351–354].

While it is conceivable that doctors in ancient times would have been reluctant to treat malformations such as clefts, and in particular those involving the palate, due to technical difficulties and the lack of an effective anaesthetic, it is less clear why such a visible and relatively common defect as the facial cleft is never even mentioned. Some have inferred from the wording of a passage by Galen in his text *De Methode* that he had treated congenital clefts: "Next we will describe a similar method for cases of defects due to colobomata, as these mutilations of the lip are called, whether on the sides of the nose or in one ear. In fact these mutilations can be treated in the following way: scarify the skin on both sides, then approximate and unite the flaps of the skin after removing the calloused part on both sides, and finally sew and glue." (Fig. 8.4)[5] In this passage the Greek term coloboma means defect, but Galen's observation that they could be found "on the sides of the nose" suggests intrigueingly that he might have been referring to the rare congenital cleft known today as the *facial coloboma* or *oblique facial cleft*, which sometimes extends as far as the lower eyelid. However, the physician also speaks of "mutilations", which would appear to denote a traumatic rather than congenital aetiology, even if it does not exclude the possibility that such an injury might be present at birth. What raises the most serious doubts that Galen was referring to clefts, or at least to congenital deformities, in this passage is his mention of "partes cal-

4 A prosthesis with four loops can be seen in the museum of the Villa Giulia in Rome, while the Etruscan Museum in Florence and the Guarnacci Museum in Volterra both have interesting collections of antique dental instruments. On display at the University of Ghent in Belgium is an Etruscan skull with a prostheses to which two teeth are still attached.

5 See *De Methode*, Chapters XVI and XXIV, in the Latin translation from the original Greek by K.G. Kuhns.

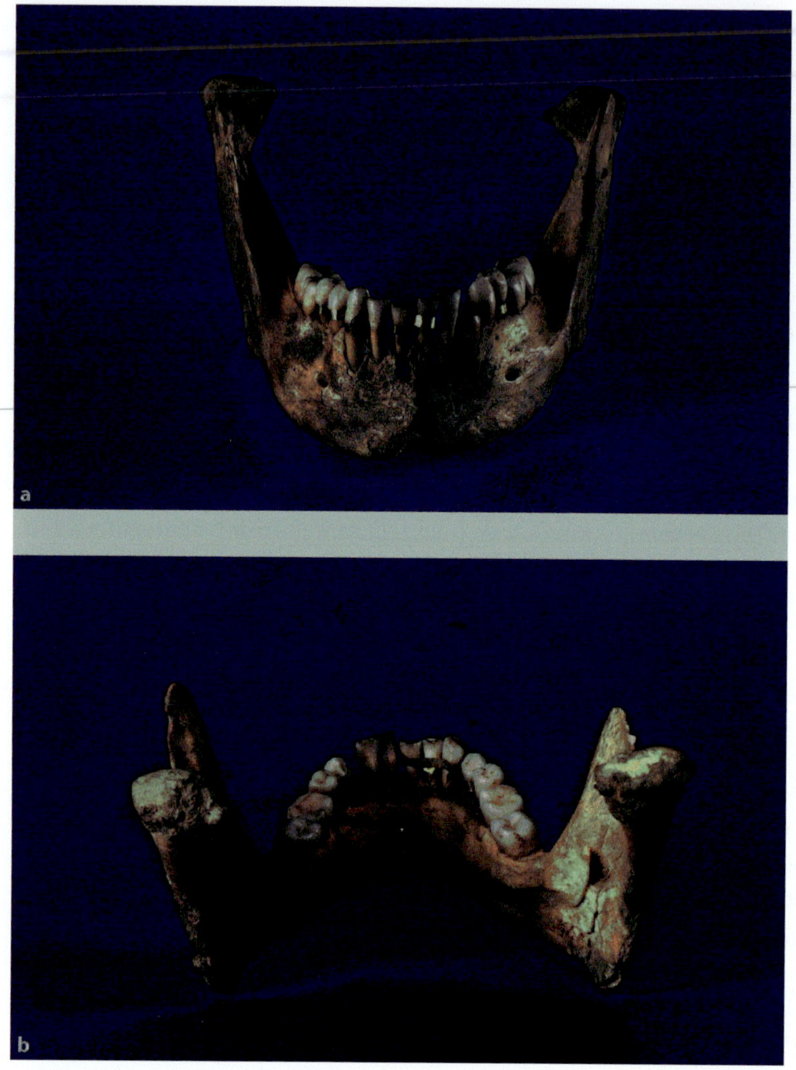

Fig. 8.2a,b These advanced dental prostheses were made by the Etruscans (c.1000 B.C.) and are in the Archaeological Museum of Florence. *By permission of the Soprintendenza Artcheologica per la Toscana, Florence*

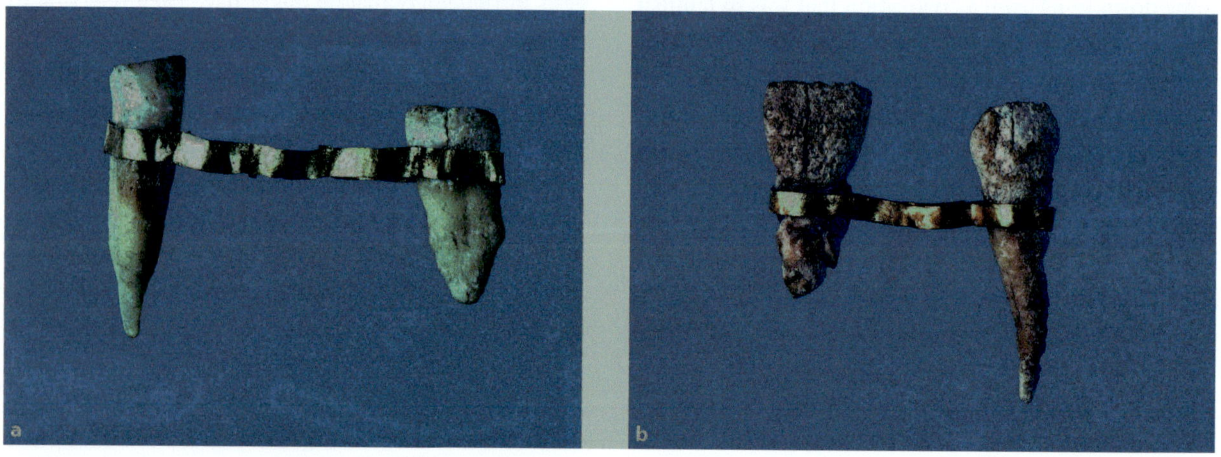

Fig. 8.3a,b Etruscan dental prostheses found in Tarquinia dating from the ninth century B.C. and exhibited in the Villa Giulia Museum Rome. *By permission of the Soprintendenza per i Beni Archeologici del Lazio, Rome*

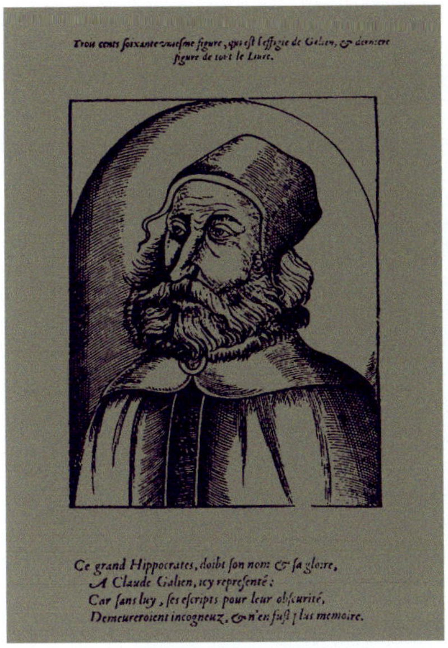
Trois cents soixante-unıesme figure, qui est l'effigie de Galien, & derniere figure de tout le Liure.
Ce grand Hippocrates, doibt son nom & sa gloire,
A Claude Galien, icy representé:
Car sans luy, ses escripts pour leur obscurité,
Demeureroient incogneuz, & n'en fust plus memoire.

Fig. 8.4 Portrait of Claudius Galen from Paré's book *Les Oeuvres*. He was one of the few who recognized the importance of the palate in speech. *Courtesy of Riccardo Mazzola, M.D., Milan*

losa" translated as scars, which would clearly imply an acquired rather than a congenital defect.

Pre-Columbian America

In contrast to this lack of information on clefts in the ancient Mediterranean civilizations, there is abundant evidence that they were known in Mesoamerica. Indeed, children born with defects were believed to possess supernatural powers and representations of human figures with various deformities have come to light, as is discussed in a study by Fernando Ortiz-Monasterio and R.A. Serrano [760]. Statuettes of figures with facial clefts can be seen at the Musée Guimet in Paris (Wagner Collection), the Museum für Folkerkunde in Munich, and in a group known as *Los Danzantes* at the archaeological site of Mount Alban in Mexico.

The pre-Colombian Americans possessed remarkable surgical skills despite the fact that they knew nothing of metallurgy and used knives made of obsidian for their operations. As R. Moodie observed [688, 689]: "No other people in an archaic or primitive phase of development have ever reached such a deep surgical knowledge as the Peruvians in the pre-Colombian age." The Aztecs and Mayas in Mexico reached a similar level of expertise. Bernardino de Sahagun [879] described with admiration in his *General History of the Things in New Spain* (c.1577) the fine sutures of human hair with which they repaired lip injuries to obtain the least noticeable scar. It may be noted that there is no evidence to support the hypothesis that they used the mandibles of ants to close the margins of the harelip.

Despite the fact that there are many references to clefts and each civilization had its own specific term for the defect—the Incas calling it *chektasema*, the Atzecs *tothcivitzy*, and the Pipils of El Salvador *sinsoste* [204]—we have no evidence that they attempted to repair this type of malformation.

From the Gods to Embryology: Interpreting the Origin of Clefts

Since in ancient times man was ignorant of embryology and morphogenesis, his explanation for the existence of congenital deformities was based on a combination of religion, superstition, invention and charlatanism. Typical of this mindset was the belief that pregnant women were so impressionable that the foetus could be influenced by the mother's emotional state. In Sparta women were advised to fix in their minds the famous statues of the gods Castor and Pollux to ensure the birth of a strong baby boy. In medieval Europe expectant mothers were told to avoid strange sights that might induce malformations in their baby, for example, looking at a monkey could cause microcephaly. Such superstitions were still current in the nineteenth century. In 1889 J.M. Keating [489] reported a series of congenital anomalies, including a harelip, provoked in each case, he claimed, by the mother looking a person with a similar deformity during her pregnancy.

Despite these myths, as early as the sixteenth century a few scientists began to explore the possibility that deformities might be caused by abnormal development in the embryo. Fabricius ab Aquapendente (1537–1619) (Fig. 8.5) was the first to suggest this hypothesis in 1600 [290], and confirmation was provided in 1651 by William Harvey (1578-1657) who had studied anatomy under

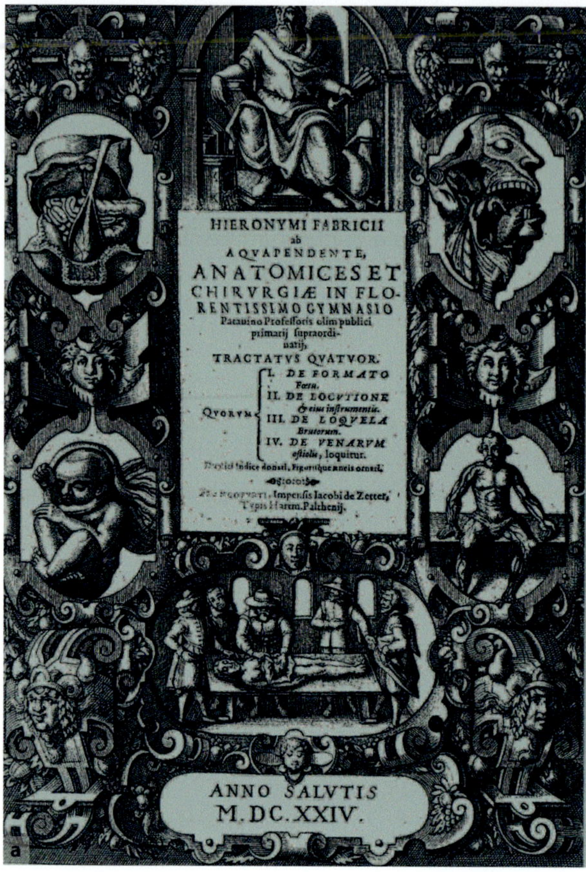

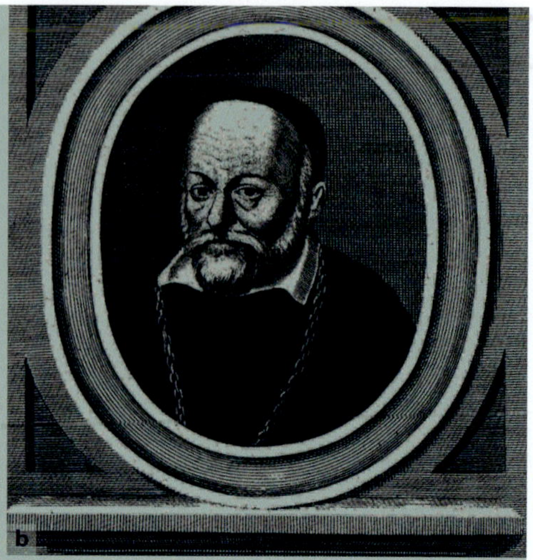

Fig. 8.5 **a** Frontispiece of Fabricius ab Aquapendente's book of 1624 and **b** his portrait. He was the first to suspect the embryological origin of congenital deformities. *Courtesy of FMN Art.spa. Bologna*

Fabricius in Padua [416, 418]. They realized that defects such as the harelip might be caused by an interruption in the normal development of the embryo. As Fabricius wrote: "This is the reason why so many are born with the upper lip divided as is seen in the hare and the camel…". He also made a new observation: "In the development of the human foetus the upper lip only coalesces along the middle line at a very late stage." Harvey supported this thesis, although he believed that the "primum movens" was an abnormally narrow uterus or the malposition of the foetus.

Their thesis, however tentative and preliminary, is all the more striking if we consider the fantastic theories that were still widely accepted in this period. For example, the learned archbishop of Uppsala in Sweden, Olaus Magnus [595], claimed in 1550: "However, there is one misfortune that many women meet with in pregnancy, either by eating or by leaping over the head of a hare; they bear children with a hare mouth, who have the lip permanently split between the mouth and nostrils, unless right from the beginning they sew a small piece of the breast of a very tender chicken, killed on the spot and still bleeding." Although he does not appear to have attempted this graft himself, curiously enough the procedure is cited by Gaspare Tagliacozzi (1545–1599) in *De Curtorum Chirurgia per Insitionem* [969].[6] Faith in the efficacy of this legend lingered in German-speaking areas until fairly recent times. Edward Zeis [1059, 1060] wrote in 1863 of a father who asked him to close the defect in his newborn son's lip with the flesh of a freshly killed chicken.

The first scientific classification of congenital deformities was proposed in 1768 by Albert von Haller (1708–1777), although systematic research on the condition, including experiments to induce malformations in animals, did not begin until the nineteenth century [409]. Several authors showed interest in deformities in general and this led to a greater understanding of their morphology, embryology and pathogenesis.

6 See *De Curtorum Chirurgia per Insitionem*, Book 2, Chapter 19, Folios 86–87.

In the middle of the nineteenth century a dispute arose between Andrea Ranzi [829], who supported Fabricius ab Aquapendente's theory of the cause of the cleft lip, and Velpeau and Cruvallier, who refused to believe that in its earliest stages the upper lip of the foetus was segmented. They argued instead that the cleft was the result of a malady affecting the lip during the gestation period. Ranzi himself did not entirely abandon the idea that impressions left on the mother's mind might influence the development of the foetus. Thus he cites a case published in the September 1822 issue of *Journal de Médecine* which described a patient, Martine of Lyon, who watched her husband skin a hare when she was five months pregnant and for the remainder of her term expressed fears that she would give birth to a child with a harelip, which she eventually did. Ranzi nonetheless concluded that there could not have been a link between the two events "since the premaxilla and the maxillary segments are united in the foetus before the fifth month".

The most convincing explanation of the origin of the facial cleft in this period was furnished by Philippe Frederick Blandin (1838–1896), who suggested that it resulted from a failure of the premaxilla and the maxillary segments to unite [108–114]. The first attempt to interpret the morphogenetic error underlying the malformation came from the German school of embryology. In 1808 J.F. Meckel [648] published his theory that the lips were formed from five separate processes which eventually united, three for the upper lip and two for the lower lip. This was confirmed by K.E. von Baer in 1828 [48] and by H. Rathke in 1832 [830]. The next breakthrough came in 1901 when William His [438, 440] of the University of Leipzig described the embryological development of the mid-face, beginning with the fusion of the five processes around the *stomodeum* or primitive oral cavity. The failure of any two of these parts to join would result in the formation of a different type of cleft, varying from unilateral and the bilateral clefts to the rare cleft of the lower lip along the median line.

Less than ten years later, in 1910, this apparently satisfactory explanation was overturned by G. Pöhlman [805]. Elaborating on an idea first proposed by A. Fleischmann [321], Pöhlman suggested that the problem did not lie in the unsuccessful union of separate processes, but rather in the failure of formation of local prominences. An indirect process was responsible for the creation of a cleft. He in fact demonstrated that during the normal course of development the mesoderm penetrates the epithelial margin of the cleft (already visible in 6- to 12-mm embryos) and coalesces with the mesoderm of the other side. If this phase is interrupted and all or part of the epithelium remains, the contact and fusion of the embryonic parts is impeded leading to an incomplete or complete cleft. The structure known as *Simonart's band* is said to be formed from epithelial residues of this process.[7]

Similar theories were developed much later, in 1971, by Richard Stark [949] and M. Patten [778] to explain the formation of the cleft palate, which was first described in detail by Victor Veau [1006, 1007] in 1934.

The Earliest Lip Repairs

The first report that we have of an operation to repair a congenital cleft lip comes from China around 390 B.C. The patient was an 18-year-old youth by the name of Wey Young-Chi [712, 1053] who was born in the city of Jen in the province of Hupeh. When he learned that in the retinue of the governor Ying Chung-Khan there was a physician with the skill to correct the defect, he decided to try and see him even though he did not know his name and was so poor that he had to undertake the journey to the capital city on foot. When Wey arrived in Nanking his story reached the ears of the governor, who asked to see him and was so impressed by his courage and intelligence that he summoned his physician and commanded him to help the young man.

The surgeon promised to do so but warned the patient that "after cutting and sewing together the margins, the part would have to remain in absolute repose for one

7 P.J.C. Simonart (1816–1846), a professor of gynaecology in Brussels described amniotic bands and although the tissue in the cleft has been given this name the effect is dissimilar from the bands producing constriction ring syndrome described by Streeter. See Simonart PJC (1846) Ueber die Simonart'schen Bänder. *Arch Med Belge* 1846:119 and also Gibson T (1977) Pierre-Joseph Cecilien Simonart (1816–1846) & his intrauterine bands. *Br J Plast Surg* 30:261.

hundred days". Wey agreed without hesitation, and for more than three months lived as a guest of the governor, eating only gruel and neither speaking nor laughing. The outcome of the operation was successful and Ying invited his protégé to remain, appointing him to a position in the state archives beginning what would prove to be a brilliant career.[8]

It had previously been believed that the operation on young Wey was not an isolated case and that similar reconstructions were carried out in China long before any such attempt was made in Europe. K. Boo-Chai [120] says that during the Tang dynasty (c.618–901 A.D.) many centuries after Wey Young-Chi's adventure, there was a surgeon, Fang Kan, who was known as "the doctor who repairs lips", but he does not furnish any evidence that these repairs involved congenital clefts. The true story of "Doctor" Fang, however, was discovered by J. Vrebos [1022] while he was researching the treatment of cleft lips in ancient China. He came to the conclusion that Fang Kan was not a surgeon at all, but a poet born with a harelip who was known as *Mr. Patched Lip*. Fang was so ashamed of his deformity that he chose to pass his life in lonely solitude by the shores of Lake Jin. His story illustrates the profound psychological distress that patients born with facial deformities must undergo. Further research by M.S. Noordhoff [738] has confirmed this version of the story of Fang Kan.

Attempts to Repair Facial Clefts in Western Civilizations

We have already mentioned Celsus (25 B.C. to 50 A.D.) and the doubts about whether the operations he described were to treat congenital deformities. After this period, there are no further references to facial clefts in the West until the fourth century. Oribasius Sardianus (325–403 A.D.) [754–757] reports that the celebrated surgeon Anthyllus (c.250 A.D.) operated on facial defects. He was the author of four books [738], of which only a few sections have come down to us thanks to Oribasius. They describe "operations for colobomata, and for defects of the eyelids, forehead, nose, ears and cheeks". We have also cited Galen [348, 349, 353, 354] whose cases were probably traumatic rather than congenital defects.

The term *divided lips* was used by Aegineta (625–690 A.D.) [427]. Like his description of their repair—"Restore them by first dissecting the skin below and afterwards bringing together the edges of the wound: then removing the callused part, and thereafter sewing and glueing them together"—that suggests that he was referring to a harelip, although *the calloused part* raises doubts as to their exact nature. Among the Arabs, the great physician and philosopher Abu Bakr Muhammad ibn Zakariya ar-Razi (known in the West as Rhazes) (c.850–923) described a treatment for the *fissura labiorum* which was probably an acquired rather than a congenital deformity [957].

It is not until the early fourteenth century in Venice that a description was published by Rolando Capelluti in 1230 in *Libellus de Cyrurgia*, of what was, according to Velpeau [1010, 1011] clearly a congenital cleft palate.[9] There is also mention of *labbra spaccate* or split lip, for which Capelluti recommended a simple topical treatment. Once again, however, the exact nature of the defect is not clear, and the physician showed no curiosity regarding its aetiology.[10]

In the past treatment was recommended on empirical grounds as knowledge of the factors which we now take for granted was very limited. Furthermore with the fall of Roman Empire surgeons no longer received any medical instruction. Their concern was to treat con-

8 Wey Young-Chi was recruited into the imperial army and quickly impressed General Lin-Yu, by helping to suppress a revolt. In due time Wey himself rose to the rank of general and then Governor of the Province of Yee. He eventually became Governor General of the Six Provinces. Throughout his life he affirmed that he would never have achieved so much if his cleft lip had not been repaired.

9 See *Libellus de Cyrurgia*, Book II, Chapter V, which Guy de Chauliac included in his *Cyrurgia* published later in Venice.

10 Rolando Capelluti, like his contemporary Ruggero, was born in Parma. In his operations on the abdomen he placed the patient with the head down and the legs up, a position that many centuries later was named after Trendelenburg. He describes the advantages of this position in his *Libellus de Chirurgia* which was so popular that it was also known by the cherished title of *La Rolandina*.

ditions without much thought for how and why they arose.

In the case of cleft deformities Fogh-Andersen [326] has demonstrated that there has been a slight rise in their frequency. If this reflects a continual process extending back over centuries, a millennium ago the number of infants born with this defect may not have been very high. Babies with clefts also stood a limited chance of survival. In his lifetime a surgeon probably had little experience of treating them and it is possible that some of the cases treated by the ancients were congenital clefts, but were not recognized as such. The exact nature of the deformity was not discovered until fairly recently. Famous surgeons in the nineteenth century still had little understanding of its origins. Philibert Joseph Roux operated on his first cleft palate and attributed the condition to an infection caused by "the severe winters" in the patient's native Canada [695].

The Middle Ages

According to Sterpellone and Salm El-Sheikh [957], the Arab Albucasis and his fellow surgeons were reluctant to use the scalpel. They preferred to use cautery for a wide range of conditions. Their instruments varied and various metals were used. Gold was recommended to stop bleeding. They realized that hot metal would cause more harm than good in the delicate tissue of a child's lip and practised a more gentle form of treatment The cure recommended by Albucasis involved cutting a tiny incision into the lip, inserting a clove of garlic and leaving it for fifteen hours. After removing the garlic, the margins of the defect were approximated with a bandage moistened with butter.

According to Cockayne [183], surgeons in pre-Norman England, who were called *leeches* because of their practice of bloodletting, operated regularly on congenital clefts. A text dating from 950 A.D. recommends: "For cleft-lip, pound mastic very small and add the white of an egg, and mingle as thou dost vermillion, cut with a knife the false edges of the lip, sew fast with silk, then smear without and within with salve. If it draws together, arrange it with the hand: anoint again soon after."

Evidently they had thoroughly mastered the procedure, for the fourteenth century surgeon John of Arderne (1307–1390) was celebrated for his reconstruction of *hairlips* [465]. This term seems to have been derived from the word *cara* used by Albucasis, which was then translated into the French word *poil* (hairs) and the Latin *pili*, always plural. Why the deformity should have been associated with the notion of *hair* is not known. The English term *harelip* was adopted in the sixteenth century and represents a literal translation of the French term *bec de lièvre* employed by Ambroise Paré. By sheer coincidence *hair* and *hare* represent homophones in English.

The first to note the congenital origin of the cleft was the thirteenth century physician Jean Yperman (1295–1351). He classified the various forms of the condition and laid down the principles for their treatment [1055]. Yperman called the deformity *sarte moude* (notched mouth) and recommended scarifying the margins with a scalpel before suturing them with a triangular needle dipped in wax. The repair was reinforced by passing a long needle through the two sides of the lip and fixing the shaft of the needle with a figure-of-eight thread over the lip. His contemporaries remained unaware of his work and it was not until the sixteenth century and the studies by Fabricius ab Aquapendente, Pierre Franco, William Harvey and others that the theory regarding the congenital nature of the condition started to be considered.

The fourteenth century was marked by a number of surgical breakthroughs and practitioners began to show some interest in facial clefts. Yperman had written scathingly of colleagues who were content to close the margins with a long pin, sometimes even making two lateral relaxing incisions to facilitate the process. As he pointed out, this left disfiguring scars that "could compromise the reputation of the surgeon" [854]. Progress was slow, but eventually professional societies such as the Company of the Barber Surgeons of London were created which helped to raise the standards of all surgical treatment.

A significant contribution was made by Heinrich von Pfolsprundt in 1460 [796]. In contrast to his predecessors, who only sutured the skin, he passed stitches through all the layers when repairing the cleft. Though he was familiar with the Branca's methods he never used flaps when repairing the lip.

In a surgical treatise by Charaf-ed Din dating from around 1465, described by Rogers as a "fascinating Turkish manuscript" [854], there is a drawing of a surgeon cauterizing a patient's lip and some have suggested that he was actually be treating a harelip. This is a tantalizing but unlikely thesis, because on closer examination it can be seen that procedure is being carried out on the patient's lower lip [451].

In 1497 Hyeronimus Brunschwig, a military surgeon from Alsace, described an operation that he carried out in Strasbourg on a patient with a harelip [139, 140]. It began with the patient being lashed to the operating table! After scarify the margins of the cleft with scissors, the surgeon applied a pinching clamp (*Zwickhafft*) or self-retaining clamp (*Telphaffen*), and then sutured the margins together with interrupted waxed stitches. The sutures and clamp were left in place for some time, after which the wound was covered with a mixture made of egg and pulverized eggshell. The author also described a complicated bandage wound around the patient's head, under his arm and back and forth across the lips; a technique he claimed was invented by Roger of Salerno.

From the Renaissance to the Nineteenth Century

During the sixteenth century surgeons began to gain a better understanding of clefts and various misconceptions were corrected. Fabricius ab Aquapendente and Harvey cast some light on the aetiology. Technical improvements were also introduced since, although former methods were undeniably ingenious, results had been poor.

A important contribution was made by Pierre Franco (c.1505–1561), a pupil of Ambroise Paré. Born in Tourniers in Provence, Franco was a typical itinerant surgeon of the period and never received a formal medical education. As a Huguenot, he was persecuted for his religious convictions, but managed to escape the massacre and sought refuge in Switzerland. After several years passed first in Bern and then in Lausanne, he returned to France where he settled in Orange and resumed the practice of medicine. Although not an academic, Franco decided to write a surgical text based on his many years of experience, which he modestly called a *Petit Traité* [332] even though it was a substantial work that contained, as the author stated on the title page, "excellent sections on surgery". The book was written in French even though he was conversant with Latin and was published in Lyon in 1556 [333].[11]

In sixteenth century France surgery was practised in urban areas by barber surgeons, while the inhabitants of the countryside had to rely on itinerate practitioners known as *inciseurs*. These untrained surgeons were ready to turn their hand to anything from hernias to cataracts, and even pulling teeth. Franco began as one of these modest practitioners, but possessed sufficient ability and charisma to rise in the world socially as well as professionally for he eventually married Claudia Borrel, a member of the aristocratic family Dauphiné, les Seigneurs d'Albon. Joseph Francois Malgaigne (1806–1865) contended that it was these skilled *inciseurs* rather than the Parisian barber surgeons who contributed most to the French school of surgery in this early period [600, 601].

The treatment of cleft lips takes up four chapters in Pierre Franco's text.[12] He states that "the entire skin of the margins which are to be joined must be cut with a razor, or a scissor, or with the cautery". If cauterization is used, he warned that after two days: "the eschar will have to be loosened with fresh butter [before suturing] … otherwise it will generally be a waste of effort and hurt the patient needlessly, especially when the margins are far apart".

His second book, *Traité des Hernies* (Fig. 8.6), was published in 1561 and includes chapters on anatomy, medicine and pharmacology. While in his first book Franco only cites Avicenna, Albucasis and Guy de Chauliac, *Traité des Hernies* contains no less than 356 citations

11 A second edition of this book was published, again in Lyon, but by another printer in 1561 and with a new title, *Traité des Hernies* [333].

12 See *Traité des Hernies*. Pierre Franco's description of clefts may be found in Chapter CXVIII. In Chapter CXIX, entitled *La cure des leures findues*, the author describes his surgical procedure for the repair of clefts lips, and in Chapter CXX various other treatments. Finally, in Chapters CXXI and CXXII Franco describes his treatment for the bilateral harelip, which he called *dents de lièvre*.

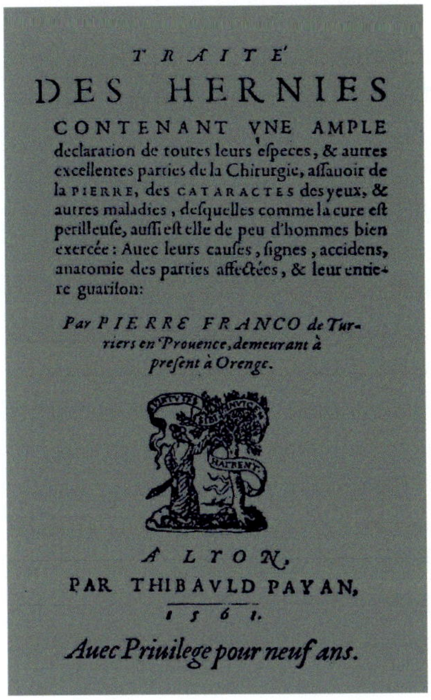
TRAITE'
DES HERNIES
CONTENANT VNE AMPLE
declaration de toutes leurs especes, & autres excellentes parties de la Chirurgie, assauoir de la PIERRE, des CATARACTES des yeux, & autres maladies, desquelles comme la cure est perilleuse, aussi est elle de peu d'hommes bien exercée: Auec leurs causes, signes, accidens, anatomie des parties affectées, & leur entiere guarison:
Par PIERRE FRANCO de Turriers en Prouence, demeurant à present à Orenge.
A LYON,
PAR THIBAVLD PAYAN,
1561.
Auec Priuilege pour neuf ans.

Fig. 8.6 Frontespiece of *Traite des Hernies* by Pierre Franco (1561). He was convinced that clefts had an embryological origin and described their repair. *Reprinted from* Surgery an Illustrated History *by Ira M Rutkov © (1993) with permission of Elsevier*

from a wide range of authorities, testifying to the remarkable learning of the supposedly unschooled author.[13] Franco discusses the cleft lip in ample detail devoting two chapters to the subject.[14] He was the first to state the congenital nature of the malformation clearly, in fact he called unilateral harelip the "lièvre fendu de nativité" (cleft lip present from birth).[15] He provides a meticulous classification of various types of clefts,[16] calling the bilateral harelip the "dent de lièvre" (hare's tooth) presumably because this condition was frequently accompanied by a marked protrusion of the premaxilla bone with its teeth. The term "bec de lièvre" was introduced by Paré.

Franco gave a meticulous description of his surgical technique. He used dry sutures, pins and a triangular bandage. He emphasized that an accurate repair produced an unobtrusive scar, an outcome which was "particularly desirable when the patient was a girl".

Surgery on the bilateral harelip was carried out in two stages due to the difficulty of closing an extremely wide cleft, often complicated by a protruding premaxilla. Franco recommended that the cheeks be mobilized in the repair, and did not hesitate to resect the premaxilla. As he wrote: "To extirpate this turpitude, we must first proceed in the manner described above, except when the teeth and maxillary segments are outside and cannot be covered by the mouth. There is no danger in cutting too much of that which serves no purpose, so one uses cutting forceps, or a saw or other instrument suitable for this, leaving the flesh which is over these teeth, if there is any, as it helps when sewing to the other parts on each side. And if there is such a distance between these lips that one cannot bring them together, it will be necessary to use dissection in the mouth similar to those in the preceding case, and proceed with the remainder of the closure as we have described."[17] This passage could not be more lucid and illustrates why Franco has been called *The Father of Lip Repairs*. Like Paré, he passed a pin or fibula across the repair and held this in place with a figure-of-eight thread, a technique invented by Henry de Mondeville (1260–1320) in 1306 for many wounds [682].[18]

Ambroise Paré (1510–1590) was one of the greatest surgeons of the sixteenth century; he conducted detailed studies on the anatomy of the lips and palate and introduced significant improvements in the technique of suturing, which he described in works published in 1564

13 Franco's accounts of his surgical procedures are admirably detailed. In his treatise he presents the principal treatments for hernias, bladder stones, cataracts, diseases of the uvula and mouth, and amputations. Among the other innovations described in his work is a surgical procedure for tumours of the parotid (Chapter CX). As we will see in the chapter on genitalia, Franco was the first to carry out a suprapubic cystostomy in a 2-year-old child.

14 See *Traité des Hernies*, Chapters XCV and XCVI.

15 See *Traité des Hernies*, Chapter XCV.

16 See *Traité des Hernies*, Chapter XCV.

17 See *Traité des Hernies*, Chapter XCVI.

18 See *Chirurgie*, Book II, Chapter 1, "De bandages et de la suture" ("On bandages and sutures").

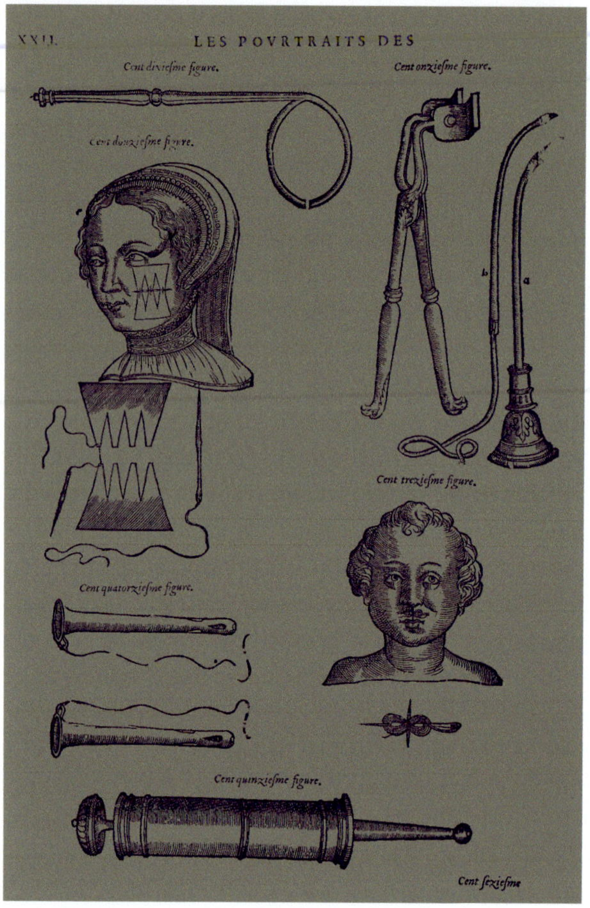

Fig. 8.7 A page from *Les Oeuvres* by Paré showing the suturing method for cleft lip repair. *Courtesy of Riccardo Mazzola, M.D., Milan*

and 1575 [768, 769]. Like Pierre Franco, Paré was a Huguenot and according to Garrison [360, 361] managed to escape the Saint Bartholomew's Day Massacre thanks to the direct intervention of the king. The sincerity of his faith is expressed in the words inscribed on his statue in Paris, "Je le pansai, Dieu le guérit." What is probably the first illustration of an operation on a cleft lip appears in a work by Paré (Fig. 8.7).[19] Although he did not have the benefit of a university education he wrote works of fundamental importance, not in Latin but in such fluent French that Garrison has suggested that he may have used the services of a pion or secretary to correct and polish his text.[20]

Jacques Guillemeau (1550–1613) was a student of Paré who, although better known for his contributions to ophthalmology, also earned recognition for his work on clefts.[21] An entire chapter of his book *Les Oeuvres de Chirurgie* [400, 401] is devoted to the treatment of this deformity (Fig. 8.8a, b). In the section *Du bec de lièvre, ou lièvres fendues*, after describing his technique the author provides specific instructions on what to do in cases of a very broad cleft: "[when] the parts cannot be put together, then we must make two incisions, one on each side of the cleft ... because the edges of the wounds must not be forced together but they must be brought in touch kindly, without violence [and] in such a way that even when we leave them they do not draw back again". Like his teacher Paré, Guillemeau recommended making relaxing incisions into the skin of the cheeks that were "full thickness but did not penetrate into the mouth". To do this, he inserted a curved lancet into the uppermost part of the cleft close to the nostril beneath the skin, and used this to make a lateral incision. In cases where the margins were under tension, they were held in place by the insertion of one or two pins with a "figure 8 suture". This is well illustrated in Le Dran's book of 1749 (Fig. 8.9a,b) [541].

During the seventeenth century surgeons also began to ask when was the best time to repair the deformity, an issue that has not been resolved to this day. Some, like Hendrik van Roonhuysen (1622–1672) of Amsterdam, declared that the operation should be carried out as soon as possible, when the patient was just 3 or 4 months of age [859]. He was supported by James Cooke of Warwick (1614–1688) who wrote: "The operation is more dangerous to perform upon a grown than young person, though happily perform'd on some of 28 years of age. The younger children are when cut, 'tis better yea while infant, unless they be sick and weak. It's more fitly done in Summer than Winter, in Spring than Fall." Cooke would abrade the margins of the cleft with a scalpel or scissors

19 See *Les Oeuvres*, chapter CCCLXXVI.

20 Collins' French-English Dictionary translates *pion* as "scholastic supervisor". In France this term is generally used to refer to a type of assistant teacher, a somewhat lowly position but usually held by a person of good cultural background and education.

21 See *Les Oeuvres de Chirurgie*, Book X, Chapter II.

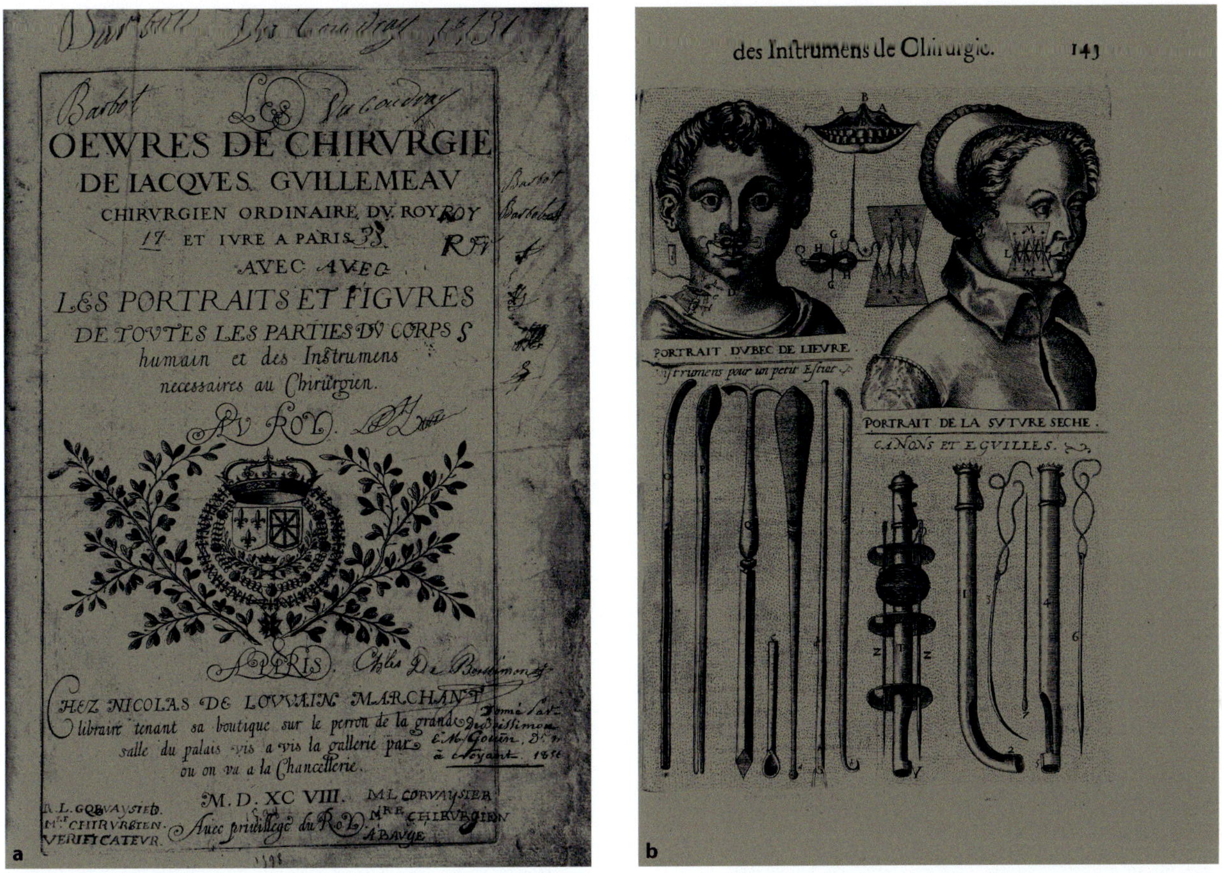

Fig. 8.8 **a** Frontispiece of the book *Oeuvre de Chirurgie* by Jacques Guillemeau, Paré's pupil. **b** His instruments and the dry suture technique are very similar to those of Paré. *Courtesy of Riccardo Mazzola, M.D., Milan*

and then close them with dry suture and figure-of-eight thread. He also suggested that the infant be kept awake for as long as possible, even up to 12 hours before the operation, in order to "increase drowsiness, perhaps administering a glass of wine, or a cordial in cases of fainting due to the loss of blood" [195].

Others preferred not to operate on very young patients; as M.G. Leclerc noted in 1701, their "continual crying would hinder the reunion". He agreed that the child should be kept awake before the operation so that he would fall asleep immediately afterwards, to help healing of the wound. He introduced a slight variation in the procedure, removing one of the pins after 3 days and leaving the second pin for no less than 8 days [539].

The debate continued, however, and in the nineteenth century Andrea Ranzi introduced an important but hitherto neglected consideration [829]. Like Roux he believed that while a simple harelip could be corrected shortly after birth, operations on more complex deformities should be postponed for up to five years. But he deserves credit for drawing attention to the psychological burden of the disfigurement as a crucial factor in the decision. In his view this usually justified operating as soon as possible. When we read his words we might be listening to the evaluation of a specialist in child psychiatry during the discussions on a modern plastic surgery ward.

It must have seemed to George de la Faye (1699–1781) and his contemporaries that the treatment for lip clefts was by now quite advanced, and in 1743 de la Faye published an overview on the subject [303]. When reading his description, however, one cannot help agree with Frank McDowell [636] who observed "… it is surprising that in two centuries [since the innovations of Pierre Franco] so little progress had been made", although he concedes that

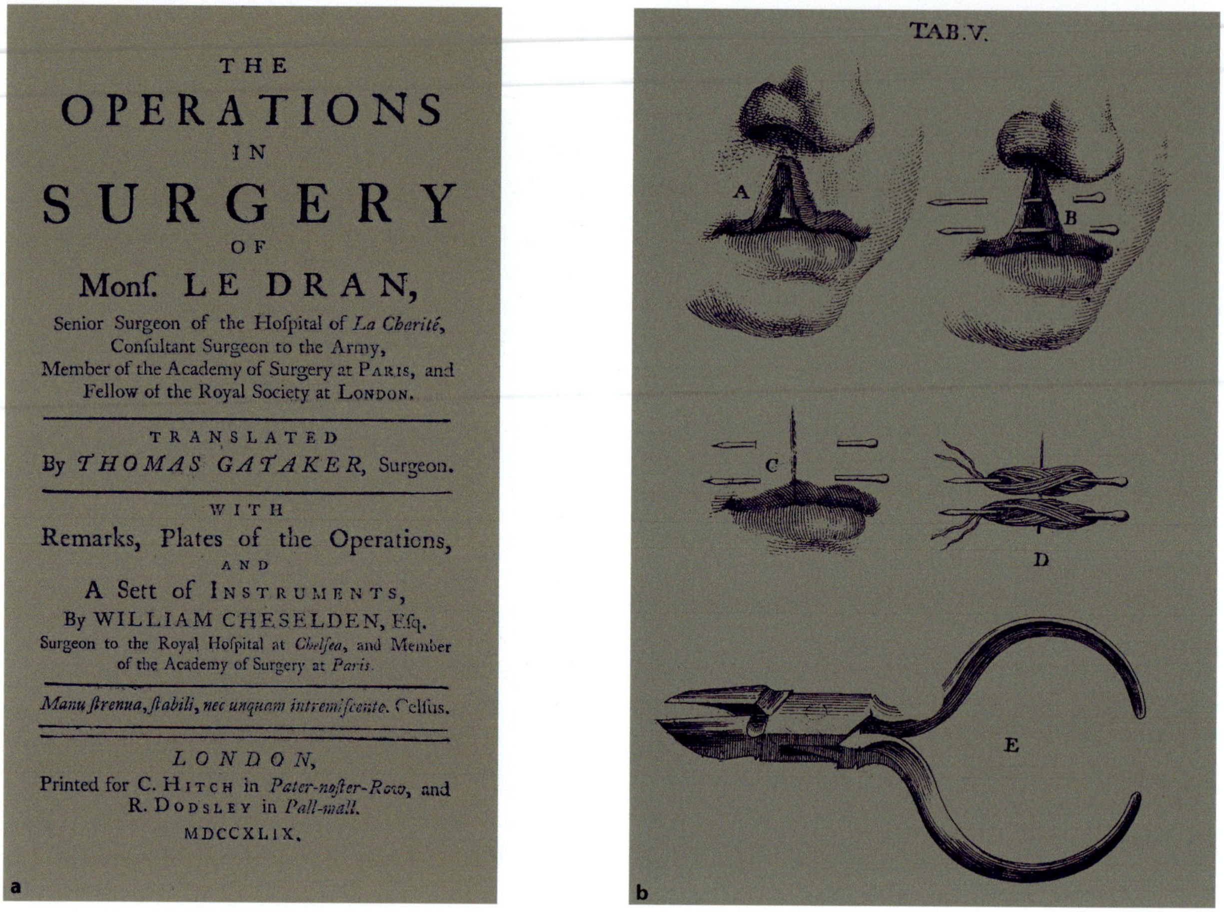

THE
OPERATIONS
IN
SURGERY
OF
Monſ. LE DRAN,
Senior Surgeon of the Hoſpital of *La Charité*,
Conſultant Surgeon to the Army,
Member of the Academy of Surgery at PARIS, and
Fellow of the Royal Society at LONDON.

TRANSLATED
By *THOMAS GATAKER*, Surgeon.

WITH
Remarks, Plates of the Operations,
AND
A Sett of INSTRUMENTS,
By WILLIAM CHESELDEN, Eſq.
Surgeon to the Royal Hoſpital at *Chelſea*, and Member
of the Academy of Surgery at *Paris*.

Manu ſtrenua, ſtabili, nec unquam intremiſcente. Celſus.

LONDON,
Printed for C. HITCH in *Pater-noſter-Row*, and
R. DODSLEY in *Pall-mall*.
MDCCXLIX.

Fig. 8.9 **a** Frontispiece of Le Dran's book *Operations in Surgery* published in 1749. **b** The closure of the lip is described in detail. *Courtesy of Riccardo Mazzola, M.D., Milan*

"… plastic surgery was awaking after the long sleep engendered by the Church's condemnation of Tagliacozzi's and all plastic surgical procedures" (Fig. 8.10).

De la Faye presented his paper, which focused primarily on bilateral clefts, before the *French Académie Royale de Chirurgie*, where it was very well received.[22] The author confessed that in one of his earliest operations he could not resist the temptation to cut away the premaxilla, believing that this would facilitate the closure of the cleft, but the outcome was so poor that he never repeated this mistake. Instead, he perfected a technique that included the prolabium to recreate the central part of the lip.

Despite the work of these pioneers and the support of prestigious institutions such as the *Académie Royale de Chirurgie*, serious obstacles continued to hamper progress and the routine practice of plastic surgery at the beginning of the eighteenth century. One example is provided by Arne Rintala [843, 844], who describes the case of a "writer of psalms"[23] living in Finland who suf-

22 De la Faye's father was also a surgeon, who died when his son was 15 years old. George went to live with an uncle who was a surgeon at the military hospital of Berg St. Vinox. Later he moved to Paris, where he eventually became a member of the *Académie Royale de Chirurgie*.

23 In Scandinavia the term *writer of psalms* was used to refer to pious members of the church who adapted verses of the Psalms so that they might be sung in church.

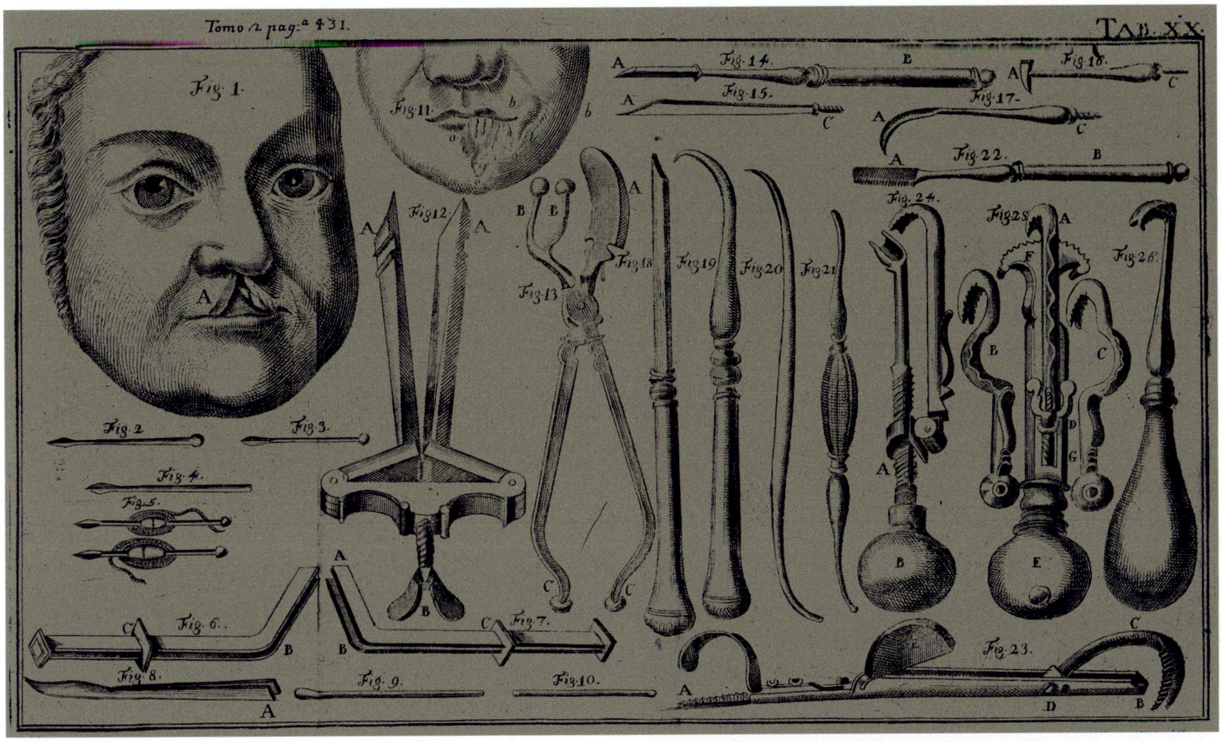

Fig. 8.10 Engraving by an anonymous artist showing a cleft lip in the early seventeenth century. The instruments shown are more like those used for cleft palate repair, an operation not attempted at the time. They may have been used on palatal fistulae. *Courtesy of Alessandro Massei, M.D., Pisa*

fered from a serious form of cleft lip. In 1763 he finally decided to consult Odenat Gerhard, a Swedish surgeon living in the city of Turku on the Baltic coast. The pious Fin had repeatedly postponed the operation, partly out of fear, but above all due to a moral dilemma. Did he have the right to correct a deformity which God had chosen to visit upon him? The patient finally laid his problem before the governing body of the Cathedral of Turku which, after thoroughly discussing the ethical and religious aspects of the case, granted permission as long as "the patient took Holy Communion before the operation" (Fig. 8.11).

In contrast during this period the repair of clefts became a fairly regular practice in America, where surgeons did not hesitate to advertise their skills and services in local newspapers. Rogers [854] has collected an entertaining series of advertisements for the correction of lip clefts published in Boston (1770), Philadelphia (May 1775), New London, Connecticut (March 1778) and other cities, by self-styled doctors of whom only one possessed any qualifications. He was a Mr. Charles Hall who was listed in the registry of the Medical Service of the English Army and who operated successfully on a child in Rosbury, Massachusetts in 1770. Rogers concludes that these "doctors could be classified by the circumstantial evidence of the newspaper advertisements in the realm of quacks, mountebanks, charlatans, and itinerant medicasters" (Fig. 8.12a, b).

In more or less the same period a certain Dr. Matthew Wilson (1734–1790) wrote a compendium entitled the *Therapeutic Alphabet* which contains the description of a method for repairing harelips using pins and like Franco two centuries earlier, extracting the protruding incisors if they interfered with the closure of the cleft. Fortunately perhaps, this work was never published.

The First Transposition Flap in Lip Repair

Most of the surgeons mentioned here, who were so bold as to attempt lip repairs, in reality did little more than

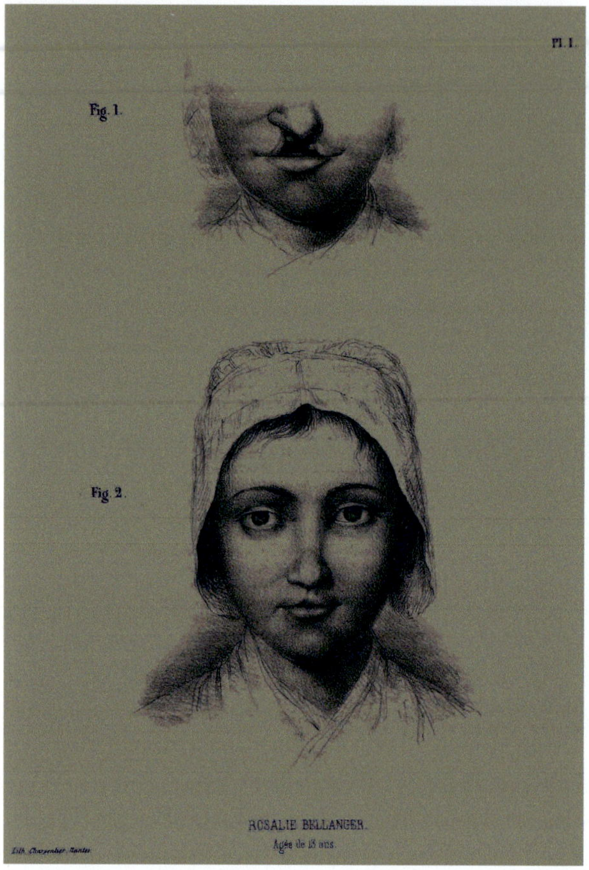

Fig. 8.11 A case of unilateral cleft included by Germanicus Mirault in the *Journal de Chirurgie* in 1844. *Courtesy of Riccardo Mazzola. M.D., Milan*

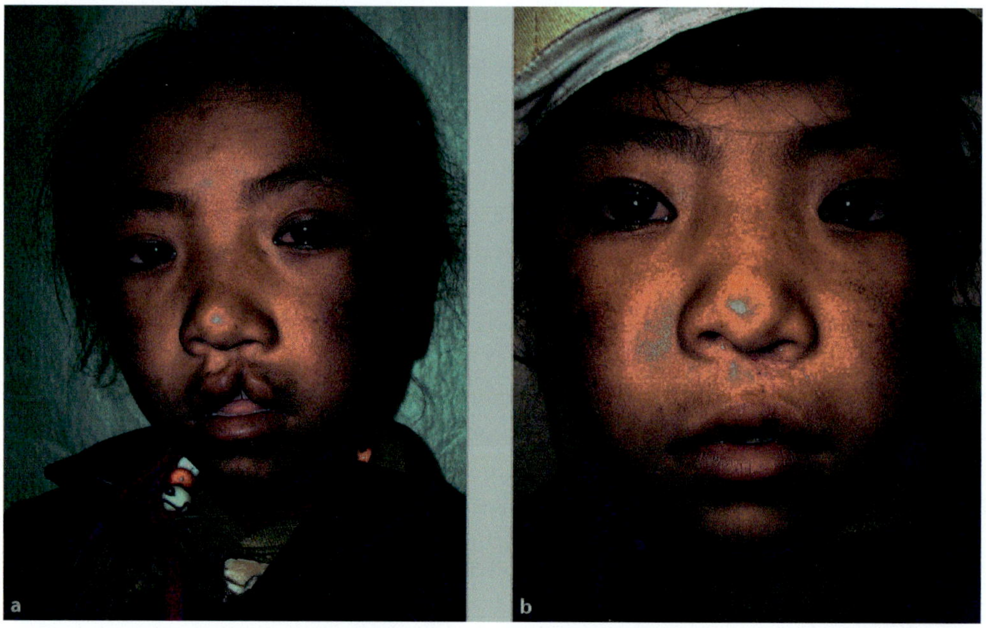

Fig. 8.12 A case of incomplete unilateral cleft lip **a** before the operation and **b** one month after the repair using the Millard method. *Courtesy of Daniele Gandini, M.D., Interplast Italy Team, Tibet*

scarify the margins and suture them together, employing various expedients to ensure good approximation of the edges. As can be imagined, the results were not always satisfactory. The vertical scar that formed invariably caused an ugly shortening of the lip.

In 1844 Germanicus Mirault (1796–1879) devised an ingenious method to circumvent this problem. He introduced a triangular flap from the lateral side into a gap created by making a horizontal incision on the medial side [679]. This broke up the linear scar and introduced some extra tissue in an attempt to lengthen the lip. It also helped create a nostril floor. More than a century later Victor Veau (1871–1949) stated that "Mirault is the genius of cleft lip surgery", and indeed his contribution was the most important since Franco's description of his two-step procedure [1006]. Malgaigne, who fully concurred with Mirault regarding the importance of interrupting the straight scar. He refined his procedure in order to achieve a more aesthetically pleasing reconstruction (Figs. 8.13, 8.14a,b).[24]

At the same time that these modifications were being introduced other surgical techniques were perfected. In 1815 Gustav Simon reiterated the need for an accurate technique practised with the greatest delicacy and precision, the least amount of scar hypertrophy being sufficient to compromise the results [928]. Johan Fredrick Dieffenbach (1794–1847), who as a specialist in urethral operations had gained considerable experience in atraumatic techniques, was equally emphatic on the subject [243]. William Rose also stressed the importance of precise incisions and meticulously executed sutures in 1891 [861].

Important developments also emerged in the area of general anaesthesia, which up to this time had been neither safe nor reliable. With the introduction of ether, operations became less traumatic for the patient and the surgeon could work with greater calm and deliberation, no longer subjected to the disturbing spectacle of the patient's suffering, which in the past had placed him under intense pressure to finish the operation as quickly as possible.

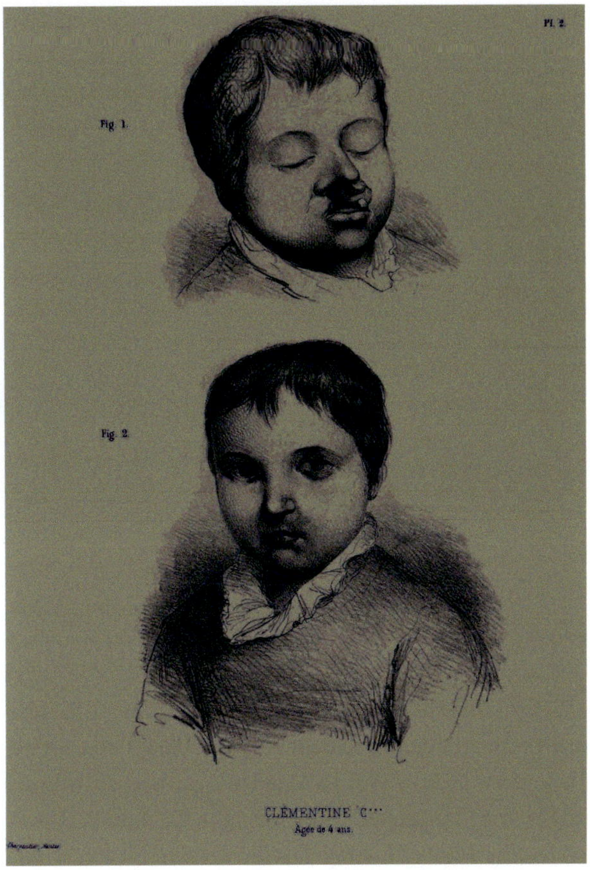

Fig. 8.13 Another case of Germanicus Mirault from his article in the *Journal de Chirurgie* in 1844. *Courtesy of Riccardo Mazzola, M.D., Milan*

Nevertheless surgeons were forced to acknowledge that the satisfactory results obtained during the operation often deteriorated over time, particularly in the case of growing children. The nostrils generally became distorted and the repaired lip tended to retrude and tighten, as V.P. Blair and J.B. Brown noted [106]. Mirault's curved scar and lateral flap technique allowed the surgeon to avoid the second problem, but only through a

24 Malgaigne was an extremely cultivated man who taught himself Hebrew, Greek and Latin in order to be able to study the Bible in greater depth. He was also a historian and in 1847 published an interesting work on the history of the philosophy of surgery from Hippocrates to his day, underlining how progress in human ideals over the centuries had always had a positive influence on the evolution of surgery. He made notable contributions to the treatment of complex scars, surgery on the lids for blepharitis and ptosis, and in the areas of otorhinolaryngology, rhinoplasty, otoplasty and urethroplast.

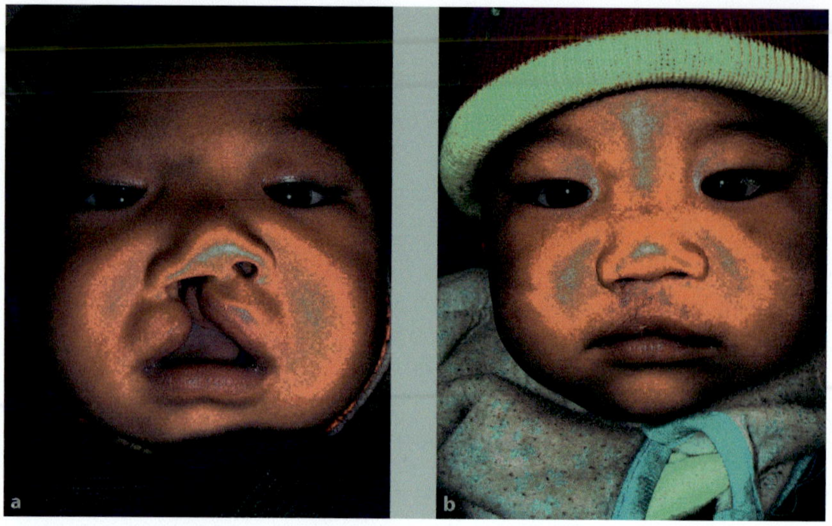

Fig. 8.14 A complete unilateral cleft **a** before surgery and **b** one month after a repair using Skoog's method with periosteal flaps to close the maxillary cleft. *Courtesy of Daniele Gandini, M.D., Interplast Italy Team in Tibet*

broad mobilization of the nostrils could the appearance of the nose be improved (Fig. 8.15a,b).

This combined approach, referred to as "Mirault's operation" [679] was widely adopted [445]. Werner H. Hagerdon (1831–1894) of Magdeburg who had studied under von Langenbeck, introduced a further improvement in 1848 [405, 406]. He recommended interrupting the vertical repair with a quadrangular rather than a triangular flap. This modification offered obvious advantages, particularly in the case of bilateral clefts, for it made the repair easier and by exerting pressure on the premaxilla helped to correct the protrusion (Figs. 8.16, 8.17a,b).

Hagerdon, together with his pupil William Rose [861], also helped to clear up the confusion between the various flaps proposed by different surgeons. They explained that a simple, straight line closure could produce entirely satisfactory results as long as the surgeon repaired the cleft with precision, accuracy and fine suturing materials. Hagerdon was an advocate of early surgery and successfully operated on two babies in the first week after birth. He was probably also the first surgeon to attempt to repair a double cleft in one operation (Fig. 8.18).

The quadrangular flap devised by Hagerdon was generally only used for bilateral clefts. A century later, in 1949, this technique was modified by Arthur Baker Le Mesurier [549] then by C.W. Tennison in 1952 [978] and Peter Randall in 1959 [827], both from the United States. Le Mesurier noted that in rare cases relaxing incisions could be cut in the mouth beneath the lateral flaps. Before Le Mesurier very few surgeons had ventured to correct the protrusion of the premaxilla. One was Levret in 1772 [667] and the other Desault in 1792 [854], but their work received little attention. Around this time some early orthodontic treatment was attempted by Giuseppe Maria Brunazzi and he wrote his *Memoria su di un Nuovo Metodo di Unire il Labbro Leporino col Mezzo di Una Macchinetta* where his method is illustrated in 1790 (Fig. 8.19a, b) [136].

In 1872 a radical method to correct this protrusion was developed by the Finnish surgeon Jacob August Estlander (1851–1881). He believed that by leaving the premaxilla intact one could avoid compromising the growth of the middle third of the face, and therefore recommended a wedge resection of the vomer which allowed the protruding premaxilla to be pushed back [284]. He published a paper in German describing this procedure, which won wide, if not universal acceptance and remained the only available method to correct severe protrusion of the premaxilla for many years.

Time would show however, that this excision impeded the growth of the middle third of the face. In 1935 another Finnish surgeon, Richard Faltin (1867–1952), published a work recommending that the procedure be abandoned because it regularly led to serious maxillary retrusion [299, 300] However, he wrote in Swedish and published in Finland, a fact which hindered the spread of his observations. Almost half a century would pass before Ralph Millard [667], in his detailed compendium of twentieth century surgical procedures for clefts, provided the English-speaking medical community with the opportunity to read Faltin's paper and understand

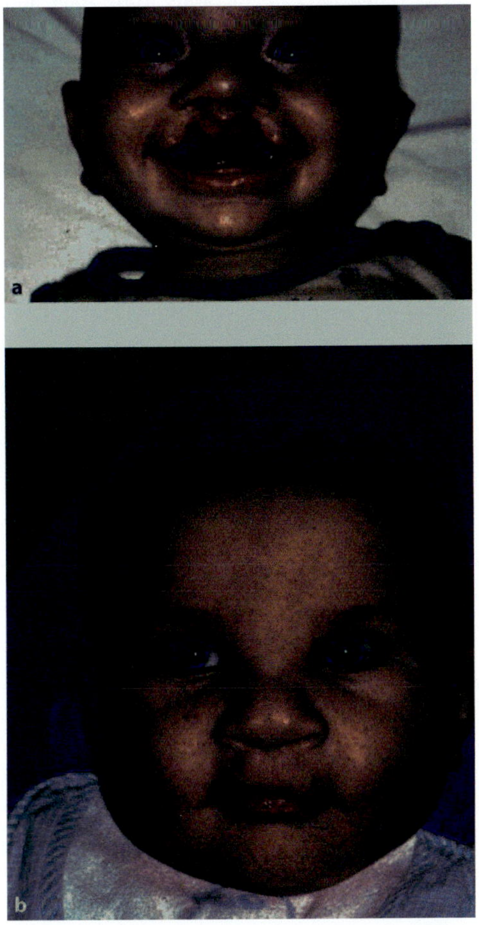

Fig. 8.15 A bilateral incomplete cleft lip. **a** Pre-operative view. **b** The result six months after repair by the Mulliken method. *Courtesy of Alessandro Massei, M.D., Pisa*

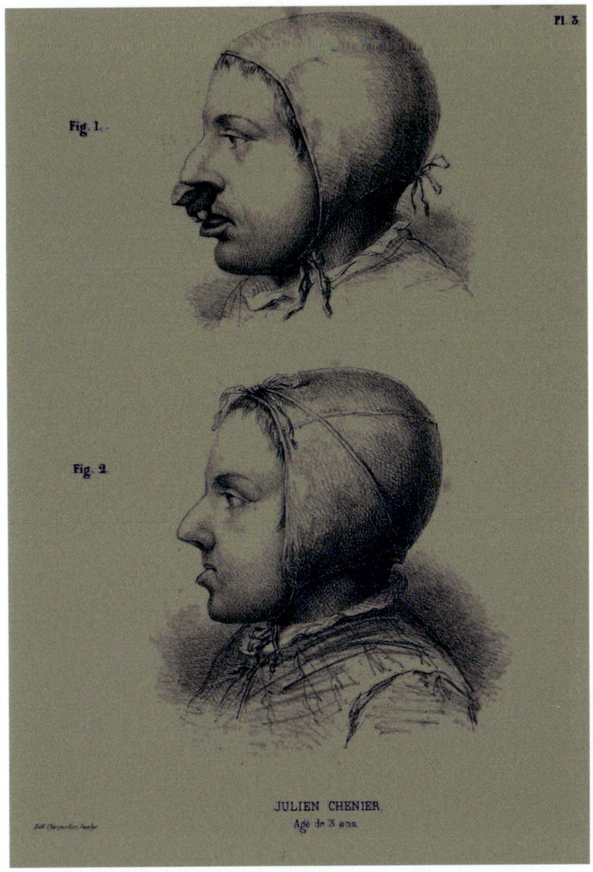

Fig. 8.16 Severe protrusion of the premaxilla in this case from Germanicus Mirault's article in *Journal de Chirurgie*, 1844. *Courtesy of Riccardo Mazzola, M.D., Milan*

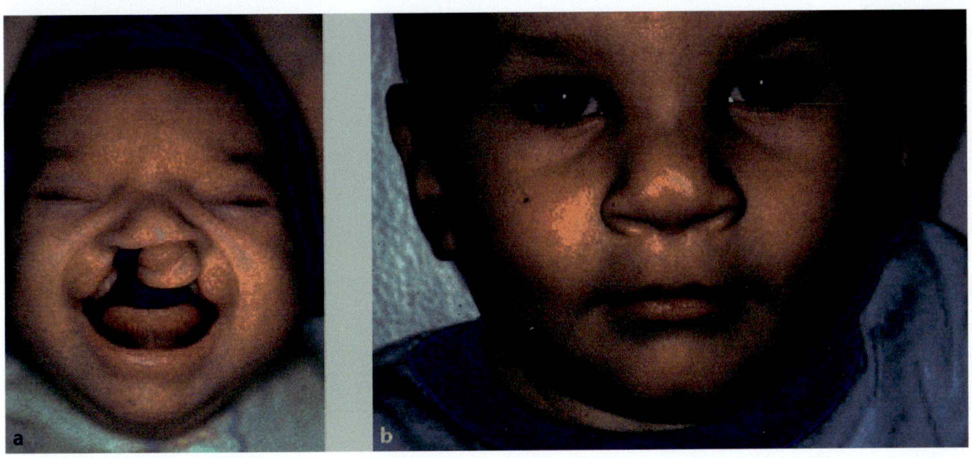

Fig. 8.17 A case of bilateral complete cleft. **a** Before surgery showing marked protrusion of the premaxilla. **b** Nine months post-operatively. The protrusion was corrected by the pressure of the lip closure and orthodontic treatment was used later. *Courtesy of Alessandro Massei, M.D. Pisa*

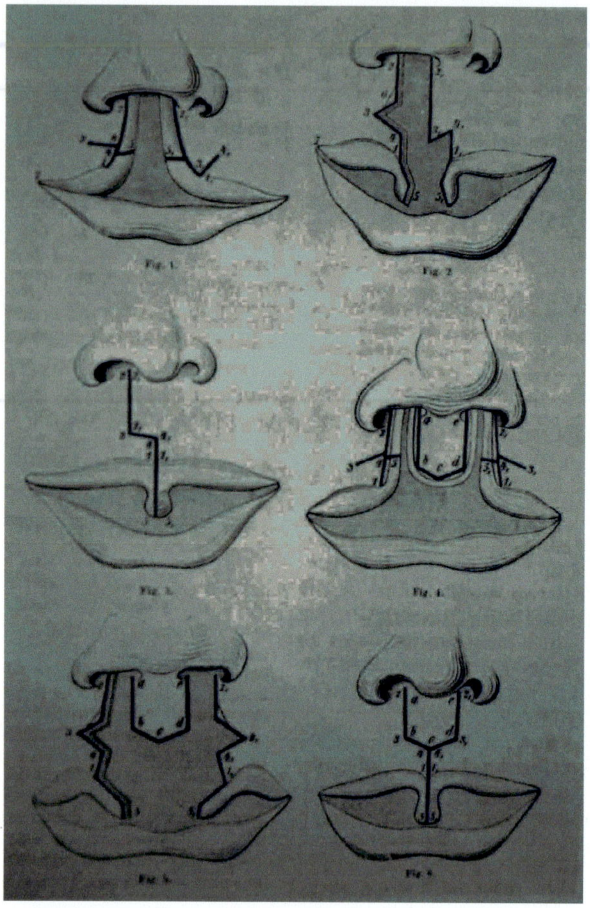

Fig. 8.18 Werner Hagerdon's lip incisions from 1884 and 1892 [405, 406]. The many cleft lip incisions that were described around this time are too numerous to include here. A useful résumé can be found in McDowell's *Source Book of Plastic Surgery* [636]

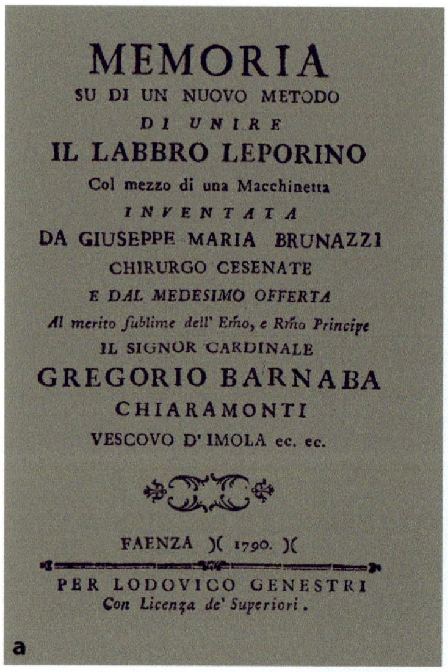

MEMORIA
SU DI UN NUOVO METODO
DI UNIRE
IL LABBRO LEPORINO
Col mezzo di una Macchinetta
INVENTATA
DA GIUSEPPE MARIA BRUNAZZI
CHIRURGO CESENATE
E DAL MEDESIMO OFFERTA
Al merito sublime dell' Emo, e Rmo Principe
IL SIGNOR CARDINALE
GREGORIO BARNABA
CHIARAMONTI
VESCOVO D' IMOLA ec. ec.

FAENZA)(1790.)(
PER LODOVICO GENESTRI
Con Licenza de' Superiori.

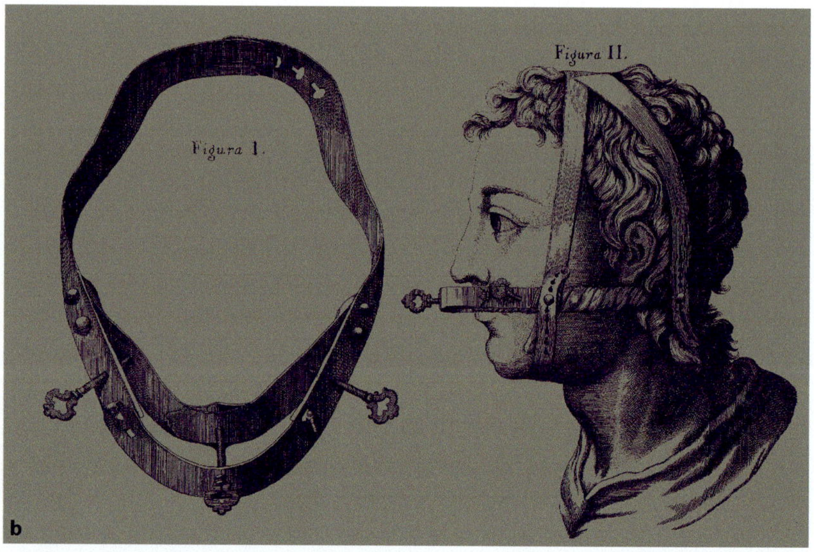

Fig. 8.19 **a** Frontispiece of the book *Memoria su di un Nuovo Metodo di Unire il Labbro Leporino* written by G.M. Brunazzi in 1790. **b** Early apparatus for orthodontic treatment of premaxillary protrusion from Brunazzi's book. *Courtesy of Riccardo Mazzola, M.D., Milan*

this late complication of Estlander's method. The delay is greatly to be regretted because innumerable class III malocclusions could have been avoided had more surgeons been aware of Faltin's study. Eventually the preoperative orthopaedic treatment devised by Ken McNeil and William Burston[25] and adopted by many orthodontist replaced the vomerine resection, and this problem was resolved [667].

Since the end of the nineteenth century surgeons have devised repairs of every type and shape, culminating in flaps raised on both sides of the cleft to improve the scar, lengthen the lip, and reconstruct the nasal floor. It is not possible to mention all of the surgeons who made contributions in this area, but the leaders were Victor Veau in the 1930s [1006, 1007], Tord Skoog who proposed a modification to Veau's approach [935, 938], Ralph Millard in the late 1950s [667], Peter Randall in the 1960s [827] and W.M. Manchester with his approach to the bilateral cleft in 1965 (Fig. 8.20) [605].

As far as the repair of the nose in unilateral and bilateral clefts is concerned, it is perhaps too early to judge the efficacy of the modifications proposed by the Bristol Study Group in 1982 [931] and 1987 [185].Their recommendations, however, include two simple methods to measure facial asymmetries that have proved extremely helpful in the planning stages, when the surgeon is deciding which procedure to use. The great advantage of these methods is that they can be carried out as routine procedures on any surgical ward. More sophisticated techniques exist, such as Rabey's morphoanalysis (1977), Larson and Nilson's anthropometric measurements (1983), Duck's stereophotogrammetry technique (1983), and Kawai et al.'s three-dimensional plotting approach (1977). All of these can produce more accurate evaluations, but require sophisticated instruments and a highly trained staff.

The Cleft Palate

Although techniques were sufficiently advanced, without the benefit of safe and effective anaesthesia and reliable control of bleeding, closure of the cleft palate was an impossible undertaking until around two hundred years ago. Misconception after the Middle Ages regarding the nature of the defect probably meant that there was little interest in treating the deformity. According to Rogers [854] "physicians and surgeons for many centuries believed that most palate defects were the direct result of syphilitic infection". Under its various names[26], syphilis was thought to interfere with the process of healing, and because it was known that the disease could affect the palate and pharynx, with calamitous effects on the voice, patients with facial clefts were automatically relegated to this category of untouchables [144]. As late as 1819 a Canadian medical student who became Roux's first cleft palate patient, underwent tests to exclude syphilis before his operation.

The term *sifilide* was introduced by Girolamo Fracastoro [331][27] in 1530 and came to be used all over Europe. It was generally treated, to little avail, with mercury preparations and medical students were taught that "one night with Venus would lead to a lifetime with Mercury". The congenital nature of the cleft palate was not demonstrated until just two centuries ago.

We have already noted that the only evidence of the deformity to come down to us from the civilization of ancient Egypt is the skull showing a cleft palate. A similar skull dating from the first century A.D. has been discovered in Peru. Since its premaxilla is missing, the somewhat unlikely suggestion was made that it had been removed surgically in an early attempt to repair a bilateral cleft. Given the innate fragility of this bone, it seems much more probable that it simply broke away at some point and was lost.

25 William Burston, orthodontist in Liverpool, pioneered early orthodontic treatment for babies with cleft deformities [see *The early orthodontic treatment of cleft palate conditions* 1958. *Dent Pract (Bristol)* 9:41]. He also invented the frame, which bears his name, for nursing babies with Pierre Robin syndrome, on their face.

26 Syphilis was known by a great many names, reflecting its symptoms and purported sources of contagion, just a few of which were: the great pox, Irish mutton, French measles, the Naples canker, Spanish gout, the Polish disease and morbus gallicus.

27 Gerolamo Fracastoro (1483–1553), a physician, astronomer and poet born in Verona, published a famous poem in 1530 entitled *Syphilis, sive Morbus Gallicus* (Syphilis, or the French Disease). In this poem Syphilis was the name of the shepherd who first caught the disease and hence was responsible for its spread.

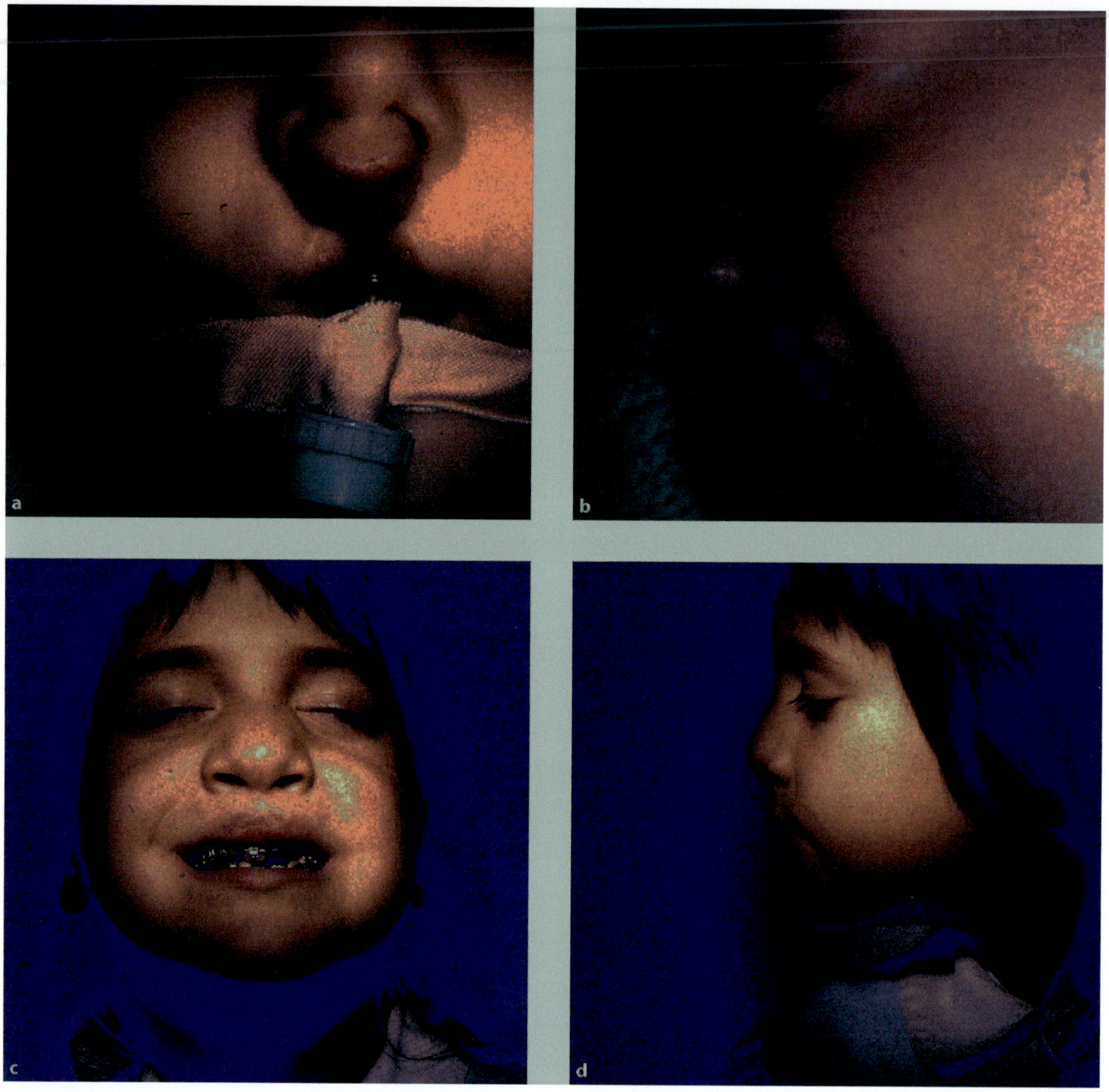

Fig. 8.20 **a,b** A complete bilateral cleft with projecting premaxilla at 8 weeks. **c,d** Result at 2 years when the palate was repaired. The patient had no pre-surgical orthopaedic treatment and the pressure of the lip repair corrected the protrusion. Orthodontic treatment was commenced prior to palatal surgery. *Operation by PSR in 1961*

Apart from these two archaeological finds, the same mysterious silence prevailed during Antiquity regarding the cleft palate as for the cleft lip. In the sixth century B.C. the Indian physician Susruta [90] described the palate and alveolar processes and nine different pathological conditions, but made no mention of congenital deformities. Hippocrates [434–437] was probably the first physician to take an interest in the role of the palate, tongue and teeth in speech, observing that irregular teeth affected the voice and those patients "could be afflicted with headaches and secretions from the ear".

While there are perhaps even fewer references to the cleft palate during Antiquity than to the cleft lip and presumably for the same reasons, there is, strangely enough, a wealth of information on the uvula. Hippocrates mentions tumours and infections of the uvula, which he treated by removing the organ. In cases of infection he warns that "... when it is red and swollen ... one must attempt to reduce the swelling by some other means" before operating.

Celsus [167, 168] discusses pathologies of the palate and uvula and prescribes specific treatments. He recommended uvulectomy in cases of recurrent infection, much like modern tonsillectomy. During Antiquity this would not have been without risk. Galen [353, 354] performed uvulectomies, as did Oribasius [754–757], although the latter noted that complete excision of the uvula could lead to speech disturbances and cause "the inhaled air reaching the lungs to be excessively cold".

The role of the uvula in speech was also recognized by Paulus Aegineta [427], who called it "the goose quill or plectrum of the organ of speech". Both he and the Arab physician Albucasis recommended chemical cauterization to destroy the organ. Albucasis adopted a curious method that consisted of immersing the uvula in quicklime, introduced into the mouth with a spoon with due caution.

Even the surgeon Lanfranchi da Milano [520], who introduced some innovations for lip surgery, limited his oral operations to the uvula and completely ignored the palate. In the translation by Fleischacher from Latin into old English he writes "the uvula is the palet of the mouth and haelp it for to make sound. For the wynd that cometh of the lungis reboundith agens the palet and makith the more soun. If the palet be rechid along and if it be so long that it lie upon the tunge, than thou muste kutte awei .... and be war that thou kutte not to myche therof, for ther mighte come greet perel therofore his vois mighte be apererid the while he livede, and continuely coughhinge, and his lungis might be the werse therfore it is greet perel for to kutte a mannes palet."

Not even Yperman (1295–1351) who was a pioneer in cleft lip surgery, mentions the cleft palate [1055].

Although surgeons may have generally disregarded this organ, the palate formed the object of detailed anatomical and physiological studies beginning in the Renaissance. The first to take an interest was Leonardo da Vinci (1452–1519), who produced accurate anatomical drawings of the palate in 1495 [551]. Not many years later Johan Dryander (1500–1560) included an illustration of the palate in his celebrated anatomical treatise (Fig. 8.21a,b) [252]. In 1603 Fabrizio ab Aquapendente published anatomical drawings which illustrated the role of the palate in the functions of speech and sucking,[28] and explained how a defective palate could lead to serious malnutrition and even death [292, 293].

The studies of Antonio Maria Valsalva (1658–1723) published in 1704 clarified the morphology of the muscles of the palate and pharynx and their interaction with the middle ear [1002]. This period culminated in the work of Wilhelm von Kampeleen (1732–1804), who described the physiology of the palate in minute detail in 1791 and even invented a "talking machine" [484].

The Palatal Obturator

We know that Ambroise Paré shed light on many aspects of the physiology of the palate [466]. He designed clever prostheses for facial defects, sometimes even including a moustache and teeth. He also made the first palatal obturator, probably in 1537 and published the details of his invention in 1564.

Pierre Franco had already noted that normal speech required an intact palate in 1556 and wrote what was probably the first description of a submucous cleft which he called a "cleft without a cleft" [332]. He had also observed that "cleft patients always talk through their noses. If the palate is only slightly cleft, and it can be plugged with cotton, or else if a plaque of silver or lead can be applied by some means, provided it holds, he will speak better." This was the best result that could be expected at a time when surgery was impossible.

Some historians contend that the true inventor of the palatal obturator was Amatus Lusitanus [585, 586] a surgeon who was born in Portugal in 1511 and narrowly escaped the clutches of the Inquisition. He invented an instrument "which is a blade in the middle of which there is a hole, and through this a piece of sponge may

28 See *Anatomia*, Part I, p 268 (*De Larynge Vocis Instrumento*), as well as Part I, p 249 (*De Aure Auditus Organo*) and finally Part II, p 255 (*De Actione Auris*).

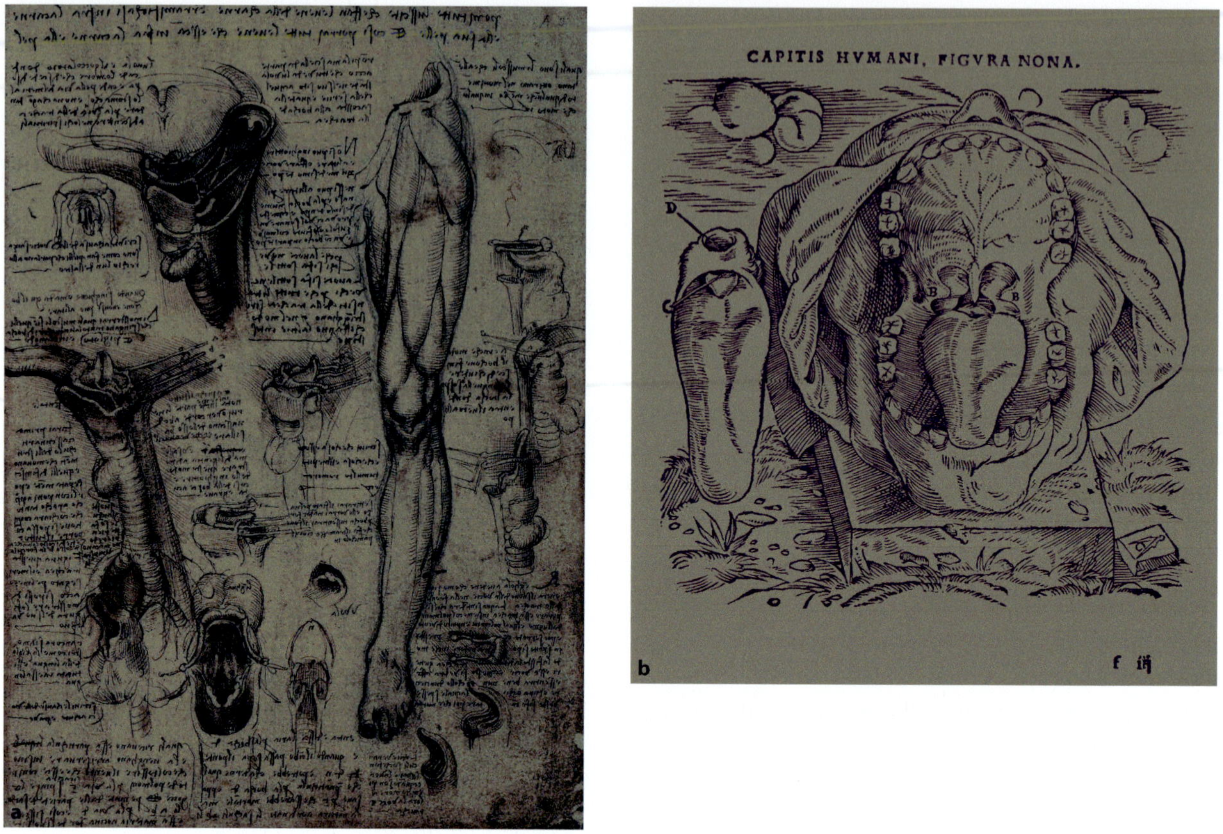

Fig. 8.21 **a** Leonardo da Vinci's drawing showing the palate and some of the muscle. (RL19002r) *The Royal Collection © 2005, Her Majesty Queen Elizabeth II.* **b** Dryander's *Anatomiae Miae hoc est Corporis Humani…* published in 1537 showing the palate. *Courtesy of Riccardo Mazzola, M.D., Milan*

be passed and fastened firmly to the metal plate. This is then applied to the perforation of the palate in such a way that as the sponge swells with humidity, the plate is held so firmly against the palate, and closes so exactly the opening, that it only can be detached with difficulty." Lusitanus had to leave Ancona hastily in 1555 and during his flight lost the manuscript of *Centutria V*, in which he first described his obturator. The publication of this work was delayed, but still appears to predate Paré's account.

It must be pointed out that Paré, unlike his rival, actually tested his prosthesis during the Italian wars of 1537–1539, when he was serving as a military surgeon in Savoy and Piedmont. The obturator[29] was made of silver and gold and he used it to close palates that had been "shortened by a gunshot or by some other [cause], as in cases of ulcers of the velum". No direct reference is made to congenital clefts, but given Paré's close ties with Franco it seems probable that he would have attempted to correct this defect as well by using his invention. Indirect corroboration may be found in his use of the term "natural defects", i.e. congenital, in the title to his publication.

Rogers suggests somewhat audaciously that the debate regarding who made the first palatal obturator is academic because the true inventor was an Italian artisan

29 See *Les Oeuvres*, Book 22, Chapter IV, *e Moyens & artifice d'adjouter ce qui defaut naturellement ou par accident* (*Ways and means of adding that which is lacking either due to nature or through accident*). In Book 22, Chapter II, various dental prostheses are described and illustrated.

who revealed his secret to both Lusitanus and Paré, but he provides no evidence in support of this thesis [854]. He is in general quite critical of Paré, accusing him of having studied the palate only "as a true Frenchman and gourmet", showing more interest in its role in the pleasures of the table than in speech. B. Bourdet introduced various improvements to Paré's obturator; for example, in 1757 he devised a way to attach the prosthesis to the patient's teeth to make it more stable [125]. Another Frenchman, Pierre Fauchard (1678–1761) also designed an ingenious obturator [587].

This discussion of the palatal obturator would not be complete without mentioning J. Guillemeau. In *Les Oeuvres de Chirurgie* (1598) [400, 401] he claims that the ancient Greeks invented the first palate obturator, calling it a *hyperoe*. Rogers refutes this thesis categorically, however, and Guillemeau certainly furnishes no evidence in support of his claim. It must be noted that it would have been strange indeed if the Greeks and Romans had exerted themselves to construct an obturator when in all other respects they showed no interest in this malformation.

Early Surgery on the Palate: Palatal Fistulae

The first surgical procedures on the palate focused on the closure of fistulas, as described first by Leonicenus in 1497 [553], later by Giacobbe of Catania [174], and finally in the sixteenth century by Jacques Houllier [450]. Houllier seems to have been the first to accept the challenge of closing the fistula surgically, although he was persuaded that the origin of the defect was syphilitic and therefore insisted that before the operation the patient "must be prepared by gargling with a mixture of guaiacum and milk in addition to the local application of Acqua Alchymistarum made with gall nuts, malicorio and rosewater". Houllier's daring was not rewarded because, as he himself admitted, the operation was rarely successful. After 1552 he recommended closing the cleft with an obturator. "[If] as a consequence of this [surgical] treatment a complete integrity of the region is not achieved, [the fistula] may be closed with wax or a sponge, and the patient can thereafter live comfortably."

The Velum

In 1706 André Myrrhen claimed to have treated a patient suffering from necrosis of the uvula by lengthening the velum [721]. This case remains something of a mystery in that he provides no information on the indications for the operation or the technique adopted. It would appear that the purpose was not to improve the patient's speech since Myrrhen expressed surprise when he discovered that, contrary to his expectations, "the voice of the patient did not suffer any ill consequences [from the operation]". The possibility that the operation might improve this function did not seem to have occurred to him.

In 1723 De Gorengoat removed a nasal polyp that was hampering both speech and breathing by incising his palate [738] and in 1747 Le Manne [548] repeated the operation, but went even further and resutured the soft palate. Le Manne believed that clefts of the soft palate might be similarly repaired, but despite his optimism thirty-five years passed before Carl Ferdinand von Graefe (1787–1840) successfully carried out the first closure of the soft palate [390].

In the meantime Eustache de Bezier in 1779 in Belgium and others continued to suture the incised velum [250]. The Belgian surgeon noted that failure to do so could lead to difficulties in speaking and swallowing. Aristide Verneuil [1013][30] recounted that Colombe, after first practising on a series of cadavers, offered to operate on a patient who was suffering from a palate cleft in 1813 but the patient refused. According to Roux a similar experience befell a Dutch surgeon by the name of Hard; he succeeded in convincing a young woman to have her soft palate sutured, but she withdrew at the last minute on the advice of a celebrated surgeon of the time.

Karl Kaspar Siebold (1736–1807) conducted detailed studies on the speech defects exhibited by a three-year-old boy with a cleft soft palate, and noted that he had

30 See Verneuil's *Memoires de Chirugie*, p 490. Here there is a letter by Eustache dated March 1783 in which the surgeon describes the case of a patient whose incisions were not sutured, and recalls the complications of this omission.

difficulty in pronouncing the letters B, R, S and Z [924]. Siebold expressed deep regret at the "impossibility" of correcting this defect surgically. The consequences of cleft deformities on speech were also being studied in America by Matthew Wilson of Delaware (1734–1802) author of the Therapeutic Alphabet cited above [339].

M. Robert [846] reported that sometime before 1764 a dentist in Rouen by the name of Le Monnier succeeded in repairing "a complete cleft from the velum to the incisors". Le Monnier had already perfected a technique for the repair of small fistulas that consisted of scarifying the margins and then allowing the fissure to close naturally as they healed and contracted. In the case of the cleft operation, he appears to have placed sutures from side to side along the margins of the cleft, and cauterized the edges after the margins had been drawn together. When the inflamed areas healed, the cleft was presumably eliminated.

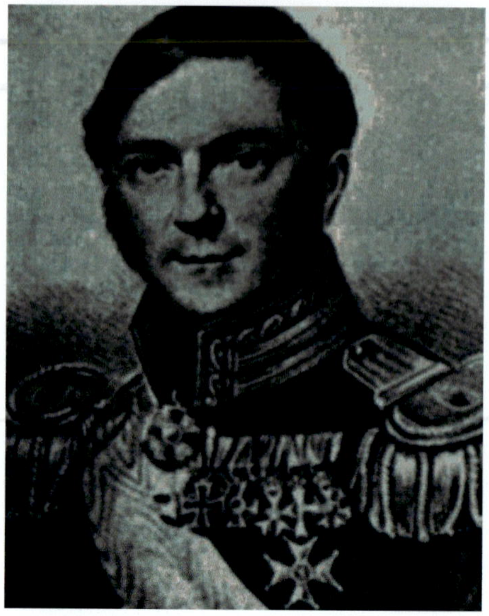

Fig. 8.22 Portrait of Carl Ferdinand von Graefe (1787–1840). *Garrison* [361]

The Earliest Operations on the Palate: Repair of the Soft Palate

It is now proved that the first documented operation on the palate was carried out in 1816 by Carl Ferdinand von Graefe (1787–1816). This achievement was a genuine milestone [390] for it marked the end of a period that had lasted for centuries during which technical difficulties, ignorance, superstition and fear, not to mention the spectre of syphilis, hampered progress in this area (Fig. 8.22).

Von Graefe presented his extraordinary accomplishment before the *Medical Society of Berlin*, and the news was published in the form of a note without any heading in a local publication with a very limited readership (Fig. 8.23).[31] His paper was then published in 1817 [390]. When almost three years later, in 1819 Philibert Joseph Roux (1780–1840) reported the details of a similar operation, he and many others sincerely believed that this was the first case to be described in the medical literature [866]. However, as McDowell observed, when Roux claimed credit for the breakthrough he "awakened a sleeping tiger". Von Graefe, who up to this time did not appear to have placed any great importance on his operation, suddenly seems to have decided that it was the most important thing in his life (Fig. 8.24).

In order to support his position, he began to operate on as many patients as he could find and in 1820 wrote a treatise on the subject [392, 394]. Roux reacted in exactly the same manner and their dispute was transformed into a question of national honour. Surgeons all over Europe were forced to take a position in favour either of Roux and France, or von Graefe and Germany. The tempest eventually subsided, because neither of the two temperamental surgeons had a very clear idea of what his rival had actually done and each had difficulty in proving his claim incontrovertibly. There is little doubt that each had managed to carry out this difficult operation successfully without the benefit of anaesthesia unaware of the others achievement.

In 1877 Verneuil made conciliatory reference to the dispute in the chapter *Historical conclusion about the invention of staphylorraphy in the 18th and 19th centuries* in *Mémoires de Chirurgie* [1013]. He concluded that "von

31 A brief note that von Graefe reported his first cleft palate repair to the *Medical Association of Berlin* on 27 December 1816 is to be found in *The Journal of Practical Theraputics* from January 1817.

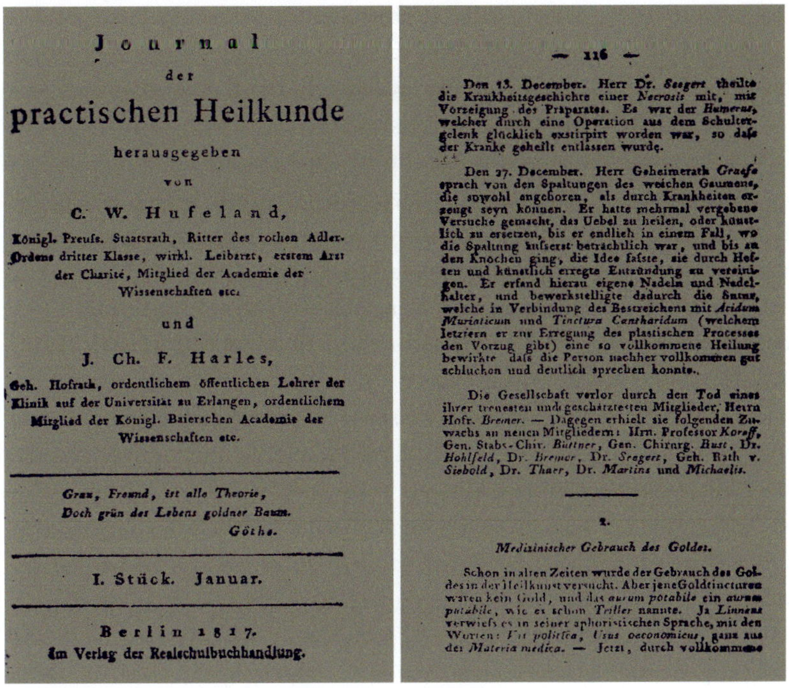

Journal
der
practischen Heilkunde
herausgegeben
von
C. W. Hufeland,
Königl. Preufs. Staatsrath, Ritter des rothen Adler-Ordens dritter Klasse, wirkl. Leibarzt, erstem Arzt der Charité, Mitglied der Academie der Wissenschaften etc.
und
J. Ch. F. Harles,
Geh. Hofrath, ordentlichem öffentlichen Lehrer der Klinik auf der Universität zu Erlangen, ordentlichem Mitglied der Königl. Baierschen Academie der Wissenschaften etc.

Grau, Freund, ist alle Theorie,
Doch grün des Lebens goldner Baum.
Göthe.

I. Stück. Januar.

Berlin 1817.
Im Verlag der Realschulbuchhandlung.

— 116 —

Den 13. December. Herr Dr. *Seegert* theilte die Krankheitsgeschichte einer *Necrosis* mit, mit Vorzeigung des Präparates. Es war der *Humerus*, welcher durch eine Operation aus dem Schultergelenk glücklich exstirpirt worden war, so dafs der Kranke geheilt entlassen wurde.

Den 27. December. Herr Geheimerath *Graefe* sprach von den Spaltungen des weichen Gaumens, die sowohl angeboren, als durch Krankheiten erzeugt seyn können. Er hatte mehrmal vergebene Versuche gemacht, das Uebel zu heilen, oder künstlich zu ersetzen, bis er endlich in einem Fall, wo die Spaltung äufserst beträchtlich war, und bis an den Knochen ging, die Idee fafste, sie durch Heften und künstlich erregte Entzündung zu vereinigen. Er erfand hierzu eigene Nadeln und Nadelhalter, und bewerkstelligte dadurch die Sutur, welche in Verbindung des Bestreichens mit *Acidum Muriaticum* und *Tinctura Cantharidum* (welchem letztern er zur Erregung des plastischen Processes den Vorzug gibt) eine so vollkommene Heilung bewirkte dafs die Person nachher vollkommen gut schlucken und deutlich sprechen konnte.

Die Gesellschaft verlor durch den Tod eines ihrer treuesten und geschätztesten Mitglieder, Herrn Hofr. *Bremer*. — Dagegen erhielt sie folgenden Zuwachs an neuen Mitgliedern: Hrn. Professor *Koreff*, Gen. Stabs-Chir. *Büttner*, Gen. Chirurg. *Rust*, Dr. *Hohlfeld*, Dr. *Bremer*, Dr. *Seegert*, Geh. Rath v. *Siebold*, Dr. *Thaer*, Dr. *Martins* und *Michaelis*.

2.

Medizinischer Gebrauch des Goldes.

Schon in alten Zeiten wurde der Gebrauch des Goldes in der Heilkunst versucht. Aber jene Goldtincturen waren kein Gold, und das *aurum potabile* ein *aurum putabile*, wie es schon *Triller* nannte. Ja *Linneus* verwiefs es in seiner aphoristischen Sprache, mit den Worten: *Vis politica, Usus oeconomicus*, ganz aus der *Materia medica*. — Jetzt, durch vollkommene

Fig. 8.23 Page from *Journal der Praktischen Heilkunde* on 27 December 1817 with a short report about the meeting of the *Medical Society of Berlin* announcing von Graefe's first palatoplasty

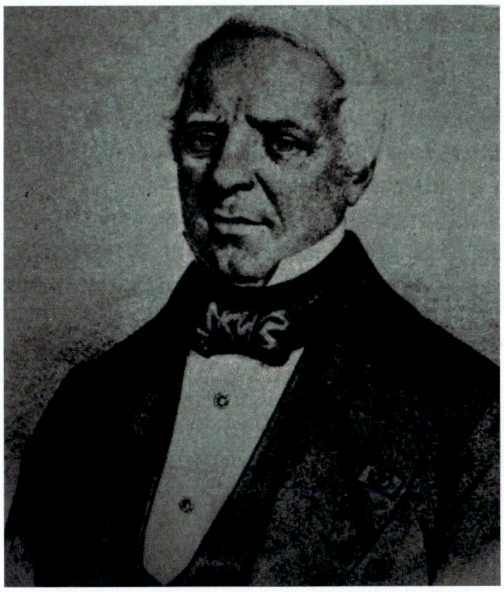

Fig. 8.24 Philibert Joseph Roux (1780–1840). He operated on his first cleft palate around the same time as Von Graefe, precipitating a long controversy about who was first

Graefe had preceded Roux. But what is also morally demonstrated is that in a sudden 'coup d'inspiration' Roux on his side conceived the staphylorrhaphy in less time than has been necessary to write this paragraph." However, he then made his own contribution to the quarrel by declaring that the principle underlying the operation had actually been conceived and applied a century earlier by … a Frenchman (of course, sic!), Le Monnier, and independently by Eustache de Bezier in Belgium. He also mentions Colombe's experiments on cadavers in 1813. Unfortunately, Verneuil does not substantiate his claim of French precedence by citing any papers presented before scientific societies or published by these surgeons.[32]

In an Addendum to his article on *the palate suture* published in 1820, von Graefe reiterates that he presented a communication before the *Medical Society of Berlin*[33] during a meeting held on 27 December 1816, and that he gave lectures on the procedure in 1817 and 1818 at the university's medical school, which was frequented

32 Verneuil's book, apart from its account of the dispute between Carl Ferdinand von Graef and Philibert Joseph Roux, is of great interest and covers for example, flaps and grafts, surgery on the genitals and on the hand.

33 See Hufelands *Journal der Practischen Heilkunde*, vol I, p 116.

by French as well as German students. Furthermore he had published a detailed description of the method. He concludes therefore that "his" operation must have been known in France and most certainly "Herr Roux could not have been ignorant of its existence". Von Graefe's treatise is indeed quite detailed and complete, explaining how to separate the mucous membrane from the margins of the cleft, insert the sutures, close the margins and keep them tight. He also provides exhaustive recommendations on post-operative care, including advice on speech therapy.

Roux's account of his procedure is equally detailed. He first explains how to position the patient with his mouth wide open to obtain an unobstructed view of the palate. His technique consisted of passing "three wax-threaded loops using a curved needle", and then drawing them together in order to unite the margins and obtain an idea of the true extent of the gap. He notes that immediately after the operation: "...the voice of the patient was almost normal ... [indicating that] the operation was a success". Roux concludes that the improvements, above all to the speech, were so great as to justify the risks of the operation. Roux wrote many papers about his procedure and used the term "staphyloraphy" to refer to repairs of congenital clefts and palatoplasty for the repair of acquired defects of the palate [867–870, 872].

Claude Bernard (1813–1878) and Charles Huette de Montargis (1820–1881) in 1860 [81], confirmed the importance of Roux's contribution to cleft palate surgery. They cite the needle holder and the coudé or elbow scissors that he invented and which facilitated the operation. Roux's first patient, as we have already mentioned, was a Canadian medical student, John Stephenson (1797–1842). Stephenson wrote a thesis on his experience entitled *De Velosynthesis*, which was presented at the University of Edinburgh in August 1820, one year after the operation [955]. In it he recounted how his mother had experienced great difficulty in feeding him when he was an infant as most of her milk escaped through his nostrils, so that his weight gain was extremely slow. The family doctor diagnosed his cleft, but not its congenital origin, attributing the defect to the extreme cold that had prevailed in Montreal during the weeks preceding the delivery.

While studying medicine in Edinburgh, Stephenson decided to spend some time in Paris and attend the course of the famous surgeon Professor Roux. In Paris he made a series of observations. He noticed that cases of cleft palate were relatively frequent even though France enjoyed a much warmer climate than his own country! One of his brothers had been born with a bifid uvula and he thought that this was not without significance. In *De Velosynthesis* he describes his speech defect, noting that although like many Canadians he was bilingual, his nasality was more marked when he spoke English. He also recalled "never being able to drink from a spring".

When Professor Roux first met Stephenson, he observed his speech defect and immediately became interested in his case, which represented an unusual congenital anomaly. After examining him and ascertaining that he had never contracted syphilis, Roux offered to operate. With Stephenson seated before a bright lamp, the surgeon passed three interrupted sutures some distance from the edges of the repair, "... in doing so, given that the fingers are too short to work at such a depth, and the needles are rendered slippery by the constant flow of saliva, [he made use] of a stylus-like instrument". This is probably the first documented report of the use of the *porte aiguilles* or needle holder. Although his uvula was not sutured, Stephenson's speech nevertheless seems to have immediately improved. His thesis describes every detail of the operation and his convalescence, down to the dietary restrictions imposed by his surgeon [1024].

Hard Palate Repair and the Role of the Periosteum

Three gifted German surgeons, Carl Ferdinand von Graefe, Johan Fredrick Dieffenbach and Bernard Rudolph Conrad von Langenbeck, form the triumvirate that contributed most to the development of surgery of the hard palate. After the introduction of procedures to repair the soft palate by von Graefe in 1816, nearly ten years passed before more radical surgery was attempted. In 1825 Sir Astley Cooper (1769–1832), who had considerable experience in the treatment of palatal fistulas, said that closure of the hard palate should be possible by means of a mucosal flap. He wrote: "A portion of membrane from the roof of the mouth might be partially pared off and turned over the opening, its circumference being placed in contact with the edges of the aperture so as to produce adhesion: but on this operation I have no experience." As this passage shows, while Sir Astely may never have operated on a cleft palate, he had an intuitive flair for reconstructive surgery and a clear understanding of the possibilities offered by a flap.

The first surgeon to successfully close a hard palate cleft was Dieffenbach in 1826 [240, 241]. He mobilized the mucous membrane, and performed lateral relieving osteotomies in the two palatal bones (Fig. 8.25). A detailed account of his technique appeared several years later in Dublin.[34] As he wrote: "The edge of each palate bone is pierced through with a strong, straight three-cornered punch and a thick, pliable silver wire is passed through the opening, the ends of which are twisted together. The mucous membrane is divided near the place where the palatal bone joins the alveolar process. A thin, smooth, concave chisel is then applied to the bone, and it is cut through on both sides. The wires are then twisted again until the edges of the bony cleft come into contact. In cases where closure is not obtained at once, one may continue gradually with the process of approximation afterwards." [244]

In the same year two Americans, Nathan Smith (1762–1829) [940] and Alexander H. Stevens (1789–1869) [959], independently announced that they had succeeded in closing a hard palate cleft. They were apparently unaware of Dieffenbach's achievement and the acclaim which he had received in Germany, but this is no surprise to us given the slowness of communication in the nineteenth century. A boat took several weeks to cross the Atlantic.

Johan Friedrich Dieffenbach was born in Konigsberg in 1794. An accomplished student, he began his studies in philosophy and letters at the University of Rostock, but in 1813 joined the cavalry in order to fight in the long war against France. The daily sight of battlefield casualties led to his decision to become a surgeon after his military discharge. After obtaining his degree in 1820 he left Rostock because, it was whispered, of an unhappy love affair with a married woman.

He went to France, where he became the personal physician of a wealthy Russian noblewoman and met many celebrated surgeons, including Boyer, Larrey, Hagendie and Dupuytren. During this time he spent several months at the medical faculty in Montpellier, attending the operating theatre of Delpech who was a well known reconstructive surgeon. In 1823 Dieffenbach returned to Germany to take up the chair of surgery in Berlin left vacant by von Graefe. Three years later he published the celebrated paper describing his procedure for the repair of the cleft hard palate.[35] Dieffenbach's technique, which included the use of special needles, was introduced into England by Robert Liston (1794–1847) [569, 570]. In 1837 he was indirectly involved in an altercation with von Langenbeck by siding with Hulke in his quarrel regarding who had been the first to include the periosteum in palatine flaps [452].[36]

In the United States Jonathan Mason Warren (1811–1867) modified the procedure by extending the bone incisions even further both anteriorly and posteriorly, occasionally as far as the pillars of the fauces [1032]. His interest in palate clefts was probably inspired by the work of his father, the renowned surgeon John Collins Warren (1778–1856) who published a paper in 1828 describing "the cure of a natural fissure of the soft palate" [1029]. As the author noted, he had heard that this operation was performed routinely in "Poland and Germany" as well as in Paris, but "had searched in vain for details of it". John Collins Warren's own case involved a middle-aged woman with a palatal defect caused by the removal of a tumour. In 1848 Jonathan Mason Warren published the results of corrective surgery carried out on a series of 24 patients with congenital clefts, reporting that the operation was sometimes followed by the formation of a fistula, but only in one case by dehiscence of the wound.

Although general anaesthesia had recently been introduced in the city of Boston and the Warrens campaigned vigorously for its general acceptance, John Collins Warren did not use anaesthesia during his palate operations, because of the risk posed by "the constant flow of blood down the throat in an unconscious patient". At this time the procedures of tracheal intubation and aspira-

34 Dieffenbach (1845) *Practical Observations on the Operation of Cleft Palate Repair. Dublin J M Sci* 28:227–249.

35 The other contributions of Dieffenbach included the treatment of urethral stenosis. He was also a pioneer in the areas of intravenous perfusion and blood transfusion.

36 Liston deserves credit for being the first to introduce general anaesthesia on the European side of the Atlantic, just one month after Morton introduced the technique in Boston in October 1846.

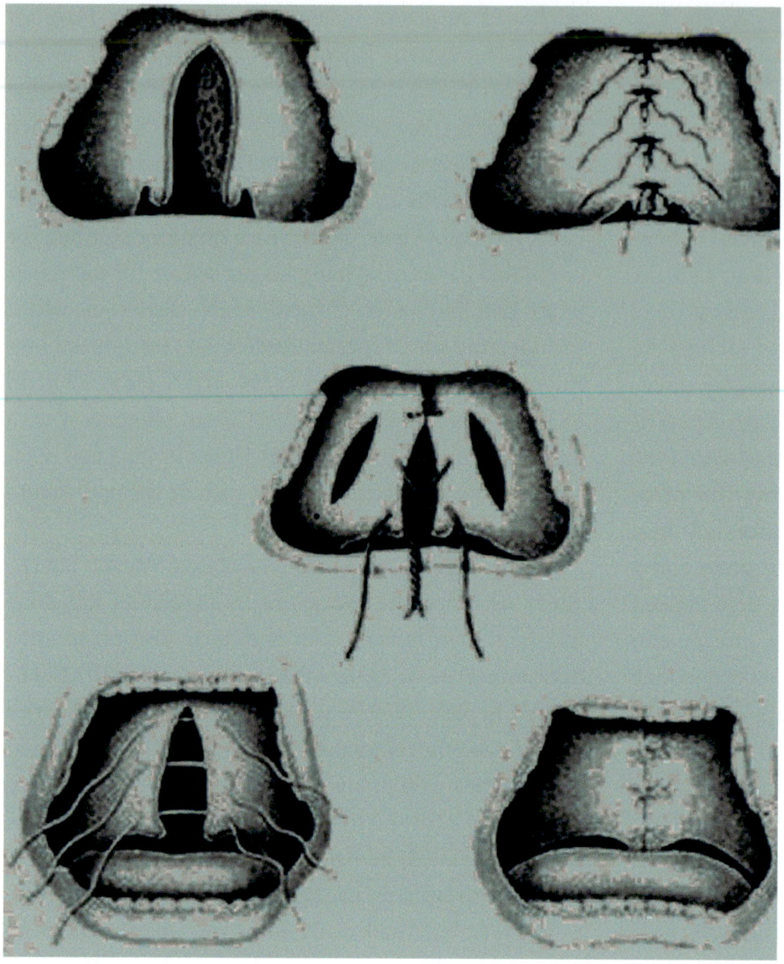

Fig. 8.25 Dieffenbach was one of the first to describe a palatoplasty technique. He used lateral incisions to relax the palatal flaps. This diagram is from *Die Operative Chirurgie* (1845). *Courtesy of Riccardo Mazzola, M.D., Milan*

tion were not yet used. Indeed, tracheal intubation was adopted as a routine procedure in cleft palate surgery only much later around 1922, after Ivan McGill perfected the technique during his work with Harold Gillies on the repair of gunshot wounds to the face during World War I [590–594].[37]

Before this time, despite the courage, ingenuity and skill of many pioneering surgeons, patients had to endure intense pain and continual bleeding which made cleft operations extremely difficult. As a consequence, the surgeon had to work quickly and the palatal flaps were often not completely undermined. This meant that the cleft was repaired under tension and dehiscence of the suture line was a fairly frequent event. For this reason the introduction of general anaesthesia has been described as one of the most important advances in the history of cleft palate repair, for it allowed accurate dissections and complete undermining. This meant that the palatal flaps could be mobilized more freely, as had been envisaged by Dieffenbach and Liston.

With these advances, by the middle of the nineteenth century surgeons felt confident enough to attempt the repair of a complete palate cleft in a single operation. At this point, although the rate of dehiscence fell, problems remained, particularly at the junction of the hard and soft palates, where breakdown of the repair remained a frequent occurrence. Liston found the correct explanation for this based on Sir William Fergusson's studies of the le-

37 An extended recapitulation is proved by Gillies and Millard in *Principles and Art of Plastic Surgery*, p 60.

vator palati and the palatopharyngeal muscles [306–308]. He suggested that the palatal sutures were literally pulled apart by the action of these muscles during speech.

Sir William Fergusson (1808–1877) made important contributions to the field of palate repair, conducting a series of dissections on bodies of people who had suffered from a cleft palate and describing the anomalies present in these muscles. From his studies he provided evidence for the theory of *arrested development* in the aetiology of clefts. He also noted and discussed the significance of the familial nature of certain clefts in his work *A System of Practical Surgery*. Fergusson advocated early surgery, generally between the third and fourth months but even as late as 8 or 10 months after birth[38].

Another fundamental breakthrough was made by von Langenbeck (1810–1887) (Fig. 8.26). He recognized the capacity of the periosteum to produce bone (see Chapter 7) exploiting this in various reconstructions (nose 1850, and jaw 1859). He did not miss the opportunity to apply this to the repair of the palate, suggesting the inclusion of the periosteum of the palatal bones in the mucosal flaps. He believed this would produce a stable repair [524].

Von Langenbeck also proposed a significant modification to Dieffenbach's bipedicle flap of mucous membrane and bone (presumably preserving nasal mucosa), converting it into an easier posteriorly based transposition flap without bone. The flap began immediately behind the incisors and extended backwards to the posterior edge of the hard palate. This gave him better access to the levator and palato-pharyngeal muscles, on which he performed a myotomy that relaxed the repair and minimized the risk of dehiscence. Von Langenbeck generally carried out his repair in a single operation, but advised less experienced surgeons to use two sessions. His modification of the Dieffenbach flap received the full approval of the *Medical Society of Berlin* when it was presented in 1861 [525]. His publications on cleft surgery are extensive. His first report [523] was followed over subsequent years by several more (Fig. 8.27a,b) [526–529].[39]

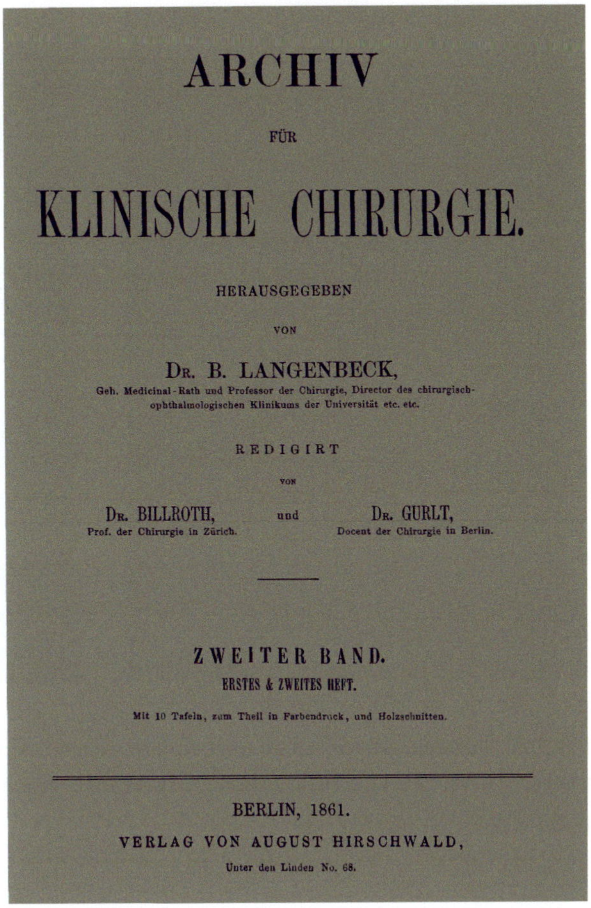

ARCHIV

FÜR

KLINISCHE CHIRURGIE.

HERAUSGEGEBEN

VON

DR. B. LANGENBECK,

Geh. Medicinal-Rath und Professor der Chirurgie, Director des chirurgisch-ophthalmologischen Klinikums der Universität etc. etc.

REDIGIRT

VON

DR. BILLROTH, Prof. der Chirurgie in Zürich. und DR. GURLT, Docent der Chirurgie in Berlin.

ZWEITER BAND.

ERSTES & ZWEITES HEFT.

Mit 10 Tafeln, zum Theil in Farbendruck, und Holzschnitten.

BERLIN, 1861.

VERLAG VON AUGUST HIRSCHWALD,

Unter den Linden No. 68.

Fig. 8.26 Von Langenbeck wrote numerous articles on palate repair and included periosteum in the flaps. He published some of these in *Archiv für Klinische Chirurgie* and used the term uranoplasty [523–529]. *Courtesy of Riccardo Mazzola, M.D., Milan*

Von Langenbeck was born in Padingbuttel on the coast of the North Sea in 1810. The son of a pastor, he went to live with his uncle, who was a famous ophthalmologist in Göttingen, with the intention of studying for the same profession. However, after spending a short period on a scholarship in England, where he had the

38 Sir William Fergusson FRS, professor of surgery at King's College, London wrote his book in the mid nineteenth century. It was published by John Churchill and ran to several editions.

39 One of the most lasting legacies of Bernard Rudolph Conrad von Langenbeck was the school of surgery that he created. In fact, for many decades surgery in Germany was dominated by his students, among whom were Bergman, Billroth, Bosa, Esmarc, Gurlt, Hunter, Kroenlein and Trendelenburg.

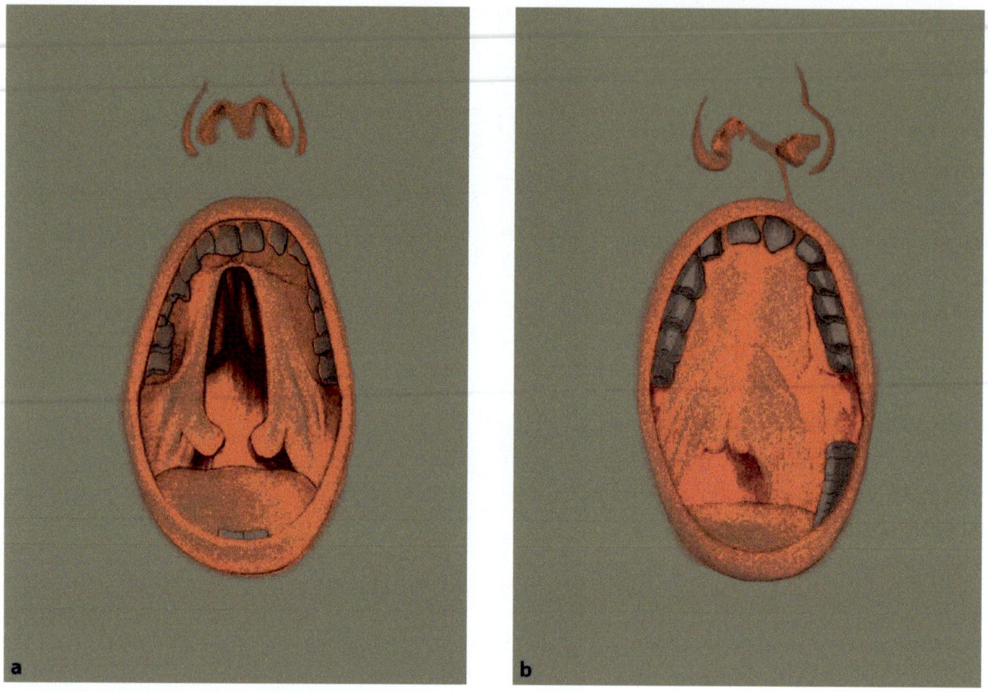

Fig. 8.27 Illustrations from von Langenbeck's book. **a** An incomplete cleft palate. **b** After closure of what appears to be a complete unilateral cleft. *Courtesy of Riccardo Mazzola, M.D., Milan*

opportunity to meet Benjamin Brodie, Lawrence Green and Astley Cooper, he decided to take up surgery. At the age of 30 he became professor of pathology at the University of Kiel. His lectures were immensely popular and he was an inspired teacher. He integrated biology, pathology and physiology into his courses. After serving as a surgeon during the War of Holstein, von Langenbeck was invited to accept the chair left vacant by Dieffenbach at the University of Berlin in 1848.His popularity among the medical students in Berlin helped his appointment and they demonstrated, demanding that the post be offered to him (Fig. 8.28a,b).

Together with Billroth and Gurlt, von Langenbeck founded the *Archiv für Klinische Chirurgie* in 1860. This remained the most authoritative surgical journal until the First World War. Von Langenbeck was not a prolific writer, but as a brilliant teacher he inspired many young surgeons. The Wars against Austria in 1866 and the Franco-Prussians in 1870 were formative experiences which gave him the opportunity to perfect his surgical techniques but also to introduce humane ethical standards on the battlefield which may be summed up in his famous phrase "A wounded enemy is no longer an enemy but a comrade in need of help." Von Langenbeck was also probably the first surgeon since Anthyllus to use tracheotomy to keep the airways clear in patients with severe facial injuries.

At one point in his career von Langenbeck, like von Graef, found himself under attack by a rival on a matter of precedence. J.B. Hulke, a surgeon at Kings' College London, contested his claim to have been the first to include the periosteum in palatine flaps for cleft repairs, in a paper published in *The Medical Times & Gazette* in 1861 [452], the same year that von Langenbeck presented his paper in Berlin. Hulke claimed that a similar procedure was already being used in England, although from his description it would appear that he sectioned the greater palatine vessels whereas von Langenbeck took great care to preserve them. Furthermore, while von Langenbeck had devised an ingenious periosteal elevator to facilitate the undermining of the flap, it appears that Hulke found an ordinary scalpel sufficient for this purpose (Fig. 8.29). In support of his claim, the English surgeon wrote that the periosteum was "always" included in the flap and

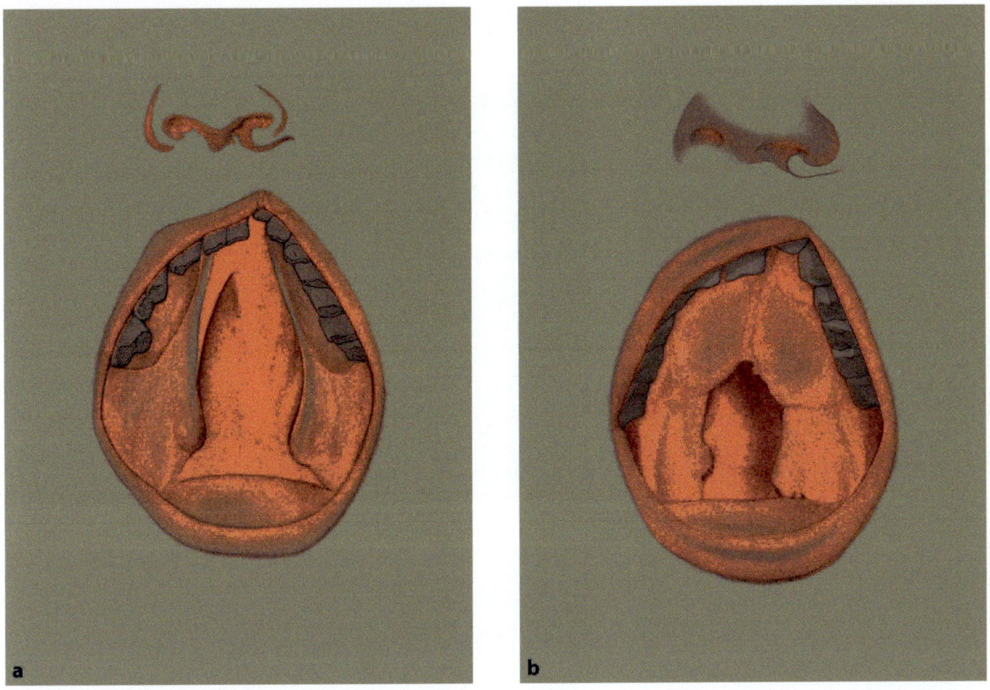

Fig. 8.28 Another case of von Langenbeck's. **a** A complete cleft palate. **b** The hard palate is closed at the first operation. *Courtesy of Riccardo Mazzola, M.D., Milan*

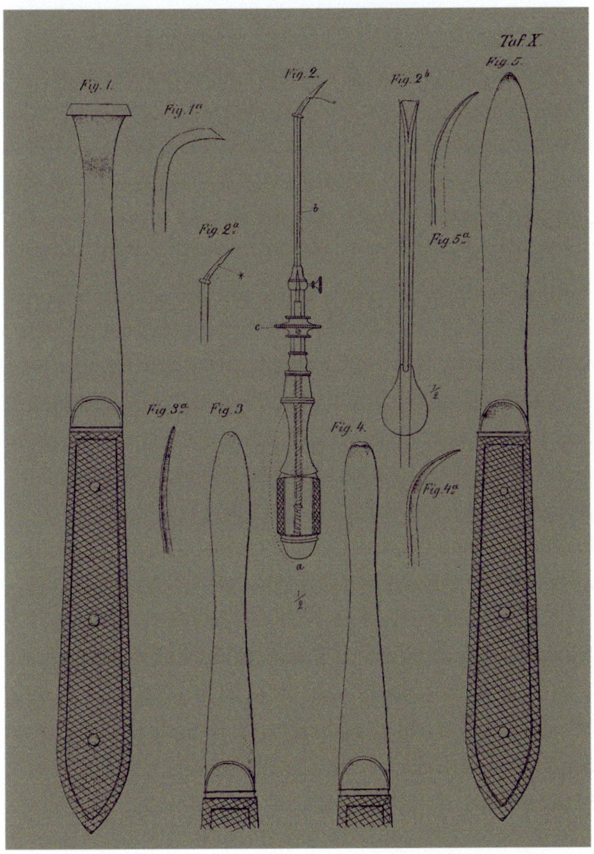

Fig. 8.29 von Langenbeck's instruments including the periosteal elevator essential for raising the flaps. *Courtesy of Riccardo Mazzola, M.D., Milan*

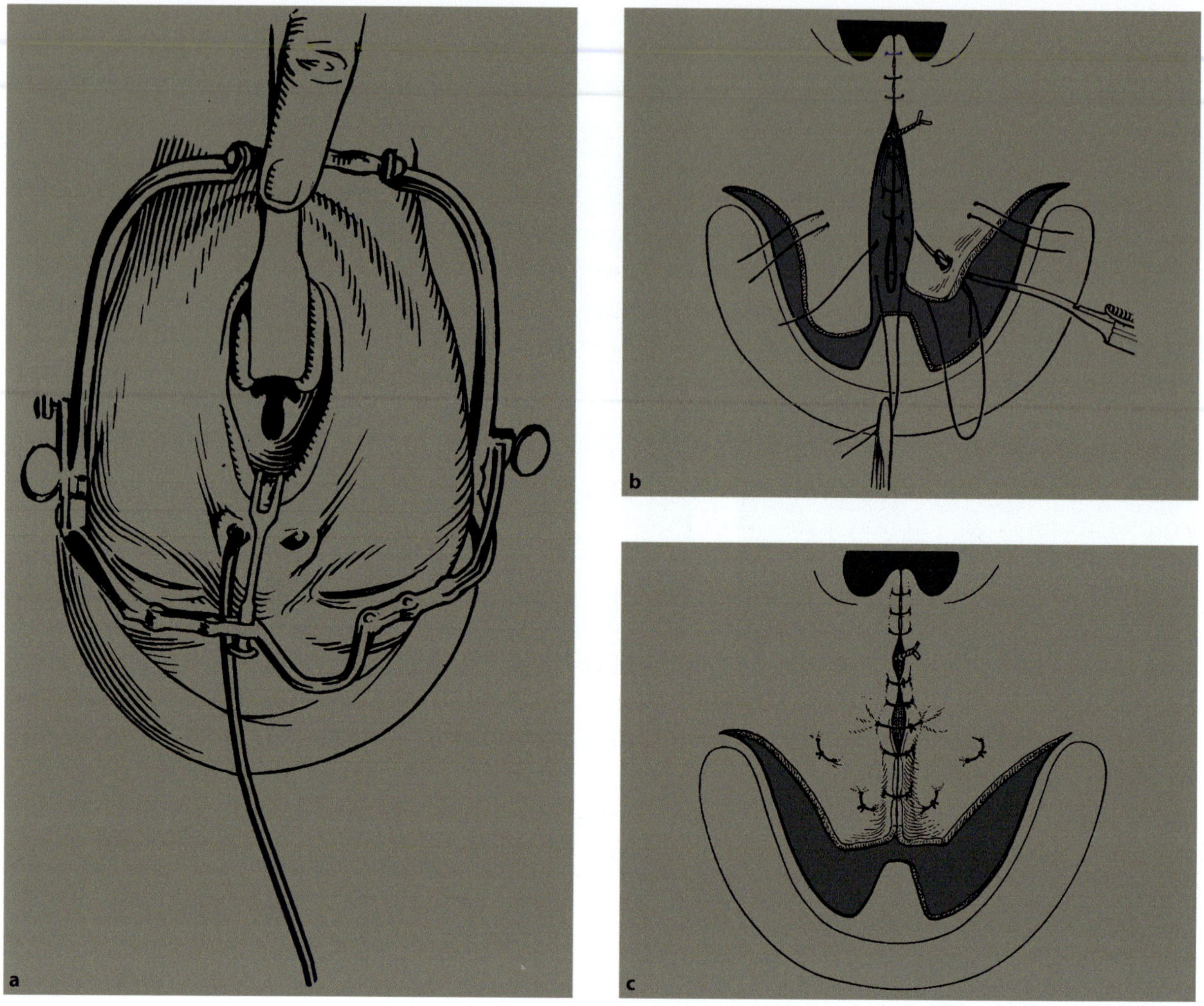

Fig. 8.30a–c Victor Veau's technique from *La Divione Palatine. Courtesy of Riccardo Mazzola, M.D., Milan*

that it was in fact more difficult to leave it attached to the bone than to include it in the mucosal flap, "even though this may not have been done intentionally".

Von Langenbeck immediately refuted Hulke's assertion and, in response to his specific point regarding the separation of the periosteum from the bone, declared that this was an almost impossible undertaking without his periosteal elevator [528]. In the following year von Langenbeck published his opus magnum *Die Uranoplastik mittelst Ablösung des mucös-periostalen Gaumenüberzuges* [526] which offered a detailed description of his reconstruction procedure, a list of the necessary instruments, as well as a discussion of the advantages of the mucoperiosteal flap and a classification of different types of clefts. This work of 92 pages amply justifies von Langenbeck's place among the pioneers of cleft surgery. His techniques formed the basis for cleft palate repair and were only refined and modified some 50 years later notably by Victor Veau (1871–1949) (Fig. 8.30a–c).

Surgical Treatment of Speech Defects

We have noted how, centuries ago, men of the stature of Hippocrates, Galen, Pliny the Elder and Lanfranchi had grasped the importance of the palate in speech. When palatoplasty became a reality, however, it was realized that corrective surgery did not always result in an improvement in the patient's articulation. Evidently, simply closing the cleft was not sufficient. In order to achieve clear speech the new palate had to be mobile and capable of making good contact with the posterior wall of the pharynx, in order to prevent the nasality caused by air escaping through the nasal passages.

Surgeons therefore turned their attention to the problem of how to obtain a longer and more mobile new palate without the concurrent development of fistulae. When this proved to be more difficult than expected, alternative solutions were considered. Palatal obturators briefly came back into fashion, while surgical advancement of the posterior pharyngeal wall to meet the short, immobile new palate was also proposed.

Gustav Passavant (1813–1893) was the first to study this problem in detail and to propose a series of surgical solutions [771]. He cleverly observed, in 1862 that the nasality which so often developed after an operation was due to the inability of the short, reconstructed palate to completely close off the velopharyngeal space. He first attempted to correct this by suturing the posterior pillars along the midline, but the results were disappointing. Nevertheless he continued his work undeterred, for although he had not yet discovered an effective solution, he knew that he had correctly grasped the nature of the problem of dysphonia.

In 1865 Passavant operated on a girl who still exhibited a severe speech defect after palatal repair and made substantial improvement by partially suturing the posterior border of the velum to the back wall of the pharynx. Although this operation was effective it never became very popular, in part due to the understandable reluctance of both patients and surgeons to undertake a second operation after the first had proved less than successful, but above all because the procedure was quite difficult to perform.

In 1878 Passavant proposed a third solution which consisted in advancing the posterior pharyngeal wall by cutting a quadrangular flap of mucosa and folded it back on itself. This significantly reduced the space through which air might escape towards the nose. Unfortunately, the impressive results obtained proved to be short-lived. As Ronald Pigott [801] noted in 1993, the repair (known as *Passavant's ridge*) tended to flatten within the space of six months, causing the narrowed space to widen once again. This is no doubt the reason why Passavant himself eventually abandoned the method.

After a long period of experimentation, Passavant concluded that the most effective procedure was to close the cleft in two steps. During the first operation the soft palate should be repaired, combining this if necessary with a pharyngoplasty operation, while the second step could be devoted to the more difficult challenge of repairing the hard palate. Passavant underlined the importance of using an atraumatic technique both to minimize the scar and to avoid compromising the vitality of the flap, which was already at risk. The first time he carried out this operation he anaesthetized his patient with chloroform and closed off the trachea by means of a Trendelenburg cannula, but thereafter he generally performed a tracheostomy.

Another surgeon who studied the problem of correcting speech defects was Karl Schoenborn (1842–1906). Based on a suggestion made by Friedrich Trendelenburg[40] he conceived "a flap about 2 cm wide and 4 to 5 cm long, with its long axis [oriented] vertically and its base caudally from the posterior wall of the pharynx. The flap was designed as high up on the posterior wall of the pharynx as possible so that it could be brought easily and without tension to the back edge of the hard palate" [905]. In his first attempt Schoenborn based the pharyngeal flap inferiorly, but he soon shifted to a superior pedicle, suturing it to the back wall of the repaired soft palate. He furthermore suggested that the flap be divided after more or less normal speech had been attained, but it is not known whether he ever carried out this second operation.

A simple, but illusory solution to the problem was suggested by Robert Gersuny (b.1844), who dedicated his career to experimenting with the use of paraffin injections for a variety of problems. These were mostly cosmetic but he thought that it should be possible to diminish the velopharyngeal gap by injecting paraffin be-

40 Friedrick Trendelenburg (1844–1924) described the *Trendelenburg position* in 1880. It is still widely used in surgery and anaesthesia. Rolando Capelluti from Parma described the position in 1230. Trendelenburg also published an account of congenital dislocation of the hip in 1885, developed the Trendelenburg test for varicose veins, and experimented with pharyngeal flaps in dogs.

hind the pharyngeal wall, but the results were disastrous [365–367]. For decades surgeons continued to tinker with this approach using more inert and better tolerated materials, but it remained controversial due to doubts regarding the tolerance the material and stability of the "repair".

It seems odd now that Passavant's solution, which was both logical and technically feasible, was ignored for more than thirty years while surgeons experimented with other, less reliable methods. Finally, the notion of reducing the pharyngeal space was revived by Friedrich Christian Rosenthal, who in 1924 proposed a caudally based flap similar to that of Schoenborn [863]. Just a few months before Rosenthal's death Trendelenburg read his paper, which reminded him of the work of Schoenborn. He contacted Rosenthal, who acknowledged Schoenborn's prior claim as the inventor of the procedure, and thus the operation came to be known as the Schoenborn-Rosenthal pharyngoplasty procedure, even though if one compares them carefully, there are significant differences between the two techniques.

In the same year that Rosenthal published his paper, the American surgeon George Dorrance approached the problem from the opposite direction, his idea being that the gap between the velum and the pharyngeal wall might be closed by lengthening the palate rather than advancing the pharyngeal wall [294]. In order to achieve this he dissected the hard palate in continuity with the soft palate and moved the entire unit backwards to meet the pharynx. This manoeuvre, which came to be known as *the push-back operation*, gained wide acceptance among plastic surgeons.

In 1931[41] Veau pointed out important drawbacks to Rosenthal's approach which he confirmed in 1935 (Fig. 8.31) [1005]. There was little mucosa available in the upper portion of the pharyngeal vault, it was difficult to include juvenile adenoid tissue in the flap and avoiding this compromised the blood supply entering the flap superiorly. The muscle tissue in the flap also atrophied due to denervation. This explains why the flap shrinks to form a cord. Some improvement occurs despite these problems, through the reduction in the circumference of the pharynx. Rosenthal's procedure helped to reduce and sometimes even to eliminate velopharyngeal insufficiency.

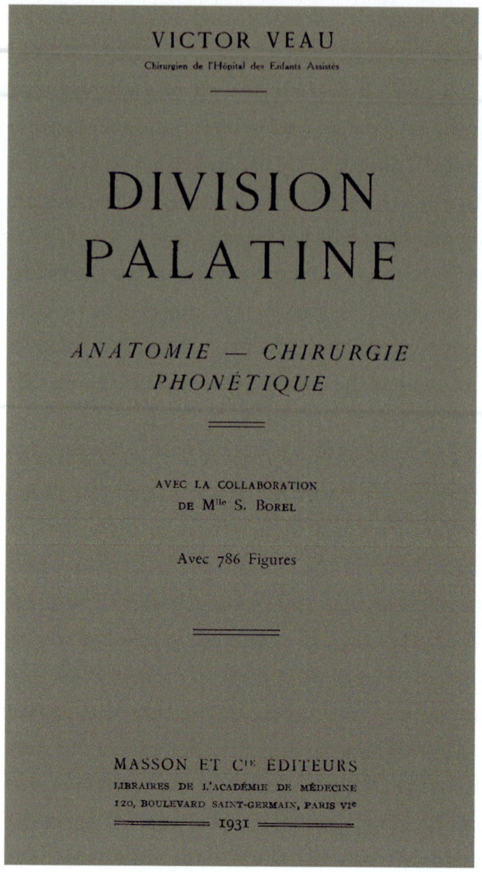
VICTOR VEAU

Chirurgien de l'Hôpital des Enfants Assistés

DIVISION PALATINE

ANATOMIE — CHIRURGIE PHONÉTIQUE

AVEC LA COLLABORATION DE Mlle S. BOREL

Avec 786 Figures

MASSON ET CIE ÉDITEURS

LIBRAIRES DE L'ACADÉMIE DE MÉDECINE

120, BOULEVARD SAINT-GERMAIN, PARIS VIe

1931

Fig. 8.31 Frontispiece of *Division Palatine* (1931) by Victor Veau written in collaboration with Madame Borel the speech therapist. *Courtesy of Riccardo Mazzola, M.D., Milan*

With regard to the problem of reducing an overly large pharynx, we should recall here the contribution of Willis who according to Pigott [800], managed to prolong the palate by carrying out a transverse incision and suturing it vertically, with impressive success.

Two years after Veau, Gustavo Sanvenero-Rosselli (1897–1974) proposed a novel flap that was based cranially and inserted, sandwich-like, between the reopened nasal and palatal layers of the velum pendulum (Fig. 8.32a, b) [897]. In 1953, following the success of these static pharyngoplasty procedures, Wilfred Hynes added a completely new dimension to the approach by introducing the dynamic reconstruction of the velopha-

41 Veau published his book in collaboration with Madame Borel a speech therapist in 1931 [1005].

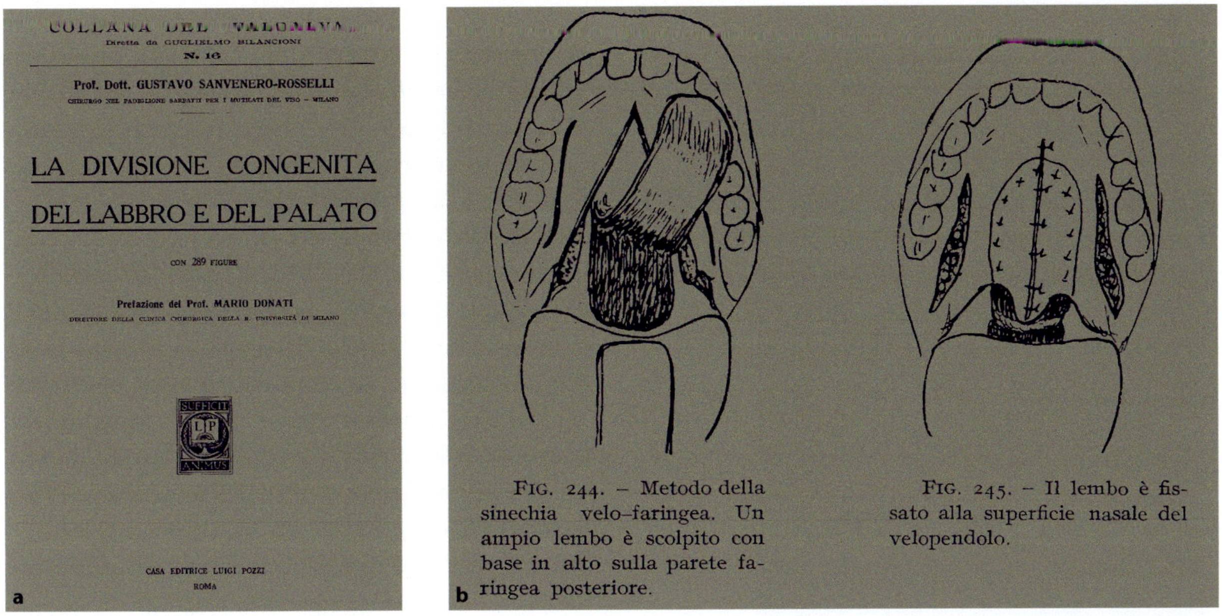

Fig. 8.32 **a** Frontispiece of Sanvenero-Rosselli's book *La Divisione Congenita del Labbro e del Palato* (1934) where he describes his pharyngoplasty. **b** His superiorly based pharyngeal flap represented a substantial improvement and overcame some of the drawbacks of previous methods. *Courtesy of Riccardo Mazzola, M.D., Milan*

ryngeal sphincter. He suggested elevating bilateral myomucous flaps based superiorly behind the posterior pillars, which he sutured transversally [458, 459]. In 1968 Mario Orticochea developed a similar procedure which incorporated a pharyngeal flap and became quite popular [759].

In 1964 R. Ruding suggested dissecting the palatal ends of the levator palati muscles from their abnormal insertion to the back of the hard palate, and sewing them across the midline in their usual alignment during soft palate repairs [874]. A modification to this procedure suggested by O. Kriens in 1967 greatly improved the mobility of the palate [510]. The development of these procedures led to the coining of the term *veloplasty* to replace the more generic *palatal repair*, thus underlining the importance of creating a long and mobile palate, and avoiding whenever possible the necessity of later pharyngoplasty.

In 1969 in effort to evaluate all these methods Pigott suggested that one might study the movement of the velum and its closure with the back wall of the pharynx by means of a paediatric cystoscope inserted into the nose [800]. Later he employed a flexible fibre optic instrument that could be used together with the videofluoroscope invented in 1970 by M.L. Skolnick [934] to obtain a dynamic, three-dimensional picture of the movement of the palate and pharynx during speech [802]. Surgeons have found this technique to be quite useful when choosing between different procedures aimed at correcting the escape of air through the nose.

Speech Rehabilitation

The importance of a functioning palate in speech was understood in ancient times as we have noted. Few studies were made over the years (Fig. 8.33) and it has only been in the last century that the mechanisms involved have been studied in detail. Speech rehabilitation is one of the primary goals of corrective surgery for the cleft palate. During the time of the first repairs in the middle of the nineteenth century, infants and children were rarely operated on and most patients were mature adults with acquired speech defects which were almost impossible to correct. However, as improvements were introduced

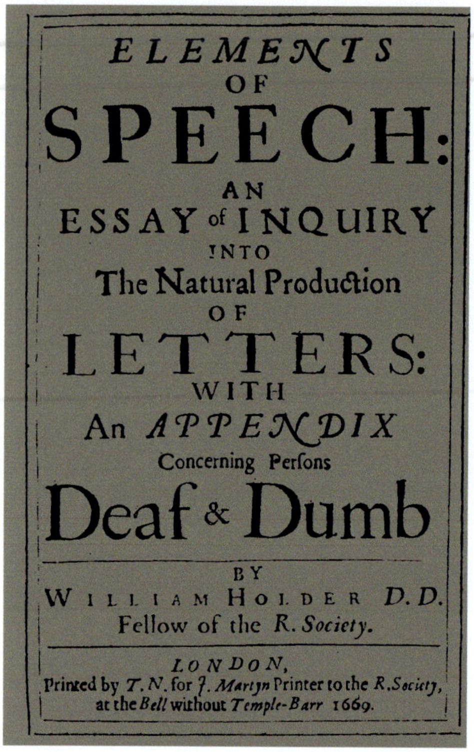

ELEMENTS
OF
SPEECH:
AN
ESSAY of INQUIRY
INTO
The Natural Production
OF
LETTERS:
WITH
An APPENDIX
Concerning Persons
Deaf & Dumb

BY
WILLIAM HOLDER D.D.
Fellow of the R. Society.

LONDON,
Printed by T. N. for J. Martyn Printer to the R. Society,
at the Bell without Temple-Barr 1669.

Fig. 8.33 *Elements of Speech* by William Holder DD, FRS published in 1669. *Courtesy of FMR Art.spa Bologna*

in surgical techniques, anaesthesia and paediatric medicine, the age of the patients gradually fell, although surgeons continued to differ regarding the best age at which to operate. During the 1860s von Langenbeck advised surgeons to wait until the child was 7–8 years of age, whereas later the Austrian Theodor Billroth (1829–1894) said that one could operate successfully on a 4-week-old infant [101]. Other surgeons recommended varying ages from 8 months, proposed in 1869 by J. Ehrman in France [275] to between 2 and 4 years as suggested by the English surgeon T. Smith in 1871 [943].

The first surgeon to recognize the importance of speech therapy was Ulisse Trelat who in a presentation to the *Académie de Médicine de Paris* in 1884 explained that therapy was useful both before and after an operation, although he complained that patients below the age of seven were too restive and uncooperative to obtain much benefit from this exercise [995].

In recent decades various methods to help patients to improve their speech following an operation for cleft palate have been developed. These measures, which range from speech therapy to orthodontic procedures and psychotherapy, have been thoroughly reviewed by Mazzola and Filippi [625]. One of the staunchest advocates of speech therapy was Billroth, who wrote "Patients must learn to use muscles for speech that they could not use voluntarily before. Speech therapy consists in making the patient read aloud and especially to accent their vowels, thus training the muscles. The sounds formed in the anterior oral cavity are pronounced more easily than the ones originating in the posterior oral cavity. The voiceless sounds are more difficult to pronounce than the voiced sounds. The explosives are less distinct than the hissing sounds. L is uttered most easily, G with the most difficulty. Adults, like children, [can] learn to speak; however, the disadvantage consists in the fact that adults have to forget their previous language and acquire the new one." [101]

It should be observed that the "training of the muscles" envisaged by Billroth was quite different from the techniques of speech therapy practised today, which were developed by Mme Borel-Maisonuy, a speech therapist and close collaborator with Victor Veau, who codified a set of phonetic rehabilitation procedures in 1930 [1005]. Her outstanding work was followed by that of Mrs. Muriel Morley [710] a therapist working with W.E.M. Wardill [1027, 1028] in England whose authoritative text was first published in 1926, extended in 1928 and reprinted several times later.

As in many other fields of reconstruction, cleft surgery has undergone a series of refinements and improvements in recent decades although the principles established by the giants of the past are still valid. The list of these innovations is too long to mention here and many surgeons have contributed. The areas which have benefited patients most are probably pre-surgical orthopaedics and orthodontics, speech therapy, bone grafting of the maxillary cleft and accurate repair of the velum for which some surgeons use the operating microscope. Perhaps the one development that has had the biggest effect on the life of the family is the establishment of multidisciplinary teams and the realization that to retain their skills surgeons have to treat an adequate number of cases each year. There is no place for the occasional operator. The complete rehabilitation of the cleft patient is now a possibility.

Chapter 9

Reconstruction of the External Genitalia

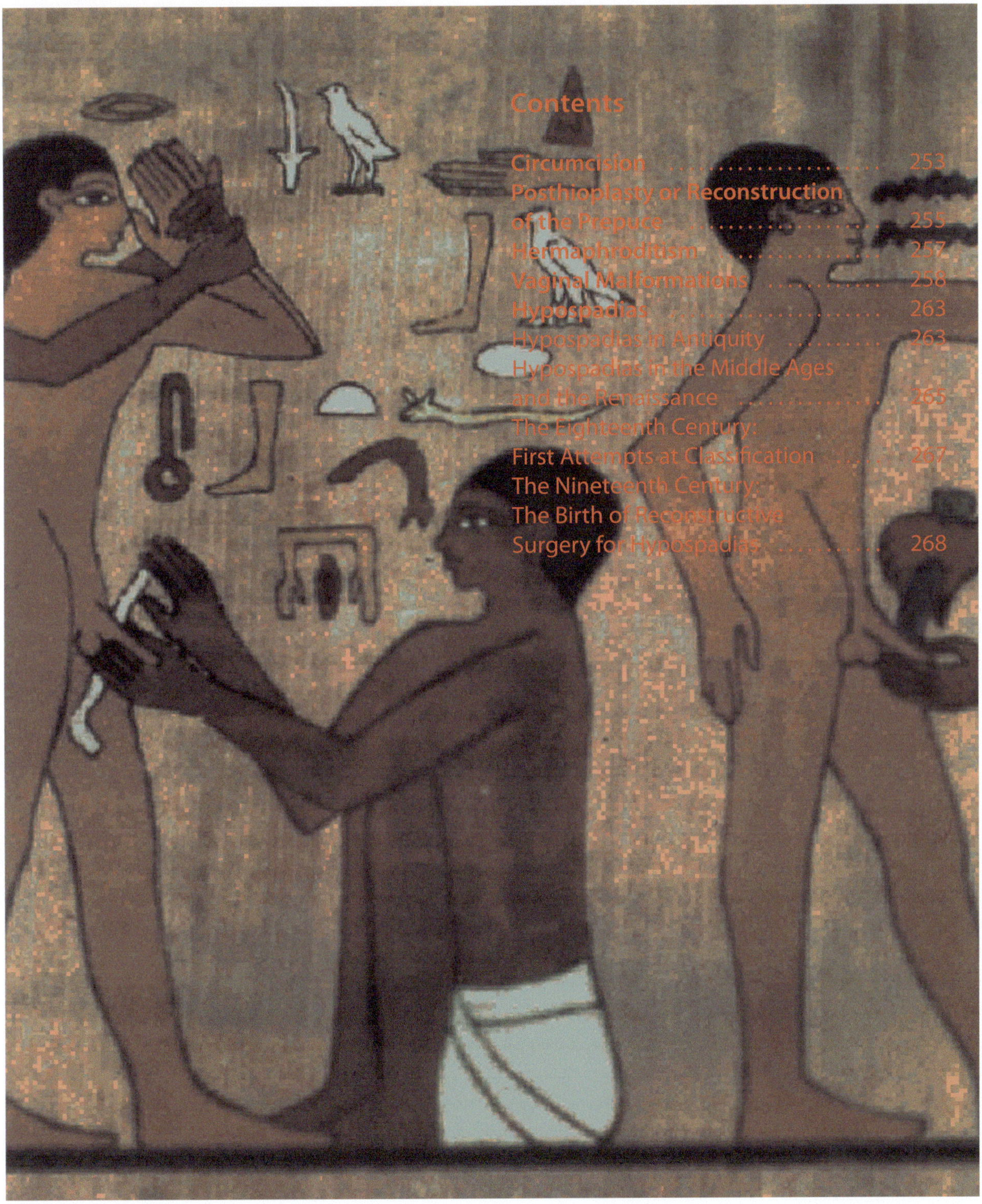

Contents

Urology is the branch of surgery to which the earliest historical references may be found, however intermittent and fragmentary. We know for example that the Chaldeans of ancient Kurdistan who seem to have been the first people to carry out circumcisions, were aware of the condition of agenesis of the penis, although they did not arrive at a medical interpretation of this malformation and certainly made no attempt to repair it surgically [51]. Many genital anomalies are described in the Old Testament, though from a religious rather than a medical perspective. For instance, a man afflicted with hypospadias could not marry a woman of the Jewish faith, while cryptorchidism excluded him from becoming a rabbi.

The British Museum possesses a collection of more than 20,000 clay tablets found among the ruins of the Palace of Nineveh, which was sacked by the Babylonians, Scythians and Medes in 612 B.C. These bear cuneiform texts on religious, administrative, literary and scientific subjects, some of which are believed to date back as far as 1600 B.C. They were collected and copied for the Assyrian monarch Ashurbanipal. On one of these tablets may be found the somewhat confused but unmistakable description of a congenital anomaly with caudal displacement of the umbilicus and absence of the penis. P.P. Rickham [840] believes this to be the oldest record of exstrophy of the bladder. Significantly, this tablet was found among others describing surgical procedures and therefore the deformity was regarded as a medical condition rather than a magical or supernatural occurrence. The literature would have to wait more than two thousand years before another, better description of the anomaly was formulated by Johann von Grafemberg Schenck (1530–1598) in *Observationum Medicorum Rerarum Novarum* in 1595 [903], while exstrophy in females was described for the first time in 1670 by van Horne [852].

Infibulation[1] and circumcision have been practised since earliest times; the latter in particular was invested with profound religious significance, and the operation was described in precise detail as early as 1550 B.C. in the Ebers Papyrus [271]. According to M.B. Assad [33] female circumcision was performed between 6 and 10 years since it was a Pharaonic belief that Gods were supposed to be bisexual. The resection of the labia minora and of either part or all of the clitoris prepared the women for marriage.

Furthermore, as we will see, other medical procedures involving the genitalia such as *cutting for stones* (urethral lithotomy) were known in antiquity, while *upadansa*, a treatment for aggressive phagedaenic balanic ulcers, was described by the Indian surgeon Susruta [90].[2]

The next significant contribution to urology was made by Hippocrates (c.460–360 B.C.), who has left us an accurate description of the anatomy of the male and female genito-urinary systems [434–437]. It is curious to note that, while he discusses various pathologies of the genitalia, he does not mention congenital malformations.[3]

Infibulation was practised in Rome to prevent coitus and masturbation, but sometimes also among actresses "to preserve the voice".[4] Aulus Cornelius Celsus (25 B.C. to 50 A.D.) describes the operation, although in

1 Infibulation is still practised today in some parts of Africa. For example in Ethiopia it is customary to suture the labia in young female children in such a way as to allow only the passage of urine. The demonstrably virgin daughter can later be given away by her father for a bride price, and only just before the marriage is the vagina reopened with a sharp knife.

2 The aetiology of *upadansa* is not clear, although the detailed explanation furnished by Susruta suggests that it is venereal in origin. For example, he writes that the ulcers may develop after: "… promiscuous and excessively frequent sexual intercourse, or lying with a woman who has observed a vow of abstinence for her entire life or one who has not been possessed by a man for a long period of time or who is menstruating, or lying with a woman who is not lovingly disposed toward the visitor or vice versa, or after knowing a woman who washes her intimate parts with unclean water and neglects the hygiene of these parts, or who is suffering from a disease of the vagina, or to engage in intercourse with a woman in every natural orifice in her body apart from the organ of copulation".

3 Like most Greeks and Romans, Hippocrates was of the opinion that the female genitalia should be kept hidden from view. It is interesting to note that the Latin word for the female genitalia, *pudendum,* derives from *puden* which means "shame".

4 In the Collegio Romano there are two statues that portray infibulated musicians. The size and weight of the ring in each case is notable and this perhaps confirms the hypothesis that infibulation was carried out not only to maintain chastity but also as an instrument of penitence.

somewhat dismissive terms; after piercing the vulva, the lips were closed with a ring using the same technique as that "to prepare the ear for pendants" [167].

In this chapter we will discussion circumcision, its history and ethnographic significance. Its relevance to early plastic surgery lies in the fact that reconstruction of the prepuce was practised in ancient times. Then we will retrace the tangled but fascinating history of hermaphroditism. Finally ending with one of the oldest problems in corrective surgery, that of congenital hypospadias, which for many centuries was mistakenly linked to hermaphroditism (Figs. 9.1, 9.2).

Circumcision

B. O. Rogers noted that: "Circumcision is probably one of the oldest forms of ritual mutilation." There are many references to this operation in the Old Testament, one of the most familiar being: "This is my covenant, which ye shall keep, between me and you and thy seed after thee. Every man child amongst you shall be circumcised. And ye shall circumcise the flesh of your foreskin."[5] Initially conceived as a religious ceremony, the practice quickly spread as the benefits for personal hygiene, particularly in warm climates, became evident.

Archaeological studies suggest that the Chaldeans from the mountains of Armenia and Kurdistan, followed by the Phoenicians and the Egyptians, were the first to carry out circumcisions. The Ebers papyrus, which dates to at least 1550 B.C., describes the procedure in considerable detail; for example, to stop post-operative haemorrhaging it recommends the application of a paste made of "honey, cuttle fish bone and the fruit of the sycamore mixed together". A bas-relief dating from the same period, on the facade of the tomb of Ankh-ma-Horshows probably constitutes the earliest surviving representation of the operation. The men portrayed in some antique sculptures have clearly been circumcised. The pharaoh in the Museum of Cairo described by Ernest Desnos is an example [237]. W.M. Krogman [511] writes about the same subject (Fig. 9.3).

Although adopted by the Egyptians and Phoenicians primarily for reasons of hygiene, the procedure of

5 See *Genesis* XVII, 10, 11.

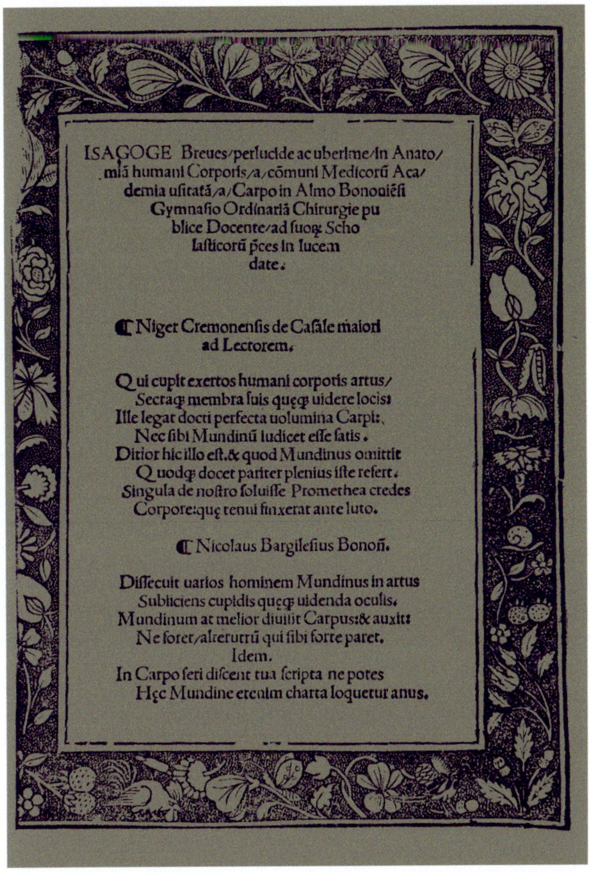

ISAGOGE Breues/perlucide ac uberime/in Anato/
miã humani Corporis/a/cõmuni Medicorũ Aca/
demia usitatã/a/Carpo in Almo Bononiẽsi
Gymnasio Ordinariã Chirurgie pu
blice Docente/ad suoꝝ Scho
lasticorũ pces in lucem
date.

Niger Cremonensis de Casale maiori
ad Lectorem.

Qui cupit exertos humani corporis artus/
Sectaqꝫ membra suis queqꝫ uidere locis:
Ille legat docti perfecta uolumina Carpi:
Nec sibi Mundinũ iudicet esse satis.
Ditior hic illo est.& quod Mundinus omittit
Quodqꝫ docet pariter plenius iste refert.
Singula de nostro soluisse Promethea credes
Corpore:quę tenui finxerat ante luto.

Nicolaus Bargilesius Bonoñ.

Dissecuit uarios hominem Mundinus in artus
Subiiciens cupidis queqꝫ uidenda oculis.
Mundinum at melior diuisit Carpus:& auxit:
Ne foret/alterutrũ qui sibi forte paret.
Idem.
In Carpo seri discent tua scripta nepotes
Hęc Mundine etenim charta loquetur anus.

Fig. 9.1 Frontispiece of Berengario's *Isogae* where the anatomy of the genitalia is described in detail. *Courtesy of Riccardo Mazzola, M.D., Milan*

circumcision was not devoid of ritual associations. In Egypt, for example, it was at first reserved for the pharaoh's family, the aristocracy and members of the temple and was carried out by a priest. However, when its practical advantages were grasped, the operation was extended to all males and was even forced on foreign visitors. When the Greek Pythagoras (c.580–500 B.C.) wished to visit Egypt to study its temple architecture, he first had to undergo circumcision. With time this directive may have been relaxed, because there is no evidence that Herodotus (c.490 to c.430 B.C.) or Diodorus Siculus (80–90 B.C.) were subjected to a similar requirement [429].

While the medical texts of ancient India do not mention circumcision, it was routinely practised by the He-

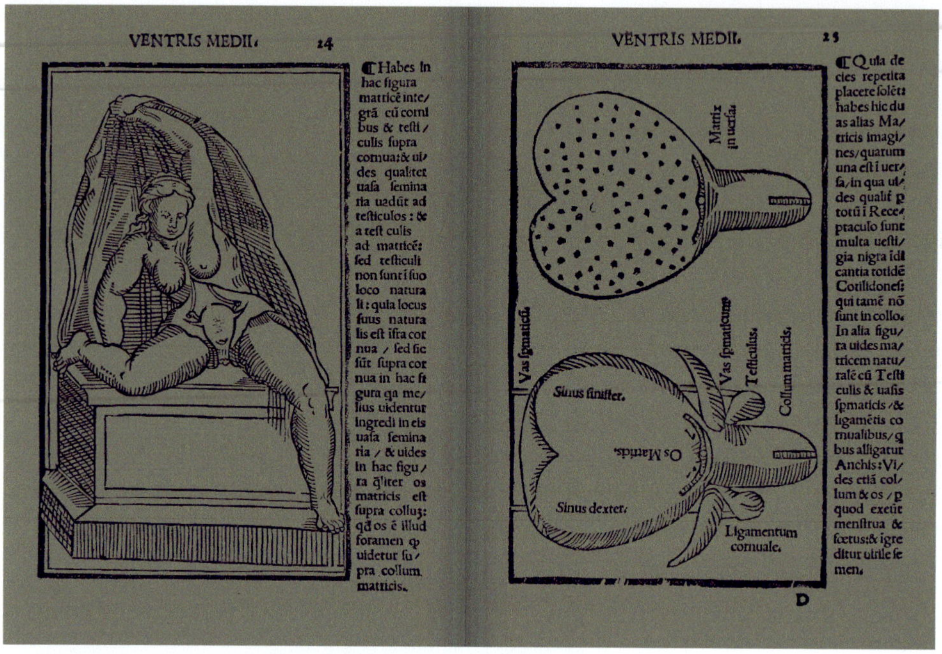

Fig. 9.2 Illustration of male and female genitalia from *Isogae* by Berengario (1460–1530). *Courtesy of Riccardo Mazzola, M.D., Milan*

brews, as stipulated in the Old Testament [835]. Regarded as a sacred ritual, this operation was presided over by a rabbi. If we consider that as a general rule the ancient Hebrews never resorted to surgery except in cases of dire necessity, the solemn significance of this practice becomes all the more striking [163].

We know from Herodotus that circumcisions were carried out in Greece in the fifth century B.C. as a prophylactic measure, and this practice was continued in ancient Rome, where knowledge of urology was quite advanced; Celsus (25 B.C. to 50 A.D.) provides a thorough discussion of the subject in his monumental work *De Medicina* [167]. The Roman surgeon's grasp of anatomy[6] was impressive and the techniques he described were quite sophisticated for the period. Celsus recognized that circumcision was medically indicated in cases "where the glans cannot be denuded",[7] i.e. when the foreskin could not be retracted to expose the glans. He wrote: "If the glans has become so covered that it cannot be bared, a lesion which the Greeks call 'phimosis', it must be opened out, which is done as follows. Underneath, the foreskin is to be divided from its free margin in a straight line back as far as the frenum, and thus the skin above is relaxed and can be retracted." However, in cases of severe constriction or hardening of the skin due to fibrosis this measure might not be sufficient and then Celsus did not hesitate to use a flap "having its apex at the frenum and its base at the edge of the prepuce".[8]

There is a widespread notion that circumcision can be linked to the advent of Islam, but in fact the practice was already common on the Arabian peninsula long before the birth of the Prophet. Mohammed himself was circumcised at the age of 13 in accordance with the customs of his tribe.

6 See Celsus, *De Medicina*, in particular Book VII, Chapters XXI–XXVII, where the anatomical differences between the two sexes are analyzed in detail.

7 See *De Medicina*, Book VII, Chapter XXV, paragraphs 1 and 2.

8 The flap must have been made on the internal layer and prevented a circular scar.

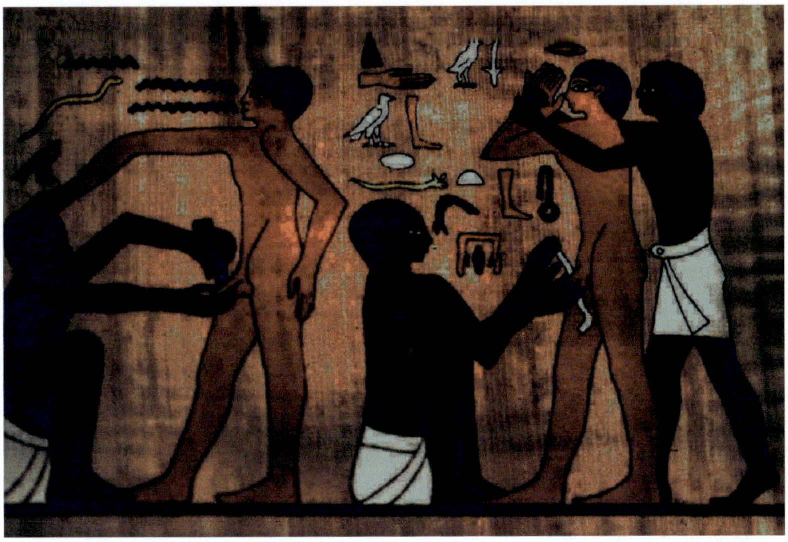

Fig. 9.3 Facsimile painting of a stone relief carving c.2350–2200 B.C., depicting a circumcision from the Mastaba of Ankh-ma-Hor, "The Doctors Tomb" in Saqqara, Egypt (Old Kingdom Sixth Century). *PSR*

In pre-Colombian America, the Aztecs and Totonacs circumcised male infants at the age of 28 or 29 days. Female babies were deflowered by the finger of a priest at the same age and this procedure was repeated when they were six.

Posthioplasty or Reconstruction of the Prepuce

In Rome the practice of circumcision was viewed in a negative light because a radical excision could result in an exposed glans; the man who presented himself at a gymnasium with such a defect was looked upon as the most unfortunate of beings! Centuries later this drawback and the largely unnecessary reason for the operation were reiterated by Gabriele Fallopius (1523–1562) [296–298].[9]

Requests for the procedure did not abate, however, and Celsus devised a corrective measure to help those men who found themselves with a deficient prepuce.[10] After observing that "When the glans is bare and the man wishes for the look of the thing to have it covered, this can be done … [although] more easily in one in whom the defect is natural than in one who, after the custom of certain races, has been circumcised." He continues: "The prepuce around the glans is seized, stretched out until it actually covers the glans, and there tied. Next the skin covering the penis just in front of the pubes is cut through in a circle until the penis is bared, but great care must be taken not to cut into the urethra, nor into the blood vessels." Celsus describes the entire operation in careful detail, concluding with instructions on how the penis should be bandaged to minimize inflammation and swelling. This procedure would be used for centuries; we know that it was adopted by Paulus Aegineta [427] in the seventh century and during the Renaissance by Fabricius ab Aquapendente (c.1533–1619) [290–293] and Fallopius.

Celsus was regarded by the ancient Romans as a demigod and men suffering from genital malformations dedicated votive statues to him in the temples of Hygieia, the goddess of health, and Aesculapius, the god of medicine. Some of these were moulded in the form of a penis complete with scrotum, while others depicted various

9 Gabriele Fallopius (1523–1562) was very interested in this subject and in Book VII, Chapters 21–27 provide a detailed description of the anatomy of the genitals in males and females. He also wrote a section on *De preputio brevitate corrigenda* (How to correct shortness of the prepuce).

10 See *De Medicina*, Book VII, Chapter XXV, paragraph 1.

pathological conditions such as ulcers or a swollen foreskin. Indeed phallic images could be seen everywhere in Imperial Rome, where morals were relatively lax and such symbols were even worn as amulets to guard against infertility or to ward off evil spirits.

Celsus also provided an accurate description of how to catheterize the bladder, including the specific indications for this procedure.[11] He used catheters made of bronze in different shapes and sizes depending upon the age and sex of the patient.

It is known that reconstruction of the prepuce (posthioplasty) was sometimes carried out by Jews, and for a specific reason. In the First Book of the Maccabees, we read that some Jews, bowing to pressure from the Selucid ruler Antiochus IV, "made themselves uncircumcised and forsook the holy covenant". In fact, when Antiochus conquered Judaea, as part of a Hellenization program he banned all Jewish practices, including circumcision. Furthermore he created the institution of the gymnasium, a meeting place for cultural and athletic activities, including hot baths; here a Jew could not hide this sign of membership of a prohibited sect.

In the New Testament Saint Paul mentions "uncircumcision", and references to this as a practice among Jews can be found in the works of Dioscorides (first century A.D.), Marcus Valerius Martial (40–104 A.D.) and Saint Epiphanias (first half of the ninth century).[12] It is doubtful, however, that the motive for the operation was the one suggested by Gabriel Groddeck [398] in 1733: "... because they imagined that their harlots and sweethearts had more pleasure in sleeping with a man who either never had the foreskin removed or had it restored artificially".

Much more convincing is the explanation offered by Peter Charles Remondino (1846–1926) in his treatise on circumcision [835]. He suggested that the reconstruction was undertaken to avoid the persecution to which Jews were subjected in various periods during their history, by eliminating this *brand* of their faith. For example, a decree handed down by Antiochus IV in 167 B.C. imposed the death sentence on mothers who had their sons circumcised. Discrimination continued under the reigns of the emperors Hadrian (74–134 A.D.) and Marcus Aurelius (121–180 A.D.). During this period, in the city of Rome any Jew could be stopped in the street and asked to show his penis. Circumcised males discovered in this manner were required to pay an exorbitant tax for the right to exercise their "freedom of conscience". Under the reign of Justinian in the sixth century, Jews were forbidden to raise their children in the faith of their ancestors and whoever refused to convert to Christianity was driven into exile after having all his worldly goods confiscated. Interestingly enough, Christians in Turkey faced similar tribulations when the fact that they had not been circumcised was exposed.

Under these circumstances it is not difficult to understand why many Jews resorted to the measure of reconstruction, which Celsus called "recutilis". This procedure gained a certain acceptance, although there were always opponents prepared to ridicule it at a later date such as Pierre Dionis (d.1718) [248, 249].

Non-surgical methods for the reconstruction of the prepuce were also developed. In the first century A.D., for example, Martial, the Roman, bound a funnel-shaped copper tube which he called a *judunm pondum* (Jew's

11 See *De Medicina*, Book VII, Chapter XXVI, paragraph 1, and also Book VII, Chapter XXVI, paragraph 1. Celsus describes the catheterization of the bladder and the indications for this operation (translation by W.G. Spencer): "Sometimes we are compelled to draw off urine by hand when it is not passed naturally; either because in an old man the passage has collapsed, or because a stone, or a blood clot of some sort has formed an obstruction within it, but even a slight inflammation often prevents natural evacuation. For this purpose bronze tubes are made, and the surgeon must have three ready for males and two for females, in order that they might be suitable for everybody, large and small: those for males should be the longest, fifteen finger-breadths in length, the medium twelve, the shortest nine; for females, the longer nine, the shorter six. They ought to be a little curved, but more so for men, and they should be very smooth and neither too large nor too small. Then the man must be placed on his back on a low seat or couch; while the practitioner stands on his right side and taking the penis of the male patient into his left hand, with his right hand passes the pipe into the urethra; and when it has reached the neck of the bladder, the pipe together with the penis is inclined and pushed right on into the bladder; and when the urine has been evacuated it is taken out again."

12 See Epiphanias, *St. Epiphanis, Constantiae sive Salaminis Cypro Episcopi. Opera Omnia Tomus Secundus*, Petavius W. Aureliensis Ed. Nove, Coloniae, 1582, (Chapter XVI, p 172).

weight) to the penis and left it there until, with time and the effect of gravity, the weight had stretched the cutis downwards to cover the glans. This method (skin expansion *ante litteram*) must have been reasonably effective because it was still being used by the Sephardic Jews during the period of the Spanish Inquisition in the 1500s.

Remondino describes a case which illustrates the climate of fear that reigned during these centuries of religious conflict. While crossing the Adriatic Sea, an Austrian sailor suffering from severe phimosis was circumcised, but when he saw the result he became quite desperate at the prospect of being mistaken for a Turk. To calm his patient, the surgeon was forced to re-graft the foreskin that he had just excised!

Hermaphroditism

The origin of the term *hermaphrodite* may be traced back to ancient Greece and the names of the god Hermes and the goddess Aphrodite (also known as Cythera). Until relatively recent times, ignorance of the nature and causes of congenital deformities meant that a person who bore any of the primary or secondary characters of the other sex—hence raising doubts as to his or her true gender—was considered to be a hermaphrodite. As a result, completely extraneous conditions such as hypospadias (particularly in its proximal form) were wrongly placed in this category of malformations (Fig. 9.4).

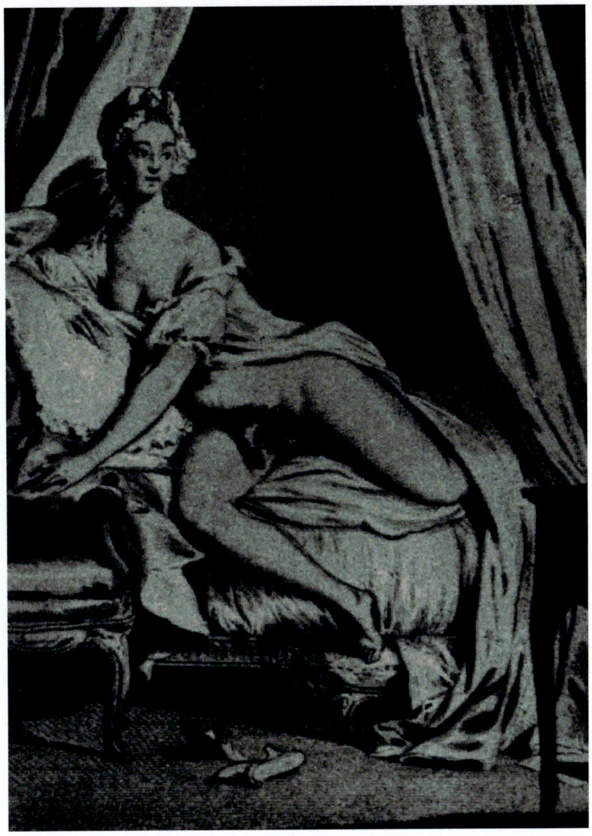

Fig. 9.4 Engraving of a hermaphrodite by Marie Angé from *Hermaphroditen in der Kunst (19th Century). Courtesy of Riccardo Mazzola, M.D., Milan*

If we study the literature over the centuries, a confusing picture emerges based on notions that bear little similarity to modern diagnostic criteria. Instead they reflect the uncertainty that reigned not only among physicians but also historians, students of law and mythology. In the seventh century Aegineta drew up a classification system and an interpretation of what was meant by the word *hermaphroditism* [3–5], but his observations show how poor the understanding of the condition was at the time: "There are four varieties according to Leonides; three of them occur in men and one in women. In men, sometimes about the perineum and sometimes about the middle of the scrotum, there is an appearance of a female pudendum with hair; and in addition to this, there is a third variety in which the discharge of urine takes place at the scrotum as from the female pudendum. In women there is often found, above the pudendum and in the situation of the pubes, the appearance of a man's privy parts, there being three bodies projecting there, one like a penis and two like testicles. The third of the male variety, in which the urine is voided through the scrotum, is incurable, but the other three may be cured by removing the supernumerary bodies and treating the parts like sores." It appears obvious to us today that most of the patients he described were actually suffering from different forms of hypospadias. At this time the anatomy of the genitalia was studied in detail by a number of authors. One of the most important, who gave accurate descriptions, was Berengario da Carpi (1460–1530) (Figs. 9.1, 9.2). Over a century later the Danish anatomist Caspari Bartholini described the glands which bear his name in his book on *Anatome* published 1678 (Fig. 9.5) [60].

Many examples of thoroughly documented, but completely misinterpreted cases can be found in the literature. H.H. Young, who wrote an exhaustive review in

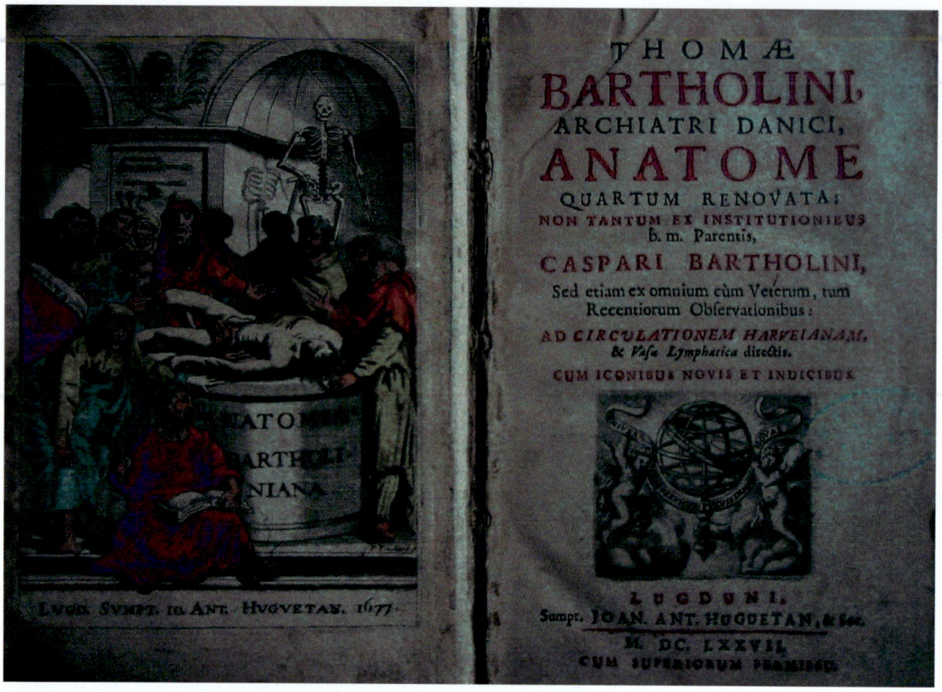

Fig. 9.5 Frontispiece of Carspari Bartholini's book *Anatome* published 1668 in Lugdunum (Lyon). *Courtesy of C.d.L. Flaminio Farnesi, Pisa*

1937, was able to list only a few cases of true, histologically proven hermaphroditism. The great majority of the other cases were listed as "Undetermined Sex".[13] Young's conclusions were confirmed by Louis Ombrédanne in 1939 when he wrote about the surgical possibilities of treating hermaphrodites (Fig. 9.6) [753]. We will discuss some of these below, limiting ourselves however to the conditions of greatest interest to the plastic surgeon, i.e. vaginal malformations such as the imperforated hymen and vaginal atresia and hypospadias.

Vaginal Malformations

One of the earliest descriptions of vaginal abnormalities was by Celsus [167, 168], who described surgical methods of treatment. For the imperforated hymen he recommended an X-shaped incision just sufficient to open the vaginal orifice, with the warning that the surgeon should take great care not to touch the urethra.

In cases of vaginal atresia he proposed that a cavity should be dissected between the bladder and the intestine, and then filled with cotton soaked in vinegar to keep it open. This bandage was to be changed every three days, eventually replacing the vinegar with an unguent, until the wound had completely healed.[14] To keep the cavity from closing up, the patient was instructed to insert a tin tube at frequent intervals into the new vagina.

This operation was used for centuries and indeed, with some modifications and refinements it was still considered the procedure of choice by Dupuytren, well into the nineteenth century. Aegineta [3–5], who made a special study of congenital deformities, introduced a slight

13 H.H. Young wrote *Genital Abnormalities, Hermaphroditism and Related Adrenal Diseases* Bailliere Tindall Cox, London, in 1937.

14 See *De Medicina*, Book VII, Chapter XXVIII, paragraph 1.

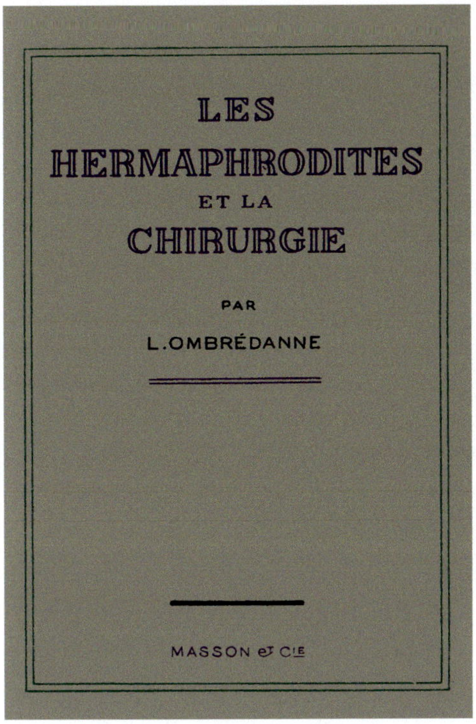

Fig. 9.6 The frontispiece of the book by Louis Ombrédanne on hermaphrodites where the indications for surgery are discussed. *Courtesy of Riccardo Mazzola, M.D., Milan*

variation; instead of a bandage he used "a priapus-shaped tent covered with an epulotic preparation". After Celsus, fifteen centuries passed before there was another description of vaginal atresia. In 1559, Matteo Realdus Columbus (c.1516–1559) produced an excellent anatomical description, although he did not discuss treatment [188].

In contrast, Fabricius ab Aquapendente's interest in congenital malformations, extended to how they might be corrected [290–292]. In his discussion of the imperforated hymen he recounts the case of "a servant maid, whom several scholars could not deflower, after having shock'd all their vigour against the ligature of her caruncules, [and who] was forc'd to have recourse to him [Fabricius] … the girl, being wholly imperforated, could not discharge her menstrual terms, they being detained by a membrane which join'd the caruncules, and entirely lock'd up the passage … A lengthwise incision in that membrane, from where issued out a great quantity of black and stinking blood, gave the patient ease, and perfectly cured her."

While it does not appear that any significant surgical advances were made between the end of the Roman Empire and the eighteenth century, during this long hiatus physicians continued to take an interest in the condition of hermaphroditism. In Turkey Charaf-ed-din (fifteenth century) [451] produced a copiously illustrated surgical text that includes a section on congenital anomalies (Fig. 9.7). Under this heading the author placed a certain number of conditions that at the time were thought to be hermaphroditisms, such as the imperforated hymen and vaginal atresia. These misapprehensions show that Charaf-ed-din probably never studied the conditions in situ; it was unthinkable that a pious Muslim might look at the intimate parts of a woman who was not his wife, and female patients could only be treated by midwives [451, 746, 887].

Although he did not make any original contributions in this area, it is interesting to read what the sixteenth century surgeon Ambroise Paré (1510–1590) had to say on the subject (Fig. 9.8). We learn that in France *hermaphrodites* were required "to choose the sexe which they will use, and in which they will remain and live, judging them to death if they be found to have departed from the sexe they made their choice of, for they are thought to have abused both promiscually, to have had pleasure with men and women" [769, 770]. In every part of Europe, persons born with genital anomalies were still being punished, in some cases quite severely, because their malformations were thought to be the work of the devil. In 1602, for example, both in Scotland and France there are documented cases of death sentences being carried out for these "crimes."

At the same time, attempts were being made to study genital malformations objectively; a description by Paré is exemplary, being the most thorough and accurate compiled to that date. Entire treatises were written on the subject; one by Jacques Duval (1555–c.1620) recounts the story of a 20-year-old woman, Marin le Marcis, and a young man, Jean Fabre, both from the town of Monstiervillor in France, who were condemned to be burned at the stake for their unnatural sexual behaviour: "Pour avoir changé d'habit et de nom, à esté en grand danger de perdre la vie" (for having changed her way of dressing and her name, was in great danger of losing her life) [269]. Both appealed this cruel sentence and before making its decision the court asked Duval to examine the young couple. He was able to testify that they were "deux

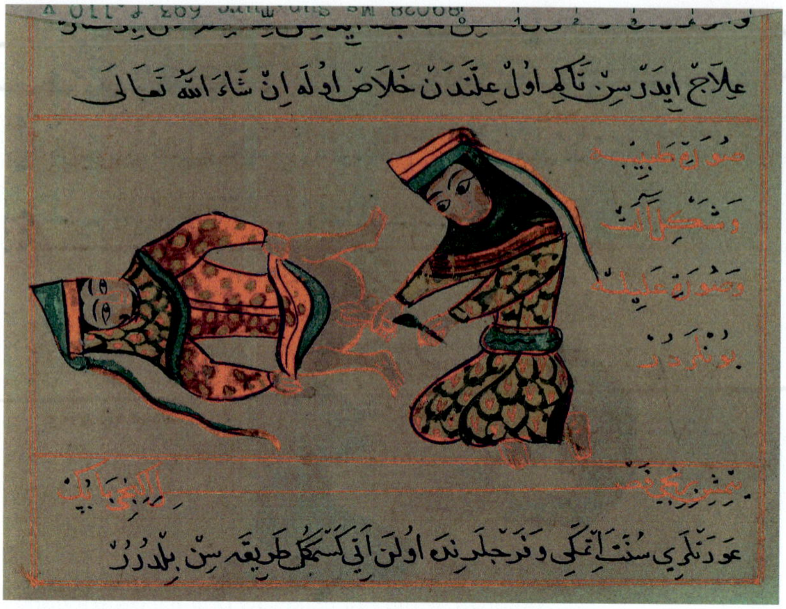

Fig. 9.7 A midwife operating on a hermaphrodite, 1466 by Charaf-ed-Din (1404–1468). *Bibliotheque Nationale, Paris, France, Archives Charmet / The Bridgeman Art Library*

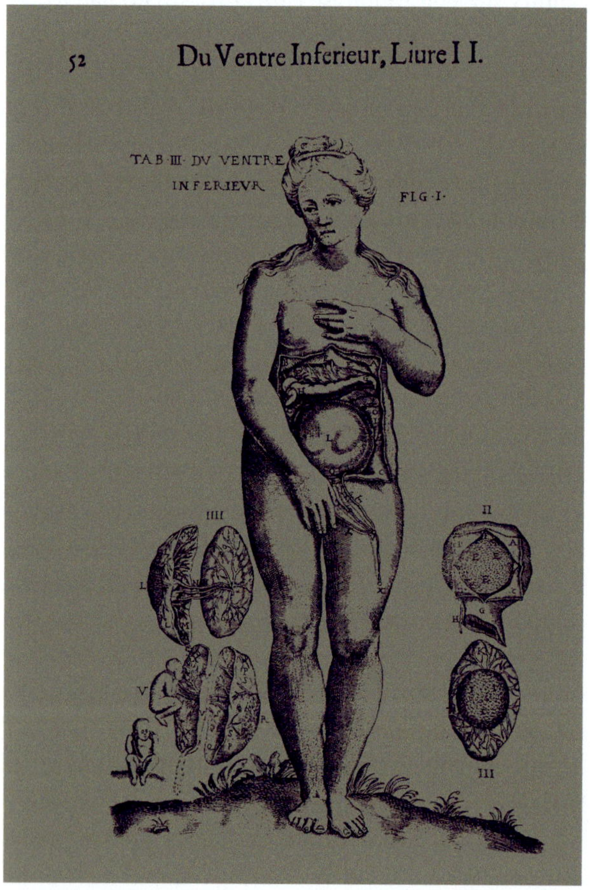

Fig. 9.8 In his *Les Oeuvres de Chirurgie* (1598) Guillemeau, like his teacher Paré, describes the genitalia in detail. *Courtesy of Riccardo Mazzola, M.D., Milan*

'Hermaphrodites Parfait' qui ont l'occasion de s'unir ensemble charnellement" ("two 'perfect hermaphrodites' who were able to unite themselves carnally"). This is the first time that we encounter the concept of the "perfect hermaphrodite", i.e. a person who is capable of both producing sperm and becoming pregnant. The concept of the "imperfect hermaprodite" also existed, referring to one who is not able to procreate and having characters of both sexes but in incomplete form.

The existence of the condition of "perfect hermaphroditism" was confirmed by other surgeons. In 1768 George Arnaud de Ronsil (b.1699)[15] described a famous case dating from 1663 in Valence, France: "Two young persons were married and some time later they were pregnant one of the other. They were persecuted as criminals, found guilty of an abominable crime and condemned to the fire, but Laurent Matheu, a Spanish doctor who was consulted about the case at the very moment that they

15 After teaching surgery in Paris at the Ecole de Saint Come, de Ronsil moved to London where he became an well-known and successful surgeon.

were being taken to the place of the execution, decided in their favour, that the Church had given them the power of being united, and of being only one body." [858]

Wolphius [269] also made the distinction between the "perfect hermaphrodite" who possessed the organs of both sexes in complete form, and the "imperfect hermaphrodite" in whom these organs were present but not fully developed. He concluded that "it is rare to find a hermaphrodite who has the perfect power of both sexes". He described the complex case of a 35-year-old patient who exhibited two testicles, one of which was normal and the other smaller and in the groin, as well as a penis-like clitoris furnished with a proximal meatus simulating an imperforate vagina and lacking any other aperture. This could have represented a case of scrotal-perineal hypospadias were it not for the fact that the patient complained of monthly perineal swelling followed by the evacuation of dark-coloured blood through the anus.

Wolphius decided to attempt surgery and, when he opened the perineum, discovered the presence of a cervix and a two-inch-long uterus. Following the construction of a new vagina the patient experienced normal menstruation, but unfortunately she neglected to use a 'tampon' to prevent stenosis and the aperture closed. When Wolphius operated again, the patient also requested that her clitoris be removed because it caused her intense pain when stimulated. A very similar case was described in 1704 in Nouvelle Literaires de la Mer Baltique.[16]

There are other interesting examples of trans-sexuality in this period, one being described by the English physician John Bulwer [143][17] in 1653 and another recorded by Licinius Mutianus at Izmir in Turkey around the same time. Bulwer's account is somewhat vague and might actually have represented a case of scrotal hypospadias. A review of the literature based on modern criteria highlights the uncertainty that prevailed, with interpretations based on erroneous clinical observations being commonplace. For example Loren Heister (1693–1758) defined a hermaphrodite as any person with an unusually large clitoris, observing that "Some woman have so large a size as to equal and resemble the penis of the male … Notwithstanding, the clitoris is without any perforation, and does not discharge either semen or urine." [422, 424] As in many such cases a more thorough examination would probably have revealed the absence of a vagina, leading to the correct diagnosis of scroto-perineal hypospadias.

Fortunately, during the nineteenth century accurate morphological descriptions of various anomalies and estimates of their frequency began to appear. Several contributed to an understanding of the deformities of the genitalia. We should mention Carlo Taruffi [972] the author of an encyclopaedic treatise in eight volumes in 1881, Thomas H. Morgan [709] in 1893 and Jacques Loeb [572] in 1907. Detailed embryological studies were also conducted by scientists such as G.M. Gould and W.I. Pylr [388], E. Schwalbe [910] and in particular Wilhelm His [438–440]. He was well known for his work on clefts and helped to shed light on the origin of many malformations (Fig. 9.9).

In the United States commendable attempts to repair vaginal malformations were already being made at the end of the nineteenth century. Perhaps the first to under-

16 Even if some doubt persists about the exact nature of these anomalies, two cases were reported in the nineteenth century. One is known as the case of Catherine (or Charles) Hoffman, born 1824, who became a mother by her thirtieth year. But after forty the sexual desires changed and acting as a man "Charles" even married with full satisfaction. Another case is that of Marie-Madeline Lefort who had well developed breasts with erectile nipples, regular menses, a large pelvis and a normal vulva from which projected a penis about 7 cm long which was also partially erectile. She grew a rich beard and mustache. This person died in 1864 and underwent autopsy which confirmed the presence of Fallopian tubes, uterus and ovaries.

17 Bulwer said that: "Nero, whom nothing in the ordinary course of Nature would satisfy, by a most prodigious conceit attempted to make such a monster of Arts and would need to have a boy of his, called Sporus, cut and made a woman, to whom he was solemnly married, which occasioned some justly to say that it had been happy for the commonwealth if Domitius, his father, had had other but such a wife." Bulwer also reported a curious practice that was quite widespread in Western India and Siam, that of implanting "… yarde balls, inserted between the penis skin and the flesh. [These were balls] of gold, silver or brasse which they put in when they reached the age to use women." One small ball was implanted for every child a man had engendered, up to a maximum of three; this was done in order to increase the pleasure of their women during coitus.

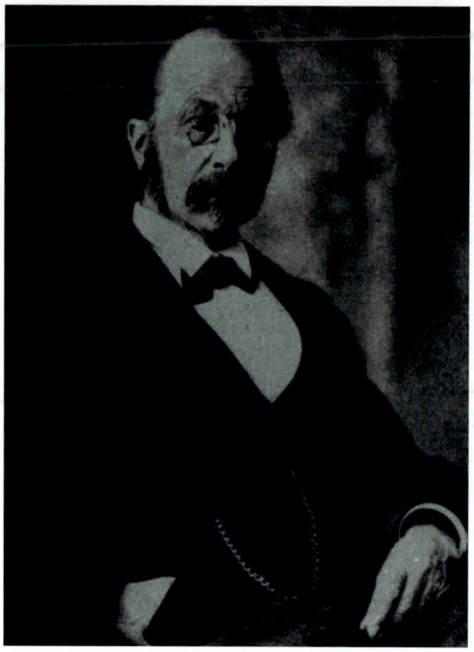

Fig. 9.9 Portrait of Wilhelm His (1831–1904) Swiss anatomist and embryologist. *Courtesy of FMR Art.spa. Bologna*

take this challenge were John Syng Dorsey (1783–1818) and his uncle Philip Syng Physick (1768–1837) of Philadelphia [250]. In 1818 Dorsey published a comprehensive surgical text that includes the description of a vaginal reconstruction carried out by his uncle. The procedure he used was not much different from the one proposed by Celsus eighteen centuries earlier, Dorsey adding that great care must be taken not to damage the bladder or rectum during the dissection and that a tampon should be used to keep the new vagina dilated to avoid secondary stenosis. Similar operations were described by De Heam (1761), Dupuytren (1817), Villame (1826), Boyer (1831) and Dubron (1851).

Apparently unaware of the work of Dorsey, John Collis Warren (1778–1856) in Boston reconstructed a "non-existing vagina" in 1833 using the following procedure: "Holding an index finger in the rectum, with a small probe bistoury one made an opening in front of the rectum and close to it, creating a passage about three inches long and wide enough to admit a finger." [1030] To stop the copious bleeding he inserted a tube during the operation and left it for four weeks in order to keep the pocket open. After this surprisingly short interval, Warren claimed that the process of dilatation was complete and there was no further risk of secondary stenosis, although he encouraged his patient to engage in frequent sexual intercourse to maintain the vaginal opening. The surgeon's son, Jonathan Warren, cites three other such operations carried out in 1851.

There was nonetheless a discordant voice amongst this optimistic chorus of surgeons. Samuel David Gross (1805–1884) [399], who has left us a perceptive commentary on developments in the area of surgery in America during the nineteenth century, wrote on the subject of vaginal atresia in 1864: "Nothing is to be done when there is an absence of the vagina. The woman is impotent and therefore disqualified from marriage." More than fifty years later J.D. Fergusson came to the same conclusion about the vaginal reconstructions carried out in the past 2,500 years, describing them as merely an "uninspired surgical exercise on the external genitalia" [305].

Certainly contracture of the new vagina was a complication that often nullified the results of the operation. At first surgeons believed the problem could be resolved by lining the new vagina with skin. According to Ricci [838] the first to attempt this was Heppner in 1870 in Saint Petersburg. He made an incision in the form of an "H" and used the two flaps thus created to partially cover the walls of the newly formed cavity. N. Owens [762] instead declared that the first successful skin graft in a new vagina was carried out no earlier than 1936 by the French surgeons Honod and Iselin, who put into practice a technique suggested by Dupuytren—that of lining the walls with free skin grafts applied by means of a probe inserted into the new vagina. Similar trials were carried out in England two years later by Archibald McIndoe and J.B. Banister [644], although they employed medium thickness grafts that in reality did little to resolve the problem of stenosis (Fig. 9.10).

The only alternative seemed to be the use of intestinal mucosa in the form of either a free graft or pedicle flap, but excessive secretions from this tissue limited the popularity of the procedure. The reconstruction of a stable and functional vagina would have to await the development of the gracilis myocutaneous flap (Fig. 9.11a, b) [632].

The problem of vesico-vaginal fistula is one that has taxed obstetricians and gynaecologists for centuries and it is worth mentioning here that the use of the gracilis muscle flap in the repair of this devastating condition has proved very effective. In developed countries with

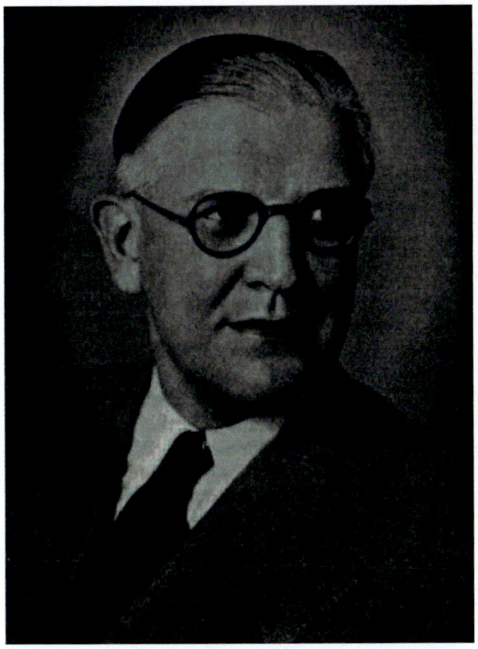

Fig. 9.10 Portrait of Sir Archibald Hector McIndoe from *British Journal of Plastic Surgery*, 1:219 © 1948 *The British Association of Plastic Surgeons*

advanced obstetrical services this consequence of obstructed labour is now thankfully uncommon.[18] However in some parts of the world it is still frequently seen in young women with a small pelvis. The pioneering work of the Hamlins at the Fistula Hospital in Addis Ababa,[19] where they have treated many cases effectively is a testament to their skill and dedication (Fig. 9.12).

Hypospadias

Hypospadias in Antiquity

The earliest reference to the commonest male malformation is in the work of Anthyllus [237], the famous Alexandrian surgeon and contemporary of Claudius Galen [353, 354].[20] Here is what he wrote "Among certain individuals the glans, because of a congenital defect, is not pierced according to nature, but the hole is found below the frenum at the termination of the glans. For this reason the man can neither urinate in front unless the penis is raised sharply toward the pubis, nor procreate children because the sperm cannot be directed in a straight line into the uterum, but [instead exits] towards the side of the vagina. Some men develop hypospadias because of an acquired defect … following an invasive ulceration or some other circumstances. Sometimes the hole is situated far from the frenum. These cases are incurable."

Anthyllus was the first to operate in some fashion on the distal malformation. The method which he proposed, although extremely painful and in reality only applicable to the glandular and very distal forms of hypospadias, certainly resolved some of the functional impediments to normal urination and ejaculation. The patient had to undergo amputation of the glans or at least that section of the penis distal to the abnormally positioned meatus, so that the end of the urethra reached the apex of the shaft, Anthyllus recommending that whenever possible the amputation should be carried out at the level of the glans, where bleeding could be more easily controlled by the application of a tightly strapped bandage soaked in

18 See Chapter 2. James M Sims was invited to Europe to describe his method of repair.

19 The Fistula Hospital in Addis Ababa was founded in 1974 by the Australian husband and wife team Reginald and Catherine Hamlin. Over the years they treated numerous unfortunate women, several of who continued to work at the hospital.

20 In his works Paulus Aegineta cites various operations conceived by Anthyllus (see *The Seven Books of Paulus Aegineta*, translated by Francis Adam, Sydhenham Society, London 1847). According to Choulant (*Handbuch der Bücherkunde für die Ältere Medicin*, Leipzig, 1841) the only edition of the works of Anthyllus extant is *Antylli Veteris Chirurgi*, Praeside Curtis Sprengel exhibit. Paniota Nicolaides (Halis, Magdeburgis, 1799), but this is not entirely accurate because other translations can be found, for example in Christian Frid de Mathaei XXI *Veterum et Clarorum Medicorum Grecorum Varia Opuscola* published in Moscow in 1898.

21 Anthyllus, like his contemporary Heliodorus, another surgeon from Alexandria, described retrovesical, retrovaginal and scrotal fistulae, phimosis, adhesion of the prepuce to the glans, preputial gangrene, and preputial fissures. He treated urethral stenosis by dilatation and re-canalization. A tube of either tin or bronze was used to keep the urethra open until the healing process was complete.

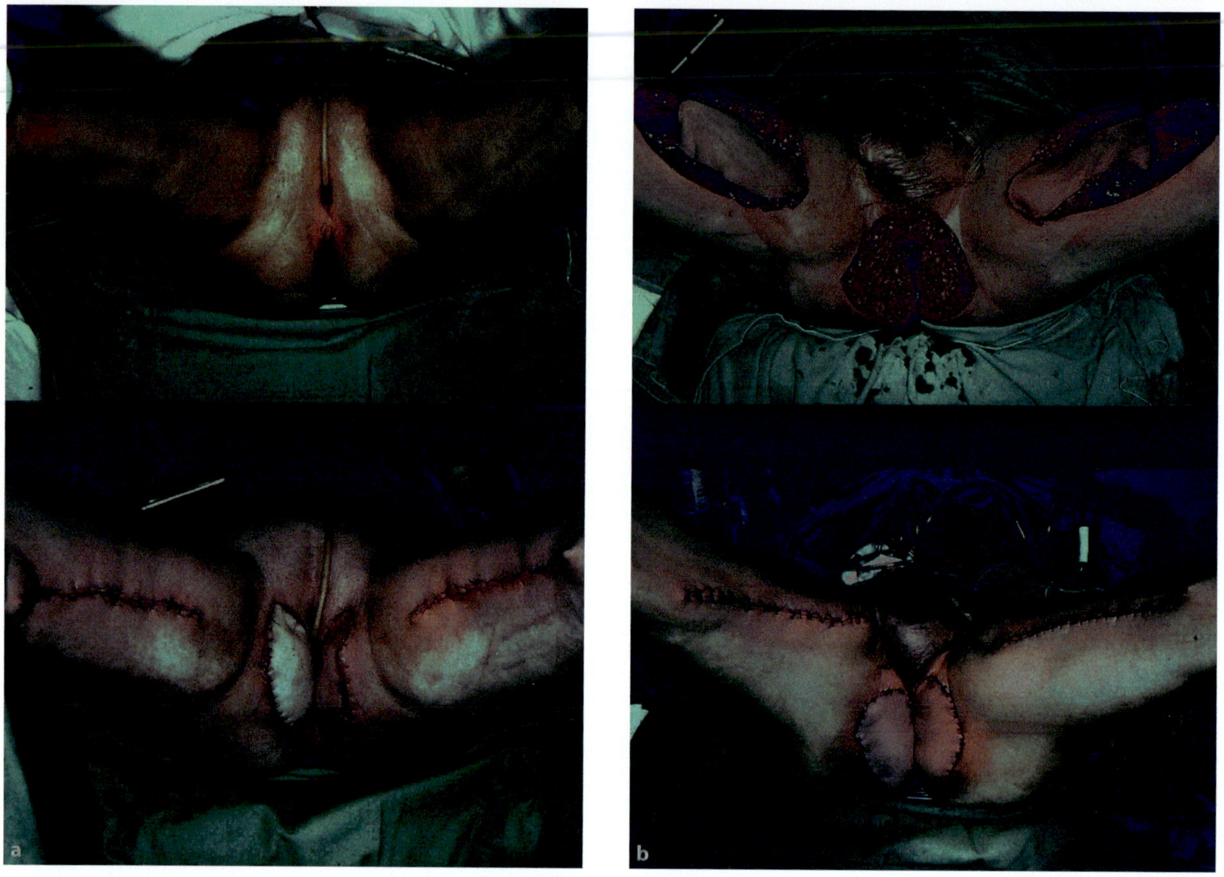

Fig. 9.11a–d Vaginal reconstruction following surgery and radiotherapy with gracilis myocutaneous flaps. *PJS*

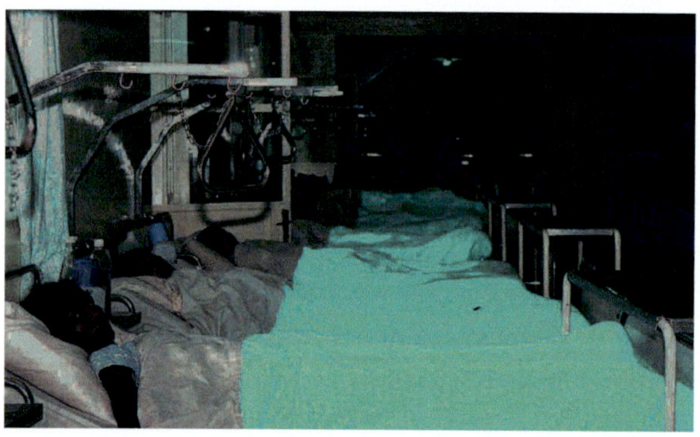

Fig. 9.12 Patients in the Fistula Hospital Addis Ababa. *© WHO/Virot*

water and vinegar.[21] The surgeon believed that cautery should only be used for the most difficult cases when absolutely necessary. Furthermore he observed: "It is necessary to understand why the resection does not pose an obstacle to reproduction: during coitus the glans does not encounter the orifice of the uterus, but the coupling takes place in the vagina, and the 'snout of the tench' being open, the sperm is directed into the uterus, whether the penis is large or small."

Despite the crude simplicity of this procedure, Anthyllus was concerned about the aesthetic outcome and in order to obtain more satisfactory results recommended that a curvilinear resection be carried out, conserving if possible a small portion of the glans, and carefully sculpting a rounded apex.

Hypospadias in the Middle Ages and the Renaissance

During the Byzantine period works by such authors as Oribasius Sardiani (325–403 A.D.) [754–757], Alexander of Tralles (525–605 A.D.), Paulus Aegineta of Alexandria (625–690 A.D.) [427] and others [988] preserved classical knowledge. In 640 A.D. Aegineta compiled a medical treatise in six volumes,[22] one of which was devoted to surgery. In it there is an excellent description of hypospadias. The works of Aegineta and Albucasis are mentioned in the book of Fabricius ab Aquapendente *Le Opere Chirurgiche* [290–293]. The Italian text describes the method of Anthyllus for hypospadias repair almost exactly (Fig. 9.13).

The surgeon Abul Qasim Albucasis of Córdoba (936–1013) was as important to the history of surgery as Avicenna was to medicine [14–18]. Like most Arab surgeons he preferred the technique of cauterization, but for delicate operations such as those on the urethra he used a very fine knife of his own design that he called a "bistoury". His technique for the correction of hypospadias was clearly based on the recommendations of Anthyllus and Heliodorus: "There are other cases in which the urinary meatus is not situated in its natural site at the apex of the glans. The surgical method [to treat this] is the following. Hold the glans firmly in your left hand; then cut the head of the glans at the eminence with a bistoury, as if you were cutting a quill or wanted to carve a piece of wood, in such a manner as to re-establish the natural shape of the glans, and in which the meatus falls into a median position where it should be. Take care during the operation against haemorrhage which happens frequently." Charaf-ed-Din, whose surgical treatise of around 1300 A.D. includes genital conditions, makes no attempt to describe reconstructive methods (Fig. 9.14).

Despite the impressive advances made by surgeons in other areas, by the end of the Middle Ages the only procedure available for the treatment of hypospadias was the one proposed by Anthyllus in the second century A.D. for the distal form of the anomaly. However, during the sixteenth century the situation began to change. New methods were introduced by Ambroise Paré, the barber surgeon who first established his reputation on the battlefield [768–770]. The following, somewhat ingenuous passage reflects his modest beginnings, although it must be admitted that many of the misconceptions expressed still linger today: "Those whose testicles are more hot are prompt to venery, and have their privities and the adjacent parts very hairy, and besides their testicles are more large and compact. Those on the contrary that have them cold are slow to venery, neither doe they beget many children, and those they get are rather female than male, their privities have little hair upon them, and their testicles are small, soft and flat."[23] Paré continues: "The action of the testicles is to generate seede, to corroborate all the parts of the body, and by a certain manly irradiation to breed or encreate a true masculine courage!"[24] In his description of the penis he observes that "The yarde is a ligament substance because it hath its origine from bones[25] and it is of an indifferente magnitude in all dimensions, yet in some bigger, in some lesse: the figure of it is round, but somewhat flattened above and beneath." (Fig. 9.15)

When Paré focuses on the practical problems of surgery, however, we immediately recognize the clear, authoritative voice of the experienced surgeon. He was, for example, the first to describe the condition of recurvatum (chordee) and suggest how it might be treated: "The band of the ligament of the yarde is too short so that the yarde cannot stand straight but is crooked, and it were turned downwards; in these cases the generation of children is hindered, because the seed cannot be cast directly and plentifully into the wombe. Therefore this ligament must be removed with much dexterity."[26]

In this period, after centuries of stasis during which the sole remedy for hypospadias was that of Anthyllus,

22 A French edition of the treatise by Aegineta was published in Lyon in 1540, while a Latin translation appeared in Basel in 1553.

23 See *De l'Anatomie de Tout le Corp Humain*, Chapter XXVIII.

24 *Idem*, Chapter XXXII.

25 One wonders whether Paré was aware of the not uncommon condition of heterotopic ossification in dogs.

26 Paré's description of the female pudendum, while quite detailed, is not much different from that of the Arabs and betrays a certain aversion towards the female genitalia. When writing about the clitoris he cites a description by Columbus, who called it the *tentigo* and another description by Fallopius, who called it "the clitoris ... whence procedes that infamous word 'Cleitorinzein', which signifies 'impudently to handle that part'."

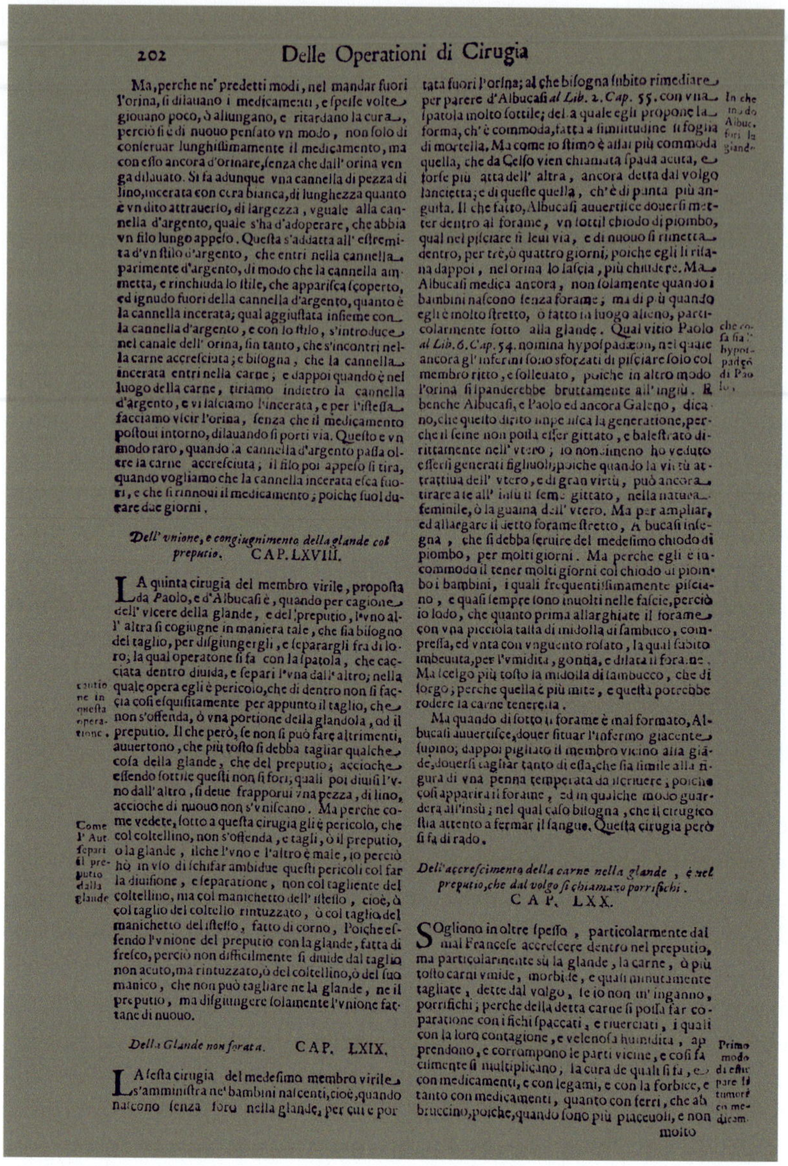

202 Delle Operationi di Cirugia

Ma, perche ne' predetti modi, nel mandar fuori l'orina, ſi dilauano i medicamenti, e ſpeſſe volte giouano poco, ò allungano, e ritardano la cura, perciò ſi è di nuouo penſato vn modo, non ſolo di conſeruar lunghiſſimamente il medicamento, ma con eſſo ancora d'orinare, ſenza che dall'orina venga dilauato. Si fa adunque vna cannella di pezza di lino, incerata con cera bianca, di lunghezza quanto è vn dito attrauerſo, di largezza, vguale alla cannella d'argento, quale s'ha d'adoperare, che abbia vn filo lungo appeſo. Queſta s'addatta all'eſtremità d'vn ſtilo d'argento, che entri nella cannella parimente d'argento, di modo che la cannella ammetta, e rinchiuda lo ſtile, che apparisca ſcoperto, ed ignudo fuori della cannella d'argento, quanto è la cannella incerata; qual aggiuſtata inſieme con la cannella d'argento, e con lo ſtilo, s'introduce nel canale dell'orina, ſin tanto, che s'incontri nella carne accreſciuta; e biſogna, che la cannella incerata entri nella carne; e dappoi quando è nel luogo della carne, tiriamo indietro la cannella d'argento, e vi laſciamo l'incerata, e per l'iſteſſa facciamo vſcir l'orina, ſenza che il medicamento poſtoui intorno, dilauando ſi porti via. Queſto e vn modo raro, quando la cannella d'argento paſſa oltre la carne accreſciuta; il filo poi appeſo ſi tira, quando vogliamo che la cannella incerata eſca fuori, e che ſi rinnoui il medicamento; poiche ſuol durare due giorni.

Dell'vnione, e congiugnimento della glande col preputio. CAP. LXVIII.

LA quinta cirugia del membro virile, propoſta da *Paolo*, e d'Albucaſi è, quando per cagione dell'vlcere della glande, e del preputio, l'vno all'altra ſi cogiugne in maniera tale, che ſia biſogno del taglio, per diſgiungergli, e ſepararglì fra di loro; la qual operatone ſi fa con la ſpatola, che cacciata dentro diuida, e ſepari l'vna dall'altro; nella quale opera egli è pericolo, che di dentro non ſi faccia coſi eſquiſitamente per appunto il taglio, che non s'offenda, ò vna portione della glandola, od il preputio. Il che però, ſe non ſi può fare altrimenti, auuertono, che più toſto ſi debba tagliar qualche coſa della glande, che del preputio; accioche eſſendo ſottile queſti non ſi fori, quali poi diuiſi l'vno dall'altro, ſi deue frapporui vna pezza, di lino, accioche di nuouo non s'vniſcano. Ma perche come vedete, ſotto a queſta cirugia gli è pericolo, che col coltellino, non s'offenda, e tagli, ò il preputio, o la glande, il che l'vno e l'altro è male, io perciò hò in vſo di ſchifar ambidue queſti pericoli col far la diuiſione, e ſeparatione, non col tagliente del coltellino, ma col manichetto dell'iſteſſo, cioè, ò col taglio del coltello rintuzzato, ò col taglio del manichetto del iſteſſo, fatto di corno, Poiche eſſendo l'vnione del preputio con la glande, fatta di freſco, perciò non difficilmente ſi diuide dal taglio non acuto, ma rintuzzato, ò del coltellino, ò del ſuo manico, che non può tagliare ne la glande, ne il preputio, ma diſgiungere ſolamente l'vnione fattane di nuouo.

Cautione in queſta operatione.

Come l'Aut. ſepari il preputio dalla glande

Della Glande non forata. CAP. LXIX.

LA ſeſta cirugia del medeſimo membro virile s'amminiſtra ne' bambini naſcenti, cioè, quando naſcono ſenza foro nella glande, per cui e portata fuori l'orina; al che biſogna ſubito rimediare per parere d'Albucaſi *al Lib. 2. Cap. 55.* con vna ſpatola molto ſottile; della quale egli propone la forma, ch'è commoda, fatta a ſimilitudine di foglia di mortella. Ma come io ſtimo è aſſai più commoda quella, che da Celſo vien chiamata ſpada acuta, e forſe più atta dell'altra, ancora detta dal volgo lancietta; e di queſte quella, ch'è di punta più anguſta. Il che fatto, Albucaſi auuertiſce douerſi metter dentro al forame, vn ſottil chiodo di piombo, qual nel piſciare ſi leui via, e di nuouo ſi rimetta dentro, per trè, ò quattro giorni; poiche egli li riſana dappoi, nel orina lo laſcia, più chiudere. Ma Albucaſi medica ancora, non ſolamente quando i bambini naſcono ſenza forame; ma di più quando egli è molto ſtretto, ò fatto in luogo alieno, particolarmente ſotto alla glande. Qual vitio Paolo *al Lib. 6. Cap. 54.* nomina hypoſpadiæon, nel quale ancora gl'infermi ſono sforzati di piſciare ſolo col membro ritto, e ſolleuato, poiche in altro modo l'orina ſi ſpanderebbe bruttamente all'ingiù. E benche Albucaſi, e Paolo ed ancora Galeno, dicano, che queſto diritto impediſca la generatione, perche il ſeme non poſſa eſſer gittato, e baleſtrato dirittamente nell'vtero; io nondimeno ho veduto eſſerſi generati figliuoli; poiche quando la virtù attrattiua dell'vtero, e di gran virtù, può ancora tirare a ſe all'inſù il ſeme gittato, nella natura feminile, ò la guaina dell'vtero. Ma per ampliar, ed allargare il detto forame ſtretto, Albucaſi inſegna, che ſi debba ſeruire del medeſimo chiodo di piombo, per molti giorni. Ma perche egli è incommodo il tener molti giorni col chiodo di piombo i bambini, i quali frequentiſſimamente piſciano, e quaſi ſempre ſono inuolti nelle faſcie, perciò io lodo, che quanto prima allarghiate il forame con vna picciola taſta di midolla di ſambuco, compreſſa, ed vnta con vnguento roſato, la qual ſubito imbeuuta, per l'vmidità, gonfia, e dilata il forame. Ma ſcelgo più toſto la midolla di ſambucco, che di ſorgo; perche quella è più mite, e queſta potrebbe rodere la carne tenerella.

In che modo Albuc. fori la glande

che coſa ſia l'hypoſpadçō di Paolo.

Ma quando di ſotto il forame è mal formato, Albucaſi auuertiſce, douer ſituar l'infermo giacente ſupino; dappoi pigliato il membro vicino alla giãde, douerſi tagliar tanto di eſſa, che ſia ſimile alla figura di vna penna temperata da ſcriuere; poiche coſi apparirà il forame, ed in qualche modo guarderà all'insù; nel qual caſo biſogna, che il cirugico ſtia attento a fermar il ſangue. Queſta cirugia però ſi fa di rado.

Dell'accreſcimento della carne nella glande, è nel preputio, che dal volgo ſi chiamano porrifichi. CAP. LXX.

SOgliono inoltre ſpeſſo, particolarmente dal mal Franceſe accreſcere dentro nel preputio, ma particolarmente sù la glande, la carne, ò più toſto carni vmide, morbide, e quaſi minutamente tagliate, dette dal volgo, ſe io non m'inganno, porrifichi; perche della detta carne ſi poſſa far comparatione con i fichi ſpaccati, e riuerciati, i quali con la loro contagione, e velenoſa humidità, apprendono, e corrompono le parti vicine, e coſi facilmente ſi multiplicano; la cura de quali ſi fa, e con medicamenti, e con legami, e con la forbice, e tanto con medicamenti, quanto con ferri, che abbruccino, poiche, quando ſono più piaceuoli, e non molto

Primo modo di eſtirpare il tumore cō medicam.

Fig. 9.13 A page from *Le Opere Chirurgiche* by Fabricius where he describes the treatment of hypospadias by the method used by Anthyllus several centuries before. *Courtesy of Riccardo Mazzola, M.D., Milan*

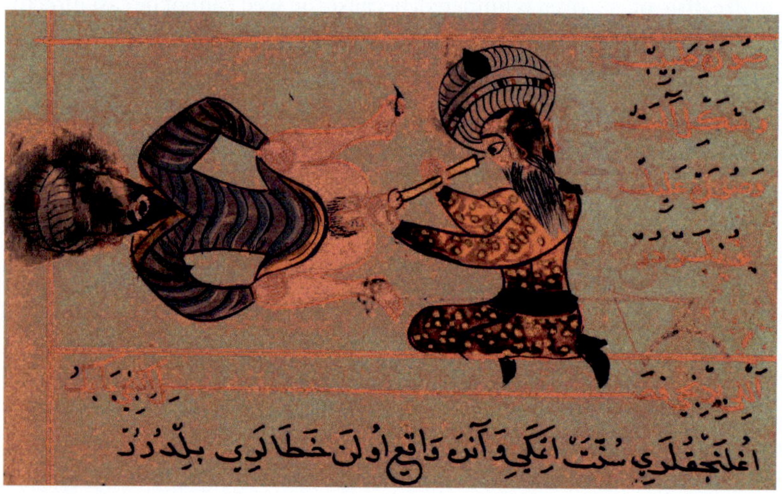

Fig. 9.14 Inspection of the male urethra, 1466 by Charaf-ed-Din (1404–1468). *Bibliotheque Nationale, Paris, France, Archives Charmet / The Bridgeman Art Library*

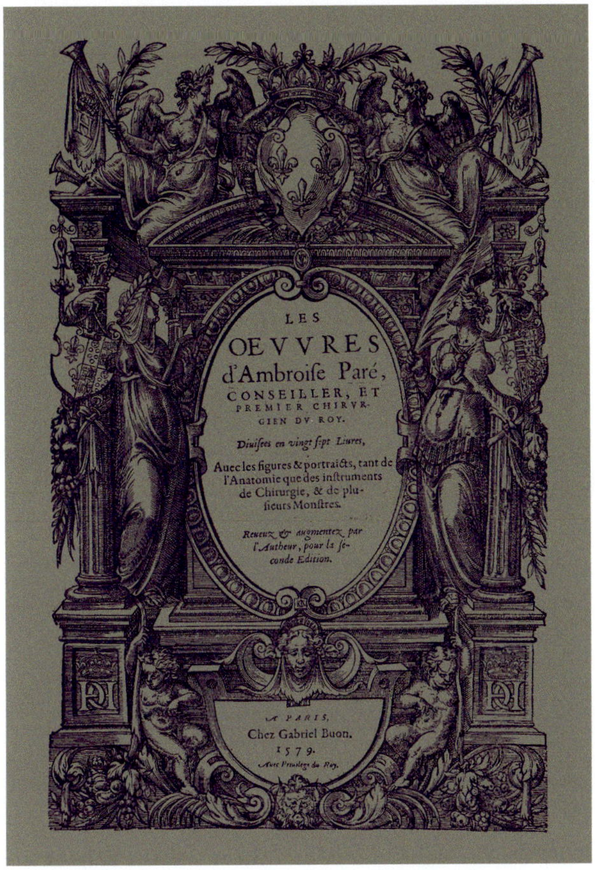

Fig. 9.15 Frontispiece of Paré's masterpiece *Les Oeuvres* where there is a comprehensive section on urology. *Courtesy of Riccardo Mazzola, M.D., Milan*

a Portuguese surgeon who had studied medicine at the Spanish University of Salamanca, Amatus Lusitanus (1511–1561), proposed a radically new approach. This consisted of extending the urethral canal by passing a trocar through the shaft from the abnormal meatus to the glans. However dubious and painful this method may seem to us today, at least it represented the first effort by a courageous surgeon (and patient!) to resolve the condition of proximal hypospadias. For the next two centuries this would remain the only alternative to Anthyllus' procedure, and the only option for the treatment of proximal hypospadias.[27]

The Eighteenth Century: First Attempts at Classification

The mystery that had surrounded the problem of congenital malformations and hampered progress in their treatment began to subside as scientific curiosity led researchers to conduct detailed studies on many anomalies. These in turn enabled surgeons to resolve some of the problems associated with hypospadias, although the reconstruction of a functioning urethra remained being an unattainable goal.

In a text published in 1710 the surgeon Dionis discussed many types of congenital malformations, focusing, like Paré, on the condition of chordee: "There are some who are born with the bridle of their yeard too short. This 'frenum' draws the glans downward, particularly at the time of erection: whence the aperture being at that time too low, if the yeard be not rei'd, the person will piss on his legs or feet, and 'twill be impossible for the seed to be darted directly into the matrix, whence the generalized way will be obstructed." The remedy he suggested was to cut "the bridle across in the same manner that we do the string under the tongue" [248, 249].

Heister, one of the greatest surgeons of the nineteenth century and the author of a textbook that was translated into many languages, also studied the condition of hypospadias, which he called "the imperforated glans". He adopted the procedure of Lusitanus, reconstructing the urethra using a trocar. In contrast, his treatment for chordee was quite conservative; unlike Paré and Dionis, he did not advocate surgery but rather "the application of emollients to the contracted side of the penis, and of astringents on the other side: assisting both with a proper bandage, and sometimes by making small incisions in the integumentum of the contracted side." Heister classified the various types of hypospadias and explained the difficulties in procreation that they caused. In 1770 he published another text containing innovative contribu-

27 The method of Lusitanus was still being used three centuries later, for example by Heister in the eighteenth century, and by Dupuytren in France and Bushe in the United States in the nineteenth century.

tions in many fields, including a six-page discussion of catheterization [422–424].

The Nineteenth Century: The Birth of Reconstructive Surgery for Hypospadias

While rudimentary solutions for some aspects of hypospadias had been found, genuine progress was not made until the nineteenth century, when the entire field of surgery was revolutionized. In England, France and Germany several surgeons began to take an interest this area, and their colleagues in the United States were soon making their own contributions.

Like the early attempts at cleft palate repair, the first operations in this area were for the closure of urethral fistulas. This exercise provided surgeons with useful experience in preparation for the more complex challenge of reconstructing the missing portion of the urethra. Up to this time the closure of fistulas had been achieved by incising and approximating their margins using a scalpel. More often, cautery with chemicals, such as nitric acid was used. This stimulated granulation tissue, fibrosis and scarring with eventual stenosis or even closure of the smallest fistulas. However, for large holes or those located in inaccessible sites, the method was rarely successful and surgeons began to consider how these defects might be closed surgically (Fig. 9.16).

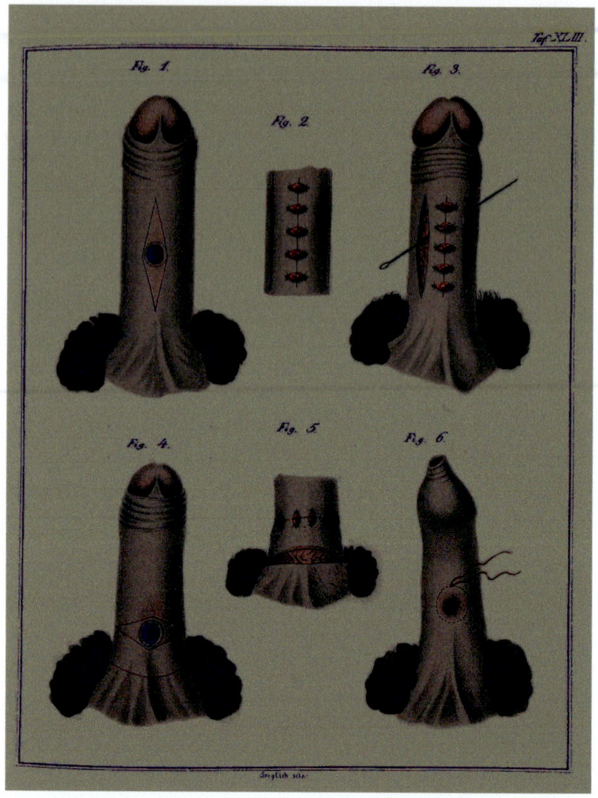

Fig. 9.16 The repair of urethral fistulae was the only reconstructive surgery attempted in the nineteenth century. An illustration of one of Dieffenbach's methods from Fritz and Reich's book *Die Plastische Chirurgie* (1845). *Courtesy of Riccardo Mazzola, M.D., Milan*

In 1819 Sir Astley Cooper (1768–1841) and B. Travers (1783–1858) [197] in a moment of inspiration devised a solution that would change the approach radically (Fig. 9.17). In a 59-year-old patient suffering from a large fistula at the peroneo-scrotal junction they used a skin flap, outside the face, for the first time. This was rotated from the scrotum to cover the defect and fixed in place with a few stitches. They then inserted a catheter, leaving it in place for about one month. This operation proved a success, and was repeated in the same year by Henry Earle [270], head of the surgical ward at Bartholomew's Hospital in London. Many surgeons in other countries copied the procedure and within a few years good results were being reported [20, 243, 279]. Surgeons were beginning to grasp the advantages of the skin flap (Fig. 9.18).

While the treatment of fistulas was relatively straightforward, a true reconstruction of the urethra was not yet possible. It must be remembered that anaesthesia did not yet exist, although surgeons, particularly in the United States, did not hesitate to carry out certain traditional operations such as Lusitanus' procedure for attempting to recreate the urethra. In Europe the surgical treatment of hypospadias was viewed by such figures as Malgaigne, Boyer and Dieffenbach with a distinct lack of enthusiasm. Understandably, most surgeons and their patients were discouraged by the fact that the outcome of this painful procedure was often unsatisfactory due to complications and as a result we find only scattered reports of such operations being carried out.

This pessimism does not appear to have affected surgeons on the other side of the Atlantic. In 1831 George McArtney Bushe of New York (1793–1856) published a report describing five operations carried out on patients with scrotal hypospadias [148]. He adopted the tech-

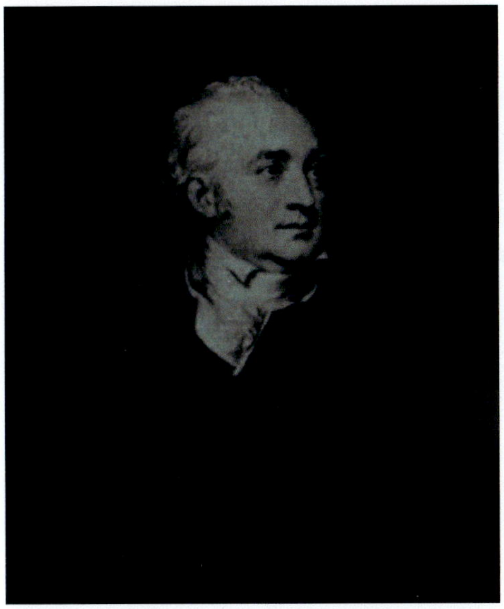

Fig. 9.17 Portrait of Sir Astley Cooper who used the first flap outside the face to close a urethral fistula in 1819. *Courtesy of FMR Art.spa. Bologna*

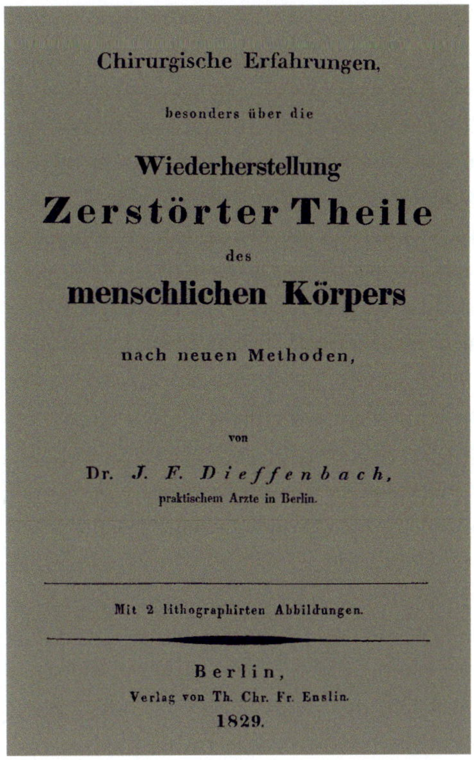

Chirurgische Erfahrungen,

besonders über die

Wiederherstellung

Zerstörter Theile

des

menschlichen Körpers

nach neuen Methoden,

von

Dr. J. F. Dieffenbach,

praktischem Arzte in Berlin.

Mit 2 lithographirten Abbildungen.

Berlin,

Verlag von Th. Chr. Fr. Enslin.

1829.

Fig. 9.18 Frontispiece of Dieffenbach's book *Wiederherstellung Zerstörter Theile des Menschlichen Körpers* (1829). He was one of the first, after Paré, to correct chordee. *Courtesy of Riccardo Mazzola, M. D., Milan*

nique of Lusitanus, afterwards dilating the new urethra repeatedly to avoid stenosis, and finally cauterizing the original hypospadic meatus as suggested by Dupuytren. He claimed that all five patients had a good outcome, and that "afterwards [one of his patients] successfully exercised his procreative powers, and [another] enlisted in the army and had a normal career". J.P. Mettauer [449, 663] in 1842 and Joseph Pancoast (1805–1882) [763] built upon Bushe's work, successfully treating cases of epispadias as well as hypospadias. In his paper Mettauer noted that "this mode of operating has been in use by us for over twelve years," that is, forty-four years before the first successful case reported in Europe.[28] The technique itself was nothing more than a variant on the procedure developed by Lusitanus three centuries earlier. After extending the urethra using a trocar, Mettauer left a rubber catheter in situ for several days, and then made certain that for a considerable period afterwards the patient dilated the new urethra three or four times a day for at least one hour using a probe.

Mettauer's most important contribution to the study of hypospadias was his observation that the corpus spongiosum was missing distal to the meatus and was replaced with fibrous tissue producing chordee. This point had perhaps eluded Dieffenbach when in 1830 he attempted to correct this aspect of the malformation.

Pancoast recommended the technique of Lusitanus to reconstruct the urethra in cases of mid-penile hypospa-

28 According to *Morton's Medical Bibliography*, Mettauer successfully carried out the first closure of a vesico-vaginal fistula in August 1838.

dias, describing the procedure in an admirable treatise furnished with lucid illustrations, which was published in 1844 [763].

Compounding the problem of surgical correction was the fact that up to this time there was confusion regarding the true aetiology of hypospadias. Hence the term was used indiscriminately to refer to fistulas, abnormal apertures resulting from venereal disease, and other conditions. Robert Liston (1794–1847) was the first to define hypospadias as a congenitally displaced meatus in 1897 and therefore as a term appropriate only to cases of an abnormal defect present at birth [569, 570]. Liston was also probably the first surgeon in England to put into practice Sir Astley Cooper's suggestion that a portion of the urethra could be reconstructed using a preputial flap sutured around a catheter.

Thanks to the development of anaesthesia, during the second half of the nineteenth century, surgeons could finally attempt reconstruction of the urethra. The first to do so was probably Theophile Anger, who presented a paper describing his treatment of a case of a peno-scrotal hypospadias to the Societé de Chirurgie de Paris on 21 August 1874 (Fig. 9.19) [27, 28]. He made two parallel incisions along the axis of the penis from the point of the hypospadic meatus down to the glans and sutured the margins in such a way as to create an extension of the existing urethra. The resulting cutaneous defect was closed by undermining the margins to obtain two advancement flaps. As he noted, it was crucial that this suture line should not coincide with that of the underlying new urethra in order to avoid, or at least reduce, the risk of fistulas. This was a milestone, for it was the first time an attempt had been made to reconstruct a urethra lined with skin. Other surgeons, such as G. Novè-Josserand [739, 740] and L. Ombrédanne [751, 752] in France, quickly followed suit and introduced further improvements. Anger's technique remained the treatment of choice for the next 120 years.

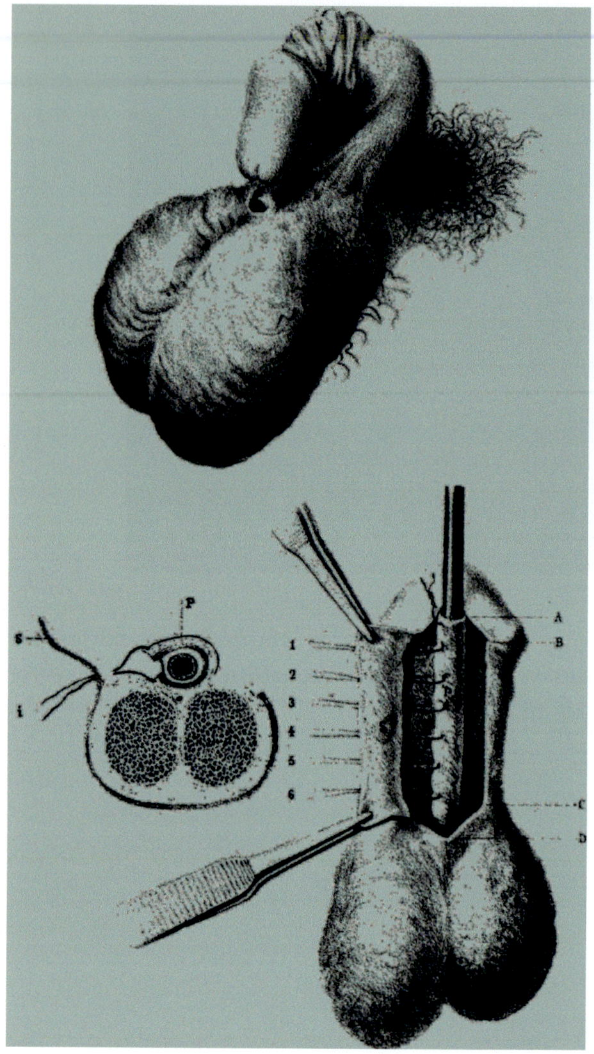

Fig. 9.19 Anger's correction of peno-scrotal hypospadias from 1874. After correction of the chordee he reconstructed the urethral tube using Thiersch's method employed in epispadias. A turnover flap of penile skin is tubed over a catheter and covered with shaft skin from one side. The suture lines were off set. *From Anger* [28]

Simon Duplay (1836–1924) another French surgeon inspired by the method used by Thiersch for epispadias [982] showed that it was not necessary to construct a tube in order to extend the urethra [264]. It was sufficient to leave the skin strip buried beneath the lateral flaps where it tended to form a tube spontaneously. All these methods relied on catheterization for varying periods once the new urethra was joined up. Duplay developed an elegant reconstruction procedure consisting of three phases. At the first step he corrected the chordee and created a urethral tube in the glans by burying a strip of cutaneous tissue and suturing the edges over it. As a second step he cut a strip of skin extending from the meatus to the glans with parallel incisions along the underside of the penile shaft but instead of suturing the margins to create a tube, he simply covered it, as Angier had done, with two lateral advancement flaps. The strip

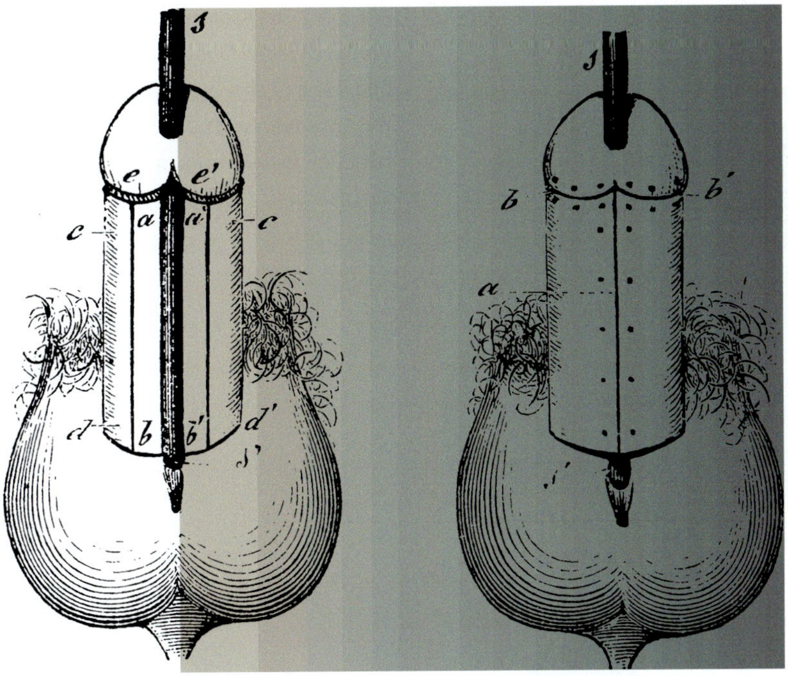

Fig. 9.20 Duplay corrected the chordee using a vertical diamond-shaped excision leaving a midline longitudinal scar and made a glandular meatus at the first stage. He later reconstructed the urethra by burying a skin strip beneath lateral advancement flaps. *From Duplay* [264]

of skin would tube itself spontaneously into an epithelial canal. In the third operation this new urethra was connected with the portion running through the glans that had been constructed in the first step (Fig. 9.20). Byars (Blair) in 1938 [107] reintroduced a modification and made a urethral tube. As with other methods the first stage was correction of the chordee which had already been recognized as an essential step in reconstruction. The suture line of the urethral repair corresponded to the skin closure with the subsequent increased risk of fistula formation (Fig. 9.21).

Duplay's procedure was further modified by the English surgeon Denis Browne [133–135] who retained the buried skin strip without making a new urethral tube. He suggested that the tension in the suture line of the advancement flaps might be lessened by the use of interrupted sutures, which he passed through the flaps and held with "beads and stops", the latter made of lead which were crushed to prevent the beads from slipping. The closure was completed by means of a fine continuous suture of the relaxed margins. The repair was protected by an indwelling perineal catheter and a dorsal relaxing incision was made (Fig. 9.22).

Cecil had his own way of compensating for shortage of ventral penile skin [166]. At the second stage he buried the penile shaft in the scrotum thus covering the new urethral tube. This necessitated a third operation to complete the reconstruction (Fig. 9.23). His technique was later modified by Culp [210].

When skin grafts was invented during the second half of the nineteenth century surgeons hoped that they might be used to line the new urethra. The first to attempt this was G. Novè-Josserand [739, 740] in 1897. He sutured a thin skin graft around a catheter that was then introduced using a cannula passed through a tunnel from the meatus to the glans. The results of this operation were often marred by the formation of scarring and stenoses around the graft. McIndoe tried to improve the procedure by suturing the graft around a catheter, which was then passed through the penis using a sophisticated instrument consisting of a trocar with a detachable tip. His technique employed a thicker split graft that was no less prone to strictures and was soon abandoned [643]. Much later and outside timescale of this book, the use of full thickness grafts from the prepuce combined with local flaps met with more success in the hands of such surgeons as Horton and Devine for more proximal hypospadias.

A significant modification was introduced by Louis Ombrédanne (1871–1956), in 1911 when he used a flap

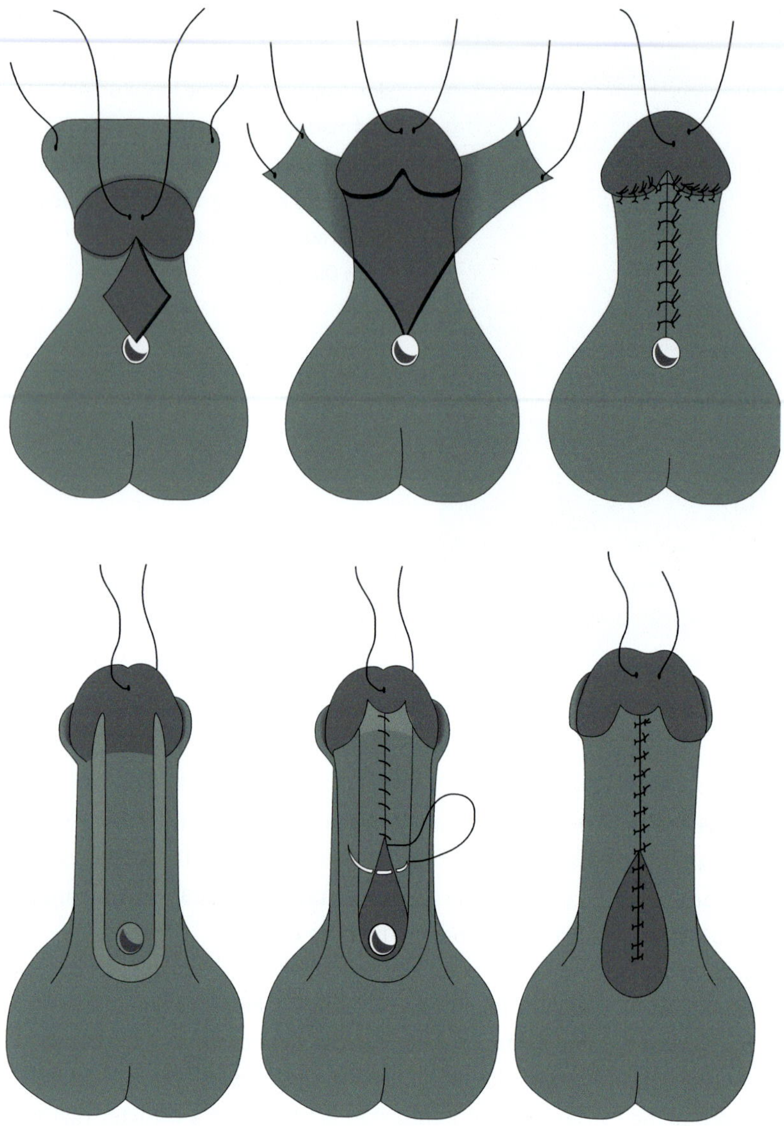

Fig. 9.21 The Byars method. Correction of chordee (*above*) which was the first stage of all the procedures used at the time, followed by urethral reconstruction (*below*) using a tube of skin. Fistulae were a problem. *PJS*

of penile skin based just proximally to the abnormal meatus to reconstruct the urethral tube (Fig. 9.24). This in turn was covered with a bipedicle flap obtained from the lining of prepuce, in which a buttonhole was made to accommodate the glans [751, 752]. Like his predecessors Ombrédanne made certain that the sutures of the inner lining and outer cover were sufficiently separated to avoid the formation of fistulas. His technique was widely adopted and further improved by other surgeons (Figs. 9.25, 9.26a,b).[29]

Until quite recently most urethral reconstructions were carried out in two steps—the first to correct the chordee and the second to reconstruct the urethra—because this seemed to be the best way to avoid the most troublesome complication of fistula formation. There has been a move in recent years to complete the repair in one operation but we will not embark on this development here.

We have made no mention of the much rarer condition of epispadias in other than a passing manner. The infrequency of this condition and its relationship with

29 Thomas Pomfret Kilner (one of the Big Four) used the technique. He was Nuffield Professor of Plastic Surgery in Oxford and Stoke Mandeville Hospital, Aylesbury having worked with Gillies at Sidcup in World War I. See obituary in *Ann R Coll Surg Engl* (1964) 35:251 and memoire in *Ann Plast Surg* (1980) 4:328.

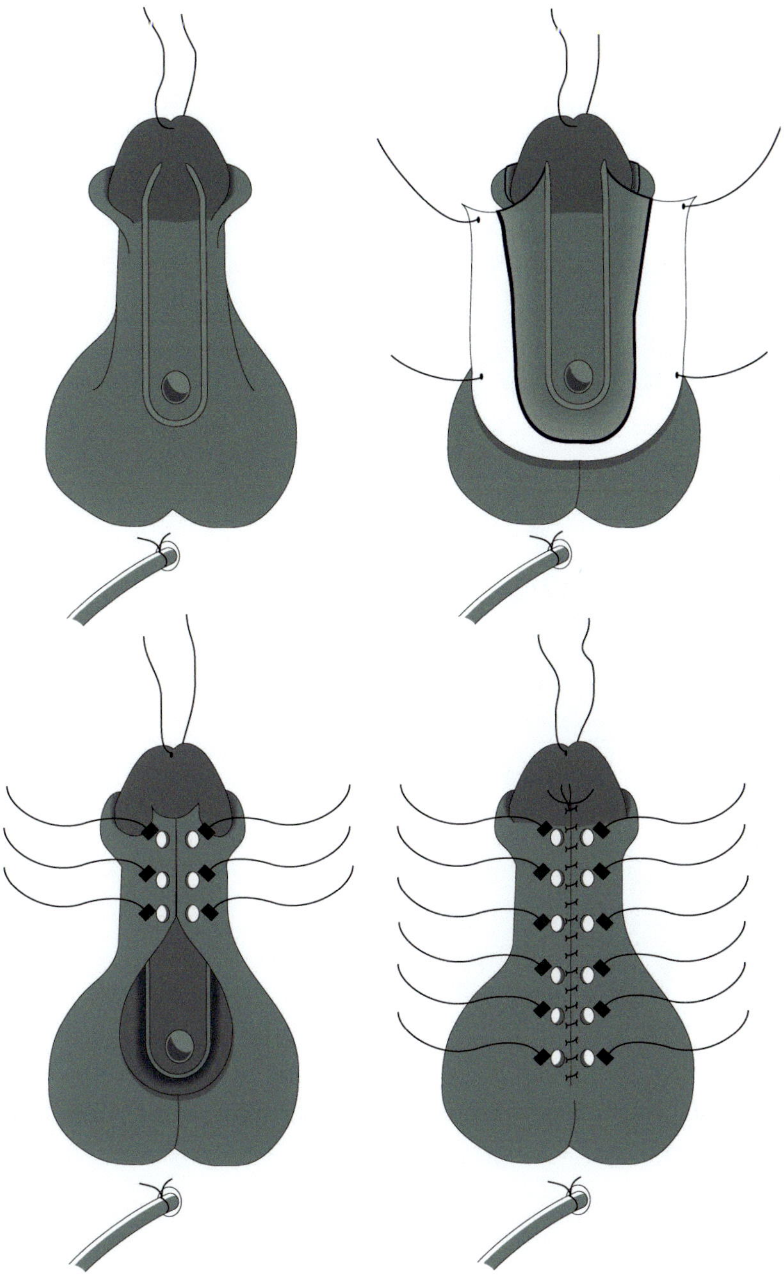

Fig. 9.22 Denis Browne used a buried skin strip to reconstruct the urethra and overcame the shortage of skin noted in other methods. The repair was protected by a urethrostomy and tension reduced with "beads and stops" together with a dorsal relaxing incision on the penile shaft. *PJS*

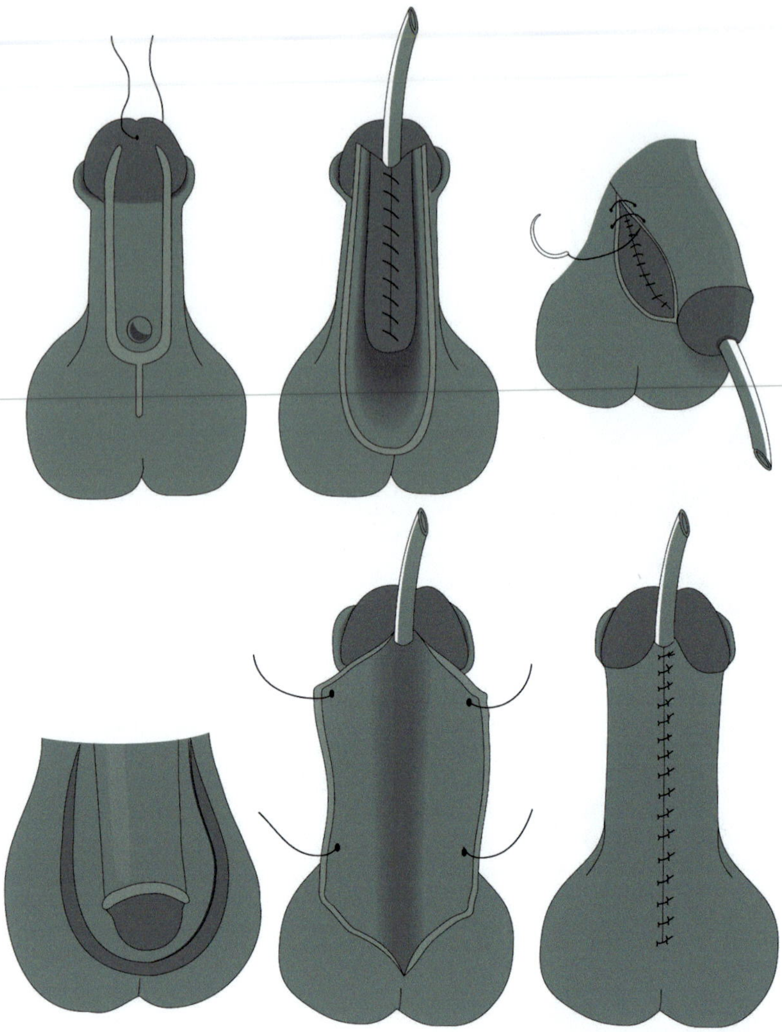

Fig. 9.23 Cecil introduced his method in the 1940s and after correcting the chordee used scrotal skin to cover the urethral tube (*top*), necessitating a third operation (*bottom*). *PJS*

exstrophy of the bladder mean that it is now treated in specialized centres by paediatric urologists but the techniques described in former years for urethral reconstruction in hypospadias were used by some of the old masters in epispadias [982].

It is impossible in this chapter to describe all the techniques and modifications of old methods that have been recommended by their inventors. Even since Horton published his book *Plastic and Reconstructive Surgery in the Genital Region* in 1973 (see Recommended Reading) the methods described in the first historical chapter by B. O. Rogers have increased greatly in number. Many of these have not yet stood the test of time so are not mentioned here. The choice of surgical techniques is numerous and surgeons will wisely persist with the one that gives them the best results.

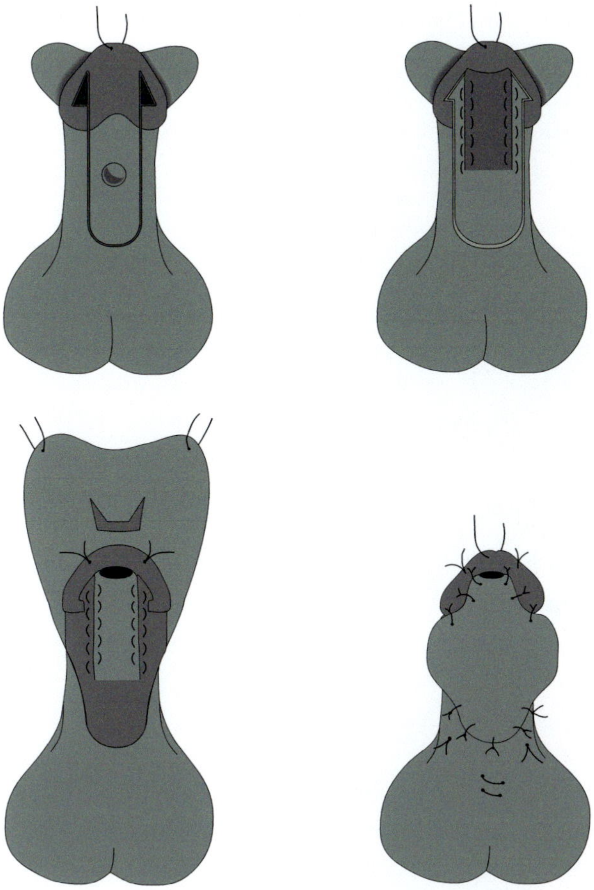

Fig. 9.24 A sketch of Ombrédanne's operation for the repair of distal hypospadias. The technique used prepucial skin and was modified by several surgeons. This shows Kilner's method. *PJS*

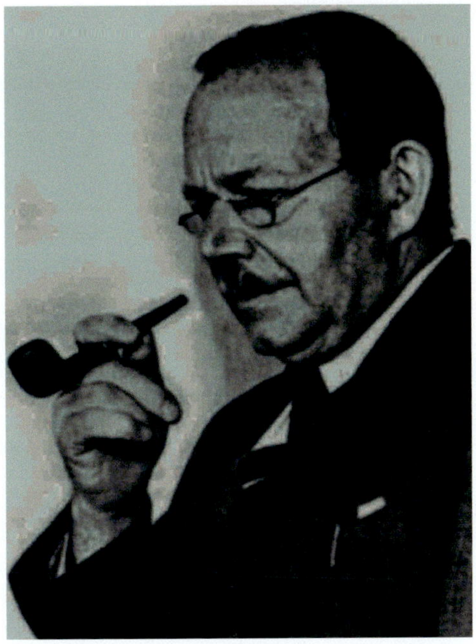

Fig. 9.25 Thomas Pomfret Kilner (1890–1964), Nuffield Professor of Plastic Surgery, Oxford. *Courtesy of The British Association of Plastic Reconstructive and Aesthetic Surgeons*

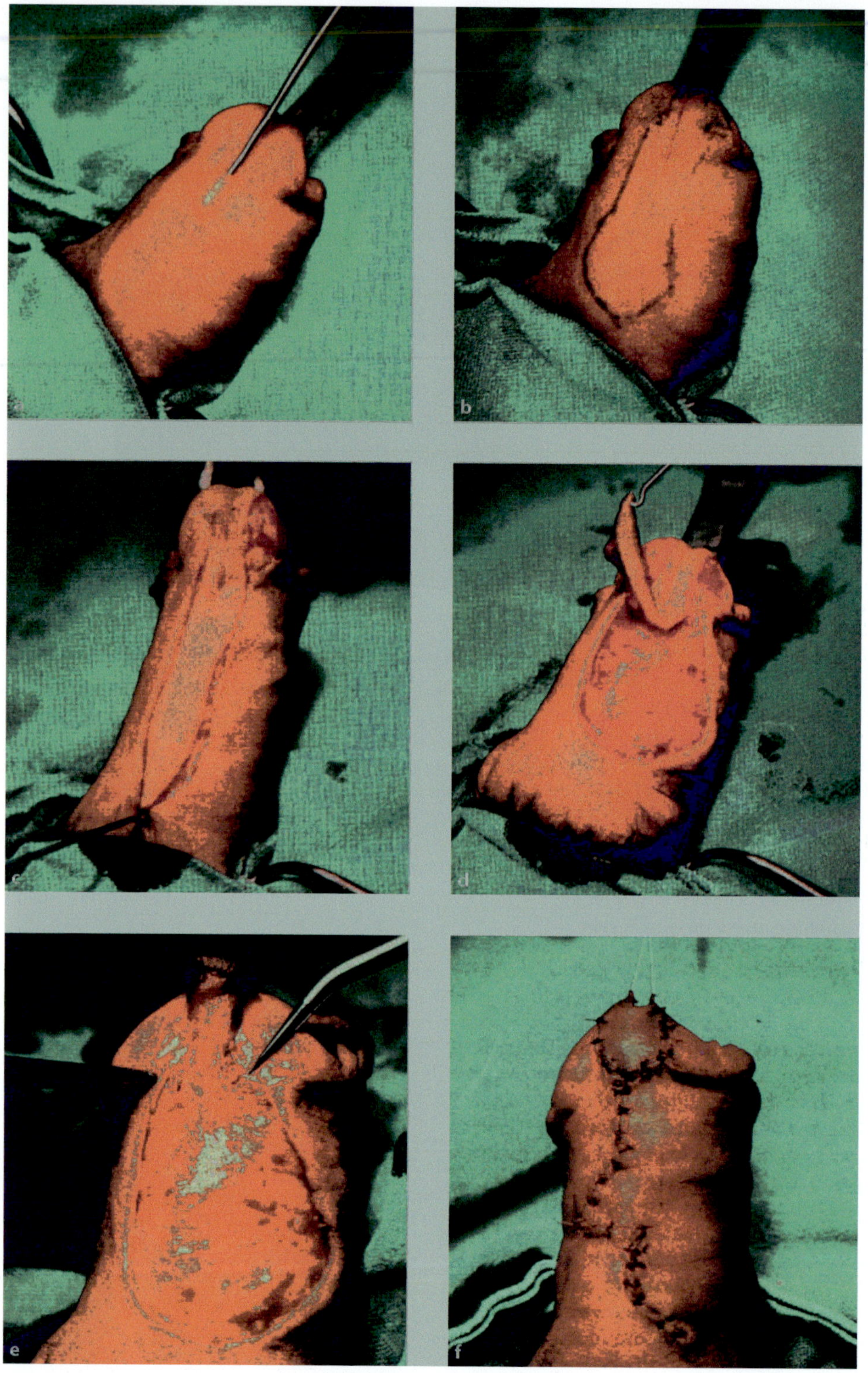

Fig. 9.26a–f Another modification of the Ombrédanne method for the repair of distal hypospadias. *PSR*

Chapter 10

Ear Reconstruction

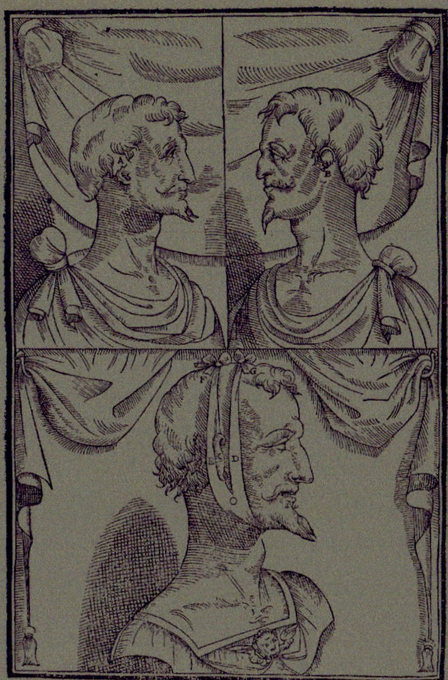

Contents

Ear Reconstruction After Trauma

In ancient times, reconstruction of the ear, or at least part of the auricle, rivalled with that of the nose, though probably it was performed less frequently.

The first report of an otoplasty appears in the *Samita* written before the sixth century B.C. in India by Susruta who we have already encountered in rhinoplasty [90]. Dhanwantary's English translation of it reads: "... a surgeon well versed in the knowledge of surgery should slice off a patch of living flesh from the cheek of a person devoid of the ear-lobes in a manner as to have one of its ends attached to its former seat (cheek). Thus, the part where the artificial ear-lobe is to be made should be slightly scarified with a knife and the living flesh, full of blood and sliced off as previously directed, should be adhesioned to it as to resemble an ear-lobe in shape."[1]

This is the so-called *Indian advancement flap* technique that is also described in nasal reconstruction. Its importance in reconstructive surgery is shown by the fact that in 1845, some 25 centuries later, Johann Friedrich Dieffenbach (1794–1847) found nothing better than this flap for a partial reconstruction of the ear [244].

Aulus Cornelius Celsus (25 B.C. to 50 A.D.) was certainly familiar with this type of facial flap, though some doubt remains as to whether he actually used the technique for nose reconstruction. In effect, when dealing with the reconstruction of various defects of the ear,[2] Celsus specifically wrote: "... the method, when there has been some mutilation, is to patch, and since this can be done in the case of the lip and nostrils as well, and the procedure is the same, the description too should be given at the same time". Then follows a detailed description of the flap with specific mention of its use not only in the lips but "... indeed in the ear and the nostrils".[3]

There are no references to reconstruction of the ear in Egyptian medical literature, or in that handed down from the Ancient Greeks or from Alexandria; neither is there any mention in the manuscripts drawn up by the ancient Arab surgeons.

There is a gap of several centuries until ear reconstruction is mentioned again, this time by Pietro Ranzano (1442–1492) [828] and Bartolomeo Fazio (1400–1457) [304] when referring to the Branca family in fifteenth century Sicily. According to both of these authors, while the principle interest of the Branca family was reconstruction of the nose it appears certain that at least Antonio performed ear reconstruction.

Talking about Antonio Branca and the method he used for reconstructing the nose, Ranzano writes: "...not only the nostrils but the lip and the mutilated ears somehow he was able to repair". In a similar manner, Fazio praises Branca by writing: "... for he conceived how mutilated lips and ears might be restored, as well as noses". It seems certain that Antonio Branca used the brachial flap for nose and ear reconstruction.

There were other surgeons in the fifteenth and sixteenth centuries who practised nasal reconstruction, such as Benedetti, von Pfolsprundt, the Vianeo brothers and Fioravanti, but there are no reports of them having ever reconstructed ears.

This is not true of Gaspare Tagliacozzi (1545–1599) and he dedicated a whole chapter, *De curtorum aurium chirurgia* (Surgery of the mutilated ear), of his book[4] to this type of reconstruction. The chapter is particularly interesting as he does not use the arm flap and, instead, employs a local flap raised "...not from the upper arm but from the area behind the ear". Two of the plates in this chapter, numbers 21 and 22, illustrate the various stages of the reconstruction (Fig. 10.1). The case illustrated had suffered an amputation of approximately half of the ear [969]. Even though the flap is not particularly clear in the illustration, what little can be distinguished and especially the explanation in the text itself suggests a close resemblance to the flap that Dieffenbach would eventually describe in 1845. Tagliacozzi, as always, supplies an abundance of details when demonstrating how "the surgeon delineates, excises and transfers the skin". He warns readers about bleeding, pointing out that it will be copious since this particular donor area has more blood vessels than the arm, and he advises surgeons to

1 The *Samita* was translated into Latin by Frans Hessler (1799–1890) and published in five volumes at Elkangen in 1844. It was subsequently translated into English by Dhanwantary and produced in six volumes in 1909 in Calcutta.

2 See *De Medicina* Liber VII, Chapter 8, paragraph 4.

3 See *De Medicina* Liber VII, Chapter 9.

4 See *De Curtorum Chirurgia per Insitionem*, Book 2, Chapter 20.

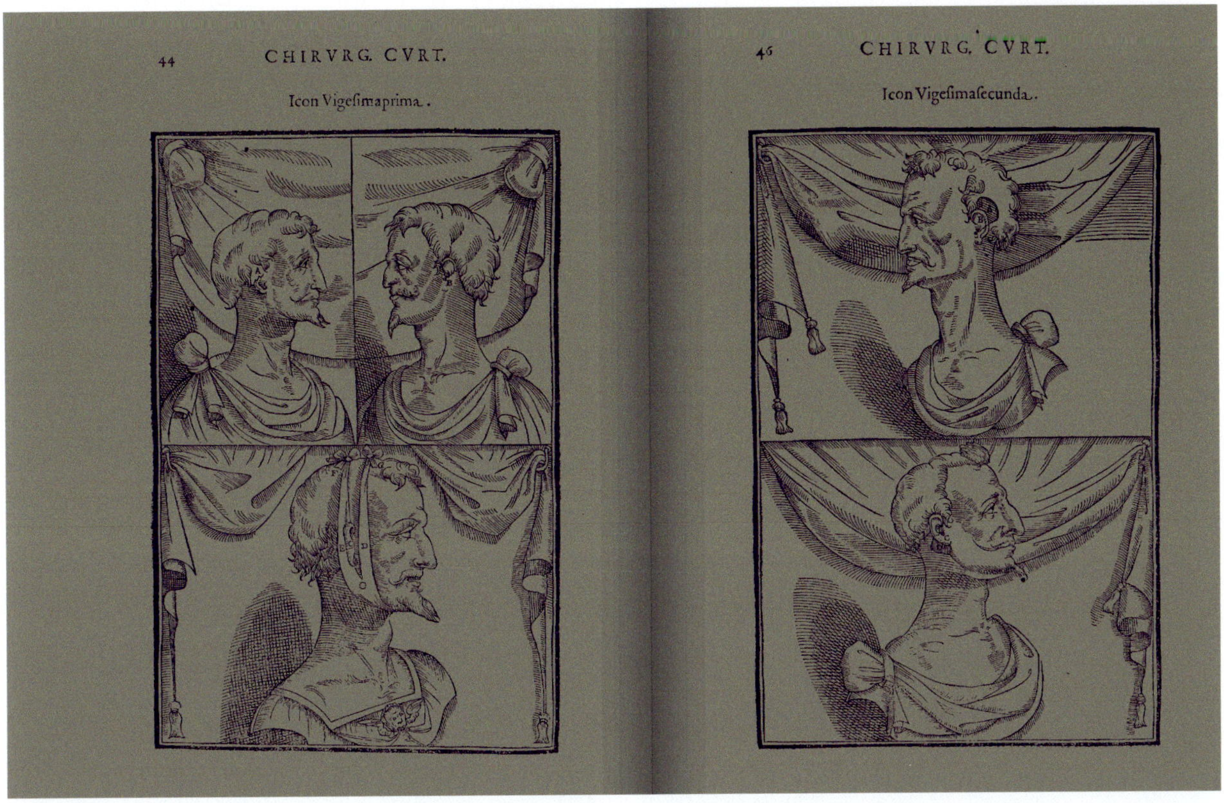

Fig. 10.1 Two illustrations of ear reconstruction from Tagliacozzi's book *Chirurgia per Insitionem*. He used local flaps instead of the arm flap he employed for nasal reconstruction. *Courtesy of Riccardo Mazzola, M.D., Milan*

have a large amount of "scorched cotton" available for controlling the haemorrhage: "When an artery is cut, there is no way to avoid a violent eruption of bleeding and unless the haemorrhage is checked the patient will be in grave danger. The assistant must therefore firmly place the tip of his finger on the vessel and gradually add bits of cotton to the area. This method is so effective that the patient will not lose another drop of blood… Once the bleeding is stopped, the surgeon grasps the flap at its apex, gently elevates it, and attempts to separate it from the underlying parts… The surgeon must try his hardest to cut in straight lines and to remove the callus evenly and consistently because if any of it remains it will impede coalescence".[5] The case described was a Benedictine monk and the author concludes saying: "I was able to restore the middle and lower parts of his ear so elegantly and beautifully that I amazed both myself and my assistants". In the same century Antonio Philippo Ciucci described a similar reconstruction in his book *Promptuarium Chirurgicum* in 1679 (Fig. 10.2a,b).

In 1907 C. Nélaton (1851–1911) and N. Ombrédanne (1871–1956) [727] wrote that they found these statements somewhat exaggerated and insisted that precedence for the reconstruction of an entire auricle must go to Antonio Branca. While this is quite true, it is nevertheless remarkable that Tagliacozzi, considered by many to be the inventor of the arm flap, should use a local flap. However the case in question was a partial reconstruction and he evidently thought that a post-auricular flap would do the job and be less uncomfortable for the patient.

Ear reconstruction does not seem to have been a common operation around this time, though Giovanni Battista Cortesi and Giuseppe Galletti, who both trained under Tagliacozzi, seem to have continued using local flaps.

5 From Robert Goldwyn's translation of *De Curtorum Chirurgia per Institionem*.

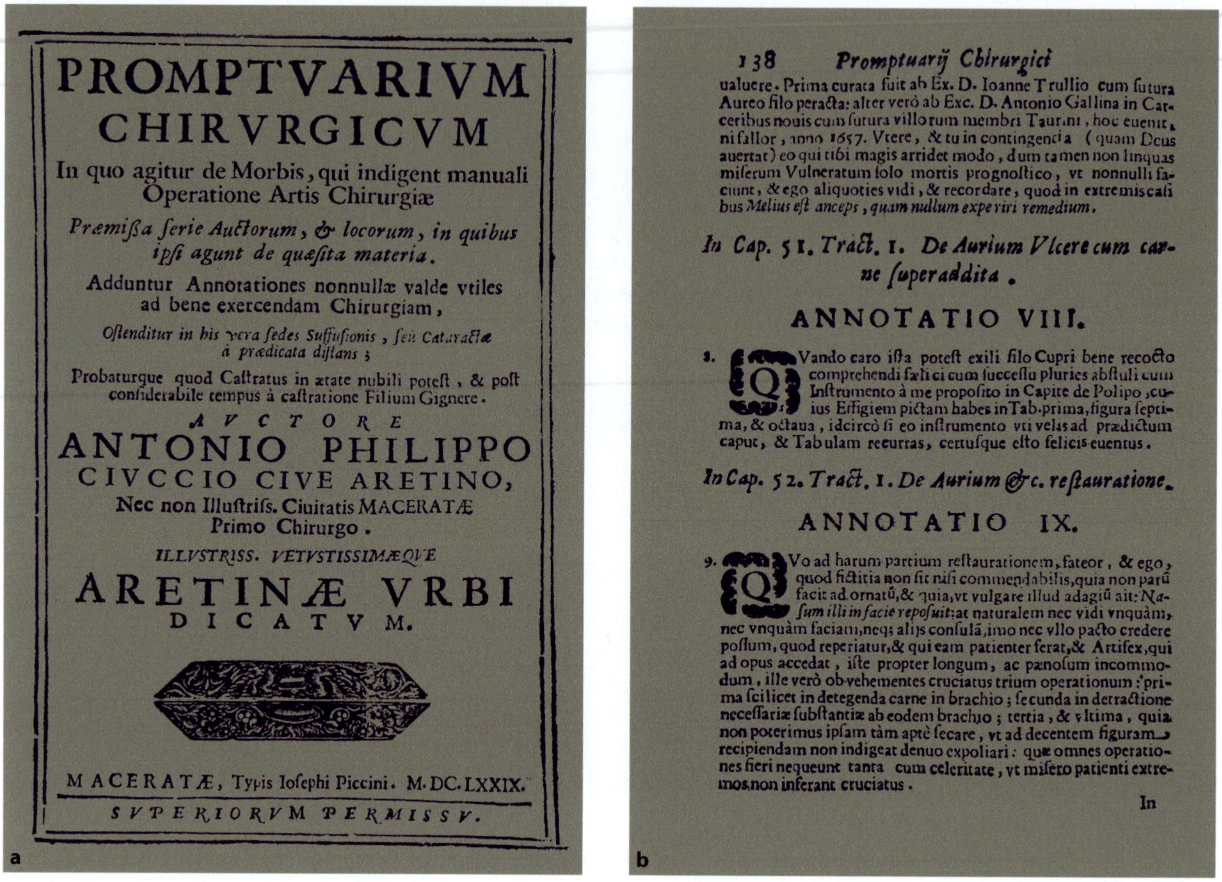

PROMPTVARIVM
CHIRVRGICVM
In quo agitur de Morbis, qui indigent manuali Operatione Artis Chirurgiæ
Præmiſſa ſerie Auctorum, & locorum, in quibus ipſi agunt de quæſita materia.
Adduntur Annotationes nonnullæ valde vtiles ad bene exercendam Chirurgiam,
Oſtenditur in his vera ſedes Suffuſionis, ſeù Cataractæ à prædicata diſtans;
Probaturque quod Caſtratus in ætate nubili poteſt, & poſt conſiderabile tempus à caſtratione Filium Gignere.
AVCTORE
ANTONIO PHILIPPO
CIVCCIO CIVE ARETINO,
Nec non Illuſtriſs. Ciuitatis MACERATÆ Primo Chirurgo.
ILLVSTRISS. VETVSTISSIMÆQVE
ARETINÆ VRBI
DICATVM.
MACERATÆ, Typis Ioſephi Piccini. M.DC.LXXIX.
SVPERIORVM PERMISSV.

a

138 *Promptuarij Chirurgici*

ualuere. Prima curata fuit ab Ex. D. Ioanne Trullio cum ſutura Aureo filo peracta: alter verò ab Exc. D. Antonio Gallina in Carceribus nouis cum ſutura villorum membri Taurini, hoc euenit, ni fallor, anno 1657. Vtere, & tu in contingentia (quam Deus auertat) eo qui tibi magis arridet modo, dum tamen non linquas miſerum Vulneratum ſolo mortis prognoſtico, vt nonnulli faciunt, & ego aliquoties vidi, & recordare, quod in extremis caſibus *Melius eſt anceps, quam nullum experiri remedium.*

In Cap. 51. Tract. 1. De Aurium Vlcere cum carne ſuperaddita.

ANNOTATIO VIII.

8. QVando caro iſta poteſt exili filo Cupri bene recocto comprehendi facili cum ſucceſſu pluries abſtuli cum Inſtrumento à me propoſito in Capite de Polipo, cuius Effigiem pictam habes in Tab. prima, figura ſeptima, & octaua, idcircò ſi eo inſtrumento vti velis ad prædictum caput, & Tabulam recurras, certuſque eſto felicis euentus.

In Cap. 52. Tract. 1. De Aurium &c. reſtauratione.

ANNOTATIO IX.

9. QVo ad harum partium reſtaurationem, fateor, & ego, quod fictitia non ſit niſi commendabilis, quia non parũ facit ad ornatũ, & quia, vt vulgare illud adagiũ ait: *Naſum illi in facie repoſuit*: at naturalem nec vidi vnquàm, nec vnquàm faciam, neq; alijs conſulã, imo nec vllo pacto credere poſſum, quod reperiatur, & qui eam patienter ferat, & Artifex, qui ad opus accedat, iſte propter longum, ac pænoſum incommodum, ille verò ob vehementes cruciatus trium operationum: prima ſcilicet in detegenda carne in brachio; ſecunda in detractione neceſſariæ ſubſtantiæ ab eodem brachio; tertia, & vltima, quia non poterimus ipſam tàm aptè ſecare, vt ad decentem figuram recipiendam non indigeat denuo expoliari: quæ omnes operationes fieri nequeunt tanta cum celeritate, vt miſero patienti extremos non inferant cruciatus.

In

b

Fig. 10.2 **a** Frontispiece of Antonio Philippo Ciucci's *Promptuarium Chirurgicum* published in 1674 in which he described **b** injuries of the ears and their reconstruction. *Courtesy of Riccardo Mazzola, M.D., Milan*

Thereafter, it is not until the nineteenth century that we encounter other surgeons interested in reconstruction of the auricle.

As William Lincoln Ballenger wrote in 1914, "…malformations of the auricle are of importance chiefly from a cosmetic point of view … and its entire absence does not materially influence the acuity of hearing" so it is likely that little interest was given to ear reconstruction [50]. The loss of the ear does not seem to have carried such a stigma as the nose, possibly because the hair hid the disfigurement. Certainly patients were not prepared to undergo painful surgery to restore an ear whatever the final appearance.

In 1868 D. Prince [817] wrote a book on reconstruction techniques, but all he had to say about ear reconstruction was "Otoplasty is chiefly required for the correction of the effects of wounds and burns, and the expedients must be varied according to the necessities of each particular malformation. The development of principles and the application of indications to other parts, renders any special attention to this organ unnecessary." The correction of congenital malformations, such as microtia or protruding ears, were not even considered, which is surprising, since fourteen of this author's scientific publications deal with other congenital malformations.[6]

6 J. Feuvrier [310] showed particular interest in malformations of the ear and published a little known book on the subject in 1865. This doesn't appear to have stimulated any concerted efforts at surgical correction.

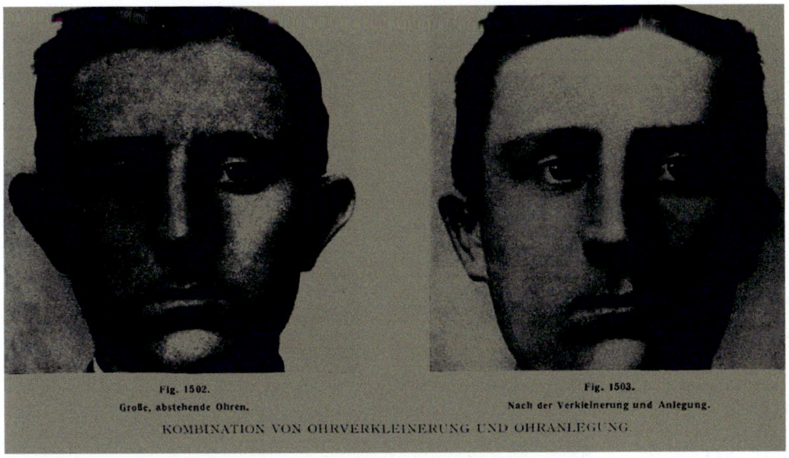

Fig. 10.3 Pre- and post-operative views of one of Jacques Joseph's cases. In 1896 he performed his first correction of protruding ears on a child. As a consequence he was dismissed from his post by Professor Wolff, Head of the Orthopaedic Clinic at Berlin University. *Courtesy of Riccardo Mazzola, M.D., Milan*

However, in 1845 Dieffenbach [244] described his famous reconstruction of the middle third of the auricle using a post-auricle flap. His book, *Die Ohrbildung* (*The Reconstruction of the Ear*), probably received more credit than it deserved around the time. It might be that surgeons just glanced at the title and the illustrations without reading it carefully and this gave rise to the misconception that he was the first to perform a complete ear reconstruction. This was a view that prevailed for many years despite the fact that the rather confused descriptions of Antonio Branca's reconstruction by others already existed. In fact all he had done was to perform a good reconstruction of the middle third of the ear. O. J. Becher [64, 65] in 1949 and George La Trenta [535] in 1980 even attributed the first correction of protruding ears to the German surgeon.

Dieffenbach's book influence many surgeons, such as Velpeau, Lamballe and others as cited by Nélaton and Ombrédanne. They all adopted the same two stage post-auricle flap for their partial reconstructions.

Congenital Malformations

In the nineteenth century there was renewed interest in congenital anomalies in general. Surgeons finally dispelled all the myths that had been prevalent in the past as they began to understand more about embryology and the origin of birth deformities.

Those malformations which interested plastic surgeons affected the size, shape and position of the ear as well as its partial and complete absence.

One method aimed at reducing the size of the ear was described by J.S. Davis [223]. In 1919, he re-introduced a technique previously described by Gersuny in Germany in 1903.

One of the first cases of correction of protruding ears reported in the literature was by Joseph in 1896 [724]. The German surgeon found himself involved with the case of a youth who refused to go to school since all his companions ridiculed him "...because of the large protruding ears".

Joseph initially told the mother that he had no remedy for this deformity, but he was so affected by the boy's psychological problem that once home he talked to his wife Leonore. She urged him to operate on the child. Despite his attempts to dissuade them by his explanation that the operation had not been done before they still persisted. Joseph simply excised and ellipse of skin from the post-auricular sulcus without remodelling the cartilage. As far as reducing the size, Joseph wrote "I carried it out in the following way: from the upper half of the auricle I ... removed a wedge shaped piece on both sides together with the corresponding cartilage, cutting through the helix, the scaphoid fossa, the antihelix, deep down into the concha ... at an angle of 50–60 degrees; then came the joining of the free wound edges." The final result was a reduction of more than one and a half centimetres (Fig. 10.3) [724].

Ten years before Joseph, a very simple method for correcting protruding ears had been suggested by Peau. His technique of excising a skin ellipse 1.5 cm wide without touching the cartilage was criticized by Nélaton and Ombrédanne. They correctly maintained that the cause of the prominence was due to the cartilage and while the initial results might be good, recurrence of

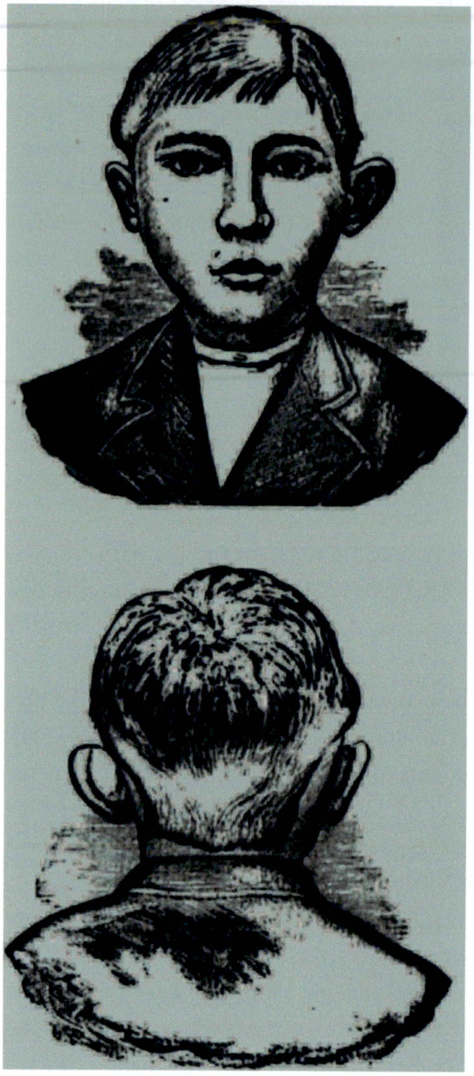

Fig. 10.4 Edward Talbot Ely (1850–1881) was probably the first to advocate the resection of cartilage to correct protruding ears. *From his article published in 1881* [278]

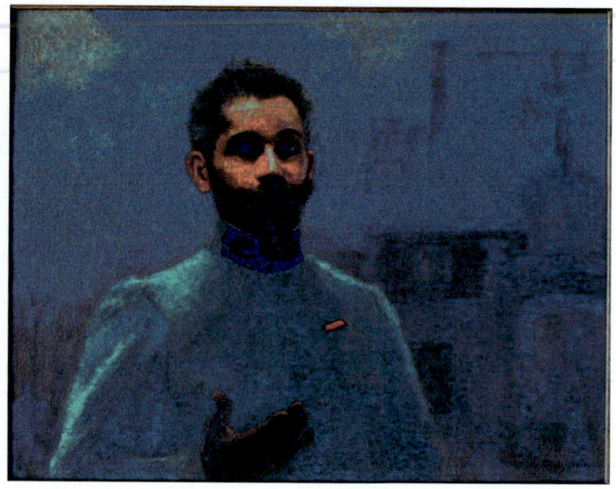

Fig. 10.5 Portrait of Hippolyte Morestin (1869–1919) by Roll. Born on Martinique he became a military surgeon. He was in charge of the Plastic Surgery Unit at the Military Hospital, Val de Grace, Paris during World War I. *Courtesy of Val de Grace Military Hospital, Paris.*

the deformity was inevitable as the abnormal cartilage caused the skin to stretch. Consequently the method gained little popularity.

The importance of the cartilage was already well understood by Edward Talbot Ely (1850–1881) in America [278]. In 1881 he published a detailed paper on the correction of protrusion by removing some of the cartilage, a method that was corroborated in Europe by Hippolyte Morestin[7] who published his work in 1903 (Figs. 10.4, 10.5) [697].

Ely[8] is universally accepted as being the first surgeon to have distinguished the true origin of protrusion of the auricle as a malformation of the cartilage framework and to have corrected it by removing a large piece of cartilage (1 to 1.8 inches long and ⅓ of an inch wide) as far as the concha. The skin excision must have been larger. Ely ad-

7 See Roger B (1982) Hippolyte Morestin (1869–1819). A brief history. *Aesthetic Plastic Surgery* 6:141. He was in charge of the Plastic Service for all French wounded soldiers from World War I at Hôpital val de Grace, Paris from 1915. He died young of tuberculosis.

8 Ely was a brilliant young surgeon. When 31 years old he published this method for correcting protruding ears. The son of a physician in Rochester (NY), he graduated MD at Columbia University, New York then spent six years at the Manhattan Eye and Ear Hospital. He wrote many papers on surgery, some in collaboration with his professor, Bennet St. John Rosa. Alas, the medical world soon lost a promising surgeon since he died of tuberculosis at the age of only 37 years.

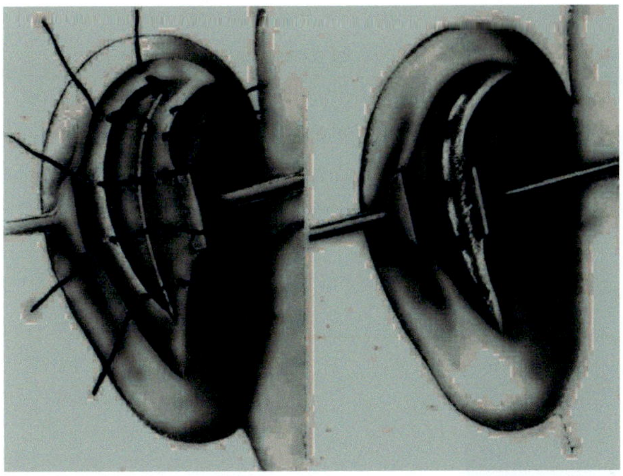

Fig. 10.6 William Henry Luckett (1872–1929) reconstructed the anti-helical fold to correct protruding ears. *From his paper of 1910* [582]

mitted not knowing whether cartilage excision had ever been performed before.

The new method produced some good results but did little to reduce the size of the ears. Another American, W.H. Luckett (1872–1929), helped in this respect. He insisted that the true cause of protrusion lay in a deformed or absent antihelix. In 1910 he published a meticulous study on the anatomy of the auricle [582], observing that "...the cartilage of the concha normally bends outwards at an almost right angle from the head until it reaches the antihelix which is formed by being folded backwards upon itself". He said that the real reason for protrusion was the abnormal development of the antihelix, or the lack of it, and that in effect "... the continuous concavity of concha and fossa of the helix" is nearly always present in protruding ears. His method was to excise an ellipse of post auricular skin as well as a piece of cartilage of similar shape and then to reconstruct the antihelix using a *Lembert* suture passed through the cartilage from above downwards and drawing it together to recreate a fold (Fig. 10.6). Luckett[9] warned that there was a risk of infection in this type of operation since chondritis appeared common following correction of malformations of the auricle.

Yet another American who devoted his skills to congenital malformations and who proposed a different technique for correcting protruding ears was F.S. Kolle (1872–1929). His method consisted of excising a large ellipse of skin from the back of the ear and mastoid region so that when sutured, the ear was draw to the side of the head. According to Kolle this was generally sufficient to correct the protrusion and cartilage should be excised only "...when seen necessary" [504]. Apparently obliteration of the sulcus was acceptable (Fig. 10.7).

Total Reconstruction of the Auricle

Total reconstruction of the absent auricle due to either congenital microtia, trauma or surgical excision, is a complex topic which only received close attention in the last half of the twentieth century. Although Antonio Branca and Tagliacozzi attempted subtotal reconstruction following trauma it appears that they did not perform complete restoration.

Microtia, the congenital absence of the auricle, was described in 1878 by F. Mason in a fine book on surgery of the face in which he deals with several congenital malformations [617]. However, he supplies no theory on the aetiology of microtia, nor does he propose any type of reconstruction.

The author appears to consider *maternal impression* as the cause of congenital malformations and describes a case where "A woman, during pregnancy, was horrified at seeing a man whose ear had been mutilated. Her child, a girl, was born with her right ear presenting a similar appearance." He also adds that the younger sister of this girl, in due time gave birth to "...a boy with his right ear deformed like his aunt's". This would suggests that even at this late stage not only where congenital abnormalities attributed to this cause but that *maternal impression* could be inherited! It is strange that in the latter part of the nineteenth century, when the aetiology of many types of malformation had already been given convincing embryological explanations, there should still be those who believed in these theories.

9 Luckett was born in Texas, USA, but completed his medical studies at Columbia University in New York. Here he worked as head surgeon at the Lutheran Hospital until his death in 1929 when he was 57 years old. During the First World War he was a military surgeon in France where his interest in reconstructive surgery began. He was also an excellent sportsman.

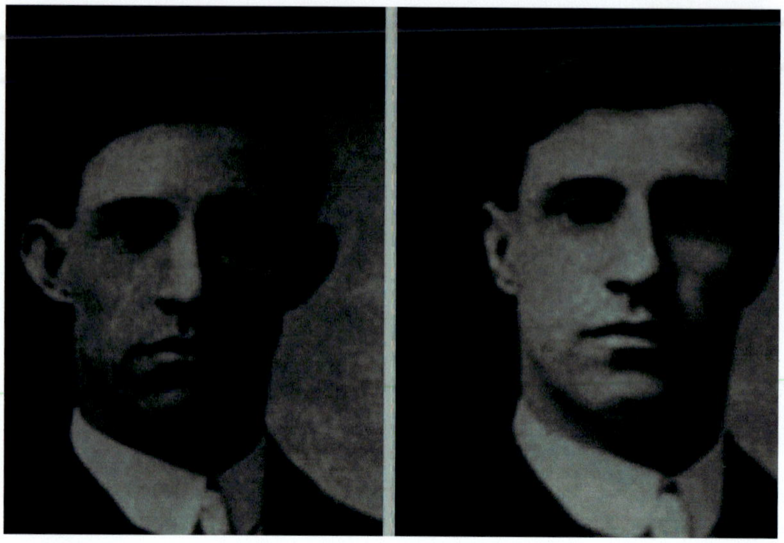

Fig. 10.7 Pre- and post-operative views of a case treated by F.S. Kolle (1872–1929). He described his method in detail and claimed that the cartilage had to be resected only "when necessary". *Courtesy of Riccardo Mazzola, M.D., Milan*

Returning to the subject of total ear reconstruction, Julius von Szymanowski should be mentioned. He dedicated a lengthy chapter in his book on surgery in 1870 to otoplasty, describing "…a rather complicated flap which was based on the pre-auricular area but elevated from the mastoid region, to be double folded on itself and with no supporting framework" (Figs. 10.8, 10.9) [968].

In spite of the large number of references available in the literature and an excellent thesis written by R.C. Cocheril in 1895, in which the author expresses enthusiastic approval of the method, Szymanowski's technique was not used very often [181]. It is hard to imagine that it would have produced an acceptable result by today's standards and the absence of a supporting framework would inevitably have led to a poor result.

In 1903, Robert Gersuny believed that "…when the entire ear or a large part of it is lacking the possibility of successful plastic reconstruction is unlikely and in the best of events, the resulting appearance is only mediocre" [367]. Nevertheless, Gersuny was the first to employ a framework and used a piece of costal cartilage for this purpose, though he concluded that a prosthesis offered better results.

In 1912, J.B. Roberts, published a fine book on partial reconstruction and cartilaginous malformations of the ear. In it, he also proposed techniques for total reconstruction. He raised two flaps supplied by the temporal and the posterior auricular arteries so that "…each of the flaps is the shape of a boy's skinny stick. They have their convex borders toward each other" [847]. This new method apparently improved the results of attempts at

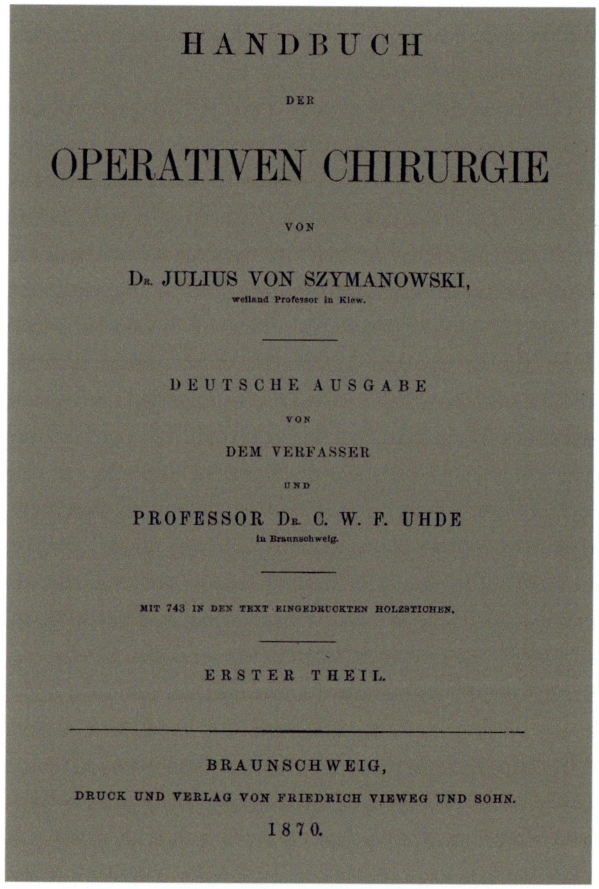

HANDBUCH

DER

OPERATIVEN CHIRURGIE

VON

DR. JULIUS VON SZYMANOWSKI,

weiland Professor in Kiew.

DEUTSCHE AUSGABE

VON

DEM VERFASSER

UND

PROFESSOR DR. C. W. F. UHDE

in Braunschweig.

MIT 743 IN DEN TEXT EINGEDRUCKTEN HOLZSTICHEN.

ERSTER THEIL.

BRAUNSCHWEIG,

DRUCK UND VERLAG VON FRIEDRICH VIEWEG UND SOHN.

1870.

Fig. 10.8 Julius von Szymanowski (1829–1868) published his book *Handbuch der Operativen Chirurgie* in 1870 and a whole chapter deals with the reconstruction of the ear. *Courtesy of Riccardo Mazzola, M.D., Milan*

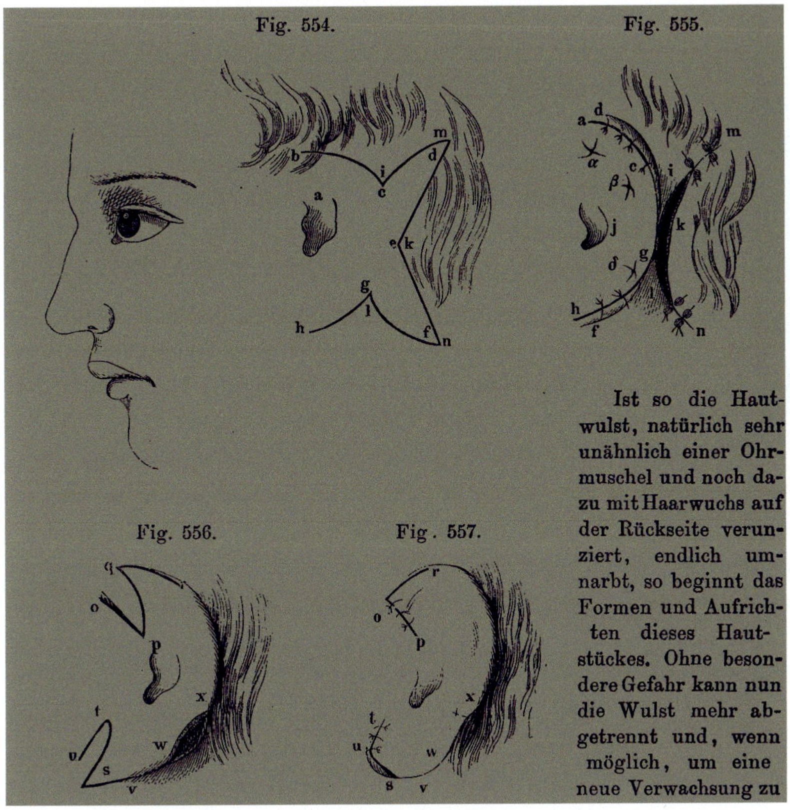

Fig. 10.9 Szymanowski described a flap from the post-auricular area to reconstruct the auricle. *Courtesy of Riccardo Mazzola, M.D., Milan*

reconstruction. In fact, he proposed inserting "...a silver filigree" between the two flaps or even "...shaping a slice of costal cartilage to be inserted so that it might offer a certain degree of stiffness to the auricular substitute".

Judging by the few surgeons who adopted it, Robert's method cannot have been considered a great success and, in effect, results only became acceptable after the First World War when Sir Harold Gillies (1882–1950) introduced his ideas [375]. One of the cases with war wounds that Gillies described was a subtotal avulsion that he treated by removing a segment of costal cartilage from the 7th and 8th ribs, shaping it accurately before slipping it under the hairless skin in the mastoid area. A flap of skin including this cartilage was later elevated and its raw surface was covered by another flap from the neck. Gillies introduced two important idea; the use of hairless mastoid skin with a similar appearance to the ear and the cartilage framework to give shape and support. According to B. Brent who might be considered an expert of the past 20 years, it was thanks to Gillies that "the concept of microtia had its beginning" (Fig. 10.10) [129].

Another technique to improve the results of total reconstruction was proposed by G.W. Pierce in 1930 [799]. He reconstructed the helix with a thin tubed pedicle flap and covered the back of the new ear with a skin graft. The thickness of the newly formed ear was then very similar to that of a normal ear.

In 1937, Gillies published a new series of 37 cases of microtia in which he used maternal cartilage. He resorted to cartilaginous homografts because it was difficult to obtain sufficient amounts of costal cartilage of good quality from the child and shaping it was frequently followed by some distortion produced by twisting. Unfortunately many of these homografts were extruded. In spite of this, 23 years later, in 1960, T. Gibson and W.B. Davis wrote enthusiastically about one of the cases Gillies treated in 1937. They discovered that not only was the cartilage still present but that it contained viable chondrocytes [371]. However, J.M. Converse [190] also had occasion to examine 21 of the 37 cases operated on by Gillies. He stated quite categorically that he was only able to trace signs of a cartilage framework in one of these, while the cartilage in the other 20 had been completely reabsorbed and the auricle was seriously deformed due to the shrinkage that had ensued. Nevertheless it was accepted that a framework of some sort was necessary although secondary shrinkage was recognized to be one of the more frequent long-term results of cartilaginous implants.

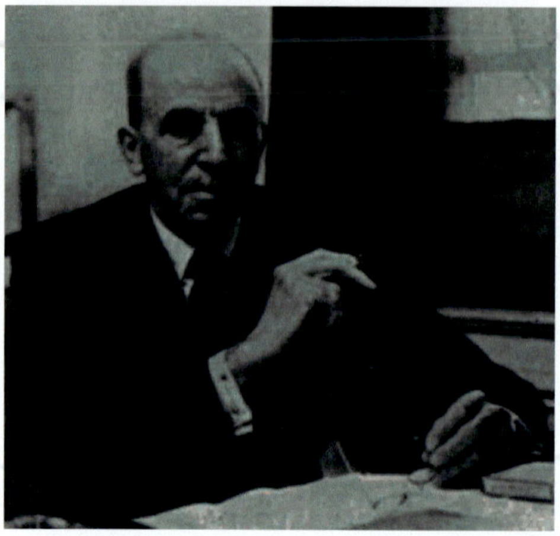

Fig. 10.10 Photograph of Sir Harold Gillies (1882–1960) who advocated the use of maternal costal cartilage to reconstruct the auricle in cases of microtia. He collected a series of 37 cases, many of which were reviewed by J. M. Converse who found almost total reabsorption of the cartilage. *From the Antony Wallace Archive, courtesy of the British Association of Plastic Reconstructive and Aesthetic Surgeons*

In order to avoid this complication, Lindon A. Peer diced the cartilage and put the pieces into a perforated Vitallium mould shaped like an auricle [786]. This was then implanted in the subcutaneous tissue of the abdomen. The idea was that by penetrating through the fenestrations the connective tissue would incorporate and vascularize the cartilage "…forming a solid but somewhat elastic structure which was an exact duplication of the ear mould". The pre-shaped cartilage was then moved at a later stage to provide the supporting framework for the new ear.

Peer had conducted experiments on rabbits over 25 years and showed that both autograft and homograft cartilage survived and was not reabsorbed. He even demonstrated that the grafts grew. He presumed that his results would be applicable to ear reconstruction in humans and many surgeons applied his theories to their patients. Unfortunately long term results were severely compromised by scar contracture from the fibrous connective tissue and the technique was not subsequently adopted.

In 1952 W.H. Steffensen proposed placing "…a sharply contoured preserved cartilage implant with multiple perforations of the scapha" under the skin in the mastoid area, so that when the cicatricial tissue penetrates these apertures it would enhance the shape of the helix when it shrank [950, 951]. The implanted cartilage together with the overlying skin was later elevated *en bloc* and its posterior surface covered with a local flap from the mastoid area with a base near the lobe and the apex reaching the upper apex of the sulcus. The immediate results were excellent, but unfortunately it was soon seen that the preserved cartilage underwent reabsorption.

A possible solution to this problem was proposed by R.C. Tanzer [971] in his multistaged procedure. After repositioning the remnants of the microtic ear in carefully chosen positions he introduced a cartilage framework beneath the skin in such a way as to use both the new cartilage and the remnants. The cartilage framework was taken from the 6th, 7th and 8th costal cartilages on the opposite side, carved to shape using a scalpel and refined with a dental drill and burr. An additional strip of cartilage was sutured to this to make a helix. The whole was then implanted under the mastoid skin and left undisturbed for at least four months before elevating the flap *en bloc* and grafting the back, usually with a full thickness graft from behind the opposite ear. Tanzer's results seemed promising, but before a sufficient number of long term results accumulated T.D. Cronin's famous article appeared [209]. He proposed the use of a silicon implant instead of cartilage and all biological obstacles usually encountered seemed to be resolved and reconstruction became technically easier. Enthusiasm for the technique was short lived as the implants were extruded. The thin skin with its limited vascularity was prone to infection and trauma and many implants failed despite attempts to overcome these difficulties with a flap of vascular temporal fascia placed between the skin and the Silastic. Surgeons fell back on a framework made from shaped, autologous cartilage and several published good results, such as E.W. Peet [788].[10] During the past decades, B. Brent [129] and O. Fukuda [343, 344] have both achieved excellent long term results with their meticulous techniques and as a consequence these are the current methods of choice.

10 E.W. Peet was an ear, nose and throat surgeon and became interested in reconstructive surgery following his experience in India during World War II. On his return he became a plastic surgeon with Patterson in Oxford and with him wrote a book on plastic surgery. His contribution to the field of ear reconstruction was this beautifully illustrated monograph on the subject. See also obituary by T.J.S. Patterson (1969) Eric W Peet (1909–1968) *Plast Reconstr Surg* 43:555.

Chapter 11

Skull Reconstruction

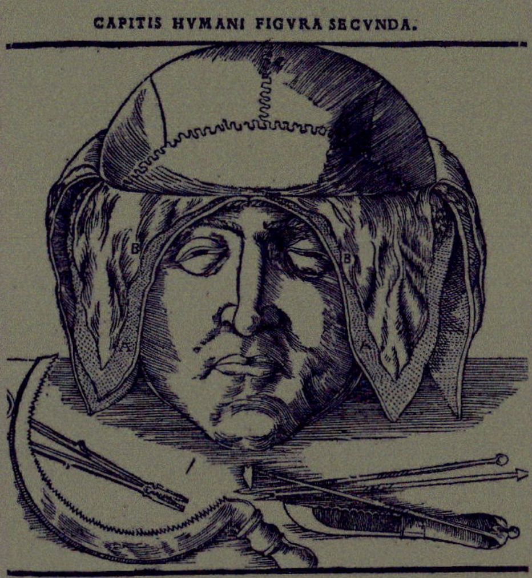

Contents

The discovery of many ancient trephined skulls in Egypt and Mesoamerican is proof that this type of surgery was practised in the distant past. There is evidence that it was not limited to these two parts of the world since single skulls have been found in other regions such as Sardinia,[1] where no other evidence of early surgery has come to light. The new bone formation seen in many of these skulls shows that the subjects survived and the surgeons were fairly skilled (Fig. 11.1).

In 1847 Pietro Sabattini produced an accurate review of the literature from the Ancient Greeks up to the Renaissance period [876].[2] Though the majority of present-day authors maintain that the most frequent reason for trephining skulls was to release evil spirits causing sickness, Sabbatini declared that at least in some of the cases the aim was neurosurgical, to relieve pressure "particularly when the cause is a fraction of bone exerting pressure directly on the brain after a fracture to the skull".

Guido Majno emphasized the fact that as many of the patients survived, the surgeons must have been very competent. He also wrote that trephination was practised as a life-saving procedure to relieve the pressure on the brain of comatose patients and therefore anaesthesia was not needed [596].

Although there is ample evidence for the practice of trephination from early times very few discoveries exist that indicate attempts at more advanced surgery. The difference between operating on a patient in a coma and on one awake is probably why. Some competent surgeons did carry out simple reconstruction. M. Auvray distinguished between *organic reconstructions* and *prosthetic filling* and this remains so today [40].

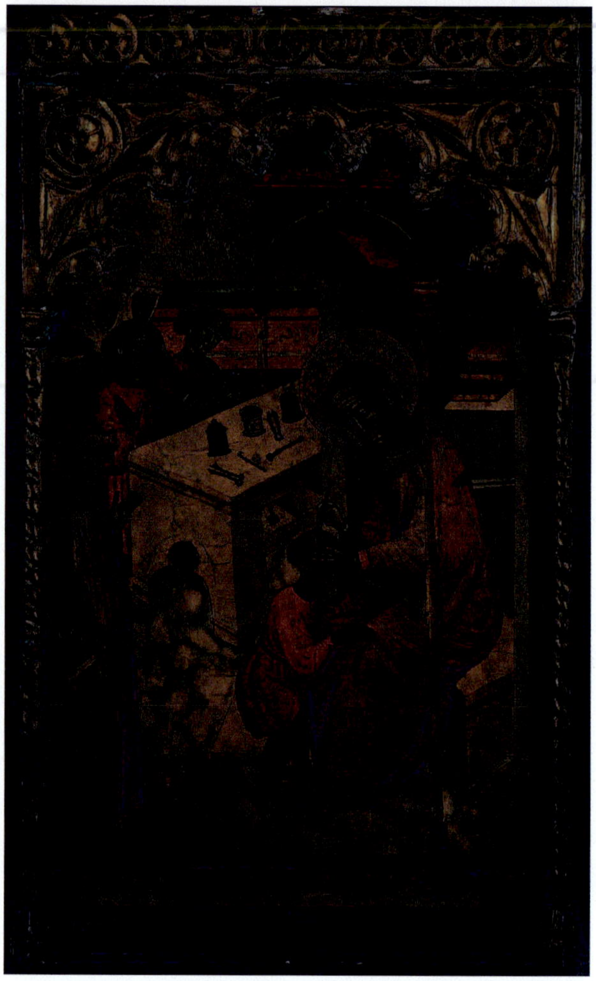

Fig. 11.1 St Luke the evangelist, patron saint of doctors said to be treating a child with a brain tumour with other patients awaiting treatment. By Juan de Sevilla (1643–1695). *By permission © Museo Nacional del Prado, Madrid*

The Earliest Corrections of Skull Defects

The oldest example of skull reconstruction is probably the Neolithic skull discovered in Peru and described by J.J. Longacre and John M. Converse in 1977 [576]. This skull from 2000–1500 B.C., which shows clear evidence of a frontal defect corrected with a finely hammered gold plate, has been described in many articles (Fig. 11.2).

Another much more recent Peruvian skull is exhibited in the Semmelweis Museum in Budapest and belonged to a man of about thirty years old who lived around 950 A.D. In this case the defect was closed with a silver plate. There

1 Two skulls showing signs of bone regeneration on the borders of the trephination are to be found in the Sanna Museum in Sassari.

2 Some of the authors mentioned by Sabattini are Heliodorus, Galen, Paulus of Aegineta, the entire Arabian School, Guy de Chauliac, Berengario da Carpi, Ambroise Paré, Guillemenau, Fabricius ab Aquapendente and Fabrice Hildanus.

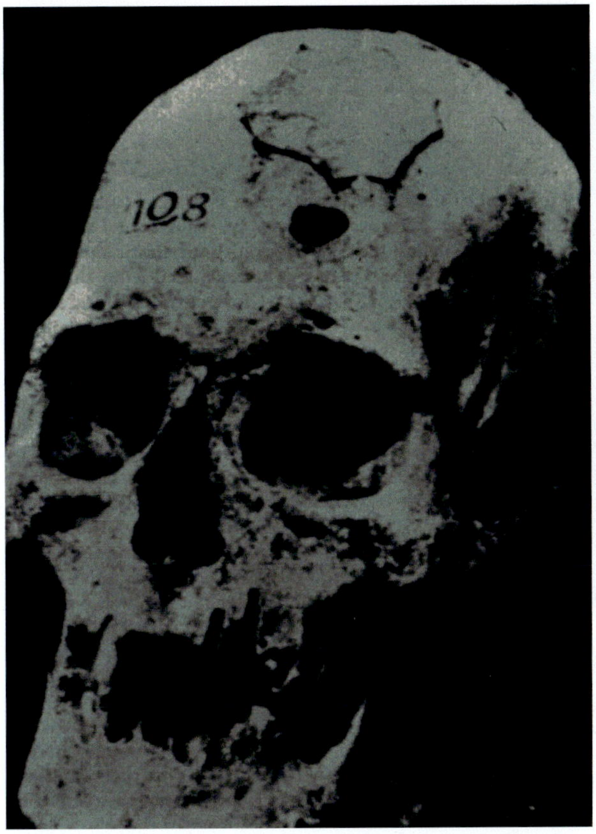

Fig. 11.2 A Peruvian skull from c.2000 B.C. with a gold plate covering a frontal bone defect. *From the British Journal of Plastic Surgery 15:121 Landazoni*: An Ancient Peruvain Skull… *©1962. Courtesy of the British Association of Plastic Surgeons*

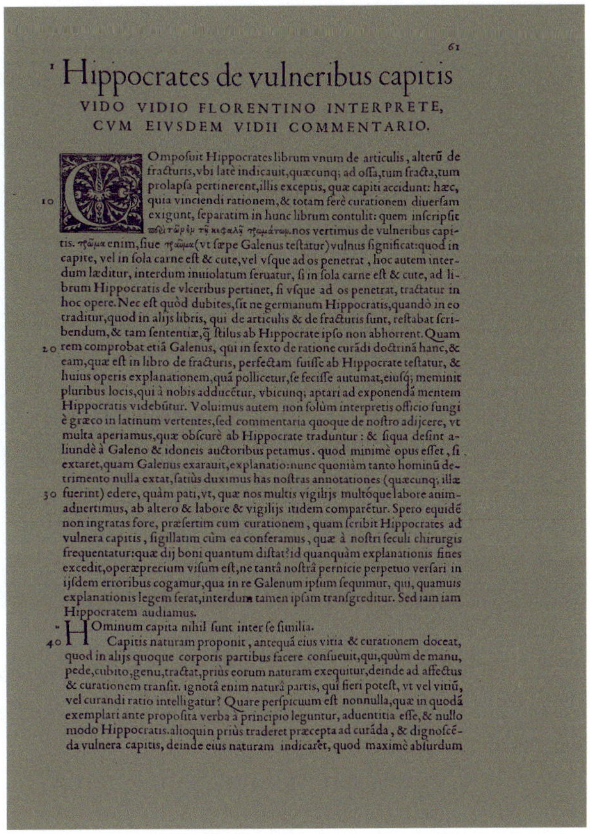

61

Hippocrates de vulneribus capitis

VIDO VIDIO FLORENTINO INTERPRETE, CVM EIVSDEM VIDII COMMENTARIO.

Ompoſuit Hippocrates librum vnum de articulis, alterũ de fracturis, vbi latè indicauit, quæcunq; ad oſſa, tum fracta, tum prolapſa pertinerent, illis exceptis, quæ capiti accidunt: hæc, quia vinciendi rationem, & totam ferè curationem diuerſam exigunt, ſeparatim in hunc librum contulit: quem inſcripſit περὶ τῶν ἐν τῇ κεφαλῇ τρωμάτων. nos vertimus de vulneribus capitis. τρῶμα enim, ſiue τραῦμα (vt ſæpe Galenus teſtatur) vulnus ſignificat: quod in capite, vel in ſola carne eſt & cute, vel vſque ad os penetrat, hoc autem interdum læditur, interdum inuiolatum ſeruatur, ſi in ſola carne eſt & cute, ad librum Hippocratis de vlceribus pertinet, ſi vſque ad os penetrat, tractatur in hoc opere. Nec eſt quòd dubites, ſit ne germanum Hippocratis, quandò in eo traditur, quod in alijs libris, qui de articulis & de fracturis ſunt, reſtabat ſcribendum, & tam ſententiæ, q̃ ſtilus ab Hippocrate ipſo non abhorrent. Quam rem comprobat etiã Galenus, qui in ſexto de ratione curãdi doctrinã hanc, & eam, quæ eſt in libro de fracturis, perfectam fuiſſe ab Hippocrate teſtatur, & huius operis explanationem, quã pollicetur, ſe feciſſe autumat, eiuſq; meminit pluribus locis, qui à nobis adducẽtur, vbicunq; aptari ad exponendã mentem Hippocratis videbũtur. Voluimus autem non ſolùm interpretis officio fungi è græco in latinum vertentes, ſed commentaria quoque de noſtro adijcere, vt multa aperiamus, quæ obſcurè ab Hippocrate traduntur: & ſiqua deſint aliundè à Galeno & idoneis auctoribus petamus. quod minimè opus eſſet, ſi extaret, quam Galenus exarauit, explanatio: nunc quoniàm tanto hominũ detrimento nulla extat, ſatiùs duximus has noſtras annotationes (quæcunq; illæ fuerint) edere, quàm pati, vt, quæ nos multis vigilijs multóque labore animaduertimus, ab altero & labore & vigilijs itidem comparẽtur. Spero equidẽ non ingratas fore, præſertim cum curationem, quam ſcribit Hippocrates ad vulnera capitis, ſigillatim cùm ea conferamus, quæ à noſtri ſeculi chirurgis frequentatur: quæ dij boni quantum diſtat? id quanquàm explanationis fines excedit, operæprecium viſum eſt, ne tantâ noſtrâ pernicie perpetuo verſari in ijſdem erroribus cogamur, qua in re Galenum ipſum ſequimur, qui, quamuis explanationis legem ferat, interdum tamen ipſam tranſgreditur. Sed iam iam Hippocratem audiamus.

HOminum capita nihil ſunt inter ſe ſimilia.

Capitis naturam proponit, antequã eius vitia & curationem doceat, quod in alijs quoque corporis partibus facere conſueuit, qui, quùm de manu, pede, cubito, genu, tractat, priùs eorum naturam exequitur, deinde ad affectus & curationem tranſit. ignotâ enim naturâ partis, qui fieri poteſt, vt vel vitiũ, vel curandi ratio intelligatur? Quare perſpicuum eſt nonnulla, quæ in quodã exemplari ante propoſita verba à principio leguntur, aduentitia eſſe, & nullo modo Hippocratis. alioquin priùs traderet præcepta ad curãda, & dignoſcẽda vulnera capitis, deinde eius naturam indicarẽt, quod maximè abſurdum

Fig. 11.3 In *De Vulneribus Capitis* Hippocrates deals with injuries of the head. The book is included in Vido Vidi's *Chirurgia a Greco in Latino Conversa* (1544, Paris). *Courtesy of Riccardo Mazzola, M.D., Milan*

was new bone around the metal implant in both of the skulls. We understand that another skull with a gold plate is exhibited in the Anthropological Museum, Mexico City and was displayed at the British Museum in 2003.

Although Hippocrates dealt in detail with head injuries he does not mention fractures of the skull (Fig. 11.3).

There is no proof that trephination was performed in either Greece or Rome despite the fact that Claudius Galen (131–201 A.D.) was so well aware of the risks arising from skull fractures that he devised a special bandage, described in his *De Fasciis* and *De Ossibus* to protect patients with fractures in the frontal region (Fig. 11.4) [350–354].

Treatment of Skull Trauma

In the seventh century, Paulus Aegineta (625–690 A.D.) wrote at length about skull trauma in his book *La Chirurgie*,[3] devoting the whole of Chapter 90 to skull fractures. The following chapter deals with "inflammation of the meninges" and the post-operative complications that arose in the cases he treated.

After the Middle Ages, many authors wrote about skull fractures. Two fourteenth century authors that deserve mention are Lanfranchi da Milano (c.1290–1315) and Guy de Chauliac (1298–1368); both described skull fractures in detail and discussed the ideal moment for

3 *La Chirurgie* was first published in Latin in Basle in 1533 and thereafter in French at Lyons in 1540.

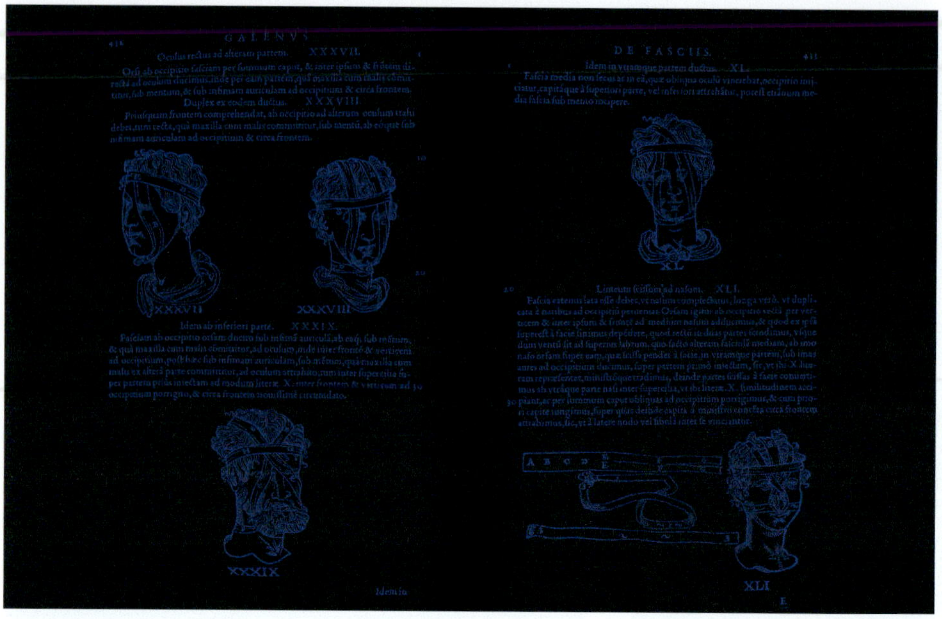

Fig. 11.4 Galen is another author who is included in Vido Vidi's *Chirurgia a Greco in Latinum Conversa*. He devoted a part of his work to head injuries and described many ways to immobilize fractures with special bandages. *Courtesy of Riccardo Mazzola, M.D, Milan*

starting treatment in order to avoid pressure on the brain (Fig. 11.5) [169–173, 520].

The First Reconstructions

The importance of restoring continuity to the skull was understood in Europe during the Renaissance. Surgeons understood the risks of a bone defects. The first to write about this was Gabriele Fallopius (1523–1564) [297] He devised a method using a gold plate when it was impossible to use local bone fragments or the dura mater and wrote at length about choosing the right moment for reconstruction. Despite the splendid account given in his *Observationes Anatomicas*, published in Venice in 1567 [297], Fallopius' idea was not well accepted by other surgeons (Fig. 11.6). Paré was one who disagreed about the use of a gold plate or of any other metal. Others, like Iacopo Berengario da Carpi[4] (1460–c.1530), maintained that every effort had to be made to put the bone fragments back into place. He wrote three books: *De Fractura Calve sive Cranei* in 1518, *Commentaria super Anatomia* in 1521 and *Isagoge* in 1522 [74–77]. The first of these is a milestone in the treatment of skull trauma and was so successful that ten editions were printed in a short time. Berengario became interested in 1517, when he was called to treat Lorenzo II of the famous Medici family (Lorenzo the Magnificent was his grandfather) who had been wounded by a gunshot while fighting for the Pope against Francesco Maria della Rovere [820].[5]

In the first chapter of this book he describes different types of fracture, the causes and the differential symptoms for reaching a logical diagnosis. The second chapter is devoted to the indications for the different surgical methods and he discusses whether or not skull wounds

4 Berengario da Carpi's real name was Giacomo Barigazzi.

5 Other illustrious patients included Giovanni dalle Bande Nere, Galleazzo Pallavicini, Cardinal Collona and Alessandro Soderini and he had the ear of the Popes Julius II, Leo X and Clement VII.

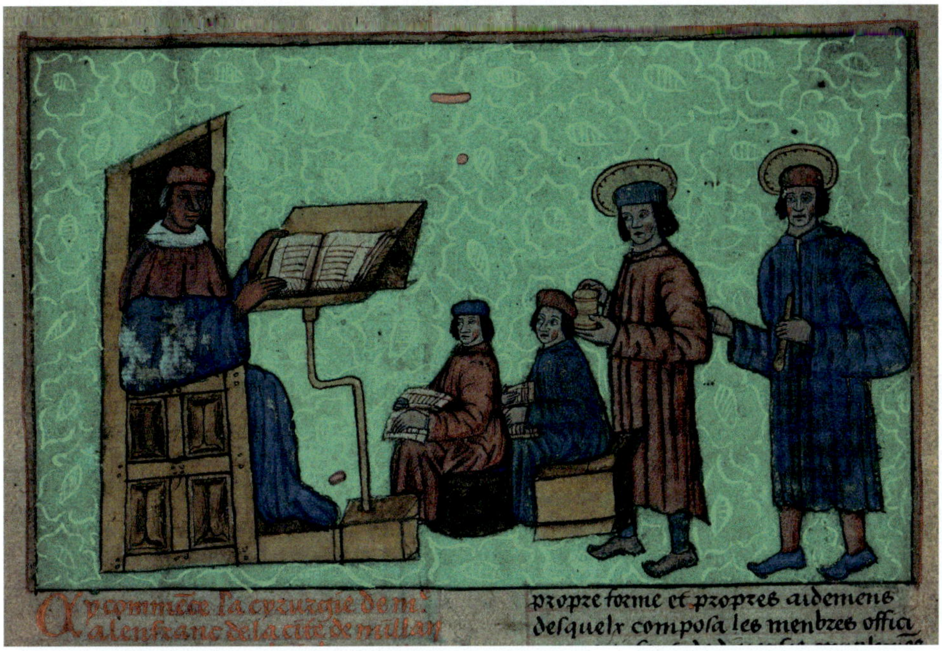
propre forme et propres aidemens
desquelx composa les menbres offici

Fig. 11.5 Lanfranchi da Milano lecturing to students while Cosmas and Damian, the patron saints of surgeons stand nearby. From a fifteenth century illuminated French manuscript of *Chirurgia*. *By permission of the Biblioteque, Nationale de France, Paris*

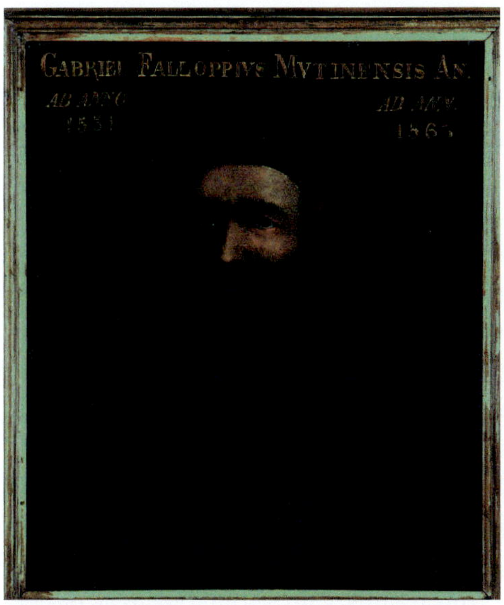

Fig. 11.6 Portrait of Gabriel Fallopius from the Faculty of Medicine at the University of Padua where he taught from 1551 to 1565. *Courtesy of the Rector of the University of Padua*

should be sutured. In the case of a fracture, Berengario suggests using a light bandage for keeping the edges of the wound together, but he also admits to having seen cases that survived after being treated without suturing.

In every case, however, he recommends using a drain. The description of a craniotomy given in Chapter 10 is very detailed and refers to the various areas of the skull. Berengario gives a description of the instruments he invented for replacing the bone fragments in their original position, but also advises the removal of fragments that are not connected with the rest of the skull or the dura mater.

Berengario's book is the first to deal with skull fractures after that written by Galen. It was the best for describing the neurological symptoms related to the site of the trauma until Ambroise Paré (1510–1590) published his book in 1562 [766–770]. In this period we should also mention Dryander who published a detailed study of the skull and the brain (Fig. 11.7a,b) [252].

Paré was definitely against the use of metals[6] for repairing cranial defects and even accused surgeons who

6 See Chapter XXII (*Des alteration de l'os de la tête*) of his ninth book (*Les Playes en Particuleur*).

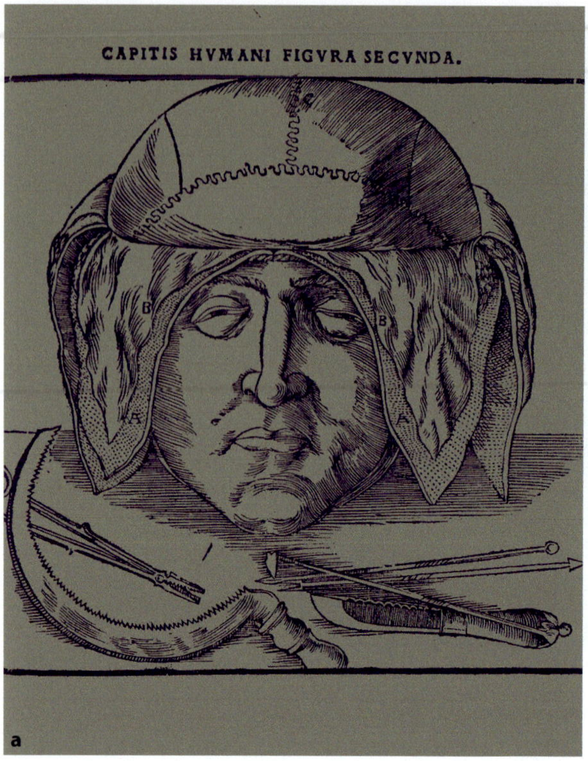

Fig. 11.7a,b Two images from a series showing the layers of the skull in Johannes Dryander's *Chirurgiae Libri Septem* (Venice, 1573). *Courtesy of Riccardo Mazzola, M.D., Milan*

performed this cranioplasty of being frauds, saying: "So called surgeons convince the patient and his assistants that, instead of the bone, a piece of gold must be placed on the defect … they hammer it, in order to make it similar in shape to the defect and apply it saying that it is going to stay instead of the bone … but then they put it in their bag."

Sarcasm apart, he declares that the real reason is that foreign bodies are ill tolerated if placed in contact with the brain, an objection that found staunch supporters even in the twentieth century. Paré was unquestionably the most famous traumatologist in the world at that time and the considerable weight of his authority tended to diminish any enthusiasm for Fallopius' ideas. Paré was another of the surgeons who recommended just the replacement of bone fragments, especially if they were connected to the surrounding tissues, such as the scalp, while any completely free fragments were to be discarded.

Knowledge of skull damage made great progress during the sixteenth century, thanks to interest shown by many authors. The first was Leone Giovanni Carcano (1536–1606), who wrote *De Vulneribus Capitis Liber Absolutissimus*, a 145-page masterpiece on skull traumas[7] published in 1583 in Milan [156].

Another author who contributed to the subject was Johannes Schultes alias Scultetus (1595–1645). In his famous *Armamentarium Chirurgicum* he referred to 19 cases of skull trauma with varying degrees of cranial depression and how he treated them (Fig. 11.8) [907–909].

7 Leone Giovanni Battista Carcano, born in Milan, became Professor of Anatomy and Surgery at Pavia University. However, it was during his term as Head of the Military Hospital in Milan that he acquired the vast experience of skull traumatology that inspired his great book. His studies on the embryological origins of certain cardiac malformations are also noteworthy.

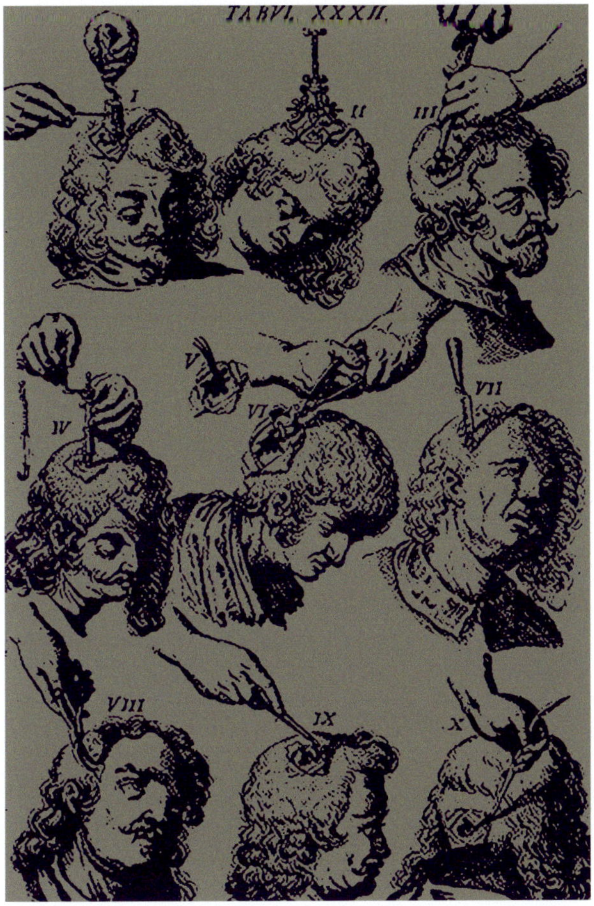

Fig. 11.8 Page from *Armamentarium Chirurgicum* (1655) by Johannes Scultetus (1595–1645). He deals with the anatomy of the skull and ways of treating fractures. *Courtesy of Riccardo Mazzola, M.D. Milan*

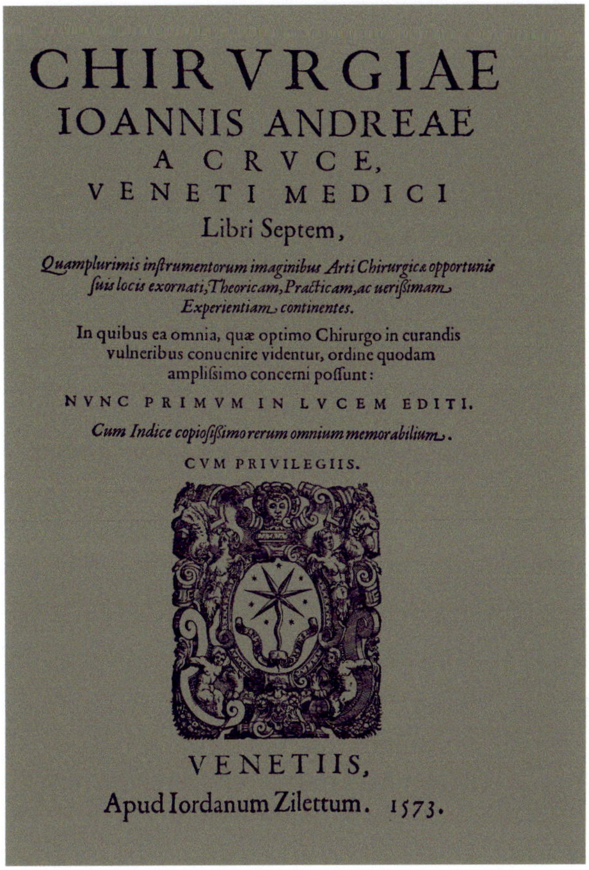

CHIRVRGIAE
IOANNIS ANDREAE
A CRVCE,
VENETI MEDICI
Libri Septem,

Quamplurimis inſtrumentorum imaginibus Arti Chirurgicæ opportunis ſuis locis exornati, Theoricam, Practicam, ac uerißimam Experientiam continentes.

In quibus ea omnia, quæ optimo Chirurgo in curandis vulneribus conuenire videntur, ordine quodam ampliſsimo concerni poſſunt:

NVNC PRIMVM IN LVCEM EDITI.

Cum Indice copioſiſsimo rerum omnium memorabilium.

CVM PRIVILEGIIS.

VENETIIS,
Apud Iordanum Zilettum. 1573.

Fig. 11.9 Frontispiece of *Chirurgiae Libri Septem* (Venice,1573) by Andrea Giovanni della Croce (1514–1575). *Courtesy of Riccardo Mazzola, M.D., Milan*

Andrea Giovanni della Croce (1514–1575) is yet another who was interested in skull trauma, devoting 70 pages of his *Chirurgiae Libri Septem* (Fig. 11.9), published in Venice in 1573, to injuries of the head and skull [231]. His description of fractures is exhaustive and he prefers the replacement of fragments rather than the use of metal plates for closing any bone defects (Fig. 11.10a,b).

The same may be said about Fabricius ab Aquapendente (1537–1619) [291, 293] and for Fabrice Hildanus (1560–1624) [433], both of whom agreed with Paré. In his second book, *Le Opere Chirurgiche*, published in Padua in 1684, Fabricius ab Aquapendente wrote ten chapters on skull fractures, distinguishing lesions involving the dura mater and penetrating the brain from simple closed fractures of the various areas of the skull (Fig. 11.11a,b).

It appears that Fallopius' suggestion of using metal plates was left in the shadows, since the majority of authors seemed to prefer replacing any fragments of bone connected to the surrounding tissues. Since this was not always applicable, a certain number of patients survived but still bore a cranial defect. The problem could have been solved by immediately replacing the detached bones as free bone grafts and for all we know this may have happened in some rare, unknown case—but it certainly did not become routine practice.

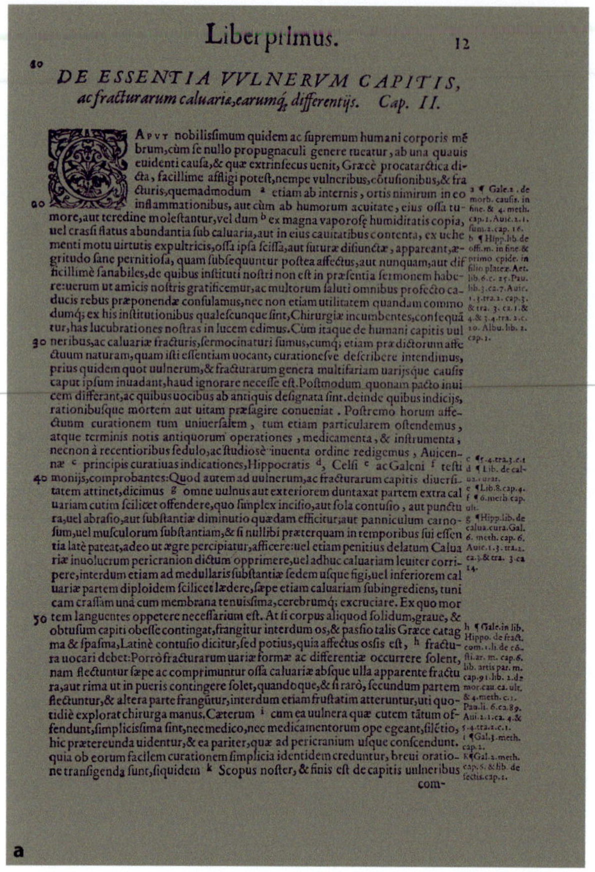

Liber primus. 12

DE ESSENTIA VVLNERVM CAPITIS, ac fracturarum caluariæ, earumq́ differentijs. Cap. II.

CAPVT nobiliſſimum quidem ac ſupremum humani corporis mẽbrum, cùm ſe nullo propugnaculi genere tueatur, ab una quauis euidenti cauſa, & quæ extrinſecus uenit, Græcè procatarctica dicta, facillime affligi poteſt, nempe vulneribus, cõtuſionibus, & fracturis, quemadmodum [a] etiam ab internis, ortis nimirum in eo inflammationibus, aut cùm ab humorum acuitate, eius oſſa tumore, aut teredine moleſtantur, vel dum [b] ex magna vaporoſę humiditatis copia, uel craſſi flatus abundantia ſub caluaria, aut in eius cauitatibus contenta, ex uehementi motu uirtutis expultricis, oſſa ipſa ſciſſa, aut ſuturæ diſiunctæ, appareant, ægritudo ſane pernitioſa, quam ſubſequuntur poſtea affectus, aut nunquam, aut difficillimè ſanabiles, de quibus inſtituti noſtri non eſt in præſentia ſermonem habere: uerum ut amicis noſtris gratificemur, ac multorum ſaluti omnibus profecto caducis rebus præponendæ conſulamus, nec non etiam utilitatem quandam commodumq; ex his inſtitutionibus qualeſcunque ſint, Chirurgiæ incumbentes, conſequãtur, has lucubrationes noſtras in lucem edimus. Cùm itaque de humani capitis uulneribus, ac caluariæ fracturis, ſermocinaturi ſumus, cumq; etiam prædictorum affectuum naturam, quam iſti eſſentiam uocant, curationeſve deſcribere intendimus, prius quidem quot uulnerum, & fracturarum genera multifariam uarijsque cauſis caput ipſum inuadant, haud ignorare neceſſe eſt. Poſtmodum quonam pacto inuicem differant, ac quibus uocibus ab antiquis deſignata ſint. deinde quibus indicijs, rationibuſque mortem aut uitam præſagire conueniat. Poſtremo horum affectuum curationem tum uniuerſalem, tum etiam particularem oſtendemus, atque terminis notis antiquorum operationes, medicamenta, & inſtrumenta, necnon à recentioribus ſedulo, ac ſtudioſè inuenta ordine redigemus, Auicennæ [c] principis curatiuas indicationes, Hippocratis [d], Celſi [e] ac Galeni [f] teſtimonijs, comprobantes: Quod autem ad uulnerum, ac fracturarum capitis diuerſitatem attinet, dicimus [g] omne uulnus aut exteriorem duntaxat partem extra caluariam cutim ſcilicet offendere, quo ſimplex inciſio, aut ſola contuſio, aut punctura, uel abraſio, aut ſubſtantiæ diminutio quædam efficitur; aut panniculum carnoſum, uel muſculorum ſubſtantiam, & ſi nullibi præterquam in temporibus ſui eſſentia latè pateat, adeo ut ægre percipiatur, afficere: uel etiam penitius delatum Caluariæ inuolucrum pericranion dictum opprimere, uel adhuc caluariam leuiter corripere, interdum etiam ad medullaris ſubſtantiæ ſedem uſque figi, uel inferiorem caluariæ partem diploidem ſcilicet lædere, ſæpe etiam caluariam ſubingrediens, tunicam craſſam unà cum membrana tenuiſſima, cerebrumq; excruciare. Ex quo mortem languentes oppetere neceſſarium eſt. At ſi corpus aliquod ſolidum, graue, & obtuſum capiti obeſſe contingat, frangitur interdum os, & paſſio talis Græce catagma & ſpaſma, Latinè contuſio dicitur, ſed potius, quia affectus oſſis eſt, [h] fractura uocari debet: Porrò fracturarum uariæ formæ ac differentiæ occurrere ſolent, nam flectuntur ſæpe ac comprimuntur oſſa caluariæ abſque ulla apparente fractura, aut rima ut in pueris contingere ſolet, quandoque, & ſi rarò, ſecundum partem flectuntur, & altera parte frangũtur, interdum etiam fruſtatim atteruntur, uti quotidiè explorat chirurga manus. Cæterum [i] cum ea uulnera quæ cutem tãtum offendunt, ſimplicisſima ſint, nec medico, nec medicamentorum ope egeant, ſilẽtio, hic prætereunda uidentur, & ea pariter, quæ ad pericranium uſque conſcendunt. quia ob eorum facilem curationem ſimplicia identidem creduntur, breui oratione tranſigenda ſunt, ſiquidem [k] Scopus noſter, & finis eſt de capitis uulneribus com-

a ¶ Gale. 2. de morb. cauſis. in fine. & 4. meth. cap. 1. Auic. 2. 1. ſum. 2. cap. 16. b ¶ Hipp. lib. de offi. m. in fine & primo epide. in filio plateæ. Aet. lib. 6. c. 25. Pau. lib. 3. ca. 7. Auic. 1. 3. tra. 2. cap. 3. & tra. 3. ca. 1. & 4. & 3. 4. tra. 2. c. 10. Albu. lib. 2. cap. 1.

c ¶ 5. 4. tra. 3. c. 1 d ¶ Lib. de calua. curat. e ¶ Lib. 8. cap. 4. f ¶ 6. meth. cap. ult. g ¶ Hipp. lib. de calua. cura. Gal. 6. meth. cap. 6. Auic. 1. 3. tra. 2. ca. 3. & tra. 3. ca 14.

h ¶ Gale. in lib. Hippo. de fract. com. 1. li. de cõſti. ar. m. cap. 6. lib. artis par. m. cap. 91. lib. 2. de mor. cau. ca. ult. & 4. meth. c. 1. Pau. li. 6. ca. 89. Aui. 2. 1. ca. 4. & 5. 4. tra. 2. c. 1. i ¶ Gal. 3. meth. cap. 2. k ¶ Gal. 2. meth. cap. 5. & lib. de ſectis. cap. 1.

a

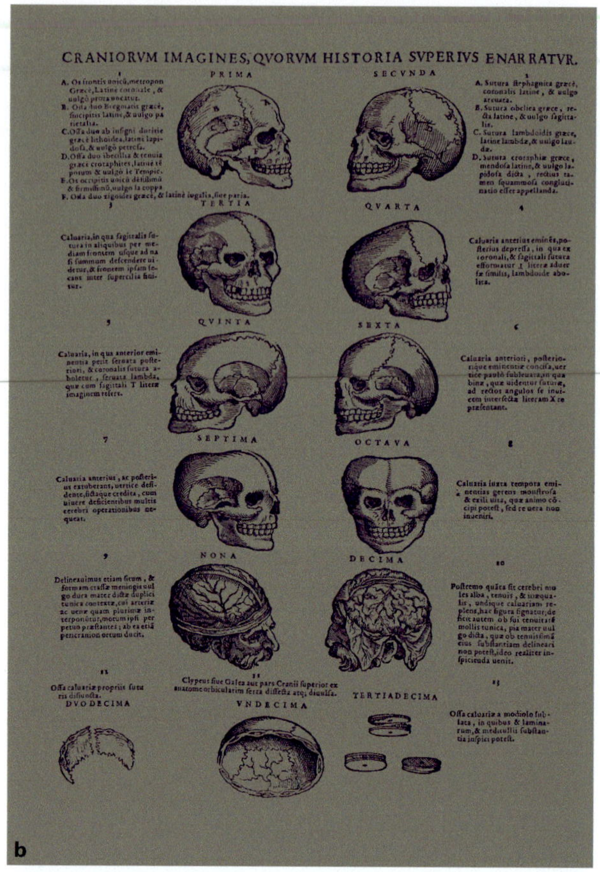

Fig. 11.10 **a** A page from *Chirurgiae Libri Septem* (1573) where head injuries are described. **b** Skull anatomy showing the cranial sutures and different shaped skulls. *Courtesy of Riccardo Mazzola, M.D., Milan*

Repair with Bone Grafts

In the chapter on bone grafts, we have already mentioned the legendary case of the Russian nobleman, Butterljin, described by Job Janszoo van Meek'ren (1611–1666). While the tale has all the aspects of a legend, it nevertheless demonstrates that the dream of surgeons was to be able to close defects in the skull bones by means of bone grafts [658]. Furthermore, the idea of using dog bone for repairing a skull was not exclusive to Meek'ren. According to P. Mauclaire, who published a study on the subject in 1922, several other authors[8] resorted to heterologous sources for their grafts in the hope that the Church might have changed its opinion since Meek'ren's times [619].

The first to use human autografts for skull repair appears to have been Henry Louis Duhamel-Dumanceau (1700–1781). He did studies on the healing of wounds in animals and plants. He was particularly interested in osteogenesis and in 1746 treated a patient for a gunshot wound which had taken off the top of the skull. He replaced the large portion of skull but because the fragment was still loosely attached by a small piece of tissue this case was not strictly a free graft. However it stimulated interest in finding the best solution for cranial defects and in that same year, Albrecht von Haller (1708–1777) disagreed with this approach [409].

Around this time interest in bone grafts was growing. Louis Xavier Ollier (1830–1900) demonstrated the role played by the periosteum in osteogenesis and

8 Naunoir (1815), von Walther (1820), Klenche (1830), Wolf (1830) and Wodemeyer (1842).

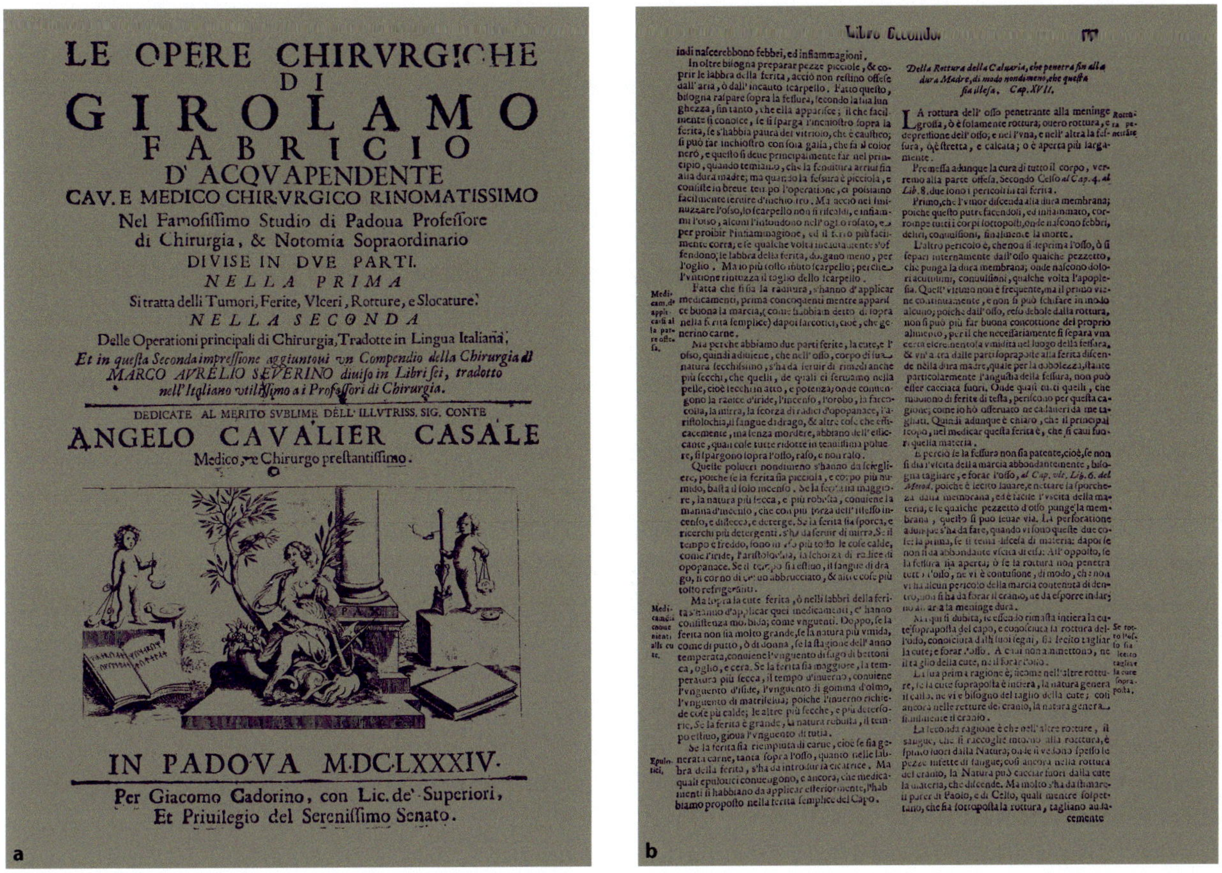

Fig. 11.11 **a** Frontispiece of *Le Opere Chirurgiche* (Padua, 1674) by Fabricius ab Aquapendente (1537–1619). **b** The page where he deals with the injuries of the head. *Courtesy of Riccardo Mazzpla, M.D. Milan*

always included it in his bone grafts [747, 749]. Clinical observations made by Pierre Flourens (1794–1867) [322], and particularly the detailed reports by Bernard R. von Langenbeck (1776–1851), encouraged surgeons to undertake the repair of skull defects with bone grafts [322, 524]. The results were not uniformly successful, probably because they used both autografts and homografts. In the former case surgeons were afraid of complications in donor site as well as the skull. Unaware of the immune response they preferred cadaver homografts or heterografts. Durand, Renier and Marchac reported that in 1891 Ricard used canine iliac bone [265] whereas G. B. Schmidt (1893) employed rabbit bone [904] and bovine bone was used by both Grekopf (1898) and Babcock (1917) [47].

Homograft failures were generally attributed to infection rather than rejection and William MacEwen (1848–1924) suggested sterilizing the homografts with mercuric chloride that must also have killed the osteocytes [637, 638].Other surgeons used different chemicals and some appear to have been successful. In the light of present knowledge, they were possibly denaturing the bone and making it non-antigenic while maintaining its capacity to act as a frame work for new bone growth. Only when anaesthesia was introduced and antisepsis became a matter of routine did surgeons begin to use autografts. In the skull use of the outer table and its pericranium carried less risk and pain.

The pioneers of this method were numerous.[9] Where possible they left the bone attached to soft tissue so in

9 W. Müller [718], Franz König [506], Hjaler von Bonsdorff [119] and Maurice Cazin [164, 165].

these instances they were not free grafts. However the availability of bone in a convenient and effective site had been demonstrated. In 1932 J. Woolfe and A.E. Walker used the outer table with the pericranium [1050, 1051] and so did Santoni-Rugiu in 1969 [891].

Others preferred to use bone without its covering. W. Kenn filled a defect with bone chips from the outer table in 1905 and this method was preferred forty years later by Mowlem.[10] H. Seydel appears to have been the first to be entirely successful with autologous free bone grafts in 1889 [919]. The sternum was used by W. Ropke [860] and P. Müller [718] and the iliac crest by P. Mauclaire [618, 619] and even a phalanx of a supernumerary digit was utilized.

H. Delangénière and P. Lewin reported on 104 cases from the First World War in 1920. They used osteoperiosteal grafts from the tibia and had only three failures [230].

After 1894 several surgeons started using cartilage instead of bone for skull reconstruction after their experience in other parts of the body.[11] In 1915 A. Kappis used the entire thickness of the 12th rib with its periosteum [485]. Others performed similar operations the following year.[12] They were soon followed by H. Morestin and A. Gosset in 1917 [701, 703] and by L. Dufourmentel in 1919 [258].

Alloplastic Implants

Gold was the material of choice in past centuries and was recommended by Fallopius but in more recent years, many other materials have been employed with variable success (Fig. 11.12a,b).

In 1917, Mauclaire used ivory in four patients. One of the implants was extruded after six months while another two remained for three years. There was no follow-up of the fourth patient [618, 619].

Gold was frequently used during the First World War and E. Estor utilized it in one hundred patients, publishing his data in 1917 [286]. However, the gold was considered both expensive and too pliable to offer suitable protection. All the same, the patients appeared to tolerate it fairly well [900].

Many types of materials were tried such as silver, aluminium, gum and lead but most were soon abandoned due to the acute toxic effects they produced.

Tantalum, Vitallium and stainless steel were used in attempts made by F. Geib in 1941 [363], R.H. Pudenz and G.L. Odom in 1942 [818], and M. Scott and H.T. Wycis in 1946 [913], but they proved to be unsuitable because of their radiopacity, the effects of heat or the tendency to induce epilepsy as well as the risk of infection.

In 1948, J.C. White [1045] compared the results of 66 cases treated with Lucite implants with 130 with tantalum. The first group had 10% complications and the second 12.3% due to infection and extrusion.

In spite of these risks, J. I. Woolf and A. E. Walker [1050, 1051] stated in 1945 that defects exceeding 8 cm in diameter could not be closed with autologous bone and should therefore be treated by alloplastic implants.

In order to avoid the problems encountered with the use of metals, O. Kleinschmidt [501] advocated the use of acrylic resins in 1941, as Zander had already proposed in 1940. More recently, the methyl methacrylate implants suggested by J.A. Subczynsk in 1977 appeared to be well tolerated [965] and J.B. Mulliken and J. Glowacki used demineralized homologous bone powder in 1980 [719]. This section would be incomplete without mention of the practical solution, related by Durand about the coconut prostheses used by aborigines in Australia! [265].

Facial Fractures

We have mentioned little about facial fractures. They are covered briefly in many of the old texts which have been quoted. Galen, for example, describes immobilization with bandages but he makes no mention of surgical treatment (Fig. 11.13). Aegineta briefly described dental wiring for treating jaw fractures in the seventh century

10 Kenn W (1905) Filling in the skull by bone chips from the outer table. *Ann Surg* 296.

11 In 1894 Sacchi used dog's cartilage in a single case but the results are not clear. *Ulteriore contributo alle plastiche del cranio. Bull Acad Med Genova* 9:71.

12 H. Weber and B.G. Schmidt in 1916.

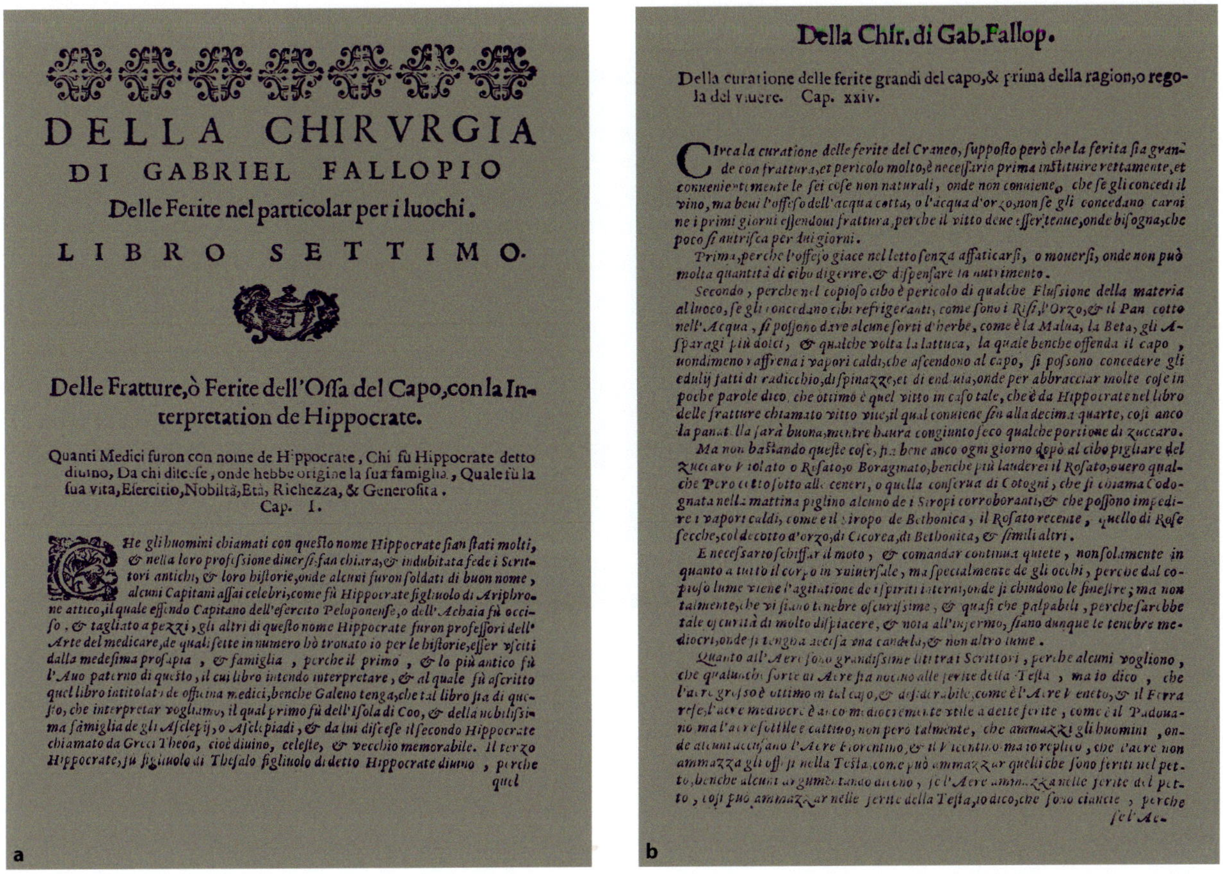
DELLA CHIRVRGIA
DI GABRIEL FALLOPIO
Delle Ferite nel particolar per i luochi.
LIBRO SETTIMO.

Delle Fratture, ò Ferite dell'Ossa del Capo, con la Interpretation de Hippocrate.

Quanti Medici furon con nome de Hippocrate, Chi fù Hippocrate detto diuino, Da chi discese, onde hebbe origine la sua famiglia, Quale fù la sua vita, Esercitio, Nobiltà, Età, Richezza, & Generosità. Cap. I.

Della Chir. di Gab. Fallop.

Della curatione delle ferite grandi del capo, & prima della ragion, o regola del viuere. Cap. xxiv.

Fig. 11.12 **a** Frontispiece of the book *Della Chirurgia* by Gabriele Fallopius (1523–1565). **b** The page where injuries of the head are described. He favoured using gold plates for skull defects. *Courtesy of Riccardo Mazzola, M.D., Milan*

but from then onwards surgery appears to have played little part in their treatment. This conservative approach continued until the end of the nineteenth century when Thomas L. Gilmer of Illinois described a way of treating lower jaw fractures by inter-dental wiring [377]. His method became widely accepted and was later used in combination with the developing techniques designed to fix complex fractures of both upper and lower jaws. With the teeth held in occlusion the jaw fragments could be stabilized by fixing them to the skull using a Plaster of Paris skull cap and metal bars. This was later replaced by a more reliable metal halo frame fixed to the skull with screws.

Our understanding of the patterns of facial fractures affecting the maxilla and consequently the best ways to treat them owes much to the experiments of René Le Fort of Lille in France. He published his work in 1901 in three parts [542]. He used cadaver heads on which he inflicted different types of injury. He then removed the soft tissue by maceration and related the different patterns of fractures to the trauma he had used. His work led to a better understanding of the lines along which the facial bones break and the well known classification into Le Fort fracture types I–III. This had practical implications for their treatment. At the time they were relatively uncommon injuries but in the age of accidents involving fast vehicles his studies acquired greater relevance. The treatment of cranio-facial deformities was subsequently influenced by his work.

Readers may feel that we have not done justice to this subheading and we acknowledge our omissions. To cover the history of facial fractures and craniofacial surgery would require another specialized chapter. This would ring with such names as Obwegeser, Killey, Rowe, Kazanjian, Tessier, Ortiz-Monasterio and many more who pioneered this work in the last century.

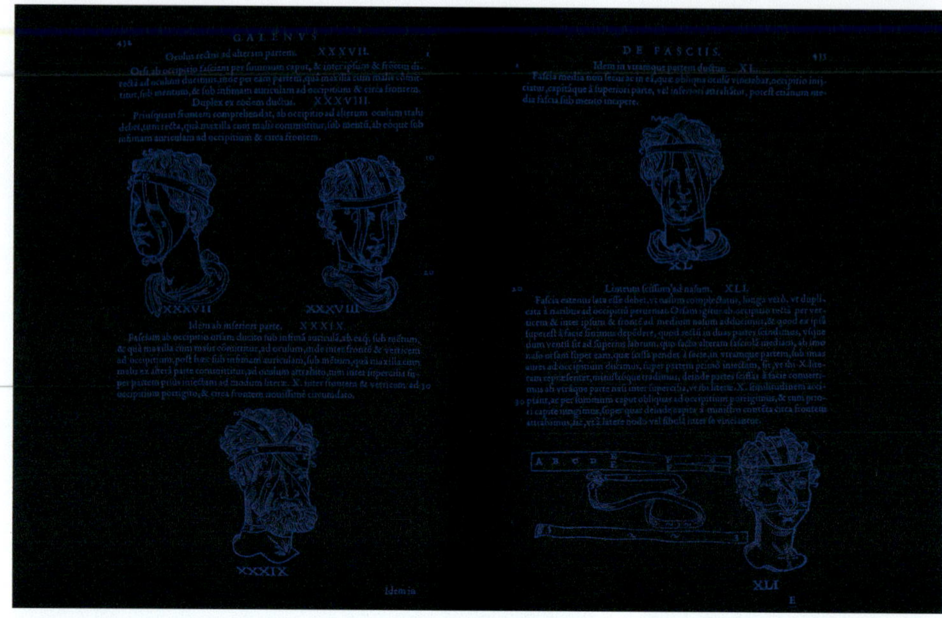

Fig. 11.13 Galen's special bandages for treating different facial fractures. *Courtesy of Riccardo Mazzola, M.D., Milan*

Chapter 12

Introduction to Cosmetic Surgery

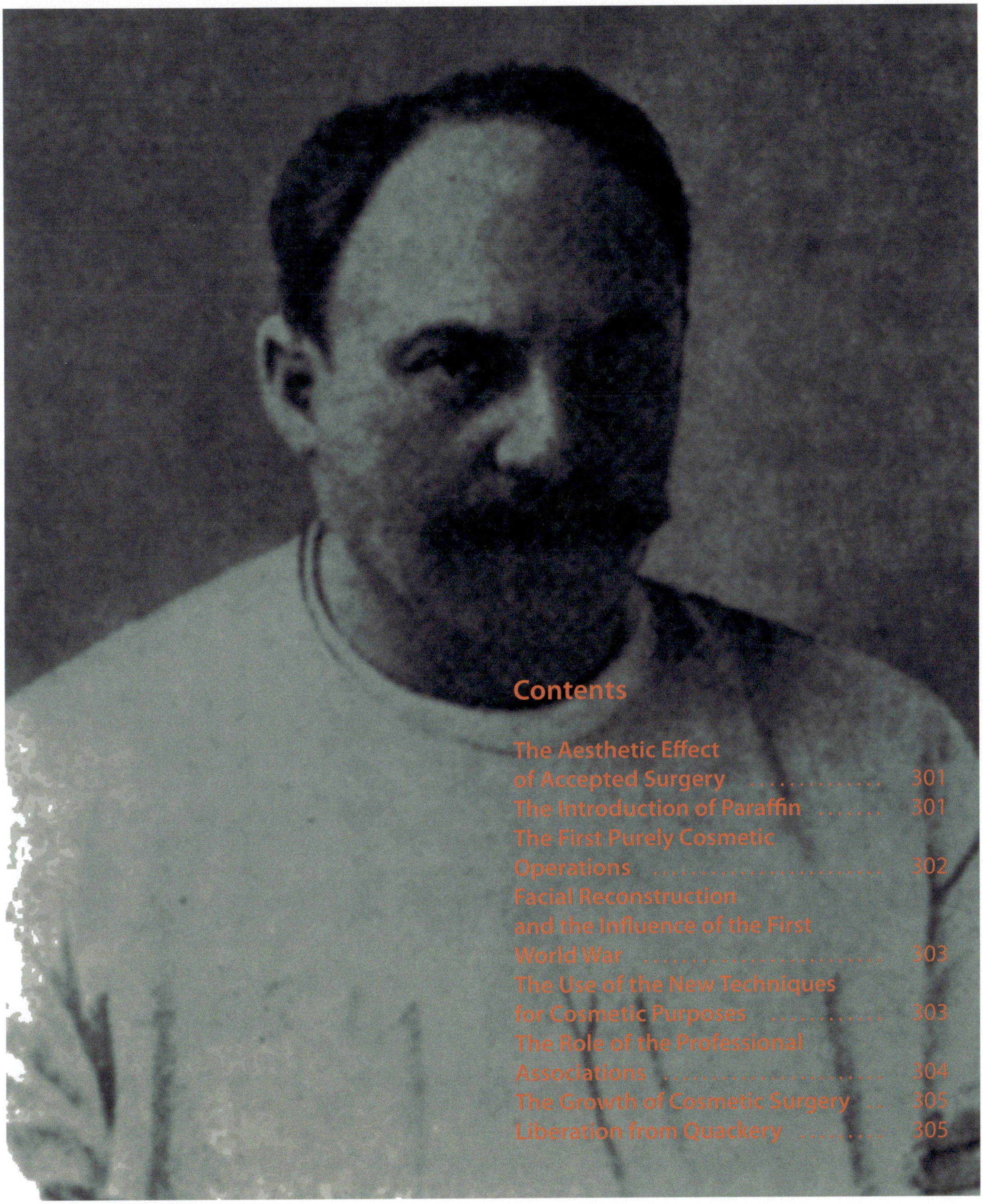

Contents

Plastic surgery did not emerge as a separated branch of surgery until the beginning of the twentieth century. This was the case with most of the specialized surgical fields while cosmetic surgery had not even been envisaged.

This does not mean that men and women had never yearned for good looks before; on the contrary, the pursuit of a pleasing appearance is probably as old as Mankind and the references on how to embellish the eyelids found in the Ebers' papyrus [271] a thousand years before Christ demonstrate that the ancients definitely sought after a beautiful appearance.

The temptation to preserve beauty as long as possible must have been very strong because, according to Pliny the Elder(23–79 A.D.) [804], women in Ancient Rome did not hesitate to use cosmetics containing lead, silver and even arsenic, fully accepting the risks of the poisons as long as they could keep their youth [596].

There are few writings from the *Scuola Salernitana* as most of the teaching were done there was by lectures. The *Regimen Sanitatis Salernitanum* represents an opus magna of the school but mention should also be made of *Trotula* a treatese on women's health compiled in the twelfth century. Despite the fact that women did not practise medicine in Salerno, there appears to be an exception since one of the authors of this book is a woman by the name of Trota.

The treatese was divided into three parts. The first two (*On Conditions of Women* and *On Womens Cosmetics*) were written by men while the third (*On the Treatment for Women*) was written by this woman. It seems that the title of the whole book (*Trotula*) was borrowed from her name. The work covers the common problems associated with women but one third is devoted to aesthetic appearance and is called *Trotula Minor*.[1]

Many years before this period, Paulus Aegineta (625–690 B.C.) suggested certain massaging ploys for improving the complexion [3–5].

At the time when southern Spain was part of the Islamic empire, Abu al-Qasim Al-Zahrawi, better known as Albucasis (c.936–1013) was one of the great pioneers of surgery in Cordoba. He wrote a medical encyclopaedia, *Al-Tasrif* (*The Method*), which contained designs of over two hundred surgical instruments. This surgical work was the first illustrated scientific textbook and was to gain tremendous popularity in Europe. Translated into Latin in the twelfth century by the Italian scholar Gerard of Cremona, *Al-Tasrif* stood for nearly five hundred years as the leading textbook on surgery in Europe.

Al-Zahrawi developed the art of plastic surgery and was particularly concerned with the cosmetic results of his operations. He stated that all incisions be marked pre-operatively and described Z-plasty for contractures. In the 26th treatise of his book, which covers surgery of the nose, lips and ears following trauma, Al-Zahrawi puts forward two important principles of surgery: primary closure and debridement and closure. This treatise also describes the surgical management of ectropion, entropion, trichiasis and symblepharon. The 19th treatise is almost entirely devoted to cosmetic surgery. Other parts describe operations for breast reduction and tendon repair.

Ambroise Paré [769, 770] and Gaspare Tagliacozzi [969][2] followed these lines at a much later date and emphasized the important rôle played by deformities and blemishes in the mental health of the patient.[3] Surgeons[4] in the thirteenth century and later were careful to stress the care of facial wounds to avoid ugly scars and were all very concerned about the effect of their operations on the appearance.

In the sixteenth century some surgeons gave more than just passing attention to the appearance. Two of these were Giovanni Minodoi [678] and Giovanni Marinello [610]. But in spite of these sporadic instances, Conley [189] states: "In the early part of the twentieth century

1 See Green M.H. (2001) *The Trotula: A Medieval Compendium of Women's Medicine*, University of Pensylvania Press, Philadelphia.

2 See *De Curtorum Chirugia per Insitionem*, Liber I, Chapter 25.

3 "...we restore, repair and make whole parts of the face which nature has given but which fortune has taken away, not so much that they may delight the eye but that they may buoy up the spirit and help the mind of the afflicted" (from the translation by Robert Goldwyn).

4 Guy de Chauliac (1298–1368), Henry de Mondeville (1260–1320), Heinrich von Pfolsprundt (c.1450), Ambroise Paré (1510–1590) and Fabricius da Aquapendente (1533–1619), to mention but a few.

there was still considerable resistance to the correction of a facial deformity or blemish, since this would constitute a cosmetic procedure and did not merit a surgeon's attention. The argument also persisted that no surgeon had the right to interfere with God's designs, regardless of their severity, and these personal tragedies were accepted as immutable situations to be borne in grief and resignation throughout life."

Despite the fact that throughout history surgeons understood the importance of minimizing the effects of their operations on the patients' looks no consideration was ever given to operating solely to improve their appearance.

It was not until relatively recent times that general surgeons and other specialists undertaking reconstructive surgery began to appreciate that appearance was an important aspect of the outcome ot the operation. Nevertheless is was never the only purpose of the procedure and this attitude prevailed.

For various reasons, these views changed during the last century but we must not forget that surgery implied quite considerable risks and that anaesthesia, when available, did not eliminate pain and anxiety completely. Under the circumstances it is not surprising that surgery was only considered necessary for restoring physical health and the time was not ripe for considering an operation on a blemish or disfigurement to improve mental health.

While medical ethics prevented surgeons from undertaking cosmetic procedures, in the nineteenth century other less scrupulous individuals performed surgery on perfectly healthy subjects to improve their appearance. This phenomenon became more frequent as the century drew to a close. The practitioners were generally referred to as *quacks* or, on the other side of the Atlantic, *beauty doctors* and these derisory names indicates the attitude of the establishment to their activities.

The Aesthetic Effect of Accepted Surgery

As already mentioned, reputable doctors occasionally achieved an improvement in the appearance when operating for some pathological condition. One typical example was the treatment of blocked noses following nasal fractures or septal deviation. Restoration of normal breathing often improved the appearance of the nose. Perhaps the first report of this benefit was in 1829 by Johan Friedrich Dieffenbach (1794–1847) who operated on a patient with post-traumatic septal deviation. He detached the septum from the hard palate with a scalpel, freed the nasal bones from the maxilla and reshaped the nose [246]. His main intention was to restore the nasal airways but he also improved the shape of the nose. Others who belong to the same category and are considered to be among the first to perform rhinoplasty operations under similar circumstances were John Orlando Roe in 1887 and 1891 [848], G.H. Monks in 1989 [686] and J.P. Clark in 1901 and 1902.[5]

The correction of a saddle nose was a different matter. This was often due to trauma, scrophula, or lupus but was also commonly thought to be the consequence of untreated syphilis, which was often true. This stigma was the reason for many patients' desire for surgery. Hence, armed with the praiseworthy intention of helping them, some surgeons operated but used inappropriate techniques, employing incompatible implant materials, such as ivory, which were usually extruded. Some tried using bone or cartilage, but the techniques were not sufficiently refined and their audacious exploits were seldom successful.

The Introduction of Paraffin

During this same period, the use of this substance spread rapidly as it was easy to use and was assumed to be harmless. Paraffin[6] had the attractions of being injectable, the procedure was relatively painless and left no scars. At the beginning it seemed to be inert and well tolerated and was used as the ideal material for correcting the contours of the face and other areas including the breast.

According to Elisabeth Haiken [407], it was considered "… absolutely harmless". Hence, saddle noses, facial

5 J.P. Clark reported in the *Boston Medical and Surgical Journal* of 1901, vol 144, p 496 and again in 1902, vol 146, p 245 on his experience correcting the Roman nose and other nasal deformities.

6 Paraffin in the UK is a thin liquid fuel which is called kerosene elsewhere. Here we refer to paraffin wax.

wrinkles, even absent testicles or small breasts were all corrected with paraffin injections. Giving an injection is such a simple matter that it is not surprising that the *quacks* and *beauty doctors* as well as outright swindlers with no basic medical knowledge made money from the procedure.[7] The practice continued until the first reports appeared demonstrating that this "absolutely harmless" substance was not what it was made out to be. As we can now imagine many complications arose including frequent *paraffinomas*, called *wax cancer* in the United States.

Despite this, many of the *beauty doctors* continued using injections, simply changing the material used. They tried different liquids like vaseline, olive oil, white wax and glycerine, sometimes boiling them in carbolic acid, which was the basis of antisepsis at the end of the nineteenth century. They believed or perhaps hoped that the cause of the numerous problems was infection. The tissue reaction to these irritant chemicals was not appreciated at a time when little thought had even been given to the true origin of the rejection phenomenon. These stories should come as no surprise when we consider more recent events and the complications that have been reported with the use of various types of breast implants but they did nothing to help those more reputable and trustworthy individuals who attempted to perform cosmetic surgery. This was especially so in the climate of dissent that prevailed in the established medical world. These predjudices were gradually overcome but this was not without the perseverance of some enlightened early cosmetic surgeons.

The First Purely Cosmetic Operations

One of the pioneers was Charles C. Miller from Chicago [668–672]. He was born in 1880 in New Albany, Kentucky and went to Chicago in 1898 to study medicine. He never disguised the fact that his ambition was to do *Featural Surgery*, correcting imperfections that from a medical point of view were not considered to be deformities. In this respect he began the practice of cosmetic surgery for its own sake and his efforts should not be scorned. Chicago, the dynamic city, always open to new ideas was a good place to begin.

In 1906 he published an article on the excision of bags under the eyes and followed this the following year with one dealing with cosmetic surgery. Unfortunately in 1908, as was the fashion of the time, he described his experience with paraffin not only for correcting saddle noses but also for inguinal hernias but like many of his colleagues, he soon had doubts. Nevertheless, his greatest merit was to bring cosmetic surgery to the attention of the medical profession who he criticized for their indifference and unwillingness to accept that even gross imperfections were worthy of treatment. In this respect he wrote: "The regular profession has disregarded the educational tendencies of thousands of columns of newspapers. When a woman or man consults the family physician regarding some defect of facial outline or fault of skin, the physician merely laughs and ridicules."

Miller was a prolific writer in the years 1907 and 1908 when he produced articles on nose, eyelid, ear and lip surgery and also devised a method for creating dimples in cheeks. In all, he wrote a total of 29 articles some of which were printed in highly regarded journals. This served to break the ice. The press had also become interested in cosmetic surgery and Miller took advantage of this. Newspapers and magazines were full of methods for improving appearance, often asserting that this could well be the passport to success.

Some years later, in 1927, he even founded a journal on cosmetic surgery called *The Dr. Charles Conrad Miller's Review of Plastic and Esthetic Surgery*. This was probably the first time that the term *Esthetic Surgery* appeared in a scientific publication.

In more conservative medical circles he was defined as a quack. This was rather harsh even in those days as he demonstrated ideas that were both valid and surgically achievable. One was the subcutaneous division of branches of the facial nerve and the facial muscles for reducing facial wrinkles. Notwithstanding being labelled, he made every effort to be accepted by the medical world. He also saw the importance of insisting that only qualified doctors should carry out this surgery so as to protect vulnerable patients and to preserve the speciality from adverse criticism.

7 It seems that the first to use paraffin injections were Leonard J. Corning in New York and Robert Gersuny in Vienna [see Robert M. Goldwyn (1980) The Paraffin Story. *Plast Reconstr Surg* 65:4].

Facial Reconstruction and the Influence of the First World War

The tragic events of the Great War had an impact on many areas of surgery. Thousands of servicemen needed treatment for devastating wounds and in Britain the Royal Army Medical Corps was formed. The Cambridge Military Hospital, Aldershot under Arbuthnot provided a comprehensive service for all the British and Commonwealth wounded but the numbers were huge and other hospitals were needed. Facial injuries, requiring complex reconstruction were very common in trench warfare and they were soon seen to require treatment by highly specialized teams of experienced doctors. Harold Gillies, then a captain, was given charge of Queen's Hospital, Sidcup and with his ear, nose and throat background and the experience gained in Paris at the Hõpital Militaire Val de Grâce with Hippolyte Morestin, he and his team developed many new methods that would eventually translate to peacetime plastic surgery. The general surgeons who were recruited became adept at the methods we now consider to be the realm of plastic surgery and some were able to adapt the techniques they had used for the treatment of cancer of the head and neck. The treatment of skull and jaw wounds were all part of the units remitt.

Unbeknownst to Gillies, Filatov [312] had already used the tube pedicle for eyelid reconstruction in Russia, but Gillies developed it coincidentally so that, together with other methods, it became one of the mainstays of plastic surgery. Operating in the region of the airway was hazardous and the contributions made by anaesthetists was of vital importance. Tracheal intubation replaced the mask and allowed better surgical access and greater safety.

Very soon, a group of young American surgeons from Harvard, Johns Hopkins and Columbia Universities, attracted by the new techniques, enrolled in the British Medical Corps and, after appropriate training in London, went to the battlefields in Europe where they collaborated with their British colleagues.

One who deserves particular mention was Varaztad Kazanjian. Born in Turkish Armenia in 1879 he emigrated at 16 and became an American citizen in 1900. He graduated from Harvard Dental School in 1905 and eventually studied medicine. He became known as the *Miracle Man of the Western Front* for the skill he showed treating soldiers with maxillofacial injuries in Hospital No. 20 at Camiers in France. He was honoured by King George V for his care of the wounded.[8] The European press reported on his achievements and the news soon reached America. His operations helped return soldiers with terrible disfigurement back to some sort of normal life after their facial rehabilitation.

The *miracles* performed on the war-wounded also brought fame to a German civilian surgeon, Jacques Joseph who was given the highest award in his country and was appointed *Professor motu proprio* by the Kaiser in recognition of his work [468–482]. It was while treating these cases that he devised and applied the famous double pedicle visor flap for reconstructing the lower third of the face of a Turkish soldier. His fame was such that although he was a Jew he managed to avoid the growing anti-Semitism that subsequently beset Germany. After the war he devoted his time exclusively to cosmetic surgery.

The Italian surgeon, Gustavo Sanvenero Rosselli was another who gained experience reconstructing soldiers suffering the deformities resulting from war wounds. He trained in Paris with Fernand Lemaitre and Ferris Smith in 1927 and returned to Milan where a special unit was established at the *Padiglione per I Mutilati del Viso*. During the 1930s and in World War II this unit began treating burns and congenital deformities and soon became a referral hospital for plastic surgery in Italy.

The war had provided the stimulus that started Plastic Surgery as a speciality in its own right and showed the importance of functional reconstruction and improved appearance.

The Use of the New Techniques for Cosmetic Purposes

The relative well-being and prosperity in the victorious countries after the war contributed to the acceptance of

8 After the war Kazanjian completed his medical training and became Professor of Maxillo Facial Surgery at Harvard, pioneering many new techniques. He wrote extensively about facial injuries [488] and published *The Surgical Treatment of Facial Injuries* with J. M. Converse.

cosmetic surgery. Although feminism had yet to take off, women became more independent and able to afford what had once been considered as frippery. The search for beauty became more overt. This was most marked in America. Over 15 years the number of hair salons quadrupled and *Beauty Parlours* became common place. These new establishments offered various cosmetic services including massage and in some, methods bordering on *quackery* were practised. Some physicians took part and these *semi-quacks* apparently became quite adept.

Many of them openly advertised their services, a practice that was considered unethical by the medical profession. Others, more intelligently and in a suitably dignified manner, publicized their activities by writing articles for newspapers. Nonetheless they offered percentages to beauty parlours and hairdressers who recruited patients for them.

All this opened up new horizons and stimulated debate among the public and within the profession. As Max Thorek said: "If soldiers whose faces had been torn away by bursting shells on the battle-field could come back into an almost normal life with new faces created by the wizard of the new science of plastic surgery, why couldn't women whose faces had been ravaged by nothing more explosive than the hand of the years find again the firm clear, contour of youth?" [992, 993]

When the war ended, many of the surgeons who had honed their skills on the battlefields of Europe found themselves with less material on which to use them. This brings to mind the story of Richard Barton, a young surgeon who introduced himself to Sir Harold Gillies because he wanted to train in plastic surgery, only to be told that there were four plastic surgeons in Great Britain already and that a fifth would probably remain without work.[9]

The Role of the Professional Associations

The situation was different in the United States where a group of former war surgeons[10] made efforts to create professional associations. The first to be established was for plastic surgeons and was founded in Chicago in August 1921 on the same day that the first Miss America was elected in Atlantic City, showing that beauty was becoming socially important. The aims of these associations, like others in Europe, were principally to raise the standards of the speciality and to admit new members only if they were fully qualified and could give proof of their competence and moral rectitude. The associations' attitude towards cosmetic surgery was ambiguous and some physicians were rather diffident. One was Blair who had gone back to St. Louis after the war and been appointed to the Chair of Oral Surgery at Washington University. Some of his students like Jerome P. Webster and James Barret Brown were to become famous. Blair had always made great efforts to promulgate plastic surgery as a serious, scientific branch of medicine and, as one of the founding members of the association, managed to get the Board of Plastic Surgery established in 1935. Although he was not openly hostile towards cosmetic surgery he was definitely against the undignified and unethical work of certain surgeons. The strict criteria for admittance to the association plus the fact that candidates had to pass Board examinations were seen as a guarantee of quality. The public soon learned this and the majority of those with cosmetic problems who sought surgery began looking to qualified surgeons. This contributed to the acceptance of this branch throughout the medical world.

In the post-war Europe of the 1920s the carefree climate, a period of elegance and appreciation of beauty together with a desire for youthfulness prevailed among the middle classes and in this environment plastic surgery thrived and cosmetic surgery became more acceptable. As Susanne Nöel [736] wrote in 1926: "… we need youth and beauty".

Another physician who contributed a great deal to the advancement of cosmetic surgery in the United Sates was Eastman J. Sheehan (1885–1951) [407]. After training under Gillies,[11] he became a member of the American Association of Plastic Surgeons and entered Columbia University in New York as one of the staff. His techni-

9 The famous four were Gillies, McIndoe, Mowlem and Kilner. It is interesting to note that while Sir Harold had quite a number of students from the United States, he taught few from Britain at that time. These Americans (Vilray Blair, Maxwell Maltz, Joseph Eastman Sheehan and many others) became famous in their field.

10 Among others: Henry S. Dunning, Truman W. Brophy and Frederick B. Moorehead.

11 Sheehan kept contact with the European military physicians he had met during the war and consequently became a supporter of General Franco during the Spanish Civil War.

cal competence earned him a good public reputation, an opinion that was not completely shared by his colleagues who criticized him for his tendency to flaunt and advertise himself. The wife of the famous actor, Walter Huston who was not satisfied with the results of a face-lift he had performed, took him to court and sued him for 100,000 dollars in damages. The lawsuit ended in favour of Sheehan because he was able to demonstrate that the bad results were due to the fact that she had already undergone a face-lifting operation which she had denied when asked specifically. The considerable press coverage inevitably gave him enormous publicity.

Another of the pioneers in the United States was Jacque W. Maliniak (1889–1976). Born in Poland, one of the provinces of the Russian Empire at the time, he studied medicine in France where he trained under Hippolyte Morestin, whose interest in plastic surgery was well known. He was decorated many times as a military surgeon in the Russian Army but after the Revolution he immigrated to the United States where he practised surgery privately [407].

The Growth of Cosmetic Surgery

Maliniak organized the first plastic surgery service in the Municipal City Hospital in New York, which became a model for the many others that were set up in the United States. He later became Clinical Professor of Plastic Surgery in the New York Polyclinic and dividing his time between reconstructive and cosmetic surgery. He contributed greatly to the growing respectability of the new branch of surgery. Since he could not become a member of the American Association of Plastic Surgeons which required university degrees both in medicine and dentistry and accepted only 40 members, he was instrumental in forming another professional body. He was convinced that plastic surgery should be performed by surgeons familiar with general techniques as well as reconstructive plastic surgery skills and waged war against those who operated in the beauty parlours. He differed from the old conservatives and believed that even purely aesthetic deformities deserved treatment by competent physicians and not quacks. Armed with these principles he founded the American Society of Plastic Surgery in 1931. This body was more accessible and less exclusive than the previous Association and soon fostered the development of a serious, skilled speciality that included cosmetic surgery.

The development of the speciality in Britain during the period between the wars slowed down only to gain momentum again during World War II. The British Association was founded at a meeting presided over by the President of the Royal College of Surgeons in London during November 1946. Sir Harold Gillies was elected as the first president. One of the Association's initial functions was to plan the provision of services throughout the country. Gillies was joined on the committee by the other members of the quartet, McIndoe, Mowlem and Kilner, all of whom worked in the southeast of England. "Second generation" plastic surgeons from other parts of the country joined them. The speciality grew from these origins and the history of the first 40 years is recorded in the monograph edited by A.F. Wallace in 1987 [1026] (see also Recommended Reading). In the early days most plastic surgeons did some cosmetic surgery in their private practices, outside the newly formed National Health Service. But in typical British fashion their diffidence and reserve meant that little was mentioned let alone discussed openly about this activity. Advertising was prohibited by the General Medical Council, a body which regulates the whole profession, and anyone who transgressed could loose his certification by being "struck off the register". General practitioners still considered requests for cosmetic surgery as unnecessary or even flippant and usually refused to refer patients to plastic surgeons. The press enjoyed the chance to write about cosmetic surgery and there were frequent "revelations". During this period it could be said that, although it continued, cosmetic surgery became almost an underground activity. The famous four founding fathers were known to do cosmetic operations and to some degree this gave credibility so that the climate slowly improved even though some other specialists looked on cosmetic surgery with suspicion. The chapter entitled *Ethics, law and the press* written by John Watson in the monograph already quoted gives an excellent picture of the atmosphere that prevailed at this time.

Liberation from Quackery

Apart from the surgeons whom we hold in regard for paving the way for cosmetic surgery, there were other undoubtedly skilled operators whose behaviour was far from ethically correct. They worked in most western countries and tales about their activities abound.[12] One of the most sensational examples was John Howard Crum (1888–c.1975) who obtained a *degree* in 1909 in an obscure institution, *Bennet College of Eclectic Medicine and Surgery* in Illinois. Even though the American Medical Association (AMA) did not accept his qualifications he was allowed to work in the State of New York 19 years after he *qualified*. Having obtained this recognition he lost no time in performing a face-lift in the ballroom of the Hotel Pennsylvania in New York City on 13 March 1931, in front of 600 people (some said 1,500) who were there for a convention of beauty shop owners. He repeated this feat a year later, this time operating on a woman who had just been released from prison after serving 20 years for murder. Freely and forcefully overturning the theories of Cesare Lombroso, the famous Italian criminologist, Crum convinced this woman to undergo the operation by assuring her that it was her appearance that had made her a criminal. These *shows* had enormous success and according to Elisabeth Haiken [407], "… in the opinion of the general public, Crum was plastic surgery personified".

He became one of the most famous surgeons in the 1930s, in spite of the fact that he had never been accepted by the AMA.

Another example that reinforced the scepticism shown in official medical circles is Henry Junius Schireson (1881–1949), who was born in Russia but immigrated to the United States as a child. He obtained a diploma at the *Maryland Medical School* but again the AMA considered this insufficient for membership. Despite this he was allowed to work in Pennsylvania in 1910 and following a series of courses at a medical school in St. Louis, Missouri, he was allowed to practise in other states in 1922. In 1923 Schireson also operated in front of an audience in the Ritz Hotel, New York, where he performed a rhinoplasty on a famous actress, Fanny Brice, who was also one of the Ziegfeld Follies. This type of operation was little known at the time and the publicity that ensued was enormous—so much so, that Schireson became the most popular surgeon in the city overnight.

Schireson got into trouble with the Law on various occasions. The first was when he failed to give his agent the agreed cut of the money from the Ritz performance. Another lawsuit involved the English actress Lady Diana Manners who he accused of not paying his fees. This turned out to be an outright publicity stunt. The most serious incident happened in 1928 when he promised to remodel the legs of a showgirl. She developed gangrene in both legs which had to be amputated. In 1939 his name appeared in a list of *quacks* drawn up by the highly respected *Journal of the American Medical Association*. Another lawsuit stemmed from this and Schireson lost his entitlement to practise in Illinois in 1930, soon to be followed in other states. He was finally condemned for fraud and perjury in 1940 [407].

This infamous case did draw the public's attention to the possibilities of cosmetic surgery. But it also served to highlight the risks of unethical surgeons and the need for regulation by a professional body.

The moral and ethical obstacles were more difficult to overcome in Britain and the moralistic attitudes of the Victorian period were slow to change. Gradually cosmetic surgery became an accepted reality all over Europe even though few were able to afford private treatment unlike their counterparts in affluent America. There was still a demand and some *quacks* thrived. Cosmetic surgery developed slowly in Europe thanks to the activities of surgeons like Joseph, Gillies, Sanvenero and Dufourmentel, to mention but a few. These surgeons practised their skills to the same high standard which they displayed in their reconstructive endeavours.

12 See Cameron K.M. and Wallace A.F. [152] for an insight into the world of cosmetic surgery in London between 1949 and 1958.

Chapter 13

Cosmetic Rhinoplasty

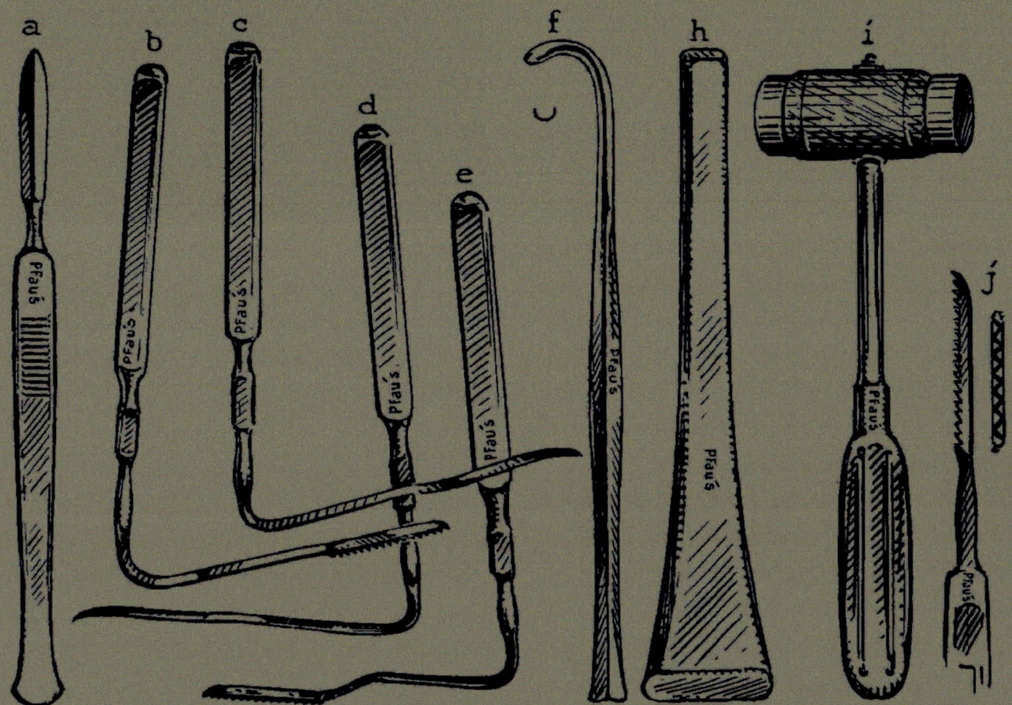

FIG. 33. Instrumentarium for correction of wide nasal bridge (Joseph). *a*, Double-edge scalpel. *b*, *e*, Right-angle saw. *c*, *d*, Right-angle periosteal elevator. *f*, Curved grooved director. *h*, Rhinoclast. *i*, Mallet. *j*, Straight saws (author's).

In the previous chapter we have noted that improvements in the appearance of the nose were seen as an additional benefit of surgery to improve breathing through the nasal airways. Johan Friedrich Dieffenbach (1794–1847) was probably the first to report this effect in 1829 (Fig. 13.1). While restoring the airways of a patient with post-traumatic deviation of the septum, he also improved the appearance of his nose [246]. In the same category falls cases of rhinophyma (Fig. 13.2) and also rhinoplasty in adults following cleft lip repair (Fig. 13.3).

The history of purely cosmetic rhinoplasty has principally an American background. In all probability, John Orlando Roe (1848–1915) from Rochester in New York State was the first to perform a rhinoplasty exclusively for cosmetic purposes [848–850]. In 1887 and again in 1891 he published reports of five cases of "bulbous nose" and described methods that had never been performed before. He made no incision on the outside of the nose and used an intra-nasal approach to excise soft tissue and some cartilage. Following this, he placed silver tubes inside the nostrils and applied a splint to the dorsum to hold the shape until the nose had healed.

This is all very familiar nowadays but before Roe nobody had attempted a nasal operation of this sort. Roe described the deformity he treated as a "pug nose", by which he meant squashed, rather like the dog of the same name. He gave a detailed account of the physiognomy and of the patient's psychological condition. He admitted that his primary intention was to improve the patients appearance but in so doing he also wished to understand the cause of the condition unlike the *quack doctors*. Having analysed the deformity he explained that it was due to the upper portion of the nasal pyramid being out of proportion to the lower. For the first time he suggested performing partial incisions through the thickness of the cartilages to add pliability and reduce their tendency to return to their former position post-operatively.

Several years later, in 1893, he described another case he had treated under cocaine local anaesthesia removing the bony hump from the nose using an intra-nasal approach. His incisions were "...just in front of the nasal bones, between it and the lateral cartilages".

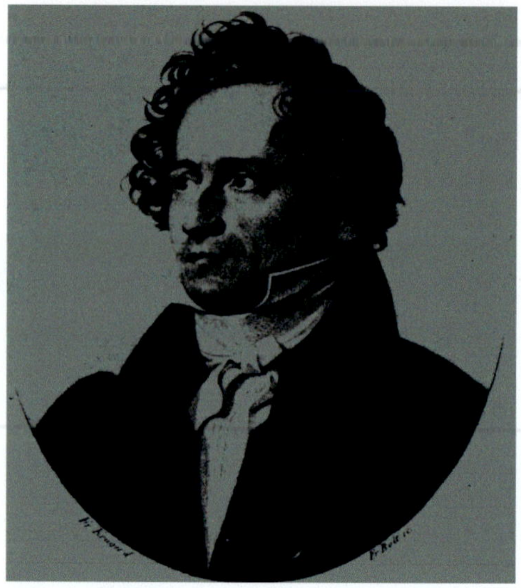

Fig. 13.1 Portrait of Johan Friedrich Dieffenbach. In 1829 he recognized the beneficial cosmetic effects of operations done primarily for pathological reasons. *Courtesy of Riccardo Mazzola, M.D., Milan*

An interesting point is that in this article Roe told colleagues how to avoid being sued for *malpractice*. This was somewhat premature, as the phenomenon arose years later, first in America before reaching the rest of the world. He must have realized that the risk of litigation was high in cosmetic surgery. When commenting on Roe's operation [636], Frank McDowell said: "It was, as can be seen, a crude and primitive procedure. But it was a beginning." Roe had invented cosmetic rhinoplasty!

While Roe, the pioneer, seems to have removed mainly soft tissues and cartilage,[1] it was another surgeon from New York who tackled the problem of reducing the size and shape of the nose by repositioning the nasal skeleton.

In 1892, Robert Fulton Weir (1838–1927) used intranasal incisions to divide the base of the nasal bones with a scalpel and shift them medially. He then held them in place with a steel needle. This was the first reduction of the transversal diameter of the nose [1041]. Even though the techniques used were somewhat primitive by mod-

1 In his first paper Roe appears to have removed "from the end of the nose that tissue which is in excess", while in the second he says "I inserted a pair of angular bone scissors and cut off the projecting piece of bone until the tip...was perfectly straight and smooth". In this paper he refers to two cases of "hump" nose.

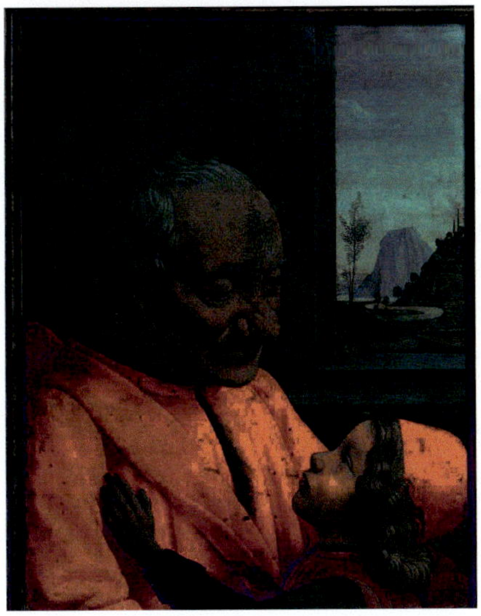

Fig. 13.2 A rhinophyma in the painting *Old Man with Grandchild* by Domenico Ghirlandaio (1449–1494). The subject was probably Count Sassetti. *Paris, Louvre 1990 © Photo SCALA, Florence*

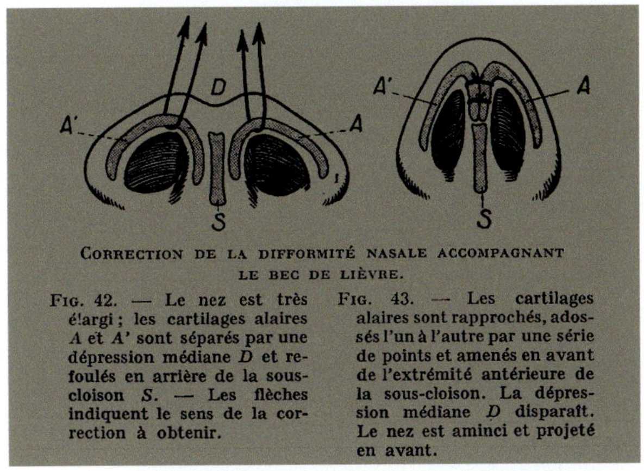

Fig. 13.3 Drawing of a technique to correct double cleft lip nose deformity by Raymand Passot in *Chirurgie Ethetique Pure* (1931, Paris). *Courtesy of Riccardo Mazzola, M.D., Milan*

ern standards, rhinoplasty had made another tentative step forward! This same American surgeon was also the first to employ the well known *nostril base excision*, that is the triangular excision of a portion of the wing of the ala of the nose that reduces the diameter of nostrils while leaving only a scar hidden in the folds of the alae nasi—nowadays referred to as the alar base excision. However, his most ambitious feat was when he corrected a saddle nose by inserting a platinum prosthesis into the defect, following an idea proposed by C. Martin, of Lyons, in his *De la Prothese Immediate*.[2] Dissatisfied with the result, he made another attempt with heterologous bone. It seems that this was with a duck's sternum and he took the fowl alive into the operating theatre so that he could use the freshest possible bone!

Vincenz von Czerny (1842–1916), who was probably unaware of Weir's work in America, described a method for correcting saddle noses in 1895 [211]. He only recommended its use in moderate cases. After elevating the skin of the nose using an incision along its whole length from the glabella to the tip, he carved a semi *elliptical full thickness flap* containing the triangular cartilages and part of the nasal bones. Their periosteal and perichondrial surfaces were rotated to face each other and they were then stitched together along the dorsum of the nose. This was probably the first cosmetic rhinoplasty carried out in Europe, but it left a very noticeable scar.

James Israel[3] (1848–1926) (Fig. 13.4) was the first to suggest correcting saddle noses by implanting autograft bone taken from the tibia [461]. The first case he described in 1896 was a 30-year-old man with a syphilitic nose who had been treated previously in Vienna with a rotation flap from his forehead. The flap necrosed and the result was disastrous. Israel used an external incision on the dorsum to create a subcutaneous pocket into which he inserted a 3 × 3.5 cm fragment of tibia. At a second

2 Weir just mentions that Martin's work "came to my notice" and that he had used it on several cases. The procedure apparently gained some support from Ollier in Lyon although he said he preferred autoplasty over the platinum (*Rev de Chir* 1890 p 828).

3 Israel was born and studied in Berlin. He trained as a surgeon under von Langenbeck and after a brief period of work in the Jewish Hospital in Vienna he was appointed Head Surgeon in Berlin. He wrote over one hundred articles and showed great interest in urology, to the extent that he is considered a pioneer in studies on the kidney and its surgery.

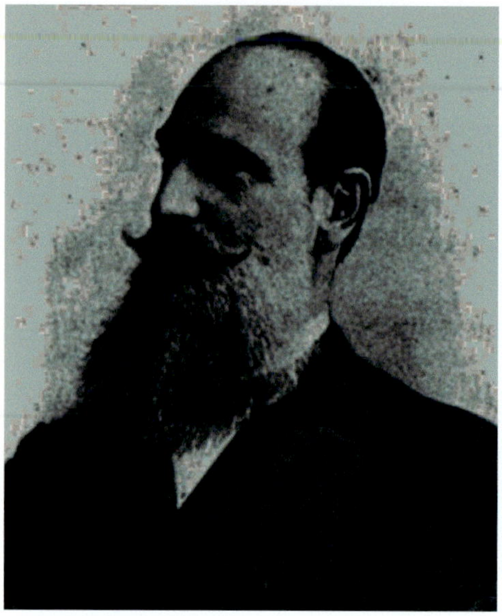

Fig. 13.4 Portrait of James Israel (1848–1926) who used a tibial autograft to correct a saddle nose in 1896 [461]

operation, mainly intended to tidy up the Viennese effort, he exposed the implanted bone and in an article on the subject remarked: "I could not see any difference between it and normal live bone."

He then operated on a second case with a syphilitic nose, a 33-year-old man with a more serious deformity since there was "…luetic exfoliation of the nasal bones, the hard palate, and gummatous ulceration of the frontal bone". The final result was unsatisfactory because the development of the middle third of the face had been retarded by syphilis.

His third patient was a 19-year-old girl who needed treatment following lupus. This tuberculous condition was prone to affect the face and nasal skeleton. Israel's solution was to use a *compound flap* of forearm skin with a piece of ulnar bone. Although Israel claimed he was the first to use autologous bone in this way others had employed the method before. In fact, Louis Xavier E.L. Ollier (1830–1900) used a flap containing periosteum and outer table from the forehead in 1860 [747, 748] and J. Hardy reported a rather unusual case in 1875 [412]. He corrected a saddle nose by stripping the soft tissue from the phalanx of the patient's little finger and inserting it in a pocket on the nasal bridge leaving it partly attached to the hand. After some weeks he separated the bone and released the remains of the finger. In truth none of these European ventures were purely cosmetic as they were designed to rectify the effects of trauma or disease.

George Howard Monks (1853–1933) was another American who devoted much of his time to nasal surgery [686]. He described many deformities like saddle noses, bent noses, rhinophyma and flat noses and operated through a small incision between the glabella and the root of the nose.

In cases where there was a hump he rasped the bone with instruments he devised himself, while in serious cases of saddle nose where scarring had pulled the tip so far upwards that "…the nostrils looked forward", he used external incisions, though smaller than those used by Dieffenbach and von Czerny. In other cases he used an incision around the base of the nose and columella so as to expose the nasal skeleton when the skin was raised. According to McDowell, resorting to this technique, as many American surgeons did, was a factor that "…unfortunately retarded the general acceptance of rhinoplasty a great deal".

Another of his important contributions was to use standard photographic views to show the pre- and post-operative results. He also treated cases of rhinophyma, which he called "hypertrophic acne". Initially he shaved off relatively thin layers of skin and allowed the raw wound to heal spontaneously. But he changed his technique after removing too much. He had to use a graft to cover a raw wound that failed to heal and the result was so good that he adopted the method for most of his patients. He was able to cover the defect created by a more radical removal of diseased skin with a full thickness graft which he believed gave a better result. The technique is still used to this day [853].[4]

However, the surgeon whose name will always be linked to rhinoplasty was Jacques Joseph (1885–1934) (Fig. 13.5). He refined his methods to suit all types of deformity and devised special instruments for the purpose [468–479]. Many of these are now in the archives of

4 Monks also dealt with the reconstruction of eyelids and the correction of protruding ears, for which he recommended the excision of portions of skin and cartilage.

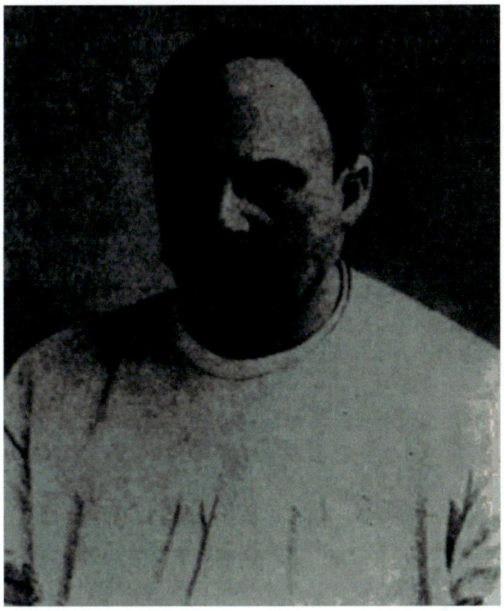

Fig. 13.5 Portrait of Jacques Joseph (1885–1934)

the British Association of Plastic Surgery having arrived there by a rather circuitous journey. After the First War Professor Joseph or Nazen Joseph as he was known developed his own speciality of nasal surgery and continued to work as the World War II approached. His fame gave him some protection against rising anti-Semitism. On his death his assistant gathered up his instruments and fled to England. When he developed Dupuytren's contracture some time later, he was so grateful to the plastic surgeon who operated on him that he gave him Joseph's nasal instruments. They were subsequently inherited by this surgeon's daughter who was persuaded to sell them by the Archivist of the *British Association* and they now rest in the collection (Fig. 13.6).

Joseph achieved remarkable results in other branches of reconstructive surgery especially during the First World War. His influence lasted for many years and to say that many—perhaps even the majority—of present-day rhinoplasty techniques are modifications of those introduced by Joseph[5] is not an exaggeration.

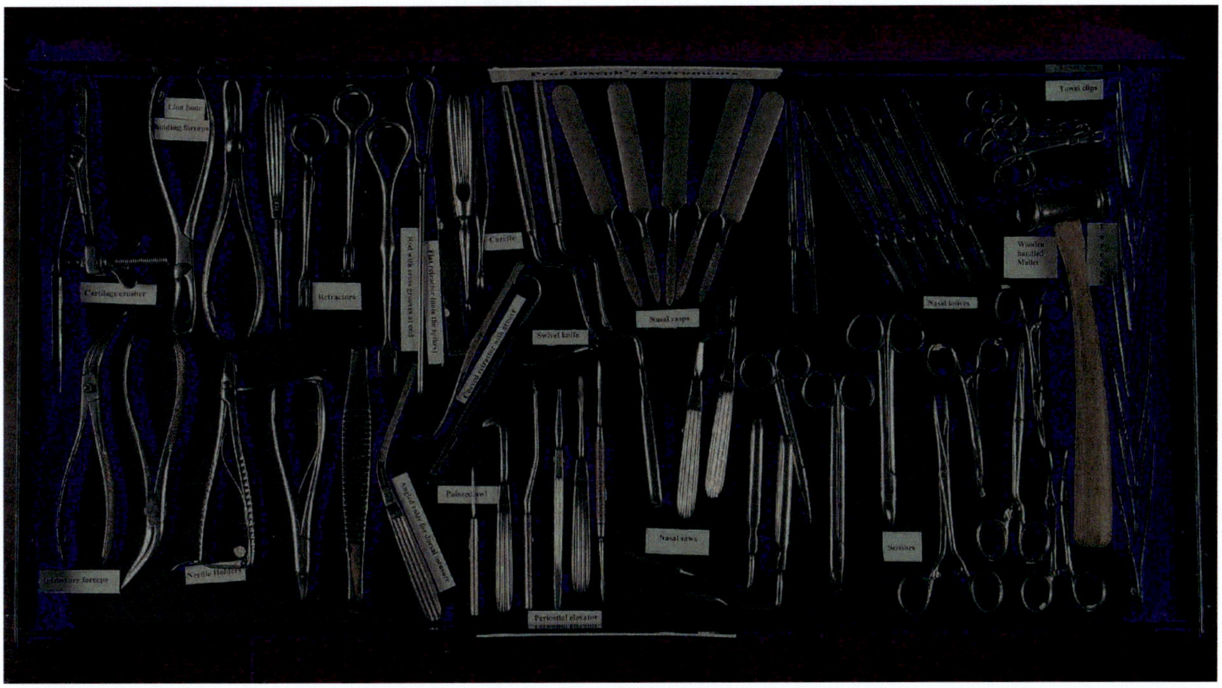

Fig. 13.6 Joseph's instruments, purchased by the archivist of the British Association of Plastic Surgeons. *From the Antony Wallace Archive by Courtesy of the British Association of Plastic Reconstructive and Aesthetic Surgeons*

5 Joseph was born in Könisberg on the 6 September 1865; he studied medicine in Berlin but graduated in Leipzig in 1890. He began his career as an assistant orthopaedic surgeon under the famous Professor Wolff, Head of the Orthopaedic Clinic at Berlin University, where he had occasion to perform numerous plastic reconstructions.

Joseph's first case of cosmetic surgery was in 1886 when he operated on a child with protruding ears. The psychological effects of this cosmetic correction were so beneficial that it encouraged Joseph to continue this work. Two years after this operation, Joseph met a 28-year-old man who asked him to reduce the size of his enormous nose. Despite the fact that he had never performed a rhinoplasty, he was fascinated by the idea and decided to plan the operation. Professor Waldayer, Head of the Institute of Anatomy, allowed him to perform operations on cadavers and once he had gained experience, he performed a rhinoplasty on that young man. Gustav Aufricht, who also made several contributions in this field [36, 37], wrote that Joseph often planned his operations by trying out various methods on cadavers in the morgue, especially when he had a difficult case where flaps were necessary.

Joseph's first cosmetic rhinoplasty took place on 11 May 1898 [37, 724]. As was the usual practice in European ear, nose and throat (ENT) surgery in those days he made two external incisions that went "…from the middle of the radix… diverging symmetrically to the nostrils". He removed the excess soft tissues between the two incisions and then shaped the hump through this exposure before suturing the wound. The patient was very satisfied even though he paid the price for an improved profile with a visible scar (Fig. 13.7).

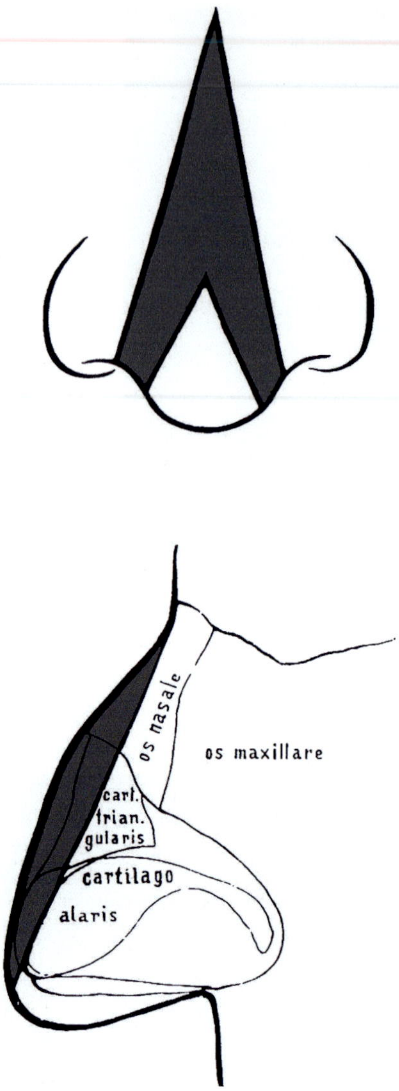

Fig. 13.7 Diagram of the method Joseph used to reduce the size of the nose in his first case. The skin and bone resection left a visible scar [469]

At this time Joseph was certain that he was the first in this field and he presented the case in Berlin in 1898. Unfortunately, he was to be disappointed by a certain Doctor Rosenstein, a visiting American physician, who reported that Dr. Weir from New York had already performed a reduction rhinoplasty in 1892 and had published the results. There was no great disquiet as the Germans were apparently unconcerned about events across the Atlantic although they did have reservations about similar progress nearer home in Paris! In fact even Rosenstein was unaware that Roe, the Rochester surgeon, had already performed and reported this type of rhinoplasty five years before Weir in 1887.

Despite not being the first, Joseph's contributions towards the techniques of cosmetic rhinoplasty were fundamental. Four years after his first report he published his famous *Nasenverkleinerungen* (*Nose reconstruction*) which included descriptions on how to reduce the width of the nose. Through small incisions both inside and outside the nose he used his specially designed saws which have remained the instruments of choice throughout the world over the years. His usual technique was to excise the hump and narrow the nose by means of a special clamp which he used to move the two nasal bones inwards after dividing them at their junction with the cheek. When he read the reports by Weir and Roe he correctly maintained that his rhinoplasty was different.

During the next six years he performed 43 rhinoplasties, 30 of which were on men. This may seem a small number by present standards but it was very significant in the surgical climate that prevailed in Europe.

In 1904 he described an intra-nasal approach and published another paper on rhinoplasty the following year. By then he had performed one hundred operations of this type and his reputation had blossomed both in Germany and abroad. In 1907 he published his *Die Korrektur der Schiefnase* (*Correction of Crooked Noses*) in which he also described the *golf-stick knife*.

Joseph introduced yet another innovation in 1912, when he modified Israel's technique of nasal bone grafting. He inserted this implant through an intra-nasal incision in order to avoid visible external scars. He subsequently revised the method in 1914 and again in 1922. In 1931, Joseph published his mammoth *Nasenplastik und Sonstige Gesichsplatik* (*Plastic Operations on the Nose and Face*). This was the summation of his many years of experience with rhinoplasty and the numerous technical advancements he had devised. In spite of the title, it also contains a description of his technique for mammoplasty.

Because of his major contributions an account of his career is worthy of mention. During the First World War he worked exclusively reconstructing mutilated faces in the ENT unit at the La Charité University Hospital in Berlin. He had charge of a section especially assigned to him. It was here that he operated on Musafer Ipar, the legendary Turkish sergeant who, after being horrendously disfigured in the Battle of the Dardanelles, was flown to Berlin by the Red Cross for reconstruction of the middle third of his face. The cheek, lips, nose, palate and right orbit were all missing. Joseph used a double pedicle visor flap from the frontal region previously lined with a free skin graft. The result was exceptional by any standards. When the case was published in 1918 it caused quite a sensation in the daily newspapers, and this contributed to Joseph's fame. However this was another example of how European surgeons ignored what was happening in America. Nicholas Senn from Chicago had already published the report of a similar case in 1903 [724]. During his first year at the *Charité* hospital, Joseph performed 201 facial reconstructions. The department was closed in 1921, but Joseph stayed on for another year to complete the reconstructions that were underway. Interestingly enough these dates are much the same for the equivalent unit at Sidcup in England where Gillies and his team treated British and Commonwealth wounded. He was awarded the Iron Cross, second class for his services, which was unique for a civilian. There is no evidence that he ever entered the armed forces and Natvig suggests that the uniform that appears in his newspaper photograph was probably borrowed for the occasion. The Kaiser himself bestowed on him an even more prestigious honour when he appointed him *Motu proprio* University Professor on 25 March 1919.[6] According to Joseph's personal account of this event, the Kaiser "…offered me the position of Professor of Plastic Surgery at the Charité but with the condition that I should deny my religious beliefs and be baptised a Christian, an offer that I refused". While Joseph was not a practising Jew and had even changed his Hebrew name from Jacob to Jacques, he had no wish to compromise himself by renouncing his religion. Natvig's comment on this incident was "He never denied his Jewish heritage but neither did he emphasize it."[7]

By the end of the war, Joseph was so well known throughout Europe that many surgeons began visiting him to receive tuition. Many of them were American. They were allowed to watch during the operations but could not ask questions in the operating theatre. The official reason for this was that the operations were performed under local anaesthesia and Joseph did not want his patients disturbed in any way during the procedure. However, Joseph rarely answered their questions after the operations. These trainees had to pay a fee in order to assist and the amount was different for the rich Americans, who were asked as much as 100 US$ while their European colleagues were only charged 10 US$. These sums were always in dollars as rapid inflation after the war led to a fall in value of the Deutschmark [37, 724].

When Hitler published his *Mein Kampf* in 1932, the fate that awaited the German Jews became evident and many of them emigrated. It seems that Joseph believed

6 At that time in Germany, the title of Professor did not necessarily involve a teaching position in a university. In special cases, as with Joseph, it was a title of distinction.

7 Among Joseph's pupils were many famous names, like Gustav Aufricht (a Hungarian who had been serving in the Austro-Hungarian Army before moving to America), Ferris-Smith and Joseph Safian from the US, Zoltan Nagel from Czechoslovakia (who was shot by the Nazis in 1938) and many others.

he was immune following his famous exploits in the war and his subsequent honours. After the fire at the Reichtag in 1933, Jews were dismissed from all public positions, Jewish physicians were excluded from the national health insurance system and Jewish university professors had to leave their posts.[8] Natvig wrote that "...none of the people in charge of the Aryan hospitals offered their resignation as a protest, nobody spoke up during a public lesson " [724]. Despite this atmosphere, Joseph was not dismissed. Martin Tram, a patient awaiting surgery by Joseph, went to the Department of Labour when he heard of the restrictions put on Jewish doctors. There an official reassured him that Joseph would be unscathed by virtue of his services to the nation and particularly to the wounded during the First World War.

Just how tragic the atmosphere was during that period is demonstrated by the case of two of Joseph's patients. Adolphine Schwarz and Hilda Strauss underwent surgery in January 1934 to change the profile of their noses in the hope of hiding their Jewish origins. Both of them perished in Dachau.

There was a great deal of mystery around Joseph's death. G.B. Fred [334] claimed that he committed suicide by shooting himself in the mouth with a revolver. This theory is supported by Blair O. Rogers [853]. But Hector Marino [612] gives another version, saying that he died in Czechoslovakia, not in the April of 1934 but at some time during the month of March. Joseph Safian [878], one of Joseph's students, wrote that he died of a heart attack when he discovered that the brown shirts had killed his son-in-law while he was attempting to flee from Germany to Czechoslovakia.[9] Safian himself also wrote of his own experience in the field of corrective rhinoplasty [877].

Natvig's well documented and accurate story discredits all these legends and explains that on the morning of 12 February 1934, when Joseph was in his home studying some documents, he was called by his nurse, Sister Grete, who said that he was to go immediately to the clinic where several patients were waiting for him. This telephone call irritated him and he replied: "I will not permit you to give me orders like this!" He then rushed out of the house, had a heart attack on the stairs and died there and then. This seems the most likely way that the maestro of rhinoplasty met his end.

Safian [878] deserves the credit for bringing Joseph's work to the attention of the English-speaking world. His clear and convincing explanations certainly facilitated the circulation of Joseph's methods (Figs. 13.8a,b, 13.9).

Eastman Sheehan (1855–1951) [922] made his own technical innovation in 1925 when he introduced the small scalpels which he initially inserted through a small incision on the columella, opting thereafter to employing an intra-nasal approach. Another advance in rhinoplasty techniques was made by Friedrick von Mangold (1857–1909). He suggested the use of cartilaginous implants for correcting saddle-noses [607].[10] He described the case of a 16-year-old boy with a syphilitic saddle nose, the tip of which had retracted upwards leaving the dorsal part of the nose very short. The boy's nostrils also collapsed when he inhaled because of cartilage destruction. Through an incision across the glabella, he created a pocket for a costal cartilage graft measuring 4.5 × 1.5 × 1 cm. The perichondrium was placed in contact with what was left of the nasal bone. At a second operation he inspected the implant and saw that there were no signs of reabsorption.

In 1920, Sir Harold Gillies [374] described another approach to expose the alar cartilages. His transverse incision crossed the base of the columella and then and upwards towards the tip of the nose on either side of the columella before turning laterally round the alar rim. Through this exposure he was able to detach the medial crura and reshape the alar cartilages accurately.

---

8 At the *Charité* hospital, the number of doctors dismissed was incredible: 47% in Internal Medicine, 30% in Surgery, 20% in Gynaecology, 45% in Psychiatry and Neurology, 33% in Dermatology. The list seems endless.

9 This is plausible because Joseph was very fond of his son-in-law, Dr. Kurt Lewinshon, a young chemist who worked for the famous Shaeter pharmacy in the Kleistrasse. Lewinshon prepared the local anaesthetics that Joseph used in the majority of his operations—a mixture of Novocain and adrenalin in sterile vials. Joseph always praised his son-in-law for this contribution towards his success.

10 Von Mangold had already used costal cartilage in 1887 for repairing a laryngeal defect. He transferred a flap, under which he had previously grafted a 3.5-cm fragment of cartilage, from the neck.

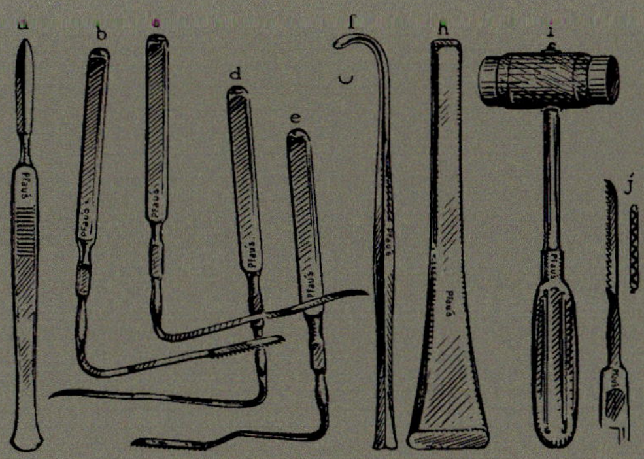

Fig. 33. Instrumentarium for correction of wide nasal bridge (Joseph). *a*, Double-edge scalpel. *b*, *e*, Right-angle saw. *c*, *d*, Right-angle periosteal elevator. *f*, Curved grooved director. *h*, Rhinoclast. *i*, Mallet. *j*, Straight saws (author's).

a

Chapter III

HYPERTROPHIES OF THE BONY PORTION OF THE NOSE

The Hump Nose

The technical difficulty encountered in the removal of a hump is in inverse relation to its size. One important point to keep in mind, however, is that no matter how small the hump

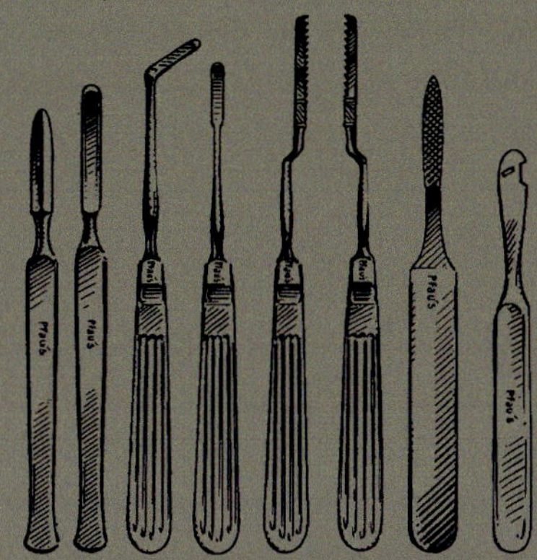

Fig. 20. Instrumentarium for correction of hump nose (Joseph).

may be, it is always necessary to narrow the nasal bridge, in order to avoid a flat appearance of the dorsum from a front view.

The removal of the bony hypertrophy is accomplished in the following manner: An incision is made along the lower border of the lateral cartilage, first on one, then on the other,

23

b

Fig. 13.8a,b Drawing of Joseph's instruments from Safian's book of 1935 [877]. He was Joseph's pupil and contributed to the popularization of his methods. *Courtesy of Riccardo Mazzola, M.D., Milan*

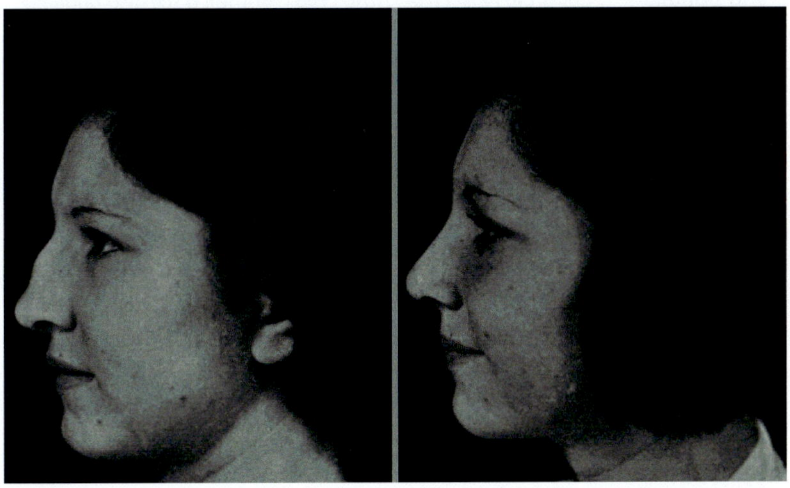

Fig. 13.9 Pre- and post-operative photograph of a case treated by Joseph's technique. [877]. *Courtesy of Riccardo Mazzola, M.D., Milan*

The various techniques of rhinoplasty were reviewed by Gustavo Sanvenero-Rosselli (1897–1974) in a comprehensive monograph published in 1931 [898]. In it he gives an exhaustive description of all the procedures for correcting nasal deformities adding his own favourites (Fig. 13.10). A. Rethi, a Hungarian surgeon, elaborated on Gillies' technique in 1934 [836]. He said that if the nose is too long and pointed [132], shortening it is not sufficient and the dorsum must be lowered as well. Using a similar incision to that described by Gillies he extended it from the columella further along the internal margins of the nostrils. He later added an incision along the caudal margin of the alar cartilages, uniting the two cuts at the columella base. By elevating the skin from the nose the exposure gave complete access to all the nasal framework including the septum and simplified complex surgery on the various components. We now call this the *open rhinoplasty* and it became very useful in complex procedures such as correction of the cleft nose. J. B. Barret Brown and B. Cannon also applied this procedure in 1940 when repairing fractures and inserting cartilaginous implants [132].

The story of rhinoplasty can end here. Modest technical details and new instruments have been devised in more recent times but the principles are essentially those that were first described by these pioneers. Today a rhinoplasty is probably the most frequent and popular cosmetic operation. The nose is seen to give the face not only harmony but the characteristics of one's origin. The terms *Roman nose* and *Jewish nose* are established in the vocabulary. The desire for acceptance in society without a label is perhaps the driving force.

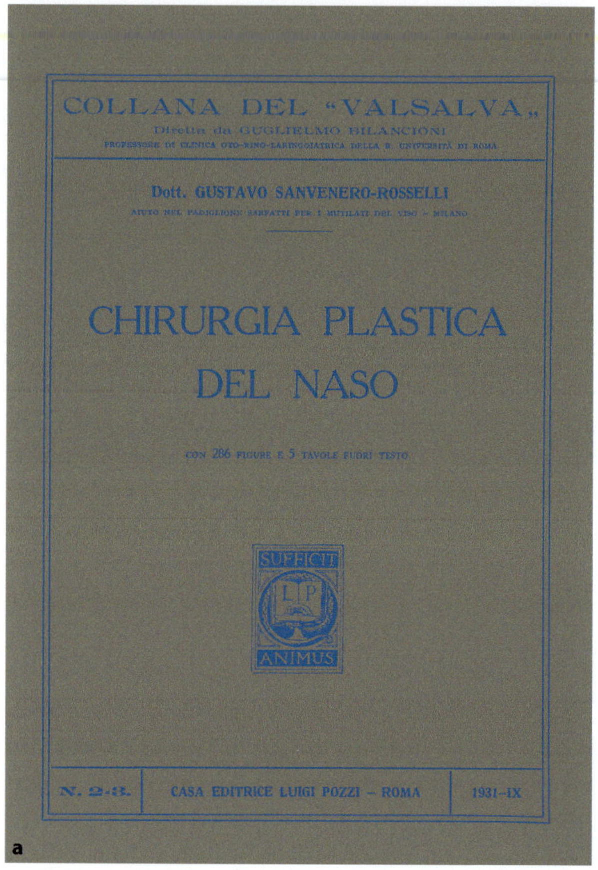
COLLANA DEL "VALSALVA"
Diretta da GUGLIELMO BILANCIONI
PROFESSORE DI CLINICA OTO-RINO-LARINGOIATRICA DELLA R. UNIVERSITÀ DI ROMA

Dott. GUSTAVO SANVENERO-ROSSELLI
AIUTO NEL PADIGLIONE SARFATTI PER I MUTILATI DEL VISO – MILANO

CHIRURGIA PLASTICA DEL NASO

CON 286 FIGURE E 5 TAVOLE FUORI TESTO

SUFFICIT L P ANIMUS

N. 2-3. | CASA EDITRICE LUIGI POZZI – ROMA | 1931-IX

a

Fig. 13.10 **a** Frontispiece of Sanvenero Rosselli's book *Chirurgia Plastica del Naso* (1931, Rome). **b** *see next page*

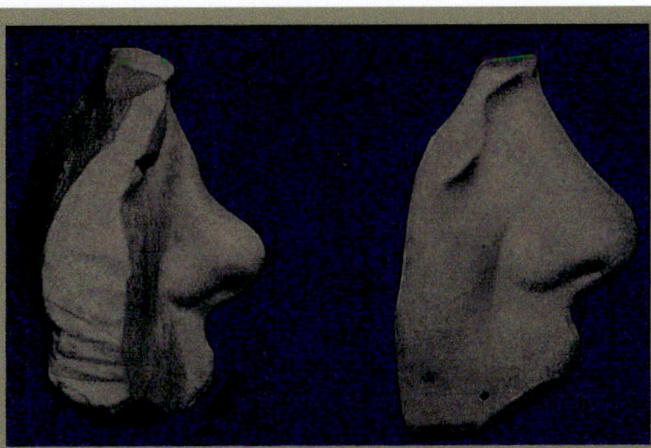

FIG. 137. – Insellatura del dorso nasale seguita a resezione eccessiva della cartilagine quadrangolare del setto.

Correzione mediante innesto di frammento duplicato di cartilagine del padiglione auricolare.

Fotografie di calchi di gesso prima e dopo l'intervento).

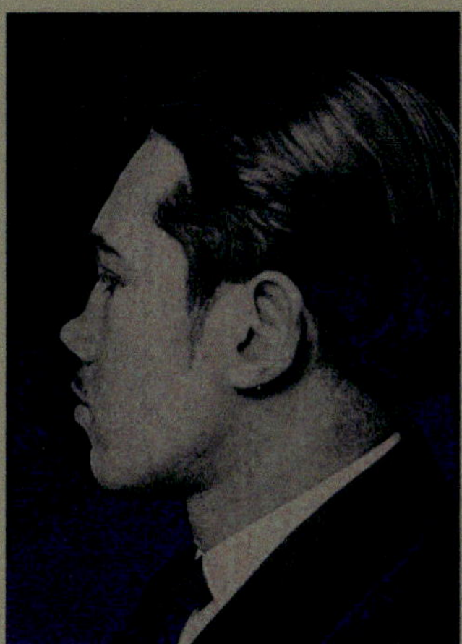

FIG. 138. – Deformazione post-traumatica del naso: insellatura accentuata del dorso con schiacciamento della punta (naso negroide).

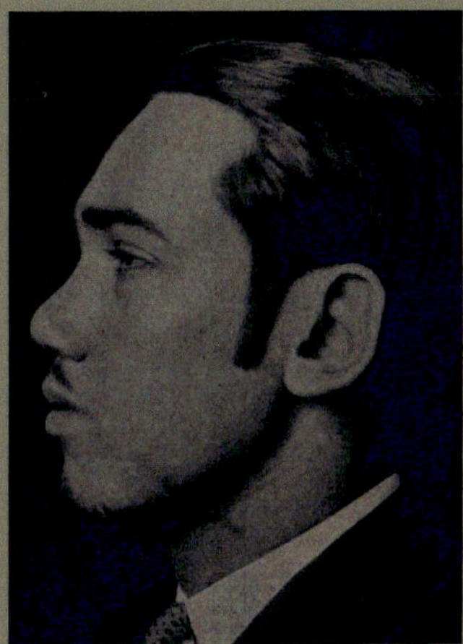

FIG. 139. – Lo stesso dopo innesto di cartilagine costale e correzione dello schiacciamento della punta.

b

Fig. 13.10 *(continued)* **b** A case of saddle nose; plaster models together with pre- and post-operative views from Sanvenero's book. *Courtesy of Riccardo Mazzola, M.D., Milan*

Chapter 14

Facial Rejuvenation

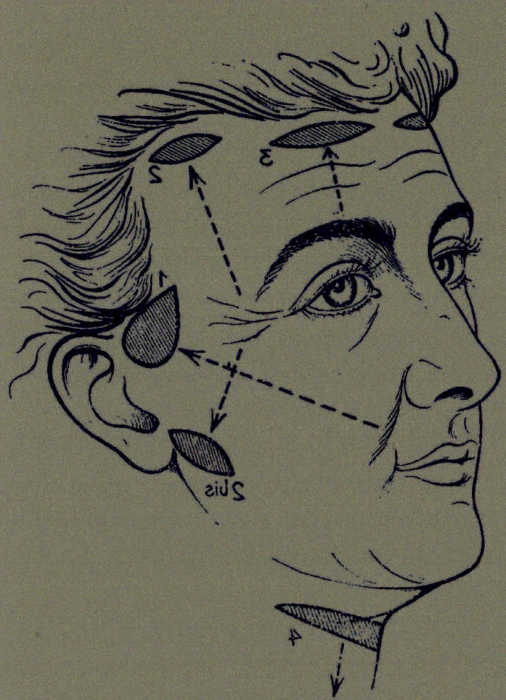

Contents

Cosmetic Treatment in the Pre-surgical Era

People were using beauty treatment and trying to keep their youthful looks long before cosmetic surgery appeared on the scene. The Ebers papyrus [271] contains instructions for women on how to paint around their eyes with green pigments and Pliny the Elder [790] later wrote that the Roman women "…smeared white lead on their face and in their hair". They also used arsenic sulphide on their faces in spite of the fact that it was known to be dangerous, for he wrote that it was "…useful for giving a woman a fair complexion but like scum of silver it is a deadly poison". It appears that women have always been willing to accept some risks in order to appear beautiful.

Facial wrinkles were a topic of interest for Paulus Aegineta [3–5]. He suggested "…rubbing the skin with a lozenge made from shavings of ivory, fish gelatine [ichthyocolla – isinglass] and frankincense".

We have already seen how certain surgeons from the thirteenth century onwards paid attention to the aesthetic effects of scars. In the sixteenth century, Gaspare Tagliacozzi who was probably the first to consider the psychological effect of an ugly scar wrote "We restore, repair and make whole parts of the face which nature has given but which fortune has taken away, not so much that they may delight the eye but that they may buoy up the spirit and help the mind of the afflicted" (translation from the original by Robert Goldwyn). Tagliacozzi explicitly mentioned eyelashes and eyebrows, as well as the consequences of age on the face, but although he had suggestions on how to improve appearance he never contemplated surgery.

Throughout the centuries much has been written on beauty and how to preserve it and the works of Giovanni Marinello (sixteenth century) and Giovanni Tommaso Minodoi (1540–1615) deserve mention [610, 678]. The former suggested recipes for the face and for keeping one's figure, declaring that a liquid extract of *eufrasia* leaves served to cure swollen eyelids while a wax preparation containing *hioscyamus* could eliminate any small wrinkles around the mouth. One hundred pages of his book[1] deal with the appearance of the facial skin, and how to counteract the effects of ageing, sunshine, illness and scarring (Fig. 14.1a,b). According to Marinello, powdered stags' horn mixed with broad beans was an efficacious remedy for facial wrinkles. Reading through his book one cannot help notice how the promises of cosmetic products have not changed much throughout the years and that female vanity has always been submitted to temptation.

In that same period, Minodoi did not consider beauty and remedies to preserve it but discussed the ugliness caused by diseases like trachoma affecting the eyelids and ageing producing senile ectropion. He suggested various remedies to hide these effects, but did not consider surgery.

John Bulwer (c.1654), while describing "the absolute perfection of the woman's face", expressed outrage at all the *cosmetic* remedies made available for avoiding the effects of ageing, trauma and various diseases, saying "It is a wonder that this corrupted custom of painting hath so long escaped general law, both of the Church and of the State, which have been very severe against the excessive vanity of apparel. And the wonder is greater how it hath escaped Ecclesiastical censure, since all the fathers of the Church have strongly enveighed against forged and feigned beauty, and the practice of introducing other than the one provided by nature." [143]

The First Operations on the Eyelids with Cosmetic Effects

From remote times physicians have understood the importance of beauty and have made attempts to help restore and preserve it but there are no traces of surgery ever being performed for purely cosmetic reasons until the late nineteenth century. We have already seen that surgical procedures on the nose undertaken to cure diseases or to correct traumatic deformities also produced improvement in appearance but the same cannot be said of the face with certainty. All the procedures performed on the eyelids illustrated in the tablets found in Mesopotamia might possibly be included in this category and they were considered so delicate and difficult that their cost was "sufficient for paying for the construction of a house" [953, 954]

In previous chapters we have seen how Paulus Aegineta [3–5] devised special "scalpels for plastic operations".

1 See *Ornamenti delle Donne*, Book III.

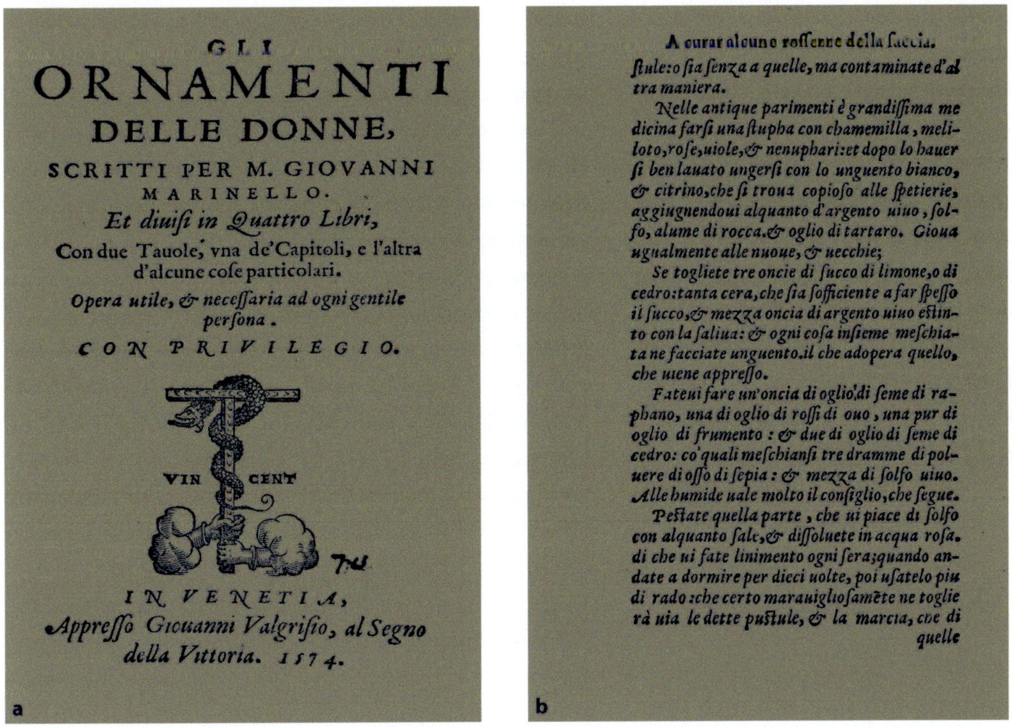

GLI
ORNAMENTI
DELLE DONNE,
SCRITTI PER M. GIOVANNI
MARINELLO.
Et diuiſi in Quattro Libri,
Con due Tauole, vna de' Capitoli, e l'altra
d'alcune coſe particolari.
Opera utile, & neceſſaria ad ogni gentile
perſona.
CON PRIVILEGIO.

IN VENETIA,
Appreſſo Giouanni Valgriſio, al Segno
della Vittoria. 1574.

A curar alcune roſſezze della faccia.
ſtule: o ſia ſenza a quelle, ma contaminate d'altra maniera.
Nelle antique parimenti è grandiſſima medicina farſi una ſtupha con chamemilla, meliloto, roſe, uiole, & nenuphari: et dopo lo hauer ſi ben lauato ungerſi con lo unguento bianco, & citrino, che ſi troua copioſo alle ſpetierie, aggiungnendoui alquanto d'argento uiuo, ſolfo, alume di rocca. & oglio di tartaro. Gioua ugualmente alle nuoue, & uecchie;
Se togliete tre oncie di ſucco di limone, o di cedro: tanta cera, che ſia ſofficiente a far ſpeſſo il ſucco, & mezza oncia di argento uiuo eſtinto con la ſaliua: & ogni coſa inſieme meſchiata ne facciate unguento. il che adopera quello, che uiene appreſſo.
Fateui fare un'oncia di oglio di ſeme di raphano, una di oglio di roſſi di ouo, una pur di oglio di frumento: & due di oglio di ſeme di cedro: co'quali meſchianſi tre dramme di poluere di oſſo di ſepia: & mezza di ſolfo uiuo.
Alle humide uale molto il conſiglio, che ſegue.
Peſtate quella parte, che ui piace di ſolfo con alquanto ſale, & diſſoluete in acqua roſa. di che ui fate linimento ogni ſera; quando andate a dormire per dieci uolte, poi uſatelo piu di rado: che certo marauiglioſamẽte ne toglierà uia le dette puſtule, & la marcia, che di quelle

Fig. 14.1 **a** Frontispiece of Giovanni Marinello's book *Gli Ornamenti delle Donne* published in 1574 in Venice. **b** A page from the book where he describes the nightly application of a herbal infusion to improve the effects of aging. *Courtesy of Riccardo Mazzola, M.D., Milan*

These were used for treating ectropion, entropion and lagophthalmos, all pathological conditions producing symptoms. The operations carried out by Avicenna (980–1035 A.D. [41, 42], Ibn Roshd (1126–1198) and Albucasis[2] (936–1013 A.D.) [15–18] would certainly have had beneficial cosmetic effects. In fact, these surgeons noticed that excess skin in the upper eyelids was a hindrance to sight, so they removed it and eliminated the bagginess.

Several centuries later, Lorenz Heister (1683–1758) performed surgical procedures to correct the effects of ageing on the eyelids, though he did not refer explicitly to aesthetic effects. He first applied various balsams (one was called *Water of the Queen of Hungary*) and when these failed, said "…then we have to rely on—and it is a wonderful effect—very cautiously cutting with the iron all excess of skin so that the skin itself is reduced closer to a natural status" [422–424]. He did not say that his intention was to make the eyelids more beautiful, but that was the result. The technique he used was very simple: "…when the eyelids were swollen and relaxed … excising the excess with either the scissors or the knife".

Another century lapsed before G.J. Beer [66, 67] proposed another similar technique for correcting baggy eyelids, and in the nineteenth century Alibert (1832), von Graefe (1836) and Ammon and Baumgarten (1842) used modified versions of this operation [24, 25].

This takes us to the period when general anaesthesia[3] and antisepsis[4] made major differences to surgical practice. Before there arrival the risks of a painful operations for purely cosmetic reasons were too much for most patients or their surgeons to contemplate. The coincidental cosmetic benefits of surgery for pathological reasons

2 Albucasis used cauterization to treat relaxed eyelids.

3 Nitrous oxide was introduced in 1819 and ether in 1848.

4 Antisepsis was conceived by Lister in the 1860s but did not enter general use until the 1870s.

were well recognized but this did not induce surgeons to attempt surgery for merely cosmetic reasons. Furthermore, this was the time when surgeons were becoming familiar with reconstruction of faces destroyed by cancer. So, when anaesthesia and antisepsis started to make surgery a safer less painful undertaking the door was opened. These factors induced Denis Montandon and his colleagues to say: "The development of cosmetic surgery for correcting blepharochalasis is closely tied to … reconstructive operations on the face " [687]. We will talk about Madame Nöel later in the chapter. She performed cosmetic surgery from the early 1920s and her eyelid operations are illustrated in her book (Fig. 14.2a,b).

The Evolution of Face-lifting

At long last, operations for the sole purpose of improving appearances came on the scene in 1906. That year, Charles C. Miller [668–672] published his first work on the cosmetic correction of eyelids. This was followed by another a year later. The indications for his operations were purely to improve the looks of his patients. The fact that Miller started these procedures in Chicago was not just by chance. As Blair O. Rogers [853] pointed out, Chicago "… has always been the epicentre of North American folklore, folk songs, folk poetry and folk medicine". Furthermore, this was the city where a series of instruments and gadgets were produced, promising outstanding results for eliminating wrinkles, reducing stout stomachs or increasing small breasts! Miller, unlike the charlatans of those days who worked the beauty parlours in various guises, had attended regular courses in medicine and had gained his MD. All the same, he was not averse to risky commercial pursuits like opening up a series of drugstores where prescriptions of a dubious scientific nature were dispensed. Patients were always willing to accept strange potions that promised to improve their looks, even if they were dangerous and sometimes lethal. This appears to have been the case of a well-known farmer who died in 1911 after taking some of the so-called *black pills* sold in one of Miller's drugstores. A court case followed and Miller was accused of selling medicines without a physician's prescription, but the prosecution was dropped.

Despite this rather shady side to Miller's career, it must be granted that his influence had the beneficial effect of encouraging American medical spheres to accept cosmetic surgery. He accomplished this not only by working vigorously but above all by publishing his experience in highly esteemed medical journals and reviews. His most productive year was probably 1907, when he published a series of 29 articles on the cosmetic correction of the nose, eyelids, lips and ears (Fig. 14.3). In the following year he published again on blepharoplasty. As already mentioned in the introduction to this section, like many others he fell to the temptation of using paraffin though he caused no more damage than his colleagues.

Eugene von Hollander (1867–1932) was one of the German surgeons who helped introduce cosmetic surgery to the scientific world [444]. Among other operations, he was a pioneer of face-lifting. He excised 5-cm-long strips of skin which curved along the hairline and the natural folds of the face so that the scarring was less conspicuous. He sutured without undermining, simply inserting oblique stitches to lift the skin laterally. At the time there were few other techniques but although he performed these operations in 1901 he failed to publish his results until much later and other practitioners were deprived of his experience.

Another author who reported on new face-lifting techniques was Erich Lexer (1867–1937). Noticing that simple excision and direct suturing of the defect brought only short-lasting benefit and the wrinkles reappeared he made S-shaped excisions in the temporal region in front of the ears and elliptical excisions along the hairline and the forehead. This was very similar to Hollander, but the important difference was that he undermined a large area of skin before suturing the wounds. In addition, he sutured the skin behind the ear to the rigid mastoid periosteum. Here again, Lexer could have promoted cosmetic surgery if only he had published his new technique and the improved results at the time. It appears that he used the technique for the first time in Würzburg[5] during 1906 when he operated

5 Before studying medicine, Lexer had been a pupil of the Sartt College of the University of Würzburg where his father was a professor of German and where he learnt sculpture and painting.

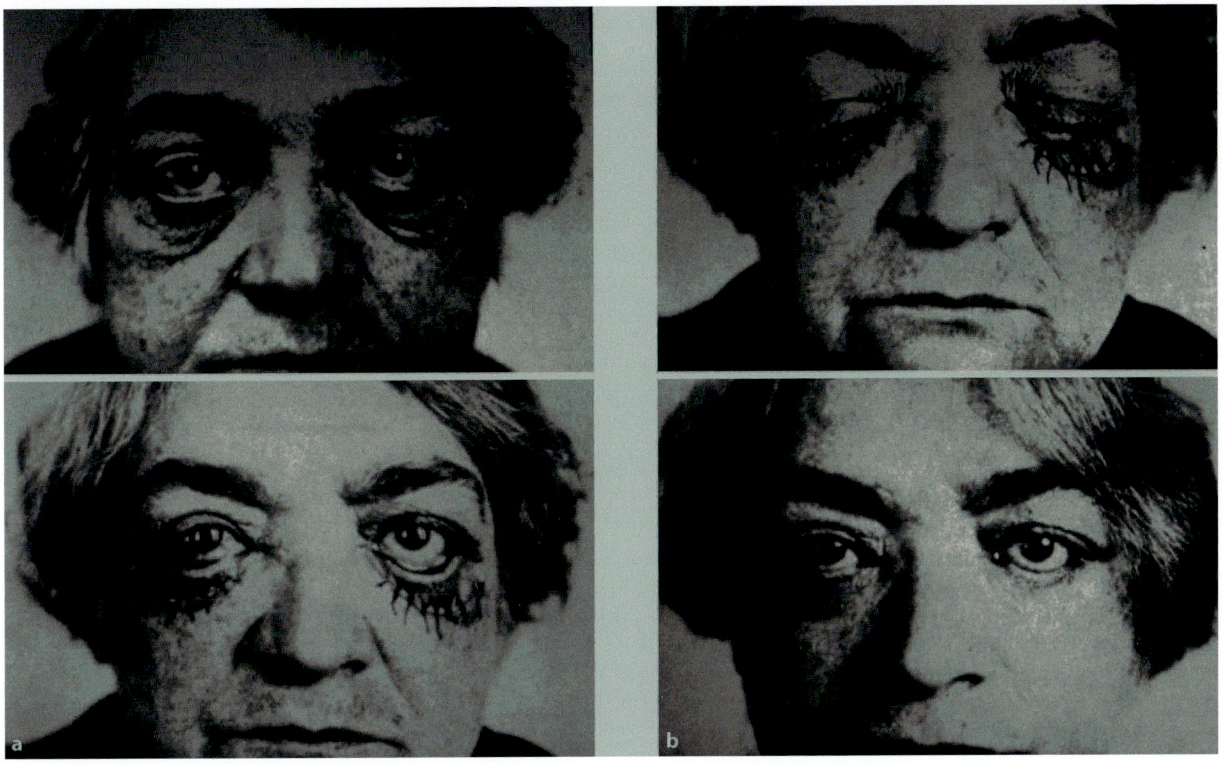

Fig. 14.2 **a** Pre-operative and **b** post-operative views of Madame Nöel's patient following a blepharoplasty. *Courtesy of Riccardo Mazzola, M.D., Milan*

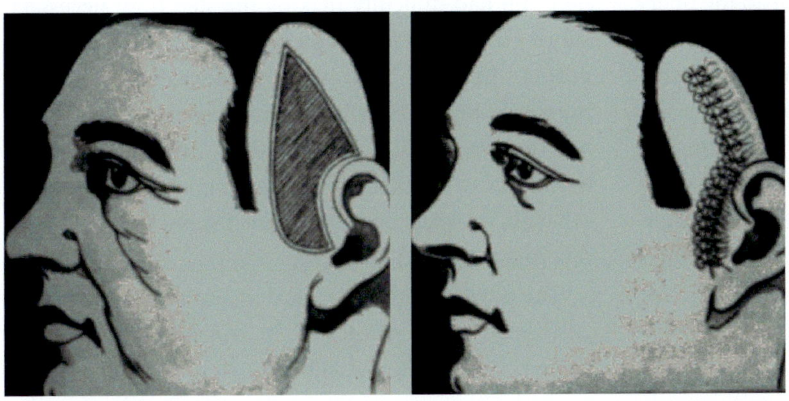

Fig. 14.3 Diagram of Carl Miller's face-lift procedure. From *Cosmetic Surgery: the Correction of Featural Imperfections*, 1907 [670]. *Courtesy of Riccardo Mazzola, MD., Milan*

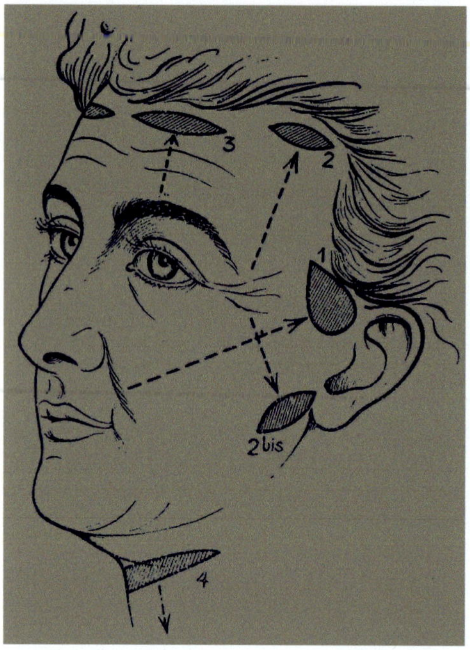

Fig. 14.4 Passot's face-lifting method using multiple skin excisions. *Courtesy of Riccardo Mazzola, M.D., Milan*

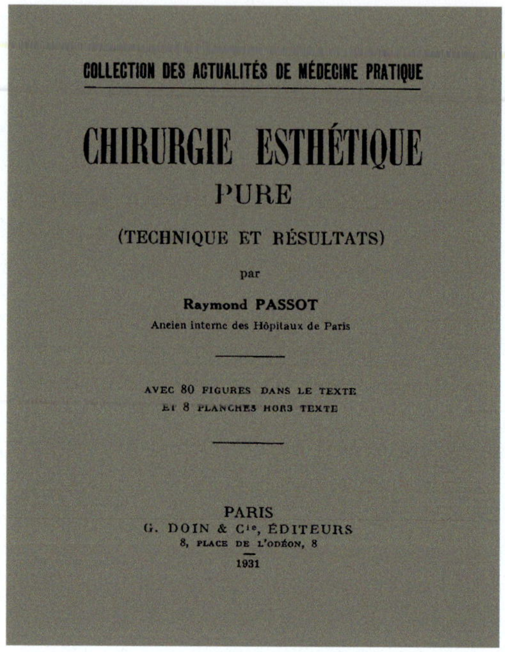

COLLECTION DES ACTUALITÉS DE MÉDECINE PRATIQUE

CHIRURGIE ESTHÉTIQUE

PURE

(TECHNIQUE ET RÉSULTATS)

par

Raymond PASSOT

Ancien interne des Hôpitaux de Paris

AVEC 80 FIGURES DANS LE TEXTE
ET 8 PLANCHES HORS TEXTE

PARIS
G. DOIN & Cie, ÉDITEURS
8, PLACE DE L'ODÉON, 8
1931

Fig. 14.5 Frontispiece of Passot's book *Chirurgie Esthétique Pure* from 1931 in which he describes cosmetic surgery for the face, nose and breast. *Courtesy of Riccardo Mazzola, M.D., Milan*

on a famous actress. She had used a complicated system of sticking plasters and elastic bands around her head to tighten her facial skin for many years prior to the operation. But Lexer delayed publishing these results until 1931, 25 years later, because he too was fearful of criticism from traditional medical spheres [561].[6] Raymond Passot (1889–1933), a pupil of Hippolyte Morestin was another who played an important rôle in establishing cosmetic surgery [772–776]. The excellent reputation that he earned working on the wounded during the First World War encouraged him to continue with facial reconstruction and he published his experiences in 1919 in *Le Presse Médicale*, one of the most important French medical journals. His technique involved excising multiple small pieces of skin from selected points on the forehead, scalp and pre-auricle regions that held up the facial skin when sutured. He used delicate fine horsehair stitches in an attempt to produce less noticeable scars (Figs. 14.4, 14.5).

At this time the general public were aware of the impressive work done on the faces of the war wounded. But they still had difficulty making the step from necessary surgery to an operation done on the face with no medical purpose in mind. Their appearance was important and the psychological benefits of this surgery was recognized but there was still a good deal of reluctance perhaps borne out of the fear of criticism. Luckily, progress in other areas, especially in the United States helped reverse this situation but it took time.

The advent of effective local anaesthesia and surgery performed in the privacy of the surgeon's private clinic helped. This was how Adalbert G. Bettman (1883–1964) worked. He employed 2% cocaine mixed with adrenalin and excised long strips of skin from the temporal region, down in front of the ears, curving below the lobes and ending behind them. He anchored the skin with very fine silver pins in the mastoid region, suturing the rest with fine horsehair [88]. He considered his bandaging

6 This delay was recorded by Converse, Morello and Guy in 1972 [193].

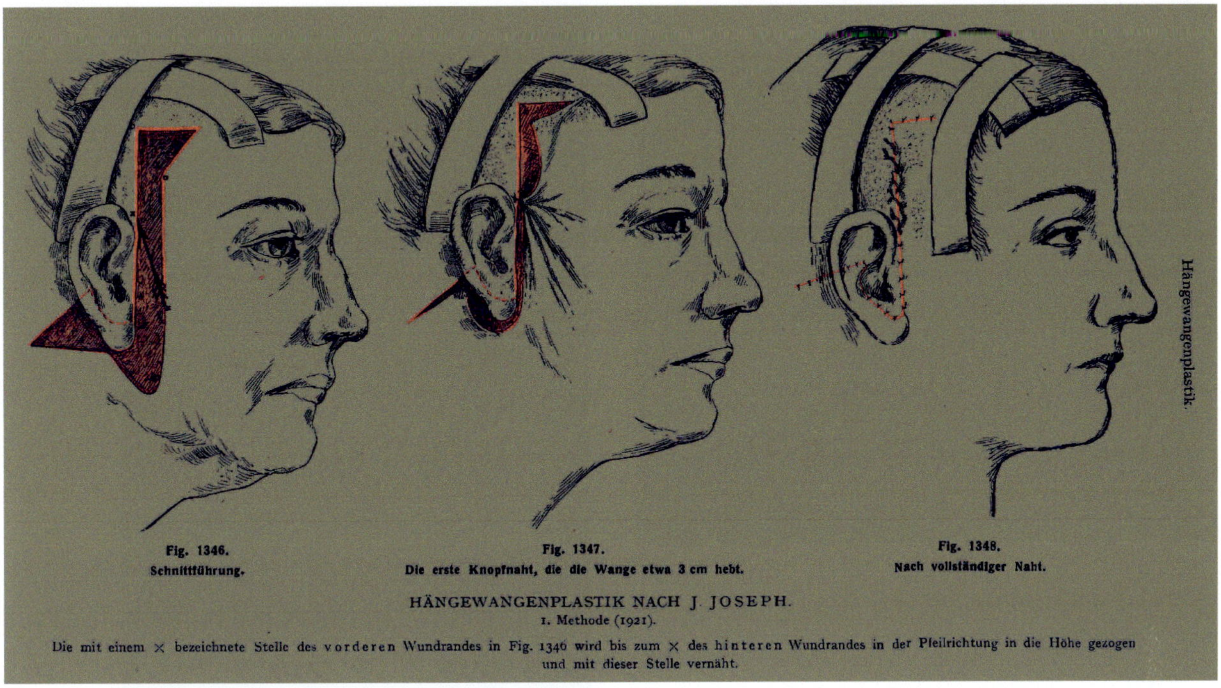

Fig. 14.6 Joseph's face-lifting technique. The incisions became widely accepted. *Courtesy of Riccardo Mazzola, M.D., Milan*

method to be very important. The results were published in the respected journal *Northwest Medicine* and demonstrated that he had standardized a technique that produced good repeatable results.

In 1919 Julien Bourguet was another surgeon who contributed in the field of blepharoplasty [126, 127]. He carried out meticulous anatomical studies on periorbital fat, describing two compartments in the upper eyelid and was probably the first to suggest the removal of herniated fat. He used a conjunctival approach, a method that was also employed and publicized widely by S. Castañares [162].

J.R. Lewis [558] however declared that Sichel [923] had already described *herniation of orbital fat* as far back as in 1844, but Bourguet was definitely the first to introduce its excision in routine blepharoplasty procedures. He also deserves credit for the accurate photographic records he compiled.

Jacques Joseph (1865–1934), besides being a famous pioneer in the field of rhinoplasty also performed face-lifting procedures [477, 482]. Unfortunately, he was another who feared public castigation and delayed reporting his first case, a 45-year-old woman on whom he operated in 1912 until 1921 (Fig. 14.6). This is surprising since Joseph was a supporter of correcting deformities to relieve psychological suffering. His firmly held beliefs led to his dismissal from the orthopaedic clinic directed by Professor Wolf, as it was in this department he had operated on the child with protruding ears.

Harold Napier L. Hunt (1882–1954), who published a book on surgery in 1926, proved to be a great help to plastic surgery because he was editor of *The American Journal of Surgery* and other prominent scientific publications [455]. His reputation gave weight to his opinion. In 1934 in *The Task of the Plastic Surgeon* he wrote "…the cosmetic branch of plastic surgery is indeed a branch in itself. Though the facial work is of great validity and value it is but a branch of an intricate, difficult and most interesting type of surgery." Some years later in 1939 he gave an interview to the *New York Times* and said "Most of us think of plastic surgery as a sop to vanity. Actually the plastic surgeon is kept busy more by the victims of accidents who need rehabilitation than by motion picture celebrities who do not like their nose or their jaws are beginning to sag."

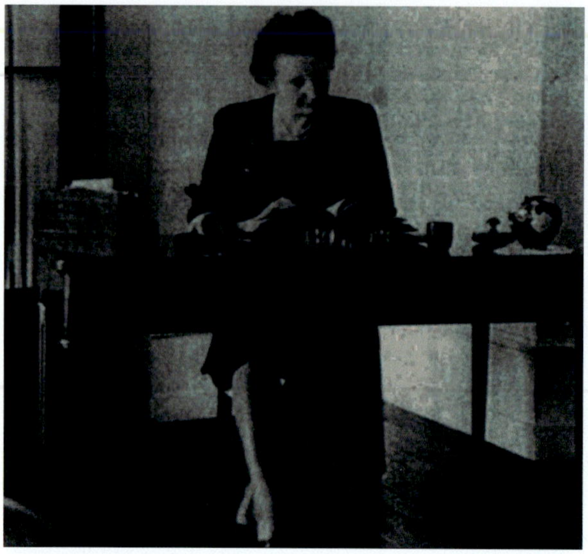

Fig. 14.7 Madame Nöel at her desk. *Courtesy of the Soroptimists' Club of Italy*

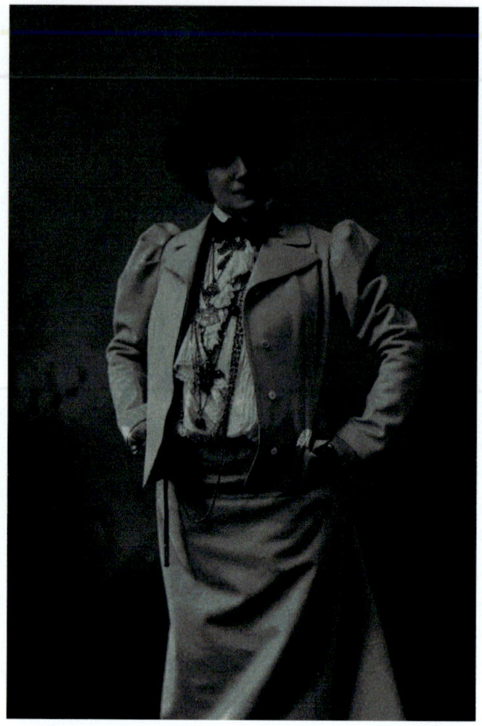

Fig. 14.8 Sarah Bernhardt by W. & D. Downey. (platino-type panel portrait, 1890s). *National Portrait Gallery, London*

In Europe during the same period a lady surgeon came to the fore. This was a great novelty at the time as women rarely practised medicine let alone surgery. Her name was Susanne Blanche Marguerite Gross and she was born in Laon in the Aisne region of France. She used the name of her second husband, Andre Nöel, a physician. With her book *La Chirurgie Esthètique et son Rôle Sociale*, which was immediately translated into German, Susanne Nöel (1878–1954) became a famous cosmetic surgeon not only in Europe but elsewhere in the world (Fig. 14.7). She pioneered the rights of women to undergo cosmetic surgery and helped establish face-lifting as an accepted technique [736, 737].

Dr. Nöel began her medical career in the dermatology department of the well-known Professor Brocq but in 1908 she began working in Hippolyte Morestin's clinic and became interested in aesthetic surgery. During the First World War she treated the wounded and developed her reconstructive skills. Her first husband, Henri Pertat, died of gas poisoning during the war and she married Dr. André Nöel, one year later. Her interest in the ageing of facial skin was kindled in Professor Brocq's dermatology clinic and in 1923 she started performing operations on tattoos, protruding ears and keloid scars.

When Susanne was 35 she learned that Sarah Bernhardt, the famous actress, had undergone a face-lift through a scalp approach in America. Mme Nöel had performed experiments on rabbits and believing their skin to be similar in elasticity and consistency to that of the human face, she began studying the effects traction had on different parts of her own face. Then inspired by the technique described by Passot she devised a series of tiny excisions that she called "interventions timides" (Fig. 14.8).

In the end she plucked up courage and called on the actress. Here is the translation of her description "After experiments on anaesthetised rabbits, I noted that their skin was similar in thickness and elasticity to the human and I decided to operate on the aforementioned actress. In a very charming way, she explained what they have done in the United States. This was different to what I had in mind. In fact they had excised a strip of skin from

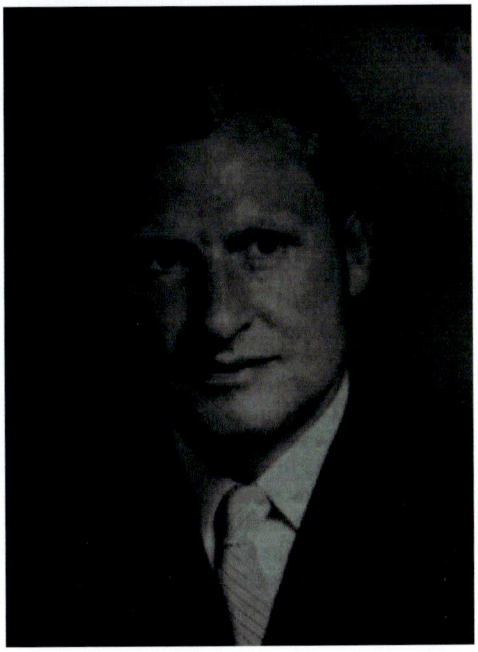

Fig. 14.9 Tord Skoog (1913–1976), Professor of Plastic Surgery in Upsala from 1960. *Courtesy of the Skoog family*

one ear to the other within the scalp. If the result had been fairly good for the upper part of the face, minimizing the wrinkles of the forehead and abolishing the crow's feet, the lower part of the face had not been modified at all." The actress "...captivated by the explanations of the means by which I hoped to correct ageing skin folds, became one of my first patients" [851].

She described her experience and techniques in her first book, published in 1926, which contains a large number of photographs taken before, during and after surgery. It also covers other aspects of plastic surgery besides the face. However, the most remarkable and revolutionary part is her psychological analysis of her patients.[7] Nobody with the possible exception of Tagliacozzi had ever considered this aspect and he expressed his opinion many years before in a simple yet sympathetic way.

It was admirable that a female surgeon, a rarity in itself, had the courage to publish her ideas at a time when, as Stephenson said "... surgeons such as Vilray Blair, Ferris-Smith, Robert Ivy, Sir Harold Gillies and others performed this surgery but did not it consider worthy of reporting... " [954].

At times during the first half of the twentieth century, many modifications were described and classified as *new techniques* [517]. A list of names referring to all of these is unnecessary since T. Rees and G. La Tenta [831] published an extensive review of the literature in 1954, concluding that only inconsistent modifications to previous techniques had been described. But there were exceptions, like Castañares' method for baggy eyelids [160–162] and others proposed by V.R. Pennisi and A. Capozzi for transposition of fat in face-lifting [789]. The most significant advances during this period were probably those made in anaesthesia and the control of bleeding which allowed wider undermining of the facial skin.

The situation was different during the second half of the century and during this period very significant advances were made. One of the first was the suspension of the muscular fascia, suggested by Fomon and then Fomon, Bell and Schattner [327, 328] in the 1950s and 1960s but carried out in 1969 by Tord Skoog (1915–1977) (Fig. 14.9). In his articles [937, 938], Skoog explains that nobody had realized the importance of J. Conley's [189] theory that "...not only are skin and subcutaneous tissue intimately related to each other to form a compound morphology structure" but, above all, this includes "the superficial fascia". The anatomy of this layer had actually been studied in 1919 by G. Sterzi [958]. He illustrated very clearly its important role but, as happened before and since, his paper on anatomy in Italian was overlooked by most surgeons. Skoog put these ideas into practice and noticed that by pulling on the orbicularis and/or platysma muscles the cutaneous wrinkles and folds were greatly minimized and the final result lasted longer. This revolutionary idea convinced surgeons that smoothing out the skin by simply excising it was no longer sufficient in the long term. Repositioning of the superficial fascia and the muscles became routine in face-lifting and the new method was

7 Dr. Susanne Nöel was one of the founding members of the Soroptimist Club in France in 1924, taking part in pioneering crusades for equal rights and female independence.

acknowledged and accepted by many surgeons. Many articles on this topic ensued, and the anatomical study by Vladimir Mitz and M. Peyronie in 1976 coined the term *Superficial Musculo-aponeurotic System* now known as SMAS [680].

Another new technique that appeared during the early 1960s which is probably attributable to several American surgeons including Frederick Grazer was the bicoronal incision in the hairline [193] a procedure borrowed from the emerging craniofacial surgeons.

Neck liposuction combined with face-lifting as proposed by B. Teimourian [976] and by C. M. Lewis [557] in the 1980s really falls outside this historical review. This technique must join other more recent developments like endoscopic dissection and subperiosteal lifting as *sub judice* for the moment.

Chapter 15

Cosmetic Surgery of the Breast

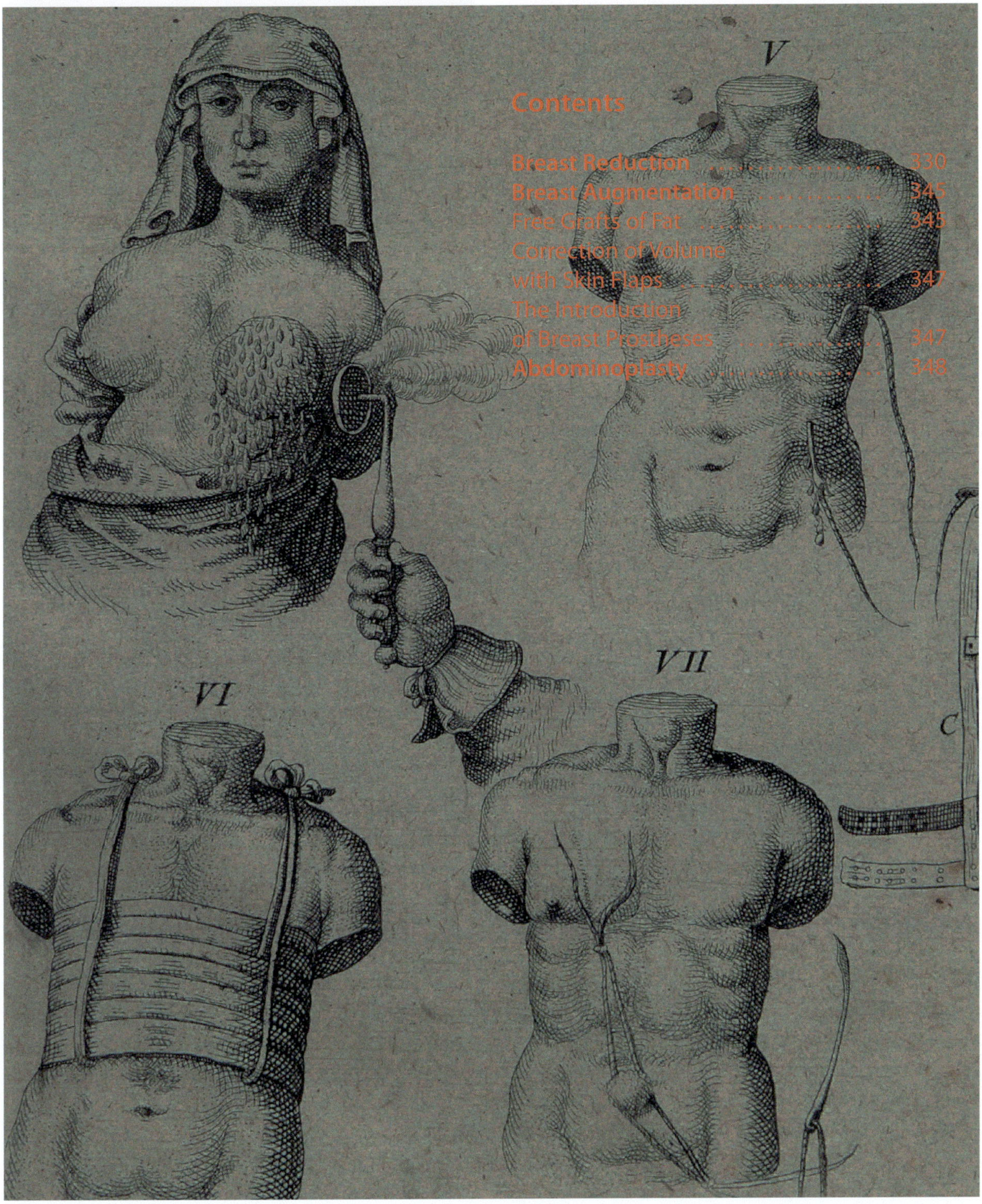

Contents

Breast Reduction

From the information in historical sources we cannot be sure if any major surgery was performed on the female breast prior to the seventeenth century. Although Hippocrates (460–370 B.C.) narrates the legend of Shi'ite women having their right breasts amputated by cauterization so that "…all their strength and power was concentrated in the right shoulder and arm", thus permitting them to handle their swords better [434–437] it seems likely that this was a myth.

Then there are other clues that reduction mastoplasty may have been performed as far back as in the seventh century. Paulus Aegineta (625–690 A.D.) operated for male gynaecomastia [3–5] and his method was adopted many years later by Albucasis (936–1013 A.D.) who described it in his *Al-Tasrif* [14–17], but both give rise to doubts as to the true surgical indications (Fig. 15.1). Francis Adams [5] translated Aegineta's description thus: "But if, as in women, the breast incline downward, owing perhaps to its magnitude, we make in it two lunated incisions, meeting together at the extremities, so that the smaller may be comprehended by the larger, and dissecting away the intermediate skin and removing the fat, we use sutures in like manner." (Fig. 15.2)

Described this way, the technique may have also served for the correction of mild cases of ptosis in moderately large female breasts but we feel we cannot agree with Ambroise Paré (1510–1590) who maintained what Aegineta had performed was none other than a reduction mammoplasty [767–770]. Coming from such an authority, Paré's opinion was however widely accepted. Nevertheless, it is improbable that Aegineta had actually aimed at reducing the size of female breasts, or that any type of reduction mammoplasty was undertaken at that time. Surgery for aesthetic reasons had been neither contemplated nor would it have been accepted due to the risks and pain involved. The ethics that prevailed and the attitude of the church also make it most unlikely, though eminent historians of breast surgery, such as Gordon Letterman and Maxime A. Schurter [554–556] are of a different opinion (Fig. 15.3).

Despite this debate we know that operations on female breasts did take place at the beginning of the seventeenth century, but even then only for pathological reasons such as cancer. In all probability, the first mastectomy

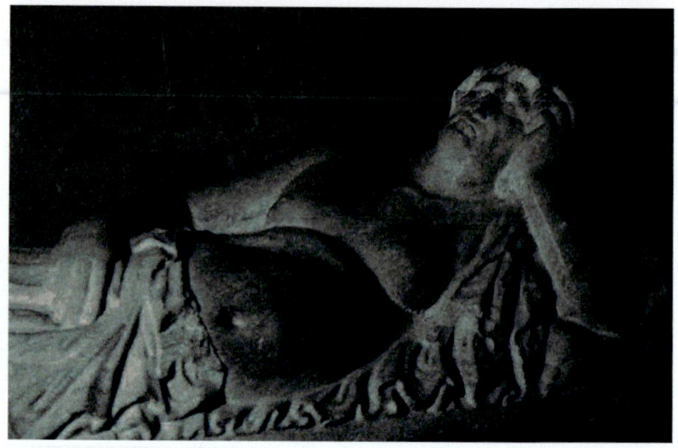

Fig. 15.1 A case of gynaecomastia on a Roman sarcophagus in the Museo Villa Giulia in Rome. *By permission of the Sopraintendenza per i Beni Archeologici del Lazio, Rome*

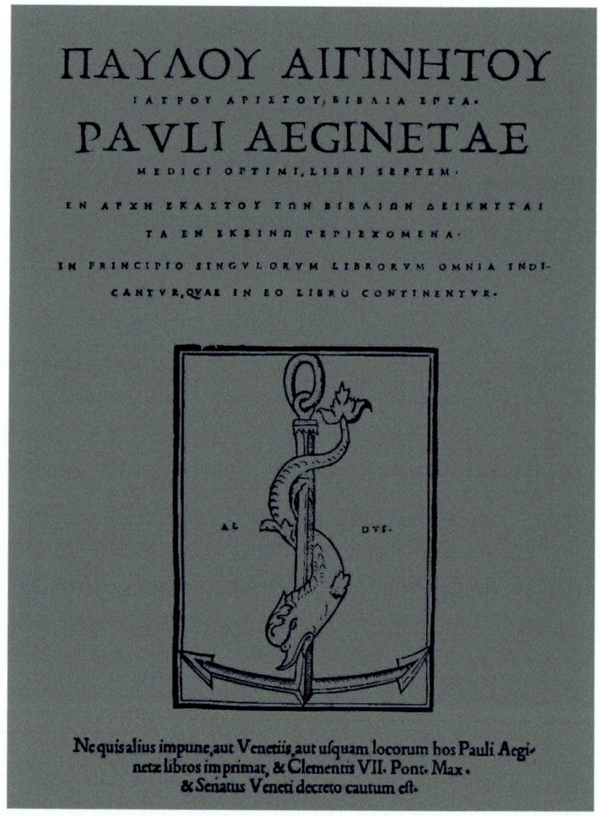

ΠΑΥΛΟΥ ΑΙΓΙΝΗΤΟΥ

ΙΑΤΡΟΥ ΑΡΙΣΤΟΥ, ΒΙΒΛΙΑ ΕΠΤΑ.

PAVLI AEGINETAE

MEDICI OPTIMI, LIBRI SEPTEM.

ΕΝ ΑΡΧΗ ΕΚΑΣΤΟΥ ΤΩΝ ΒΙΒΛΙΩΝ ΔΕΙΚΝΥΤΑΙ ΤΑ ΕΝ ΕΚΕΙΝΩ ΠΕΡΙΕΧΟΜΕΝΑ.

IN PRINCIPIO SINGVLORVM LIBRORVM OMNIA INDICANTVR, QVAE IN EO LIBRO CONTINENTVR.

AL DVS.

Ne quis alius impune, aut Venetiis, aut usquam locorum hos Pauli Aeginetæ libros imprimat, & Clementis VII. Pont. Max. & Senatus Veneti decreto cautum est.

Fig. 15.2 Frontispiece of Aegineta's book where reduction of the breast is described. This Greek edition was first published by Aldine, Venice in 1528. *Reprinted from* Surgery an Illustrated History *by Ira M. Rutkov © (1993) with permission from Elsevier*

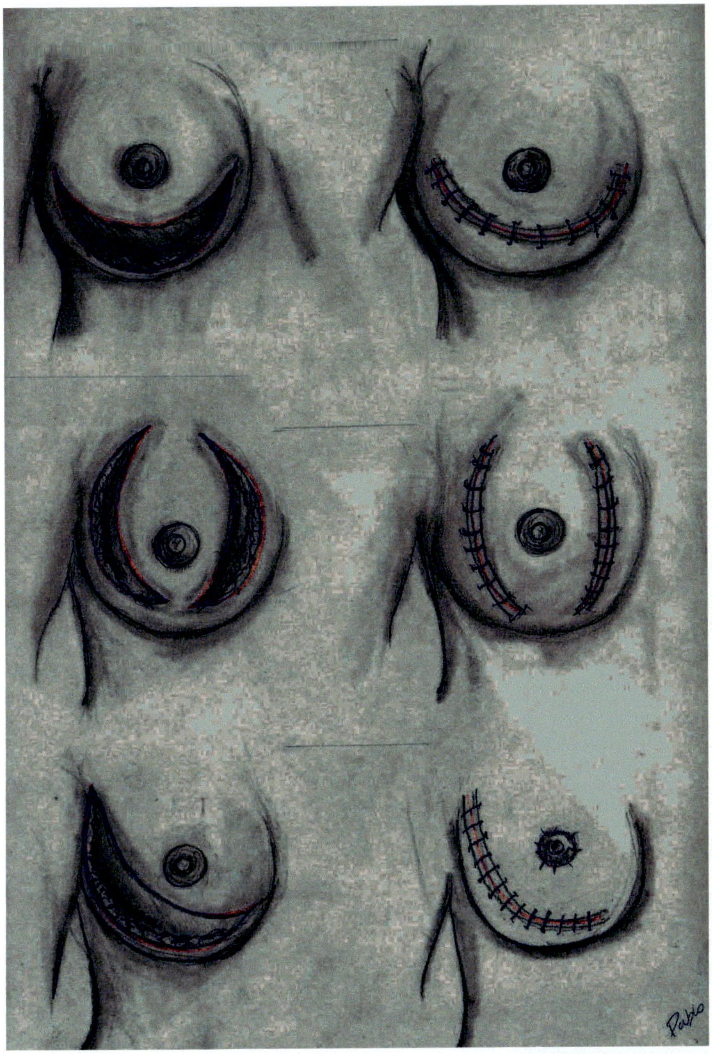

Fig. 15.3 Diagrammatic representations of the methods of Aegineta (*top*), Kausch (*middle*) and Dartigues (*bottom*). *Drawing by Pablo Patanè, Pisa*

to be performed was by Johan Schultes *alias* Scultetus (1595–1645) and a detailed description was printed posthumously in 1665 (Fig. 15.4) [908, 909]. Thereafter there was a gap of over a century until 1774, when two brothers, Luigi and Benedetto Bindi, published their experiences with tumours and what was probably chronic mastitis [103]. They were from Tuscany and deserve some attention as they predicted that rhinoplasty would eventually be performed for aesthetic reasons. But their apparent sympathy for appearance did not extend to breast surgery and their solution for breast disease was mastectomy!

During the seventeenth century, at the time when the first surgical operations were being tentatively tried, the female breasts was receiving attention in much more diverse areas. Jacques W. Maliniak (1889–1976)[1] wrote that the female breast had great influence "…in maternity, in sexual roles,…[with] religious significance in different cultures … and the profound influence on art, folklore and customs". The aesthetic appraisal of breasts was affected by "…the ambivalent religious attitude toward breasts throughout the centuries" [602–604].

1 See *Breast Deformities and Their Repair*, Chapter 1. In this same book, Maliniak says that in ancient China the feet had greater sexual appeal than the breasts, and this opinion was shared much later on by Napoleon.

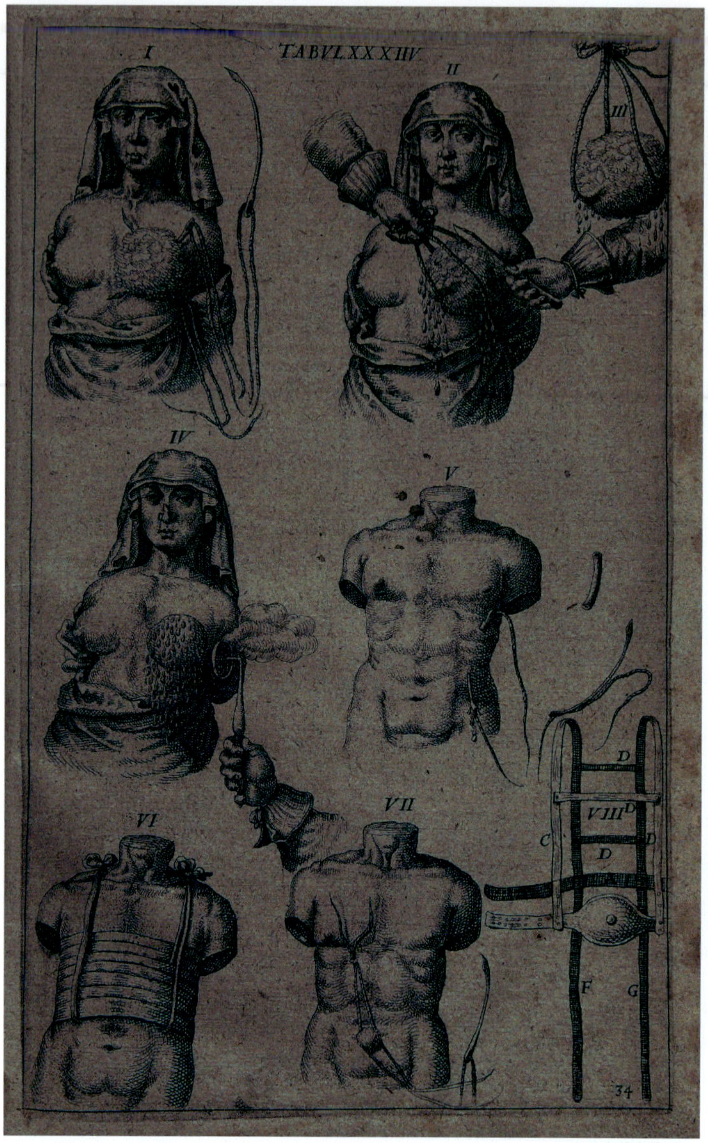

Fig. 15.4 Illustration from the book *Armamentarium Chirurgicum* by Johan Scultetus published in 1655 in which he describes what was probably the earliest mastectomy. *Courtesy of Riccardo Mazzola, M.D., Milan*

At a later date, prejudice against cosmetic surgery in general was reinforced by these attitudes and constituted another obstacle. Maliniak felt that women's fashion had always focussed on the female bosom by trying to highlight it and said "The breasts are the starting point for fashion. Modes vary as the bosom is accentuated or disguised", and that "...primitive corsets and brassieres were in use among the Minoans to emphasize the bosom and diminish the waist". This was in the year 3,000 B.C.! But the women in Greece and in Ancient Rome also dressed so that their breasts were enhanced and Marcus Valerius Martial (39–104 A.D.) wrote that the ideal female breast was one that "ut capiat nostra tegatque manus" ("one that could rest in our hand").

So, in the seventeenth century there were physicians who studied the breast and made observations about its importance. One was Giovanni Marinello who pronounced his medical and philosophical views on feminine beauty and gave advice on how to preserve it and even improve on it [610].[2] On the subject of breasts,

2 See: *Gli Ornamenti delle Donne*, published in Venice in 1562, a real treatise on female cosmetic medicine, with a second edition in 1574. The second part is entirely devoted to the beauty of the hair and how to preserve and fortify it.

in his first book he affirmed: "The breast of a beautiful woman should be wide and full of meat so that no sign of [underlying] bone be detected and the skin colour should be 'snow-white'. The beautiful neck is like snow but the breast is like milk … the best breasts are small ones, round, firm, like the round and beautiful apple; they should neither be too attached nor too small … two raw apples looking like ivory."

In his second book published a year later, Marinello deals with treatment for preserving beauty and in the case of the breasts, provides remedies for increasing or reducing their size. For example one chapter is entitled *How she who is without a bosom can make it beautiful,* and another is *How to have small breasts for the rest of one's life*. He also suggests remedies for drooping breasts, though his recommendations would not pass the approval of modern pharmacology.[3] Nevertheless, it goes to show just how important female beauty was both to the public and to the physicians of the day.

A contemporary of Marinello's, Giovanni Minodoi (1540-1615)[4] wrote a similar book in the seventeenth century, but he differed in opinion about surgery [678]. For breasts that were too large he wrote "The diminution of too fat or too large breasts is to be accomplished by suturing … therefore, concerning the surgical corrections our ancestors suggested in order to make large breasts smaller, to perform large dissections with the iron and to extract the fat." Doubt remains as to whether Minodoi actually put into practice these suggestions made by our anonymous ancestors.

Another seventeenth century author who devoted a whole chapter of his book to the beauty of the female breast was John Bulwer [143].[5] He also includes an interesting comparison of the breasts of different racial groups.[6] But Bulwer is against all types of treatment, condemning "…those who want to alter the natural features. Divine Providence hath gone beyond the rules …, they were blows of his Divine hands, a testimony of his omnipotency he affordeth us beyond our order or forces."

It is not surprising, then, that some surgeons began to be concerned about the unsightliness of the scars left after the first breast operations. In this respect, Angelo Nannoni (1715–1790), stressed that these scars should be as inconspicuous as possible and suggested spreading a glue-like substance containing "… aloe, cooked chalk, Armenian bolus, viscous materials and white of egg" on the edges of the wounds before drawing them together with a bandage [723].

Of the various methods proposed for correcting deformed breasts, one that deserves mention was suggested by Pierre Dionis (1643–1718) for inverted nipples, which he called *mammellons non formés* [248, 249]. The remedy was simply to have the breast sucked not only by a newborn baby but also by a strong infant several months older.[7] A few years later, Lorenz Heister (1683–1758) describes in his book[8] how to "…extract and extend the nipples of the breasts and how to extract milk from them" [422–424]. He is another who suggests getting an older infant or an adult to suck the nipples. For the more resistant cases he even suggests "… a newborn puppy without teeth".

The first reduction mastoplasty was attributed to Aegineta, as we have seen. The erroneous information which led to this false attribution was a recurrent factor. Almost a thousand years later, Will Durston, who was born in Plymouth, England and died in 1680, was said to

3 Marinello openly declares that one of the effects of his remedies for preserving beauty… is the prevention of cancer!

4 Minodoi, born in the North of Italy, spent seven years as physician to the government of the Republic of Venice in Constantinople and in Syria. At a later point he became Professor of Medicine at Padua, where he showed great interest in all types of deformities, meticulously classifying them and indicating the most commonly applied repair for damaged noses, ears and lips.

5 See *Anthropomorphis*, Chapter 19.

6 "In Ethiopia they have breasts that are so long they reach down upon their wastes, and they goe naked to show them for a bravery. The Egyptian women have such great breasts in being almost incredible …". Juvenal writes of them "… that their papas reach under their waste and neere under even down to the knees and when they run they bind them about their waste".

7 See *Cours d'opération de Chirurgie*, published in Brussels in 1708 and reprinted in Paris in 1740. In this, Dionis also describes nose reconstruction using a modified Tagliacozzi method.

8 See *Instituzioni Chirurgiche*, printed in Venice in 1770 and describing operations both for cancer (total mastectomy) and for benign tumours (partial resection).

have performed a reduction mammoplasty by means of *Partial Amputation* [266, 267]. In 1670 he wrote no less than three letters to the *Royal Society of Medicine* in London referring to the case of a young girl with enormous breasts. In one of these letters he made vague reference to a *surgical operation*, and this was interpreted as being a reduction of the size of the breasts. This remained unsolved until 1974, when G. Letterman and M.A. Schurter demonstrating that instead of being a reduction operation it was merely a simple biopsy [555, 556]. In effect, the incision Durston had made was only two inches long and he wrote that all he had discovered was "…the outstanding size of the breasts but with tubules and parenchyma that were simply white and solid". Hence, it appears that he found neither tumours nor cysts. In a subsequent letter to the *Royal Society* he reported that the girl had died when only 24 years of age. The right breast, removed after her death, weighed 64 pounds but was free from disease. How the rumour that Durston had performed a reduction mastoplasty began, remains a mystery. Massive breast hypertrophy was studied at a later date by Alfred Armand Louis Marie Velpeau (1795–1867) but only from an anatomico-pathological point of view [1011]. Others reported on their efforts to reduce the symptoms caused by this form of breast hypertrophy but none of these operations were performed for cosmetic reasons.[9]

The first true attempt at a reduction mastoplasty with mastopexy seems to have been performed by M. Pousson who reported to the *Société Chirurgicale de Paris* in 1897 in an article entitled *Mastopexie* [806, 807]. He used half-moon excisions of skin and mammary tissue in the upper quadrant of the breast, similar to those described by Aegineta cutting down to the muscles and subsequently connecting the residual part of the gland to the pectoral fascia with three sutures (Fig. 15.5).

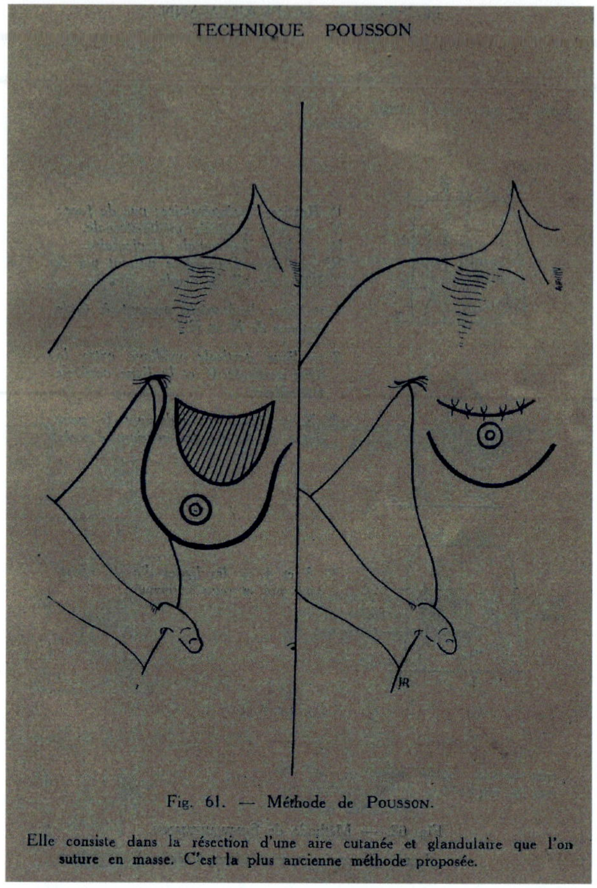

Fig. 15.5 Illustration from Pousson's *Mastopexie* published in 1897. This was probably the first description of a real breast reduction. *Courtesy of Riccardo Mazzola, M.D., Milan*

F. Verchère in 1898 used a similarly triangular excision in the superiolateral quadrant and closed the wound as a Y-shape [1008]. The scars were in a prominent position and must have been hard to hide in the fashions of the day.

Hippolyte Morestin (1868–1919) overcame this problem cleverly, with a remedy that was to become a milestone on the path to modern mastoplasty [696]. In 1905 he described an approach via the submammary sulcus so that the scar remained hidden. He may have been inspired by one of his French colleagues, A. Guinard, who two years previously had used this approach to remove a benign mammary tumour [402]. But it appears that they were each unaware of the others work. The precedence for this approach must go to Theodore G. Thomas who had already described the method in 1882 in a paper published by the *New York Obstetrical Society* [986]. He used it for removing benign tumours.

Morestin removed disks of tissue from the depths of the mammary gland to reduce its size. He came from

9 Ashwell operated on other gigantic breasts in 1842, when he removed as much as 10 kilos from each side. The same author writes that in 1901, a certain Dr. Garcia, a surgeon in a military hospital in Mexico City, removed 40 kilos from one breast alone [1046]. All these operations were undertaken for other than aesthetic reasons.

the Island of Martinique, finished his medical studies in Paris in 1894 and very quickly reached the heights of a brilliant career, taking much interest in plastic surgery from the beginning of the 1900s. His scientific reputation helped to broaden the horizons of both plastic and cosmetic surgery. His submammary approach was only one of his contributions and J.C. Warren adopted it in 1907 when he performed his first reduction mastoplasty in the United States [1031].

These operations were beginning to be accepted with muted enthusiasm largely because there was a tendency for some ptosis to recur. In 1908, J. Dehner hoped that fixing the gland to the second rib with catgut sutures might prevent the weight of the breast from causing recurrent ptosis and he gained access through a long elliptic incision in the upper portion of the breast [229]. R. Goebel [383] had the same idea in 1914 but used a strip of fascia lata to fix the gland to the fascia pectoralis in the hope that this would outlast the catgut. Unfortunately both the methods left visible scars and only delayed the return of the ptosis.

During the first twenty years of the twentieth century the basic principles of mammoplasty were improved as surgeons found out what worked best. But they remained cautious especially about undermining tissue for fear of losing the skin or even the areola. The complicated procedures that were devised to secure the gland in a new skin envelope and prevent ptosis frequently resulted in the breasts being different in shape and position.

W. Kausch developed new techniques in 1911 and in 1916 [486] (see Fig. 15.3). He made lunate shaped excisions to the sides of the areola according to how much tissue he wished to remove and reduced the size of the breasts through them. The resulting elongated shape was less than satisfactory and the blood supply to the areola was sometimes problematic. In spite of these shortcomings many surgeons adopted the technique.[10]

Kausch's suggestions were not very satisfactory and Erich Lexer (1867–1937) was probably the surgeon who tackled the problem from another angle [559]. He reported to the *Medical Society of Jena* in 1912, describing the case of a girl of twenty with bilateral hypertrophy. He had operated on her by excising a triangular piece of skin and gland from the lower portion of the breast with its apex at the nipple and the base in the submammary fold. The novelty lay in the fact that by enlarging the angle he could remove as much tissue as required. The method showed some improvement compared to previous techniques but a wedge of the areola, and even of the nipple, was always included in the excision. This could interfere with normal suckling. In 1921 he tried to avoid this problem by transposing the entire areola intact.[11]

The simple solution to this problem was described by Hans Kraske in 1923. He started the triangular excision at the lower margin of the areola instead of at the nipple and left the areola untouched [507]. The incisions continued upwards from this point, going round the areola as far as its new site higher up. In this way extra tissue was also excised from the new site of the repositioned areola. When the wound was closed it had an inverted T-shape, with the longer limb running vertically from the areola to the sulcus and the shorter lying along the sulcus. Before closing the skin, the gland was firmly sutured to the pectoral fascia to prevent ptosis. The main problems had been approached logically and recurrent ptosis was less of a problem. The technique became very popular among surgeons and was known as the Lexer-Kraske Technique (Fig. 15.6).[12]

10 A few of the surgeons who adopted this method were E. Weinold [1040] in 1926, E. Küster [512] in 1926, A. Nöel (1878–1954) [734, 736, 737] in 1928 and A. Nöel again with H. Lopez Martinez [735] in 1928.

11 Credit for priority in areola transposition is still undecided. It has been suggested that Thorek was the first but while his free grafting of the areola is well documented, as far as transposition of the areola and nipple is concerned Maliniak insists that the first was Lexer in 1912. Others give precedence to Villandre who seems to have done it one year earlier, in 1911. Transposition of the areola was also performed by Dufourmentel in 1916 but he did not publish his technique until 1926. Passot always used areola transposition when operating using the technique of Thomas, i.e. a submammary incision through which he undermined the mammary gland and suspended the posterior surface of the gland to the second rib.

12 Lexer was a pupil of Professor Bergman in the Berlin Clinic for Surgery and his great interest in plastic surgery was probably due to the fact that fine arts and sculpture had appealed to him in his youth when he attended the College of Arts at Würzburg University for two years. In 1905 he became Professor of Surgery at Königsberg University, then Freiburg in 1918 and lastly in Munich in 1928. He died in 1937 when 70 years old.

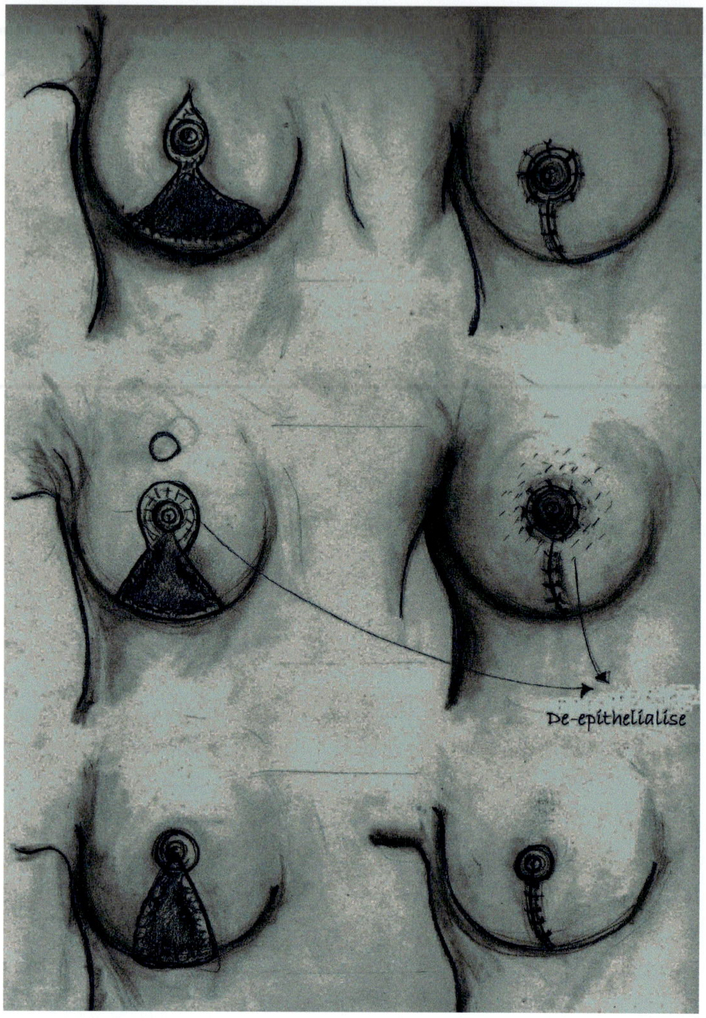

Fig. 15.6 Diagrams of three breast reduction techniques. Kraske (*top*), Aubert (*middle*) and Lexer (*bottom*). *Drawing by Pablo Patanè, Pisa*

Transposing the areola presented surgeons with new problems of necrosis especially if a large amount of breast tissue was removed and the skin was widely undermined. Max Thorek (1880–1960) attempted a solution by employing a free graft of the areola–nipple complex. He used this technique for the first time on a young girl with marked hypertrophy in Chicago during 1921 [992, 993]. He found that a free graft was the only option for placing the areola–nipple complex in the right position after excising a large volume of breast tissue and skin. The method relied on the take of the graft and inevitably had functional implications for the nipple. V. Aubert [35] again suggested transposing the areolar, but this time by making a buttonhole in the upper portion of the newly modelled breast at the pre-planned site (see Fig. 15.6). Many surgeons adopted these techniques and their subsequent modifications so that areola transposition became routine throughout the world–another milestone in the history of mastoplasty. Then, as usually happens once the principles and efficacy of a technique have been established, it was refined and modified repeatedly. Many surgeons developed their own versions of the transposition method. One of the most popular was Morestin's technique. According to his fellow countrymen Louis Dartigues [213–215] and P. Mornard [711], he had already raised a flap containing the areola–nipple complex for transposition upwards in the buttonhole in 1909. Dartigues (see Fig. 15.3), who also gave some credit to Petit, refined the technique in 1924. L. Dufourmentel also used a similar method in 1932 [259, 260].

Dartigues also developed new methods [216–218]. He made a half-moon shaped excision of skin and mammary tissue from the superiolateral quadrants of the breast and rotated the tail of the residual gland and secured it to the pectoral fascia. He modified his technique in 1925 and in addition excised skin, fat and glandular tissue from below the areola to reduce the volume in moderate to severe ptosis. The areola was then transposed subcutaneously. In 1928 he recognized the problems associated with very large breasts and recommended using a free graft of the areola–nipple complex for selected cases.

Thorek claimed that he had used similar methods before Dartigues. Apparently he had described a technique very like Dartigues' to the *Chicago Medical Society* in 1921 and had published an article in the *New York Medical Journal and Records* in 1922 [992, 993]

Raymond Passot was another who moved the areolar upwards. He described his technique in 1923 [774]. He excised the usual triangle of tissue from beneath the areola and incised round the areolar. He then removed another piece of breast tissue from above though a circular incision at the site into which he moved the nipple areolar complex on top of the breast mound. In 1930 he modified this technique by securing the gland to the fascia pectoralis (Fig. 15.7a,b). In Mme Nöel's book of the 1920s she describes Passot's method and added her own (Fig. 15.8).

Modifications of this basic method were common and it is hard to decide who were innovators and who simply plagiarized others techniques, adding their own small modifications [518]. Fritz Lotsch was one who shifted the areola into an appropriately created buttonhole at the apex of the new mammary cone in 1923. He developed a new technique in 1928 which left an inverted T-shaped scar beneath he areolar [578].

Areola transposition was recognized as a method that gave a satisfactory shape to the breast and restored the prominence of the nipple areolar complex on top of the breast mound. However there was a very real risk of areolar necrosis. Working on an idea suggested by Pousson and Verchère in 1898 [806, 807], von Hollander adopted a lateral peri-areolar incision in 1925, but he came up against the same problem of areolar necrosis [442–444] To avoid this complication, Jacques Joseph performed the operation in two stages. He first followed the Lexer-Kraske model and at the second operation used the Hollander lateral approach in order to remove more skin and glandular tissue [479, 480]. His technique was never popular with other surgeons (Figs. 15.9, 15.10).

F. Schreiber also proposed a two-stage technique in 1929, combining the Dehner technique from 1908 [229] with the Lexer-Kraske method (see Fig. 15.6). He secured the gland to the ribs and moved the areola upwards, dissecting the skin and the gland according to Lexer's suggestions at the second stage of the operation [906].

Others operated in two stages in more recent times (Maliniak in 1938 [602–], Ragnell in 1946 [825] and Aldulnate in 1948 [19]). Some returned to the Hollander method in 1965 (Marc [609] and Dufourmentel [256, 257]). Contemporary surgeons used slightly different techniques to try to preserve areolar circulation. At the first operation they used a modified version of the Passot technique, transpositioning the areola and only dissecting the gland minimally. Ragnell dissected in the upper portion while Aldulnate, following Maliniak's method, dissected the lower part of the breast. At the second operation they both removed large portions of skin and gland through an incision in the submammary sulcus.

The number of techniques and modifications which abounded during this period only serves to show that none were ideal and the complications of necrosis of skin and areolar, malposition of the nipple, poor shape and asymmetry continued to give great cause for concern. Those surgeons who mastered their own methods and stuck to them seemed to have faired best [642].

Herman Biesenberger (1885–1947) introduced a technique that was to solve many of the problems [95–97]. He had already modified the Lotsch method in 1928 and published articles on a series of cases. His book was published in 1931. It contained 160 very detailed illustrations and circulated far and wide. The modifications he proposed were to make mastoplasty an operation that was far safer than ever before. To reduce the risk of necrosis he left a disc of intact de-epithelialized dermis at least 2 cm wide round the areola which preserved the subdermal vessels. He made careful measurements and standardized the best position for the nipples. He placed them about 18–19 cm below the midpoint of the clavicle, approximately 22 cm apart and each 22 cm from the suprasternal notch (Fig. 15.11a,b). A vertical incision from beneath the areola to the submammary sulcus allowed undermining of a large portion of the breast skin. An S-shaped excision was then made on the lateral part of the gland and the excess skin was removed from the margins of the incision leaving the usual inverted T-shaped scar. Many surgeons adopted this method as it gave good results with

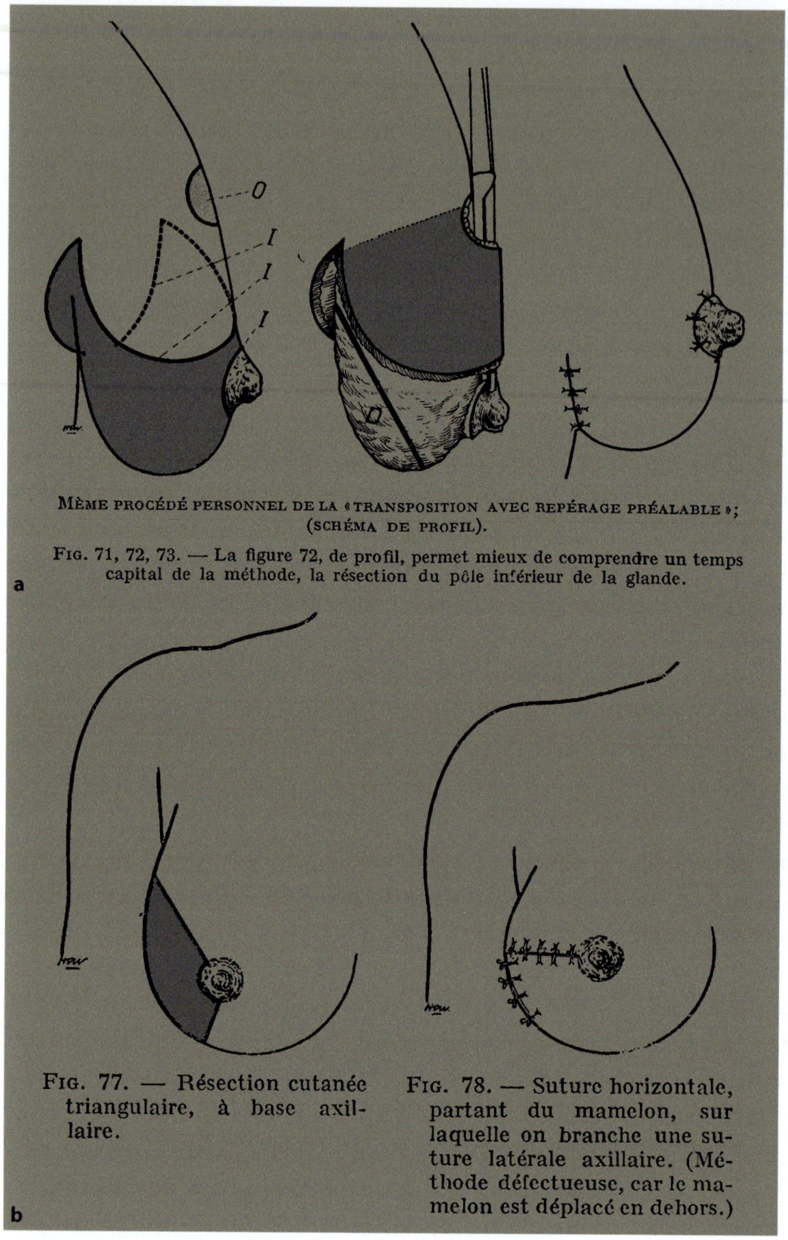

Fig. 15.7 In 1923, Passot added to previous techniques by **a** fixation of the gland to the pectoral fascia and **b** triangular excision placed laterally, allowing upward repositioning of the whole gland. *Courtesy of Riccardo Mazzola, M.D., Milan*

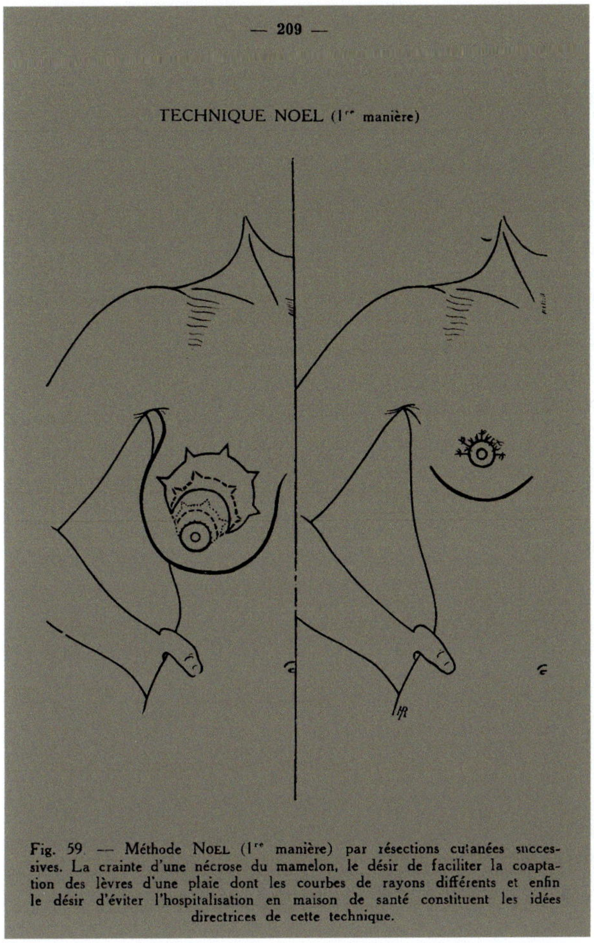

Fig. 15.8 Susanne Nöel modified Pousson's method (see Fig. 15.5). Her technique was based on repeated excisions at intervals in order to preserve the blood supply. The diagram is from her book *La Chirurgie Esthetique*. *Courtesy of Riccardo Mazzola, M.D., Milan*

less risk although necrosis was still a problem because of the extensive undermining (Fig. 15.12).

In 1930, E. Scharzmann tried to avoid these vascular complications by preserving a superomedial dermal pedicle which left the areola attached the skin of the new breast envelope [911, 912]. Biesenberger's lateral dissection endangered the lateral mammary artery and by leaving this pedicle Scharzmann hope to enhance the circulation to the areolar. Care had to be taken to prevent it twisting as the wounds were closed and it offered some safety. In 1939, Gillies and McIndoe [376] also applied modifications to the Biesenberger technique, making an incision higher than that originally suggested. Experienced surgeons found the Biesenberger method satisfactory but for learners it still held risks (Fig. 15.13).

In 1958 McIndoe and Rees [645] felt that necrosis was not only due to a precarious areolar blood supply but followed inexpert traumatic surgery and haematoma formation. They believed that gentle handling of the tissues was essential if the circulation was to be preserved. Again it would seem that those with a good technique were able to produce consistently good results. However there was obvious anxiety in the minds of all those who performed breast reductions. Despite its shortcomings Biesenberger's technique and adaptations of it became the standard procedure for around 30 years.

A safer alternative did not emerge until 1960, when Jan Olov Strömbeck proposed a method for maintaining the circulation to the nipple by preserving both the lateral and medial dermal pedicles, following one of Schwarzmann's principles [961–964]. Strömbeck's technique was an immediate success and criticisms were few–the harshest coming from the author himself in his constant attempt to improve the results! Problems of necrosis no longer bedevilled the operation and there was a collective sigh of relief from surgeons. After 13 years he reviewed the result in 570 cases and found that for extremely large breasts it was hard to produce an aesthetically acceptable shape (Fig. 15.14). One of his fellow countrymen, Tord Skoog (1913–1976) attempted to solve this problem. He left the areola on only one pedicle. He started the operation in the Strömbeck fashion and if the areola was hard to move, which was frequently the case in big breasts, he divided the lateral pedicle after testing the effects of this on its circulation using a soft clamp. He was then able to transpose it upwards with less difficulty [938]. Both of these Swedish methods were modified in various ways and the only serious criticism was that the vertical scarring was sometimes too visible.

On the whole there were few alternatives to Strömbeck's technique but one of these was devised by Claude Dufourmentel and Roger Mouly in 1951 [256, 257]. Their approach was from the lateral aspect and left a scar that was more acceptable to some. However the method was not suitable for large breasts and was more acceptable for a mastopexy procedure.

In 1960 Ivo Pitanguy [803], used a superior vertical pedicle to support the areola and nipple. The areola could be moved upwards quite easily on a short pedicle

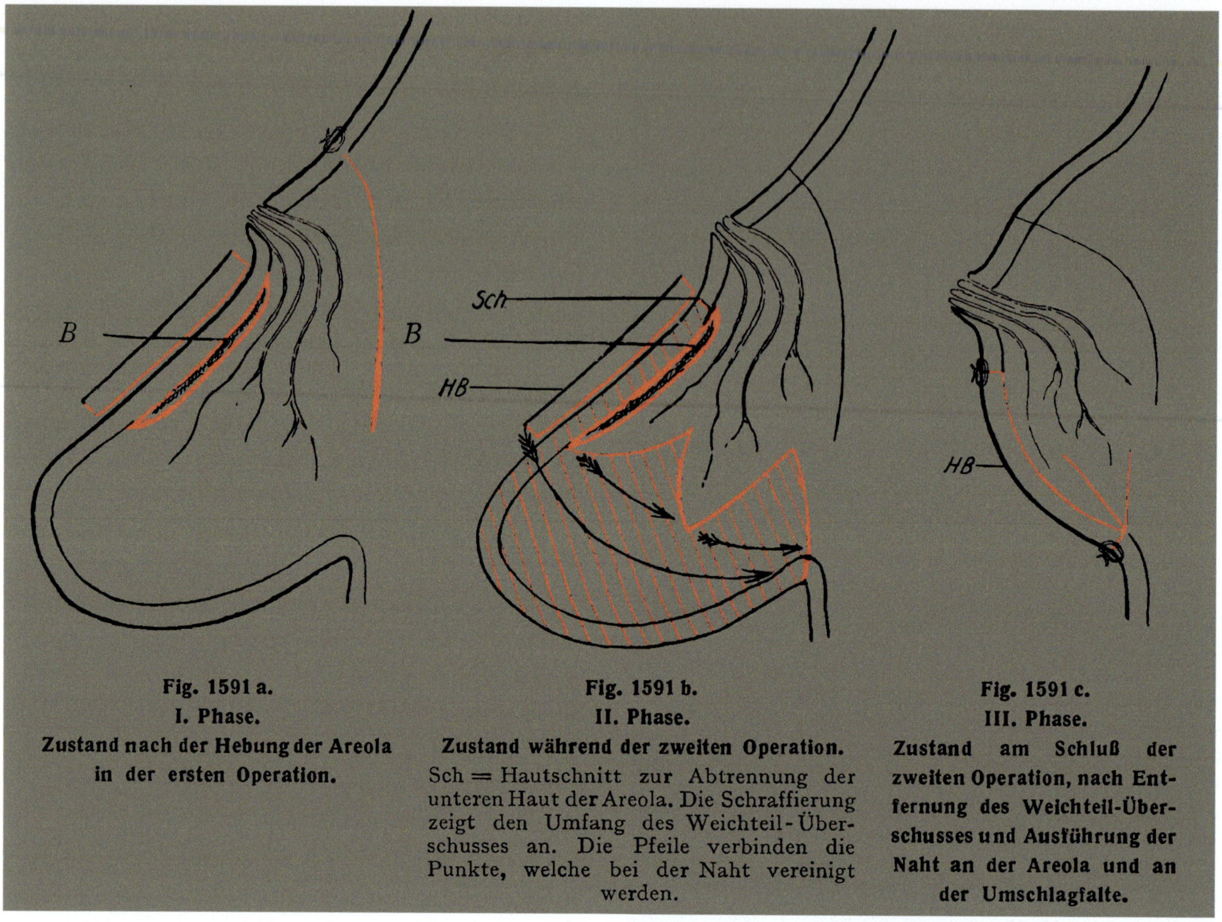

Fig. 15.9 The method of Jacques Joseph published in 1925 in his article *Zur Operation der Hypertophischen Haengebrust. Courtesy of Riccardo Mazzola, M.D., Milan*

without kinking but when this was longer (some said more than 7 cm) the dermal flap had to be folded on itself and this impaired the circulation. In 1967, Wiener et al.[13] followed a similar course. Then in 1973 P. K. McKissock suggested two vertical peduncles, one above and the other below the areola [646, 647]. The upper peduncle could be made thin enough to fold easily. This not only made it easier to transpose the areola to its new site but made the method safer for a large pendulous breast when the total length of the pedicle could safely be as long as 40 cm. The scars were similar to those produced by the Swedish surgeons (Fig. 15.15a,b). Another safe and simple method that gave consistently good results was the one devised by Tom Robbins [845]. He used similar incisions to those devised by Strömbeck but left the areolar on a de-epithelialized, wide mound of residual breast tissue attached to the chest wall and the lower line of the incision in the sulcus. This could be moved easily up to its new position after excising breast tissue from medial lateral and superior aspects.

In more recent years, Madeleine Lejour and her coworkers [543–547] adapted an idea described by Claude

13 Wiener D, Adrien EA, Aiache E, et al (1973) A single dermal pedicle for nipple transposition in subcutaneous mastectomy, reduction mammoplasty and mastopexis. *Plast Rec Surg* 51:176.

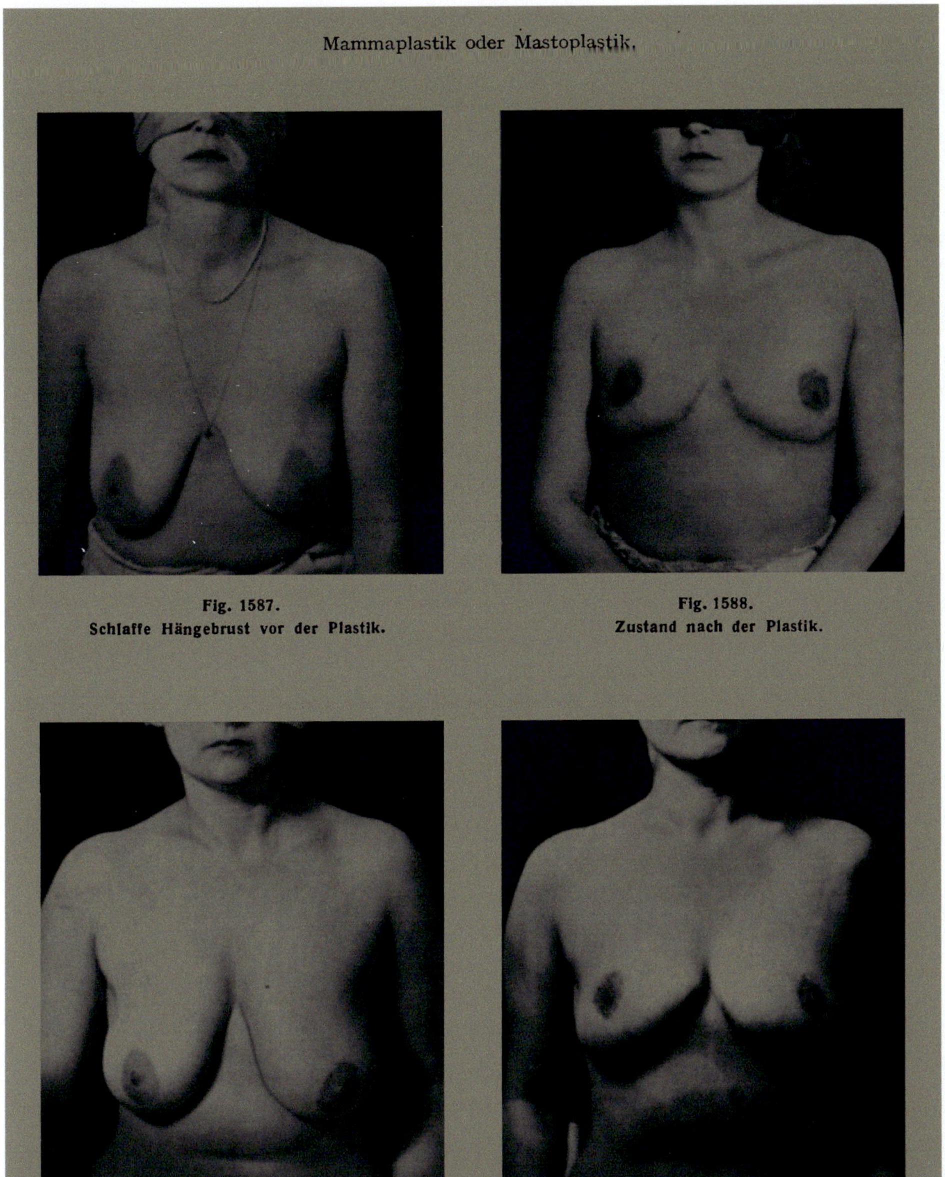

Fig. 15.10 Two of the earliest cases of mammoplasty to be published. They were reported by Jacque Joseph in 1925. The excision was performed above the areola. *Courtesy of Riccardo Mazzola, M.D., Milan*

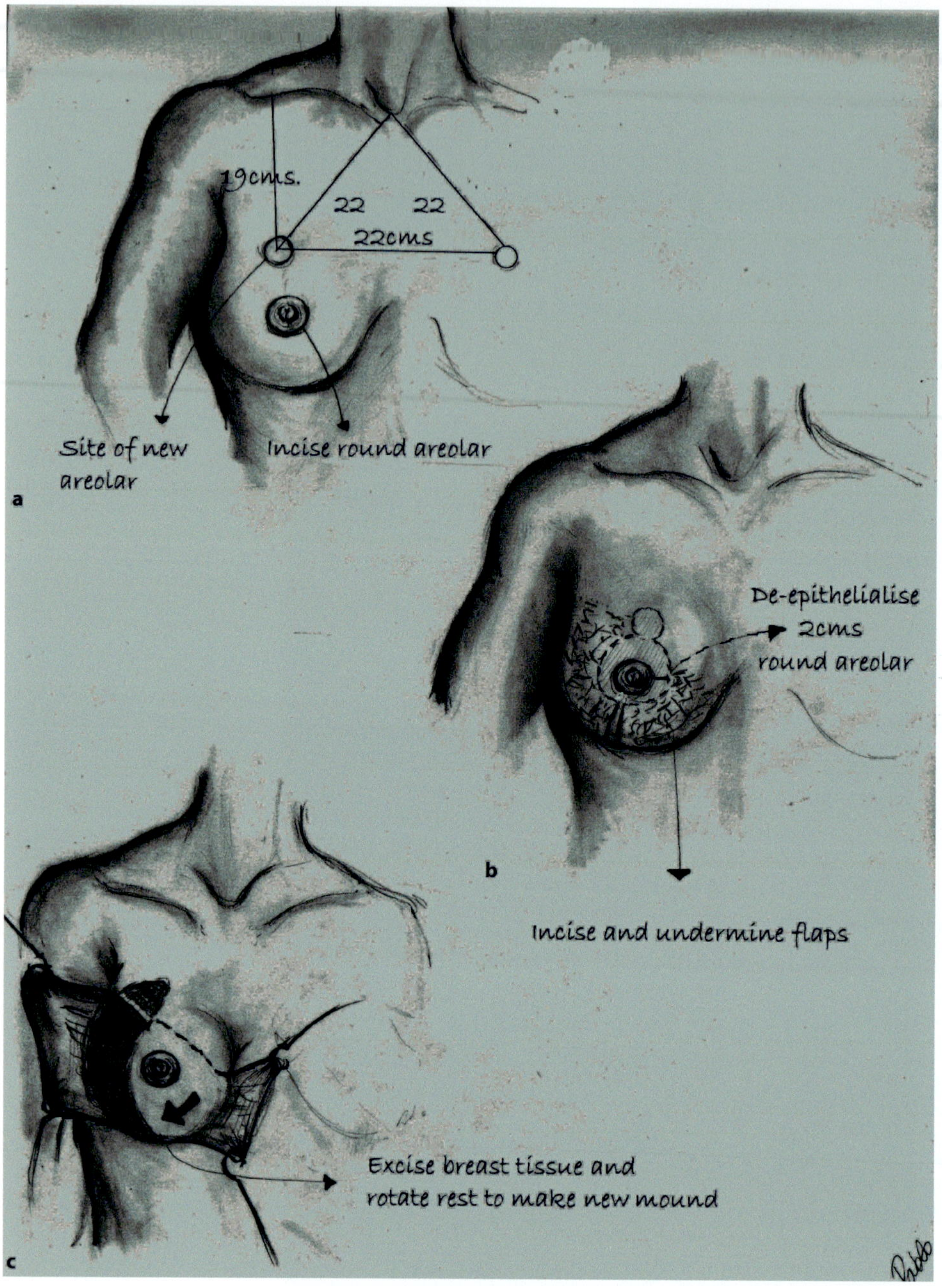

Fig. 15.11a–c Herman Biesenberger (1885–1947) modified the Lotsch method in 1928 and three years later published his technique. The operation was safer, produced pleasing results and became popular for about 30 years. *Diagrams by Pablo Patanè, Pisa*

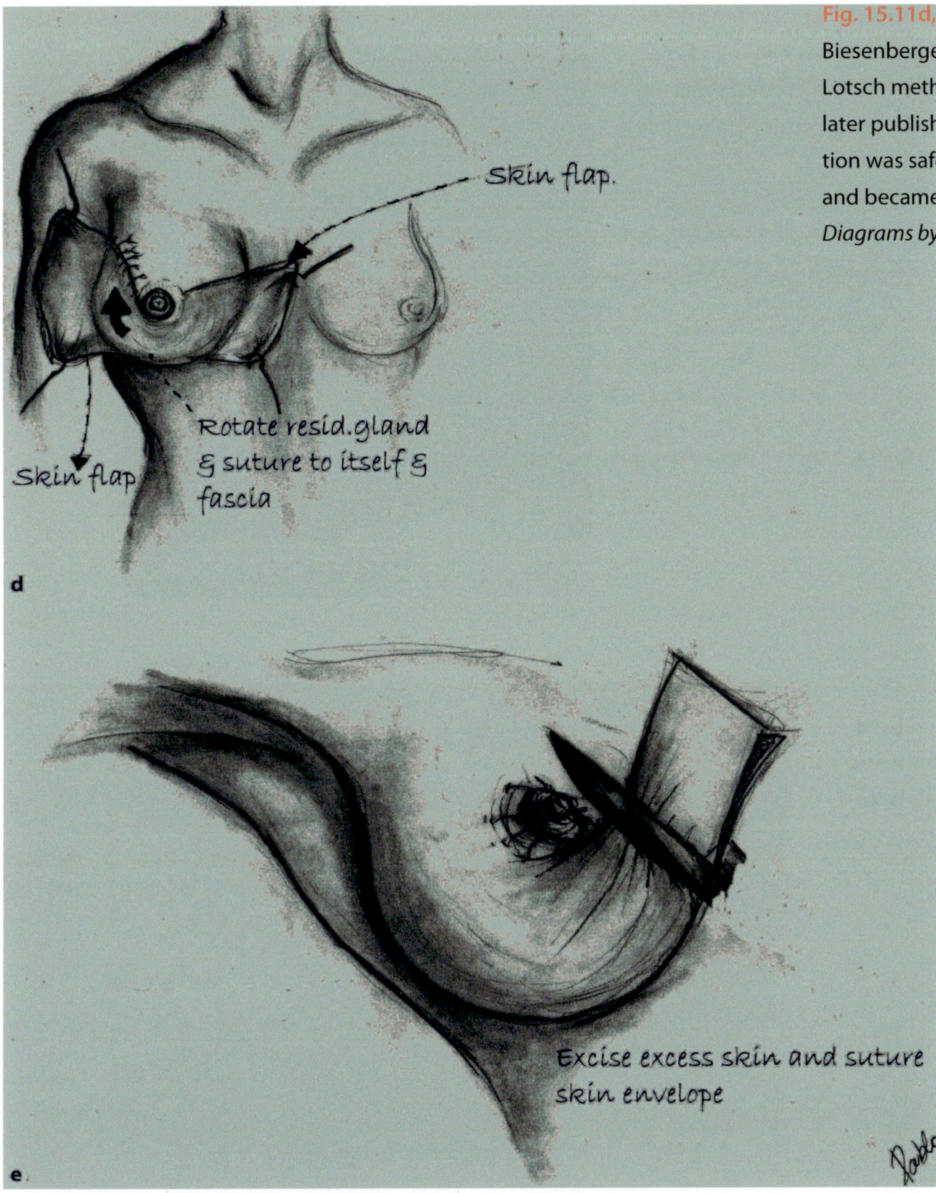

Fig. 15.11d,e *(continued)* Herman Biesenberger (1885–1947) modified the Lotsch method in 1928 and three years later published his technique. The operation was safer, produced pleasing results and became popular for about 30 years. *Diagrams by Pablo Patanè, Pisa*

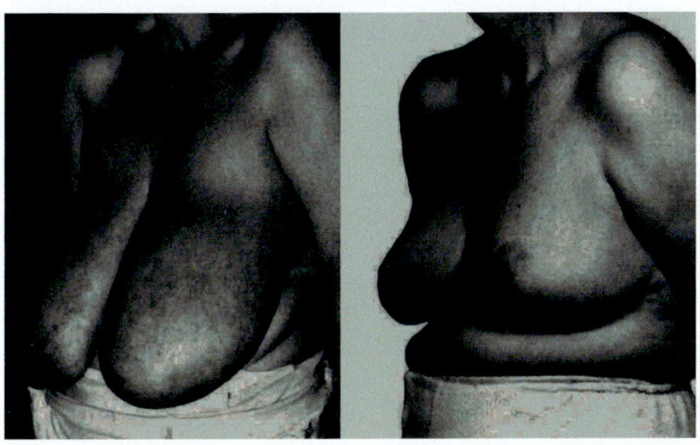

Fig. 15.12 Pre- and post-operative results of a Biesenberger reduction mammoplasty. *PJS*

Fig. 15.13 Cartoon of Sir Harold Gillies by Stig from 1926. It was presented by Gillies to Prof. Thomas Kilner and then by the latter's family to the Department of Plastic Surgery in Oxford. *Courtesy of Mr T. Goodacre, FRCS, Plastic Surgery Unit, Radcliffe Hospital, Oxford*

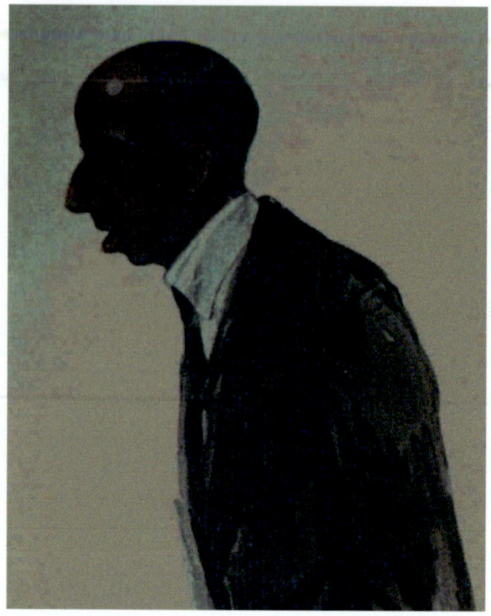

Fig. 15.14 The technique devised by Jan Olov Strömbeck in 1960. It proved reliable and gave good results but was not appropriate for very large breasts. *Diagrams by Pablo Patanè, Pisa*

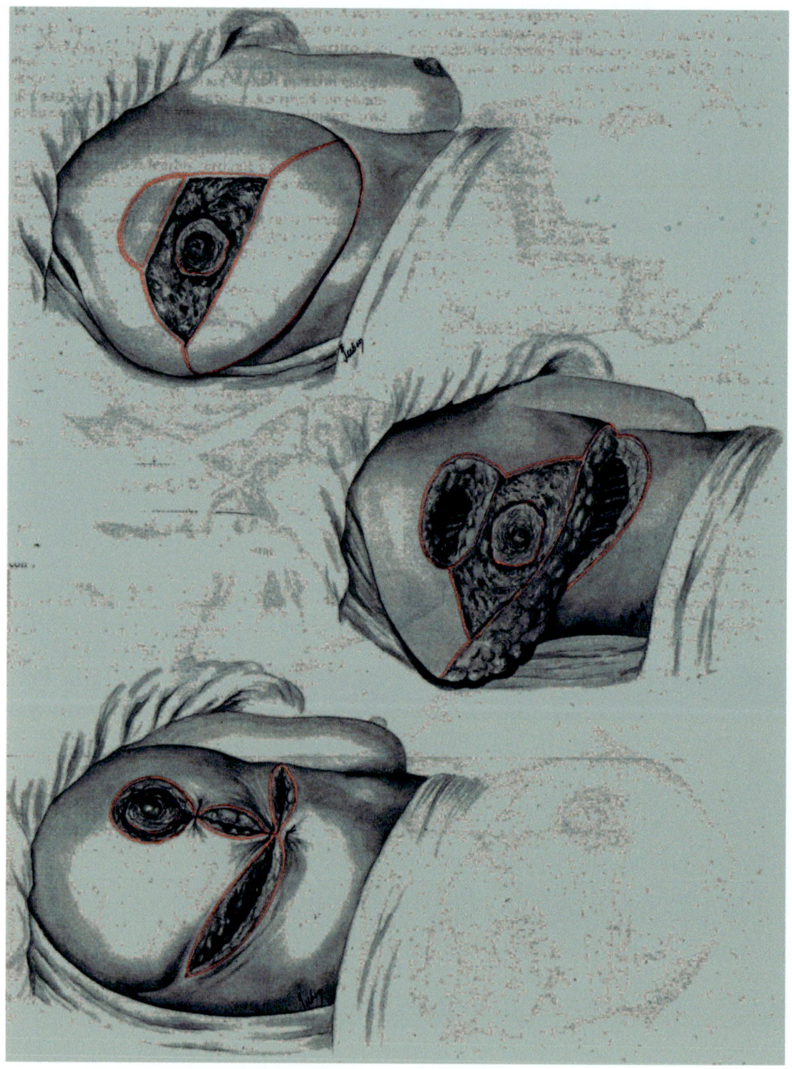

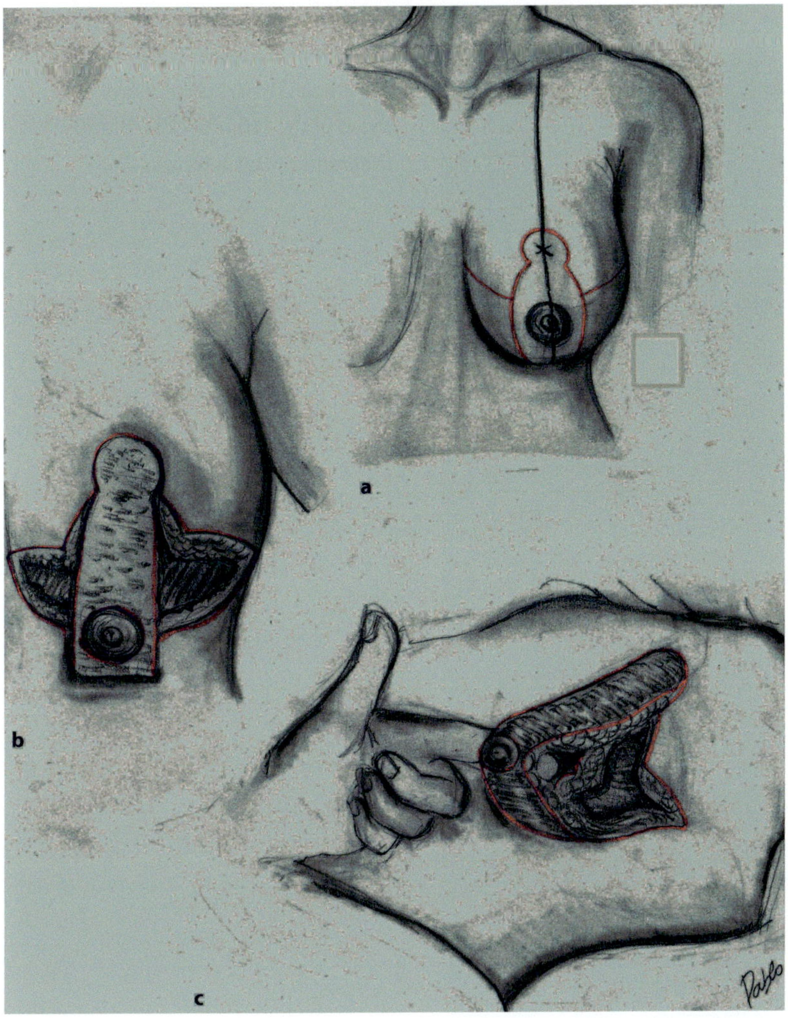

Fig. 15.15a–c McKissock used vertical pedicles, above and below the areola. The scars were similar to those of the Strombeck technique. *Diagrams by Pablo Patanè, Pisa*

Lassus [532–534]. Between 1970 and 1985 she developed a technique for mammoplasty which left a vertical scar below the areola with only a small fine scar in the submammary sulcus. With the introduction of liposuction this became an alternative to the long list of breast reductions which had accumulated in the twentieth century. However good results with this technique were limited to cases where only a moderate reduction was needed.

Breast Augmentation

Surgical techniques for increasing the size of breasts were not introduced until the latter part of the nineteenth century. Before then, the alternative for correcting asymmetry was to reduce the larger of the two breasts, but this was not always acceptable if this was the breast that was considered normal.

Asymmetry of the breasts was recognized in ancient times and several famous women in history were affected. G.J. Witkowski recounts in his book of 1913 that Queen Christine of Sweden—whom he called *The Messalina of the North*—was quite badly affected [1046].

Free Grafts of Fat

When Czerny [211] removed an enormous mammary adenoma from a patient in 1895, he filled the space with a lipoma taken from her shoulder. This does not appear to have undergone necrosis, although it grew no further

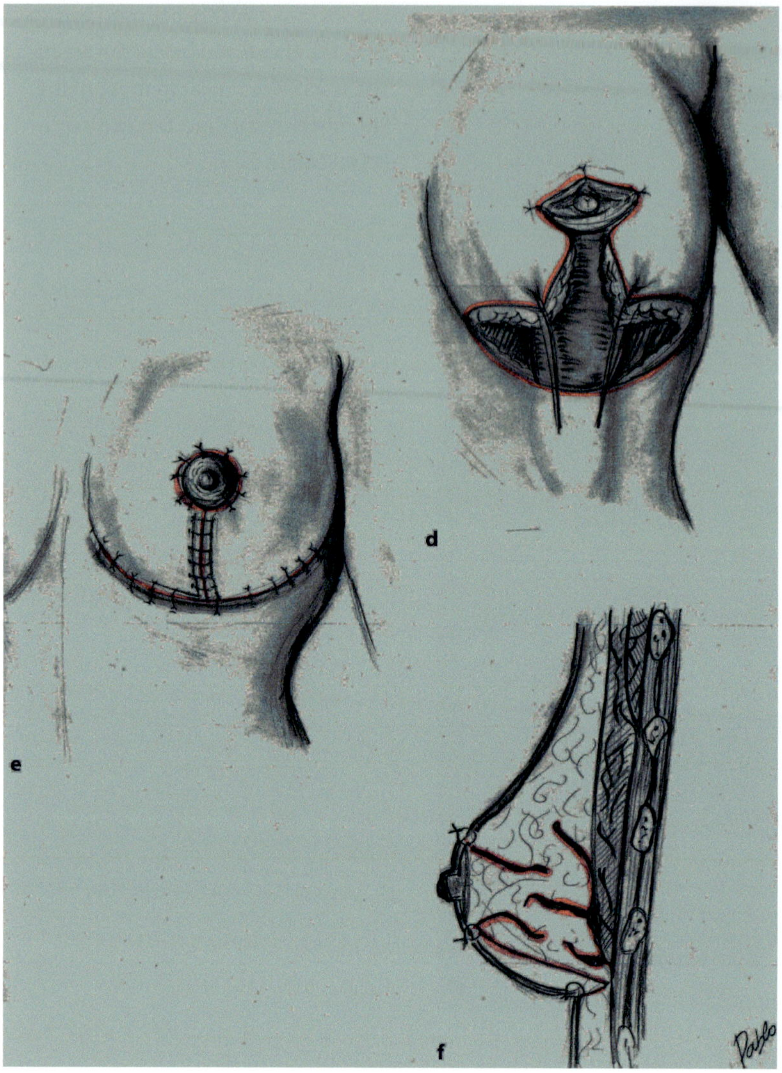

Fig. 15.15d–f *(continued)* McKissock used vertical pedicles, above and below the areola. The scars were similar to those of the Strombeck technique. *Diagrams by Pablo Patanè, Pisa*

after its removal. Similar cases were reported by August Karl Gustav Bier in 1910 [94] and by Rigollot-Simonnot in 1913 [841]. If nothing else these demonstrated that free grafts of fatty tissue were possible.

The first free graft of normal fatty tissue for correcting hypotrophic breasts, was probably performed by Gustav Adolf Neuber [728]. He had already used these grafts in 1893 for correcting hollows in the face.

Neuber's solution was also adopted by L. Wrede in 1915 [1052], and by W. Bartlett in 1917 [61], but it did not become popular until Lexer published his 20 years of experience in 1925 [560]. He reported a series of augmentation mammoplasty operations accomplished with free grafts of fatty tissue which produced pleasing effects. However, in 1950 he recommended that the correction should be 50% more than the desired volume because of the reabsorption that took place, particularly during the first year after surgery.

As the use of free grafts of fatty tissue increased, surgeons soon became aware that these underwent considerable reabsorption. In 1930, Passot [774] described his experience with grafts taken from the abdomen or buttocks. Initially he used two or three large grafts, until he realized that not only did they reabsorb but they produced a higher incidence of necrosis and extrusion than smaller grafts. R.P.G. Sandon confirmed this when he reported similar disasters [888].

Proof that only 45% of large grafts survived compared to 75% of small ones emerged in 1950, when Lindon Peer published the results of his experiments in *The Behaviour of Autogenous Human Tissue Grafts* [783–785]. Poor vascularization of the large grafts was incriminated.

H. May had already noticed this difference in 1915 so in 1943 tried to avoid it by including the fascia in the graft to increase the blood supply [621, 622]. M.T. Berson suggested including dermis for the same reason [82]. Fascia and dermis both have a richer blood network and by placing this in contact with a vascular bed there was some improvement. After 1950, fat was rarely grafted without dermis or fascia but unpredictable reabsorption remained a draw back.

The buttock crease was generally used as the best donor area although some surgeons persisted with the abdomen. Much debate also ensued about the positioning of the dermis or fascia. Contact with the most vascular surface was the sensible answer but opinions differed. Fascia was generally placed next to fascia and dermis next to glandular tissue. H.O. Barnes used the buttocks and placed the dermis in contact with the gland, giving the graft a cone shape [52]. His grafts were at least a third larger than what was to be the final size and he accepted that as much as 50% would be reabsorbed. In spite of all these attempts to reduce reabsorption, C.R. de Haan and R.B. Stark concluded in 1964 that reabsorption was an inevitable process that could continue for many months or even years [228]. G. Lupo and G. Boggio-Robutti [584] confirmed this in 1970. Reabsorption also occurred in an irregular fashion, affecting parts of the same graft unequally. This resulted in the breasts undergoing changes in shape and symmetry. Eventually it was recognized that free fat grafts, even with dermis were not the solution.

Correction of Volume with Skin Flaps

As a consequence of these failures surgeons began searching for alternatives to increase breast size. In 1950 Maliniak, inspired by the dermis-adipose flap used by F. Burian in 1934 [145, 146], employed a similar de-epithelialized flap from the submammary area and rotated it upwards to enlarge the breast [602–604]. J.J. Longacre reported his systematic study on the use of de-epithelialized skin in 1956 and other surgeons soon followed [575].[14] But this technique was unreliable because of necrosis and absorption so it did not stand the test of time

The Introduction of Breast Prostheses

We have already discussed the disastrous results of paraffin injections. The first to use them to increase the size of the breast was probably Robert Gersuny. He was also the first to describe *paraffinomas* in 1899, followed by Buck and Brockaert in 1903 [992, 993]. The lesson learned from using paraffin was so serious that many years passed before other materials were even contemplated. It was not until 1950 that J.H. Grindlay and his colleagues [397] used polyurethane sponge, but this very soon gave rise to severe fibrosis, calcification and shrinkage to the extent that the breasts took on grotesque shapes.

In 1965 H.G. Arion [31] employed siliconized rubber (called Simaplast) prostheses that were inflated with a physiological solution. These were implanted through small incisions, mainly round the areolar, a route planned to facilitate removal if required. This proved necessary after a very short time because between 3.5% and 15% of them deflated and at least 30% of them became stiff and hard.

During the Second World War silicone gel was discovered and used in industry, e.g. as a lubricant at high temperatures. Silicone rubber also became valuable for making inert tubes which were used medically, e.g. as shunts in hydrocephalus. Injectable industrial liquid silicone was probably first used to enlarge breasts by Harvey D. Kagan and he was followed by others. They encountered similar problems to those who had injected paraffin.

All these problems induced surgeons to look for alternatives and in 1961 T. Cronin and F. Gerow involved Down Corning to find an alternative. The result was the invention of the *sac* which was first reported at the Third International Congress of Plastic Surgery in Washington DC in 1963 and was universally adopted for breast

14 Maliniak (1950), Marino (1952), O'Connor (1964) and Goulian and McDevitt (1972) were a few of those who used de-epithelialized flaps.

augmentation in 1964. A thin, flexible and appropriately shaped silicone rubber shell (Silastic) filled with silicone gel was implanted as a prosthesis to increase breast size [206, 209]. These were very similar to human breast tissue in looks and to palpation. They seemed ideal and their success was immediate. They also appeared to be completely harmless and many designs appeared on the market and numerous women underwent breast augmentation. Over the years however some unsatisfactory results were reported. These appeared with increasing frequency with time and were mainly caused by firmness or outright rigidity produced by contraction of the tissues around the implant. Various modifications were made to the outer casing and other fillings were tried but the problem which led to a very unnatural appearance and feel occurred in a percentage of cases. Microscopic leakage of silicone was identified as a cause of the problem and J. Hartley designed a double lumen prosthesis [414] to prevent this. Physiological saline solution was used to fill the outer lumen and silicone gel the internal one. Another suggestion, that fibrosis around the prosthesis occurred because the shell was too smooth, resulted in the design of textured implants. However, the case against silicone prostheses exploded in the United States at the beginning of the 1980s with a series of lawsuits brought by unsatisfied patients. They complained not only of the unpleasant appearance of their breasts but also of systemic reactions. This caused many manufacturers to take their prostheses off the market. Implants filled with physiological saline solution come back into fashion (Fig. 15.16).

Despite the efforts of many manufacturers a perfect prosthesis has yet to be found. Results are generally satisfactory and complications occur in a percentage of patients. Despite this they continue to ask for augmentation and surgeons are prepared to perform the operation not withstanding the risk of litigation (Fig. 15.17).

Abdominoplasty

We have not mentioned the origins and all the different methods of abdominal reduction surgery or what is now sometimes referred to as *body contouring* when surgeons include liposuction. The list of eponymous methods is long and somewhat boring to embark upon at this late stage of the book. The paper written by Jens Foged in 1948 [325], which is a résumé of the many techniques available at that time, will prove rewarding. It will also give anyone who has got to the very end of this book something to smile about! (Fig. 15.18)[15]

15 The paper by Foged in 1948, was ready to send to the publishers when a passing trainee noticed the illustrations on his chief's desk. He could not resist the temptation to modify two of the drawings and nobody noticed. The Küster *Triby Hat* and the Weinhold *Wasp* designs must have puzzled surgeons who attempted these operations from the page of the journal. The story is related by Michael Tempest, a former editor of the journal but not the one who suffered the hoax! [977].

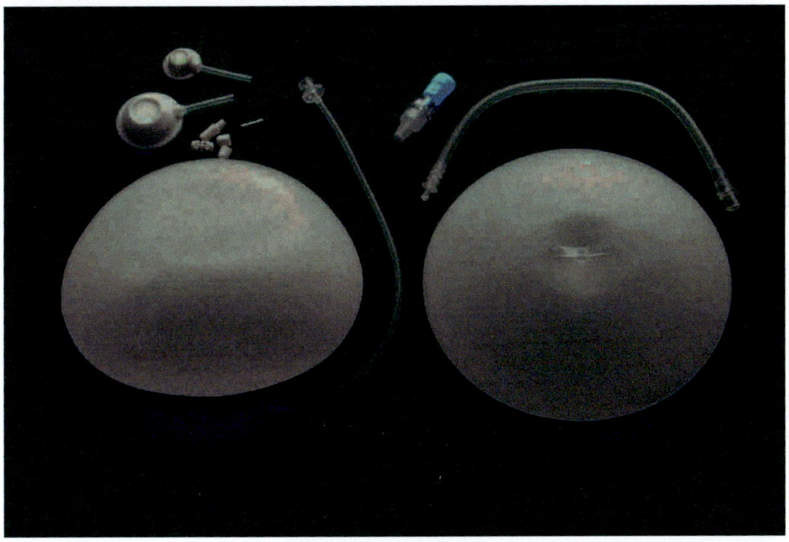

Fig. 15.16 Mammary prostheses. These are examples of the saline filled type. One has a filling tube and injection port for subcutaneous placement and gradual post-operative inflation. A self-sealing valve allows the tube to be removed later. The other has a valve on top of the silicone rubber shell for ease of inflation during surgery. Both can be folded up and inserted through small incisions

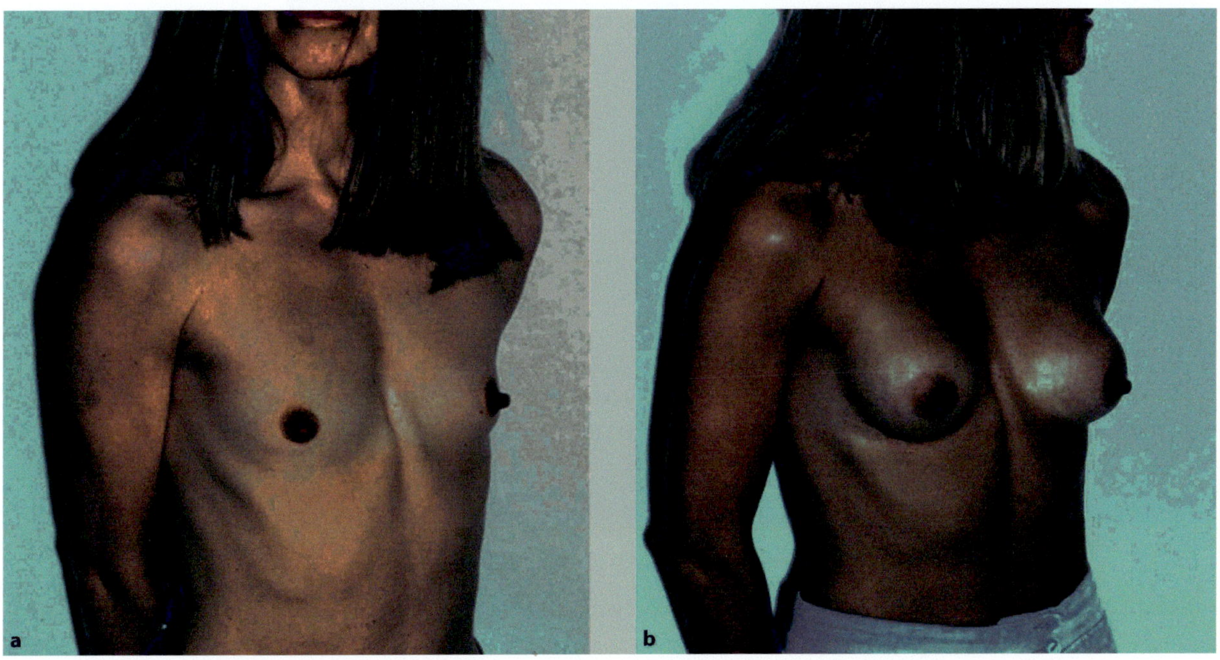

Fig. 15.17 **a** Pre-operative and **b** post-operative augmentation mammoplasty with silicone implants

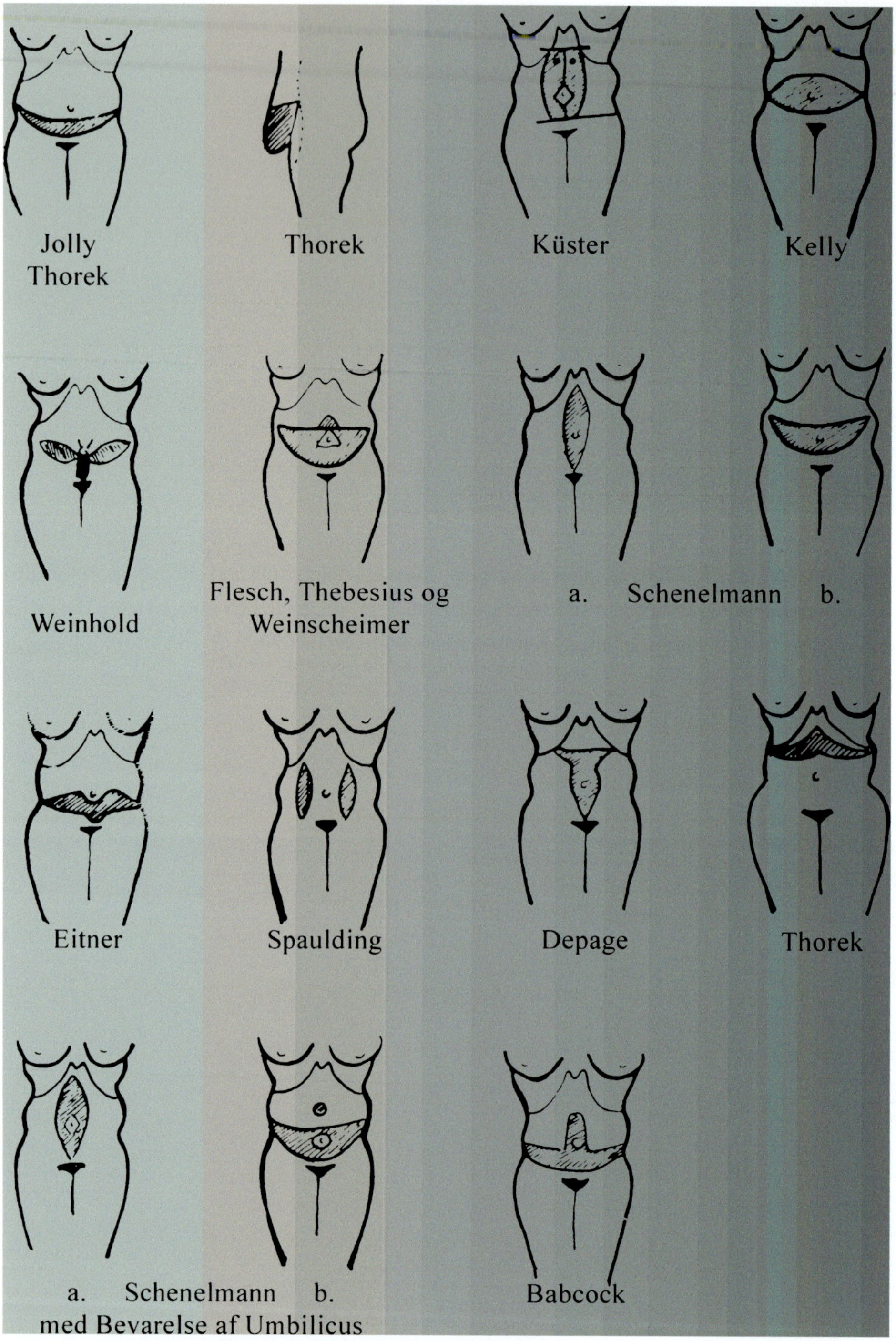

Fig. 15.18 Diagram from *Operative treatment of abdominal obesity, especially pendulous abdomen* by Jens Foged, Fig. 8.6 from the *British Journal of Plastic Surgery 1:274 © 1948 the British Association of Plastic Surgeons*

References

The authors have found the following excellent reference works indispensable. Readers will also discover that the *Zeis Index* contains fascinating comments about early texts. They are mentioned in the reference list in abbreviated form to avoid repetition:

The McDowell Series of Plastic Surgery Indices. William & Wilkins, Baltimore

Volume I The Zeis Index and History of Plastic Surgery 500BC to 1863AD (1977) compiled by Edward Zeis MD, translated with additions by Patterson TJS

Volume II The Patterson Index 1864AD to 1920AD (1978) Patterson TJS

Volume III The Leuz Index 1921AD to 1946AD (1977) Leuz CA

Volume IV The Great Index 1946AD to 1971AD (1977) McDowell F, Kramer B, McDowell M

Volume V The Honolulu Index 1971AD to 1976AD (1977) McDowell F

1. Abano P de (1496) "Conciliator" (conciliator contraversiarum quae inter philosophos et medicos versantur). Ottaviano Scotto, Venezia
2. Abbe R (1898) A new plastic operation for the relief of deformity due to double harelip. Med Rec 53:477
3. Aegineta P (1540) La chirurgie qui est la sixsieme livre de seses oeuvres. Estiene Dolet, Lyon
4. Aegineta P (1554) Paulus Aegineta Opera. In: Joanne Guintero Anderniaco interprete. Lugdum Batavor, Venice
5. Aegineta P (1844–1847) The seven books of Paulus Aegineta. Translated from Greek by Francis Adams, Sydenam Society, London
6. Agoty GJ d' (1748) Anatomie de la tete en tableaux imprimes d'apres les pieces disseques & prepares par M Duverney, Paris
7. Agoty GJ d' (1773) Anatomie des parties de la generation de l'homme ed de la femme, Paris
8. Agoty GJ d', Fabian J (1752) Anatomie generale des viscère en situation, de granduer et couleur naturelle, avec l'angeologie, et la neurologue de chaque partie du corps humain, Paris
9. Albee FH (1916) Bone graft surgery. Saunders, Philadelphia
10. Albinus BS (1734) Historia muscolorum corporis homini, apud Theodorum Haak et Henricum Mulhovium, Leiden
11. Albinus BS (1747) Tabulae sceleti et muscolorum corporis humani. J & H Verbeek, Leiden
12. Albinus BS (1747) Icones ossium foetus et muscolorum corporis humani. J & H Verbeek, Leiden
13. Albinus BS (1753) Tabulae ossium humanorum. J & H Verbeek, Leiden
14. Albucasis (Abu el Qàsin al Zahrawi) (1500–1501) Cyrurgia Albucasis cum cauterus et aliis instrumentis. In: Guy de Chauliac's Chirurgia Parva. Bonetus Locatellus for the heirs of Octavianus Scotus, Venice
15. Albucacis (1519) Liber Theoricae necnon practicae Alsaharanii. Sigismundi Grimm & Marci Vuirsung, Ausburg
16. Albucasis (1541) Methodus medendi quae ad chirurgiam requiruntur, libris III, expones cum instrumentis ad omnes fere morbos. Petrus, Basilea
17. Albucasis (1778) Albucasis: De cirurgia Arabica et latine cura. Translated by J Channing, Clarendon, Oxford
18. Albucasis (1992) La Chirurgia. Versione occitanica della prima metà del trecento. El-sheikh MS (ed) Edizioni Zeta, Firenze
19. Aldunate PE (1948) Algunas considerationes a proposito de interventiones plasticos mammarias. Boll Soc Chir Chile 26:549
20. Alliot MF (1834) Observations Cliniques. Gaz Méd Paris p 348
21. Allgower M, Blocker TG (1952) Viability of skin in relation to various methods of storage. Texas Rep Biol Med 10:3
22. Almast SC (1966) Rhinoplasty in Kangra. Punjab Med J 16:287
23. Almast SC (1969) History and evolution of the Indian method of rhinoplasty. In: Sanvenero-Rosselli G (ed) Transaction of the 4th International Congress of Plastic and Reconstructive Surgery, Rome. Excerpta Medica, Amsterdam
24. Ammon FA, Baumgarten M (1840) Plastic Surgery, cricitcally examined as to what it has hitherto accomplished; a prize essay of the Med Soc of Ghent. In: Bull de la Soc Méd de Gand, p 194
25. Ammon FA, Baumgarten M (1845) La Chirurgia plastica criticamente esposta giusta le prestazioni sue sino al di d'oggi (1704). Translated from German by Ghiminell, Cecchini e Norativich, Venezia

26. Anderl H (1973) Reconstruction of the face through cross face nerve transplantation in facial paralysis. Chir Plast 2:17
27. Anger T (1874) Hypospadias. Bull Soc Chir Paris, p 32
28. Anger T (1875) Hypospadias péno-scrotal, compliquéde coudure ed la verge: redressement du pénis et urethraplastie par inclusion cutanée: guerison. Bull Soc Chir Paris, p 179
29. Antia N, Daver B (1981) Reconstructive surgery for nasal defects. In: Blair R (ed) Reconstruction of the nose. Clin Plast Surg 8:535
30. Argelata P d' (1499) Cirurgia. Venezia
31. Arion HG (1965) Prosthesis Retromammaires. C R Soc Fr Gynecol 35:427–431
32. Aristotle (1476) De generatione animalium. Translated by Theodore Gaza. Ludovicus Podeatharus (ed) Johan de Colonia & Johannes Mauthews, Venezia
33. Assad MB (1890) Female circumcision in Egypt: social implications, current research and prospect for change. Stud Fam Plann 11:3
34. Atkins AG (1954) Ramayana of Tulsidass, vol 2. Hindustan Times, New Delhi
35. Aubert V (1923) Hypertrophie mammaire de la puberté. Resection partielle restaurative. Arc Franco-Belge Chir 26:284
36. Aufricht G (1940) Dental moulding compound cast and adhesive strapping in rhinoplasty procedure. Arch Otolaryngol 32:333–338
37. Aufricht G (1977) Commentary on operative reduction of the size of the nose (Rhinomiosis) by Jospeh J. In: McDowell F (ed) The Source book of Plastic Surgery, Williams and Wilkins, Baltimore, p 167
38. Auria V (1704) La Sicilia inventrice con li divertimenti geniali di Dr Mongitore. Marino, Palermo
39. Austad ED, Rose G (1982) A self inflating tissue expander. Plast Reconstr Surg 70:588
40. Auvray M (1931) Maladies du crâne et de l'encephale. In: Le Dentu et Pierre de Bet: Nouveau Traité de chirurgie clinique et opératoire, Librairie. Bailliére, Paris
41. Avicenna (1498) Canon (4 vols). Joannes Trechsel, Lyons
42. Avicenna (1506) Avicenna Medicorum arabum principis Liber Canonis Demedicinis cordialibus et cantica. Johannes Hieregros, Basilae
43. Axhausen G (1908) Die pathologischanatomischen Grundlapen der Lehre von derfreien Knockentransplanation beimMenschen und beim Tier. Med Klin Berlin 4:23
44. Axhausen G (1911) Kritische Bemerkungenund neue Beitrage zur freien Knockentransplanation. Arch Klin Chir 94:241
45. Aymard JL (1917) Nasal reconstruction. With a note on nature's plastic surgery. Lancet 2:888
46. B L (1794) Letter to the editor. Gentleman's Magazine, p 891 (*see also Freshwater F, McDowell F & Patterson TJS*)
47. Babcock WW (1917) Soup bone implant for the correction of defects of skull and face. JAMA 69:352
48. Baer KE von (1828) Ueber Entwicklungsgeschichte der Tierre: Beohactung und Reflecxion, part 1. Koniesberg
49. Bakamjian VY (1963) A technique for primary reconstruction of the palate after radical maxillectomy for cancer. Plast Reconstr Surg 31:103
50. Ballenger WL (1914) Diseases of the nose, throat and ear; medical and surgical. Lea & Febriger, Philadelphia
51. Ballantyne JW (1894) Case of hypospadias in a new born infant. Teratologia 1:96
52. Barnes HO (1953) Augmentation mammaplasty by lipotransplant. Plast Reconstr Surg 11:404
53. Baronio G (1786) Lettera del Dott. Giuseppe Baronio al Sig. Michele Girardi "Intorno alla regenerazione di tutto il gran tendine d'achille osservata in un uomo". Opuscoli Scelti sulle Scienze ed Arti 9:313
54. Baronio G (1804) Degli innesti animali. Stamperia e Fonderia de Genio, Milano (*this was translated in 1985 by Joan Bond Sax with a historical introduction by RM Goldwyn. The Boston Medical Library, Boston*)
55. Barri G (1600) De antiquitate et situ Calabriae. In: Italiae illustratae seu rerum urbiumque italicorum scriptores varii, notae melioris. Fol 991–1218, Frankfurt
56. Barth M (1894) Ueber histologischen Befunde nach Knocken implanation. Verh Dtsch Ges Chir 23:201
57. Barth M (1896) Kuenstliche Erzengung von Knochgewebe u. die Ziele der Osteoplastik. Berl Klin Wchnschr 33:8
58. Barth M (1897) Nochmals zur Frage du vitalitäet replantinter Knocheustueche. Arch Klin Chir 54:471
59. Barth M (1908) Ueber Osteoplastik. Arch Klin Chir 86:859
60. Bartholini C (1678) Anatome. JA Hugweten & Son, Lugduni
61. Bartlett W (1917) An anatomic substitute for the female breast. Ann Surg 66:208
62. Baschkirzew NJ, Petrow NN (1912) Bone grafts. Dtsch Z Chir 113:490
63. Baskaradoss VK, Jose RM (2006) Life and times of Susruta: fact and fiction. Indian J Plast Surg 39:109
64. Becher OJ (1949) Surgical correction of the abnormally protruding ear. Arch Otolaryngol 50:541
65. Becher OJ (1952) Correction of protruding deformed ears. Br J Plast Surg 5:187
66. Beer GJ (1792) Lehre der Augenkran heiten. CF Kappler, Wien
67. Beer GJ (1817) Lehre von den Augenkrankeiten als Leitfaden zu seinen offentlichen Vorlesungen Entworsen, vol II. Lamesina Heubner & Wolke, Wien
68. Bell C (1806) Essay on the anatomy of expression in painting. Longman Reese Hurst & Orme, London
69. Bell C (1824) The Anatomy and Philosophy of Expression. Longman Reese Hurst & Orme London
70. Benedetti A (1502) Anatomiae sive Historia Corporis Humani. Guerraldo, Venezia
71. Benedetti A (1502) Breves Perlucide ac uberrime in Anatomiam Corpori Humani. Guerraldo, Venezia
72. Bennett JE, Miller SR (1970) The evolution of the electric dermatome. Plast Reconstr Surg 45:131
73. Bennett JP (1974) From noli-me-tangere to rodent ulcer: the recognition of basal cell carcinoma. Br J Plast Surg 27:144
74. Berengario da Carpi J (1518) Tractatus de Fractura calve sive cranei a Carpo. H de Benedicitis, Bologna

75. Berengario da Carpi J (1521) Carpi commentaria cum amplissimis additionibus super anatomia mundini. H de Benedicitis, Bologna
76. Berengario da Carpi J (1523) Isagogae breves perlucidae ac uberrimae in Anatomiam Humani Corporis a comuni Medicorum Academia usitatam. Benedetto di Ettore, Bologna
77. Berengario da Carpi J (1529) Anatomia mundini castigata ab eximio atrium et medicinae doctore de Magistro Jacobo de Carpo in Almor Studio Bonon. Empresa Ottaviano Scotti e soci, Venezia
78. Berger P (1904) Autoplastie par dedoublement dela palmure et echange des lambeaux. In: Berger P, Banzet S (eds) Chirurgie Orthopedic. Steinheil, Paris (*see also numerous writings of Berger P between 1880 and 1904 pp 25–26, Patterson Index*)
79. Bernard C (1853) Cancer de la lèvre inférieure: restauration à l'aide de deaux lambeaux latéreaux quadrilatére. Bull Soc Chir Paris 3:357
80. Bernard C (1857) Leçons sur les effets des substances toxiques et médicamenteuses. JB Bailliére, Paris
81. Bernard C, Huette C de Montargis (1860) Sommario iconografico di medicina operativa e di anatomia chirurgica. Agostino Pollerano, Napoli
82. Berson MT (1945) Derma-fat transplants used in building up the breast. Surgery 15:451
83. Bert P (1864) Greffe animale. J Anat Physiol Paris 1:69
84. Bert P (1864) Transplantation: re-establishment of the circulation and propagation of sensation in the opposite direction to normal. C R Soc Biol (1863) Paris 3.s., 5:179
85. Bert P (1865) Expérience de greffe animale. C R Soc Biol 1:172
86. Bert P (1866) Recherches expérimentales pour servir à l'histoire de la vitalité propre des tissues animeaux. Paris
87. Bertocchi A (1923) Innesti di tessuti fissati. Tipografia Sociale Torinese, Torino (*see also writings of Bertocchi P, The Leuz Index p 80*)
88. Bettman AG (1920) Plastic and cosmetic surgery of the face. Northwest Med J 19:205
89. Bettman OL, Hench PS (1956) A Pictorial History of Medicine. Thomas, Springfield
90. Bhishagratna KK (1963) The Sushruta Samità, English translation of the original Sanskrit. Text XI The Chowkhamba Sanskrit Series, Varanasi (*see also pp 87–88 Zeis Index*)
91. Bichat MFX (1802) Anatomie générale appliquée à la Médicine. Brosson Gabon et Cie, Paris
92. Bidloo G (1685) Anatomie humani corporis gentum. Joannis Someren, Amsterdam
93. Bidloo G (1700) Gulielmus Cowper criminis literarii citatum coram tribunali nobiliss ampliss. Societatis Britanno-Regiae, Leiden
94. Bier AKG (1910) Fettransplantation. Chir Kong Verhandl 1:189
95. Biesenberger H (1928) Eine neue method der mammarplastik. Zentralbl Chir 55:2382
96. Biesenberger H (1930) Eine neue method der mammarplastik. Zentralbl Chir 57:2971
97. Biesenberger H (1931) Deformitaten und Kosmetische Operationen der verblichen Brust. Wilhelm Mandrich, Wien
98. Bigelow HJ (1846) Insensibility during surgical operations produced by inhalations. Boston Med Surg J 35:309
99. Bigelow HJ (1848) Ether and chloroform: a compendium of their history, surgical use and dangers. David Clapp, Boston (*reprint: Boston Med Surg J pp 1–27*)
100. Bigelow HJ (1876) A history of the discovery of modern anesthesia. In: A century of American Medicine, 1776–1876. Am J Med Sc 71:
101. Billroth TH (1889) Ueber Uranoplastik. Kl Wchschr Wien 2:241 (*see also writings of Billroth TH. Patterson Index p 80*)
102. Billingham RE, Medawar PB (1952) The freezing, drying and storage of mammalian skin. J Exp Biol 29:454
103. Bindi L, Bindi B (1774) Trattato chirurgico sopra la semplicità del medicare i mali curabili coll'aiuto della mano, Siena
104. Birch T (1756) The History of the Royal Society of London for improving of natural knowledge from its first rise. Reprinted with new introduction and biography by Hall AR, Hall MB(1968) Johnson Reprint, New York
105. Blair VP, Brown JB (1929) The use and uses of large split skin grafts of intermediate thickness. Surg Gynecol Obstet 49:82–97
106. Blair VP, Brown JB (1930) Mirault operation for single harelip. Surg Gynecol Obstet 51:81–98
107. Blair VP,Byars LT (1938) Hypospadias and epispadias. J Urol 40:814
108. Blandin PF (1836) De l'Autoplastie ou Restauration des Parties du Corp qui ont èté Detruites à la Faveur d'une Emprunt fait à d'autres Patries plus ou moins Eloignées. Thesis, Urtubie, Paris
109. Blandin PF (1836) Staphylorophie: Diction de Médic et de Chir Pratique 15:8
110. Blandin PF (1842) Bec-de-Lièvre double avec division double de la voute palatine. Opération par un procédée particulier. Gaz des Hosp Paris 2nd 5:22
111. Blandin PF (1842–1843) Cheiloplastie. Bull Acad R Tom 8:670
112. Blandin PF (1846–1847) Uranoplastie. Ann de Thérap Paris l 4:346
113. Blandin PF (1847) Autoplastie. Jour de Conn Méd Chir 14:45
114. Blandin PF (1848) Operation to remedy a division of the velum palati or cover of the palate. New York J Med 10:203 (*see also writings of Blandin PF, Patterson Index pp 124, 199, 218*)
115. Blasius E (1842) Neue Methode der Blepharoplastik. Med Ztg (Preuss.Vereinsztg) 11:43
116. Blasius E (1848) Beitrage zur prakistschen chirchurgie p 157 Forstner, Berlin (*Blasius wrote extensively on reconstructive surgery and the references are too numerous and detailed to include here. See Zeis Index, pp 124–125, 174, 119*)
117. Blegny N de (1682) Zodiacus medico-gallicus. Annus Secundus. Genevae (*see also note 11 pp 17–18, with footnote by TJSP in Zeis Index*)

118. Bonham Carter V, Lawson M (1968) George Lawson: surgeon in the Crimea. Constable, London (*see footnote p 14 McDowell F (1977) The Source Book of Plastic Surgery Williams & Wilkins, Baltimore*)
119. Bonsdorff H von (1894) Ett fall of osteoplastik operation på pannbenet. Finska Läk-sällsk Handl 36:304
120. Boo-Chai K (1966) An ancient Chinese text on a cleft lip. Plast Reconst Surg 38:89
121. Bordenave (1728–1782) Memoire dans lequel on propose un nouveau procèdè pour traiter le renversement des paupieres, vol V. Delaguette, Le Prieur, Lambert, Didot, Paris, p 97
122. Borgognoni T (1955) The Surgery of Theodoric. Translated from Latin by Campbell EC & Colton JB, Appleton Century Crofts, New York
123. Botallo L (1660) Opera Omnia Medical et Chirurgica. D & A Gassebeek, Ludguni
124. Bouisson P (1826) Cheiloplastie. Diction Encyclop Sci Med 15:625
125. Bourdet B (1757) Recherches et observations sur toutes les parties de l'art du dentiste. JT Hèrissan, Paris
126. Bourguet J (1919) La disparition chirurgicale des rides et polis du visage. Bull Acad Med Paris 82:183
127. Bourguet J (1928) Notre traitment chirugical de "poches sous les yeux" sans cicatrice. Arch Franco-belg Chir 31:133
128. Breasted JH (1930) The Edwin Smith Surgical Papyrus. University of Chicago Press, Chicago
129. Brent B (1950) Reconstruction of the auricle. In: McCarthy J (ed) Plastic Surgery, vol 3. Saunders, Philadelphia
130. Brewer EP (1882) On the limit of skin vitality. Med Rec 21:483
131. Brian DJ (1993) The early history of rhinoplasty. Facial Plast Surg 2:81
132. Brown JB, Cannon B (1947) Composite free grafts of skin and cartilage from the ear. Surg Gynecol Obstet 82:153
133. Browne D (1949) An operation for hypospadias. Proc R Soc Med 42:466
134. Browne D (1949) Hypospadias. Postgrad Med J 25:376
135. Browne D (1953) A comparison of the Duplay and Denis Browne techniques for hypospadias operation. Surgery 34:787 (*see also Nixon HH, Waterston D and Wink CAS (1983) Selected writings of Sir Denis Browne, Farnborough, England*)
136. Brunazzi GM (1790) Memoria su di un Nuovo Metodo di Unire il Labbro Leporino col Mezzo di Una Macchinetta. Genestri, Faenza
137. Bruns V von (1857–1860) Chirurgischer Atlas. Bildilche Darstellung der chirurgischen Krankheiten und der zu ihrer Heilung erforderlichen Instrumente, Bandagen und Operationen (Tables XIII, XIV, XV). Laupp, Tubingen
138. Brunschwig H (1477) Das ist das Buch der Chirurgia. Johan Grueninger, Strasbourg
139. Brunschwig H (1497) Dis ist das Buch der Chirurgia: Hautwirckung der wund artz. H Schonsperger, Ausburg
140. Brunschwig H (1561) A most excellent and perfect homishapothecarthye or homerly physick booke for all the grefes and diseases of the body. Arnold Bichman, Cologne
141. Buncke HJ, Daniller AI, Schulz WP, et al (1967) The fate of autogenous whole joints transplanted by microvascular anastomosis. Plast Reconstr Surg 39:333
142. Bünger HC (1823) Gehungener versuch einer nasenbildung aus einen vollig getrenuten haustuck aus dem beine. Gr u W Jour d Chir U, Augen
143. Bulwer J (1653) Antropometamorphosis: man transform'd or artificial changing. scripsit J B Cognomento Chirosophus MD, William Hunt, London
144. Buret F (1892) Syphilis in ancient and prehistoric times. In: Davis NS (ed) Diseases of the lungs, heart and kidneys. FA Davis, Philadelphia
145. Burian F (1934) Plastic surgery of the breast. Cas Lek Cesk 73:373
146. Burian F (1938) Our experiences with mammaplasties. Rev Chir Struct 8:35
147. Burow CA von (1856) Beschriebung einer neuen Transplantations-Methode zum Wiederersatz verloren gegangener Theile des Gesischts. Nauck, Berlin
148. Bushe G (1831) Hypospadias. New York Med Chir Bull 2:1
149. Bussmaker and Daremberg (1851–1876) Oevres d'Oribase. Texte Grec en grand partie inédit, vol 6. Imprimérie Nationale, Paris
150. Cabanes A (1918) Chirugiens et blesses a travers l'histoire. Albin Michel, Paris
151. Calentius E (1503) Opuscola. De Besicken, Roma
152. Cameron KM, Wallace AF (1991) "Dr Willi" (1882?–1972?) disciple of Jacques Joseph. Plast Reconstr Surg 88:363
153. Campanella FT (1620) De sensu rerum et magia, libri quatuor. Francofurti
154. Canano GB (1541) Muscolorum humani corporis picturata dissectio. Ferrara
155. Capparoni P (1933) Le Vincenda della tomba di Gaspare Tagliacozzi. In: Extracts from the proceedings of the 4th Congress of the Italian Soc for the History of Science, Medicine and Nature. Rome, May 11–12, XI.3 (*see also in Rass.di Clinica, Terapiae e Scienza 4. July/August*)
156. Carcano LGB (1583) De vulneribus capitis liber absolutissimus. Pietro Tino, Milano
157. Carpue JC (1816) An account of two successful operations for restoring a lost nose including description of the Indian and Italian methods. Longman, London
158. Carrel A (1912) The preservation of tissues and its application in surgery. JAMA 59:523
159. Casserio C (1600–1601) De Vocis Auditusque Organi Historia Anatomica. Victorius Baldinus, Ferrara
160. Castañares S (1951) Blepharoplasty for herniated intraorbital fat. Anatomical basis for a new approach. Plast Reconstr Surg 8:46
161. Castañares S (1964) Baggy eyelids. Physiological considerations and surgical techniques. Transaction of 3rd Int Congress of Plast Surg in Washington DC, 1963. Excerpta Medica, Amsterdam
162. Castañares S (1977) Classification of baggy eyelids deformity. Plast Reconstr Surg 54:629
163. Castiglioni A (1956) A history of medicine, 2nd edn. Alfred A Knopt, New York

164. Cazin M (1916) La cranioplastie consécutive aux large trépanations. A Malone et Fils, Paris
165. Cazin M (1916) Cranioplasty by skin and bone flaps. Paris Chir 8: 427 and ibid (1917) 9:102
166. Cecil AB (1932) Surgery of hypospadias and epispadias in the male. J Urol 27:507
167. Celsus AC (1478) De Medicina, Laurentii, Firenze (*see notes pp 1 and 20 of The Zeis Index, commentary by TJSP*)
168. Celsus AC (1989) De Medicina with an English translation. Spencer, Harvard University Press, Cambridge, Mass
169. Chauliac G de (1478) La pratique en chirugie du Maistre Guidon de Chauliac. Barthelemy Buyer, Lyons
170. Chauliac G de (1481) Chirurgia magna. Braem, Louvain
171. Chauliac G de (1513) Cyrugia. Gregorio de Gregori, Venezia
172. Chauliac G de (1521) Guidon en chirurgie. Cesare Arrivabene, Venezia
173. Chauliac G de (1890) La grande chirurgie. Nicaise, Paris
174. Chaveau C (1902) Histoire des maladies du pharynx, vol 2. Ballière et Fils, Paris, p 292
175. Cheselden W (1713) The anatomy of the human body. Cliff & Jackson, London
176. Chick LR (1988) Brief history and biology of skin grafting. Ann Plast Surg 21:358
177. Chopart F (1799) Mémoires sur la meilleure forme des aiguilles propres a les reunion des plaies. Mém Soc Med Emulation 3:79
178. Choulant L (1920) History and Bibliography of Anatomic Illustration. Translated and edited by Mortimer Frank, University of Chicago Press, Chicago
179. Clark AJ (1938) Aspects of the history of anaesthetics. BMJ 2:1031
180. Cobbett JR (1969) Free digital transfer: report of a case of transfer of a great toe to replace an amputated thumb. J Bone Joint Surg 51(B):677
181. Cocheril RC (1895) Reconstruction de l'oreille. Rev Laryngol 15:81:145
182. Cochrane T (1968) The low temperature storage of skin: A preliminary report. Br J Plast Surg 21:118
183. Cockayne TO (1865) Leechdoms, Wortcunning and Starcraft of Early England, vol 2. Longman, London
184. Codivilla A (1905) On the means of lengthening in the lower limbs, the muscles and tissues which are shortened through deformity. Am J Orthop Surg 2:353
185. Coghlan BA, Matthews B, Pigott RW (1987) A computer based method of measuring facial asymmetry. Results from assessment of the repair of cleft lip deformities. Br J Plast Surg 46:440
186. Cognatus GN (1567) Narrationum Sylva, Lib. III, Fol. 276. Basel
187. Coiter V (1573) Tractatus anatomicus de ossibus foetus abortivi et infantis dimidium amnum nati. Typis Johannes Colleni, Grönigen
188. Colmbus R (1559) De Re Anatomica, Lib. XV. Nicvolai Bevilacquae, Venezia
189. Conley J (1968) Face-lift operation. Thomas, Springfield, Ill
190. Converse JM (1977) The absorption and shrinkage of maternal cartilage used as living homograft: follow up report of 21 Gillies patients. In: Converse JM (ed) Reconstructive Plastic Surgery. Saunders, Philadelphia
191. Converse JM, Hogan VM, McCarthy JG (1977) Cleft lip and palate. In: Converse JM (ed) Reconstructive Plastic Surgery, 2nd edn. Saunders, Philadelphia, p 1930
192. Converse JM, Duchet G (1947) Successful homologous skin grafting in a war burn using an identical twin as donor. Plast Reconstr Surg 2:342
193. Converse JM, Morello DC, Guy CY (1977) Esthetic surgery of the aging face. In: Converse JM (ed) Reconstructive Plastic Surgery, vol 3, ch 7. Saunders, Philadelphia
194. Conway H, Reid WH, Beaton JJ (2006) Tom Gibson, plastic surgeon, 1915–1993. J Med Biography 14:192
195. Cooke J of Warwick (1693) Mellificium Chirurgiae: or the Marrow of Chirurgery. With the Anatomy of Human Bodies, 4th edn. Printed for W Marshall at the Bible in Newgate Street, London
196. Cooper A (1824, 1825, 1827) The lectures of Sir Astley Cooper FRS on the principles and practices of surgery, 3 vol. Underwood Lectures IV, XXIX & XXXV, London
197. Cooper A, Travers B (1820) Surgical essays, 2nd edn. Cox & Son, London
198. Cormack GC, Lamberty BGH (1984) The Arterial Anatomy of Skin Flaps. Churchill Livingstone, Edinburgh
199. Corning JL (1873) On the prolongation of the anaesthetic effects of the hydrochlorate of cocaine when subcutaneously injected. An experimental study. N Y Med J pt I 19:323
200. Corning JL (1885) Spinal anaesthesia and local medication of the cord. N Y Med J 42:483
201. Corning JL (1886) Local anaesthesia in general medicine and surgery. Appleton, New York
202. Corradi A (1877) Dell'Antica Autoplastica Italiana. Mem R Istit Lombardo Sc. e lettere, Bernardoni, Milano
203. Cortesi GB (1659) Miscellaneorum medicinalium decades denae, Messanae
204. Coury C (1969) La Médicine de l'Amerique Precolombienne. Roger Dacosta, Paris
205. Cowper W (1694) Myotomia Reformata: or an Anatomical Treatise of the Muscles of the Human Body. Sam Smith and Benj. Walford at the Princes Arms in St Paul's Churchyard
206. Cowper W (1724) Myotomia Reformata: or an Anatomical Treatise of the Muscles of the Human Body. R Knaploch & J Innys, London
207. Creause M de la (1834) Mémoires sur un nuoveau procèdé opératoire pour prevenir la recidive du cancer. Gaz Méd Paris p 657
208. Cronin TD (1964) Augmentation mammaplasty: a new "natural feel" prosthesis. In: Transactions of the Third International Congress of Plastic Surgery, Rome. Excerpta Medica, Amsterdam
209. Cronin TD (1966) Use of a Silastic frame for total and subtotal reconstruction of the external ear. Preliminary report. Plast Reconstr Surg 37:399

210. Culp OS (1967) Struggles and triumphs with hypospadias and associated anomalies: review of 400 cases. J Urol 96:339
211. Czerny V (1895) Plastische Ersatz der Brust-druse durch ein lipom. Chir Kong Verhandl 2:216
212. Daniel RK, Taylor GI (1973) Distant transfer of an island flap by microvascular anastomosis. Plast Reconstr Surg 52:111
213. Dartigues L (1924) Le traitment chirurgical du proplapsus mammaire suspension et mastopexie par voie axillotomique. Paris Chir 16:145
214. Dartigues L (1925) Le traitment chirurgical du prolaxus mammaire. Arch Franco-Belge Chir 28:313
215. Dartigues L (1928) Quelque points de chirurgie esthétique du sein. Soc Méd Paris 28:55
216. Dartigues L (1929) De la greffe autoplastique aréola-mammaire combinée à la mammectomie bilateral totale. Paris Chir 21:287
217. Dartigues L (1929) De la mastopexie costale transpectorale par voie péri-aréolaire. Bull Mem Soc Chir Paris 21:287
218. Dartigues L (1936) Chirurgie réparatrice plastique et esthetiqe de la poitrine et de l'abdomen. Bull Soc Méd 130 Paris (*see also several papers on like subjects by Dartigues L in The Leuz Index*)
219. Darwin C (1859) On the Origin of Species. John Murray, London
220. Daviel J (1755) A dissertation upon the cancer of the eyelids, nose, outer angle of the eye etc called nolé me tangere. Philos Trans R Soc 49:186
221. Davies N de G (1900) The Mastaba of Ptahhetep and Akkethetep at Saqquareh, London (*see also The Theban Tomb Series (1915) Davies N de G and Hendeson JJ, Egyptian Exploration Fund, London*)
222. Da Vigo G (1514) Practica in arte chirurgica copiosa. S Guillireti et H Bonoiensem, Roma
223. Davis JS (1913) The transplantation of rib cartilage in pedunculated skin flaps: an experimental study. Bull John Hopkins Hosp 24:116
224. Davis JS (1917) A comparison on the permanence of free transplants of bone and cartilage. Ann Surg 65:170
225. Davis JS (1919) Plastic surgery. Its principles and practice. Blakiston, Philadelphia
226. Davis JS, Traut HF (1925) Origin and development of blood supply of whole thickness skin grafts: an experimental study. Ann Surg 82:871
227. Davy H (1800) Researches chemical and philosophical: chiefly concerning nitrous oxide or dephlogisticated nitrous air and its respiration. J Johnson, London
228. De Haan CR, Stark RB (1964) Transplantability of large composite grafts improved by histamine iontophoresis. Plast Reconstr Surg 34:547
229. Dehner J (1908) Mastopexy for ptotic breast. Munchen Med Wchnschr 55:1878
230. Delangénière H, Lewin P (1920) A general method of repairing loss of bony substance and of reconstructing bones by osteoperiosteal grafts taken from the tibia. Surg Gynecol Obstet 30:441
231. Della Croce GA (1573) Chirurgiae, Libri Septem. Giordano Ziletti, Venezia (*also known as Cruce JA*)
232. Della Croce GA (1583) Della Chirurgia Universale. G Ziletti, Venezia
233. Delpech JM (1823–1828) Chirurgie de Montpellier ou Observations et Reflexions tirée des Traveaux de Chirurgie Clinique. Gabon et Cie, Paris et Montpellier
234. Delpech JM (1824) Plastic operation performed with success at the hospital St Eloi de Montpellier. Lancet 4:1123
235. Denis JB (Denys) (1667) Lettre touchant deux expériences de la transfusion faites sur des hommes. J Cusson, Paris
236. Dénonvilliers CP (1863) Nota sur le bolletin general de thérapie 65:257
237. Desnos E (1914) Historie de l'urologie. Doin, Paris
238. Dibbell DG (1974) The use of long island flap to bring sensation to the sacral area in young paraplegics. Plast Reconstr Surg 54:220
239. Dieffenbach JF (1822) Nonnula de regeneratione et transplanatione. Herbipoli. typ. Richterianius, Wurtzberg (Doctoral thesis)
240. Dieffenbach JF (1826) Beitrage zur Gaumennath. Litt Ann D Ges Heilk 4:145
241. Dieffenbach JF (1826) Uber das Gaumensegel des Menschen und der Sacugethiere. Litt Ann D Ges Heilk 4:298
242. Dieffenbach JF (1842) Ueber die Schielen und die Heilung desselben durch die Operation. Albert Forstner, Berlin
243. Dieffenbach JF (1836) Memoirés sur quelque nouvelle methods obtenir la guéisondes ouvertures contre nature a l'extremité antérieure libre de l'uréthre chez l'homme. Gaz Méd Paris p 802
244. Dieffenbach JF (1845–1848) Die Operative Chirurgie. FA Brockhaus, Leipzig
245. Dieffenbach JF (1883) Surgical observations on the restoration of the nose and on removal of polyps and other tumours from the nostril. Translted by JS Baushnam, Samuel Higley, London
246. Dieffenbach JF (1929–1934) Chirurgische Erfahrungen Besonders uber die Wiederherstellung Zerstorten Theile des Menschlichen Koerpors nuch neuen Methoden. TCF Enslin, Berlin (*see also comprehensive reference lists for Dieffenbach in The Zeis Index pp 68–69 and Patterson Index pp 129–129*)
247. Digby K (1668) Choice and experimented receipts on physick and chirurgery collected by Sir Kenelm Digby. Published by author, London
248. Dionis P (1708) Cours d'opérations de chirurgie. D'Honey,Bruxelles
249. Dionis P (1710) A course of chirurgical operations in the royal gardens at Paris. J Tomson, London
250. Dorrance GM (1933) The operative story of cleft palate. Saunders, Philadelphia
251. Dorsey JS (1818) Elements of surgery for the use of students, vol 2. Parker & Warner, Philadelphia
252. Dryander J (1537) Anatomiae hoc est corporis humani dissectionis pars prior… Eucharium Cervicornum, Marburg
253. Dubois SJ (1533) De re medicina, libr.tres. Sylvio Medico Interprete, Paris

254. Dubois SJ (1554) De febris commentarius ex libris aliquot Hippocratis & Galeni, Petrum Dronart, Paris
255. Dubrueil A (1909) Greffe cartilagineuse auriculaire pour ailes du nez. J Med Bordeaux
256. Dufourmentel C, Mouly R (1965) Development récent dans la plastie mammaire par la methode oblique latéral. Ann Chir Plast 10:227
257. Dufourmentel C, Mouly R (1968) Modification of "periwinkle shell" operation for small ptotic breasts laterale. Plast Reconstr Surg 41:523
258. Dufourmentel L (1918) Les principales méthodes des cranioplasties: un procédé d'obturation métallique exacte. Paris Med 27:503
259. Dufourmentel L (1932–1939) Comment obtenir une forme satisfisante dans l'operation de rélevement du sein par déplacement. Bull Méd Paris 46:194
260. Dufourmentel L (1939) Chirurgie rèparatrice et corrective des téguments et de formes. Masson, Paris
261. Duhamel du Monceau HL (1746) Recherches sur la réunion des plaies des arbres sur la facon dont la greffe s'unit sur sujet sur lequel on l'applique sur la reunion des plaies des animeaux et quelque example des greffes appliquées sur les animeaux. Hist Acad R Sci Paris
262. Duhamel du Monceau HL (1751) Sur le dévelopment et la crue des os des animeaux. Mém Acad R Sci Paris 55:345
263. Dunham T (1893) A skin flap from the scalp with a permanent buried vascular pedicle used to cover the defect left by excising an epithelioma of the face. Ann Surg 17:677
264. Duplay S (1874) De l'hypospadie perineo-scrotal et de son traitement chirurgical. Asselin, Paris
265. Durand JL, Renier D, Marchac D (1997) L'histoire des cranioplasties. Ann Chir Plast Esthet 42:75
266. Durston W (1670) Concerning a very sudden and excessive swelling of a woman's breast. Philos Trans R Soc Lond IV:1047 and 1049
267. Durston W (1670) Concerning the death of the big breasted woman. Philos Trans R Soc Lond IV:1068 (*see also Letterman G and Schurter M*)
268. Dutrochet HM (1817) Classic reprint from Gazette Santé 35:91 "Example of reunion of parts totally separated from the rest of the body" re-published in 1969, Plast Reconstr Surg 44:285
269. Duval J (1880) Traité des hermaphrodites. Isidore Liseux, Paris
270. Earle H (1821) On the re-establishment of a canal in the place of a portion of the urethra which has been destroyed. Philos Trans part II, p 300
271. Ebers GM, Stern L (1875) Papyrus Ebers: Das hermeische buch ueber die arzneimittel der altern aegypter, vol 2. Leipzig (*see also Ebbell B (1937) The papyrus Ebers. The greatest Egyptian medical document, Levin & Munksgaard, Copenhagen*)
272. Eden R (1913) Tendo-und neurolisis mitt fettplastik. Dtsch Ges Chir Verh 42:125
273. Eden R, Rehn E (1914) Die autoplastiische Fettransplantation zur Neurolysis und Tendolysis. Arch Klin Chir 104:65
274. Edgerton MT (1951) Replacement of lining to oral cavity following surgery. Cancer 4:110
275. Ehrman J (1889) Des opérations plastiques sur le palais chez l'enfant. Leurs resultants eloignès. Alcan, Paris
276. Eimas R (1990) Heirs of Hippocrates. University of Iowa Press, Iowa City
277. Eloy NFT (1755) Dictionaire historique de la médicine. Bassompierre, Liege
278. Ely ET (1881) An operation for prominence of the auricle. Arch Otol N Y 10:97
279. Erichsen J (1853) The science and art of surgery. Walton & Maberly, London
280. Esser JFS (1917) Studies on the plastic surgery of the face. Ann Surg 65:297
281. Esser JFS (1918) Die rotation de Wange und allgemeine Bemerkungenbeichirurgischer Gesichtplastik, Leipzig
282. Esser JFS (1929) Artery flaps. de Voos van Kleef, Antwerp (*see also The Patterson Index p 188 for numerous other papers by Esser*)
283. Estienne C (alias Stephanus) (1545) De dissectione portium corporis humani, libri tres. Simon Colinaeus, Paris
284. Estlander JA (1872) Eine method aus der einen lippe substanzverluste der anderen zu ersetzen. Arch Klin Chir 14:622
285. Estlander JA (1879) Total blepharoplastik genom hudtransplantering a färsk sâryta. Nord Med Ark 11:16
286. Estor E (1917) Cent cas de prosthése cranienne par plaque d'or. Bull Mem Soc Chir Paris 43:463
287. Eustachius B (1564) Opuscula anatomica. Vincenzo Luchino, Venezia
288. Eustachius B (1714) Tabulae anatomica. JM Lancisi, Rome
289. Fabricius ab Aquapendente G (1600) De visione, voce, auditu, 3 partes. Franciscum Balzettam, Venezia
290. Fabricius ab Aquapendente G (1600) De Formatio Fetu. Pasquali, Padua
291. Fabricius ab Aquapendente G (1619) De Chirurgicis Operationibus. In operationes chirurgicae in duas partes divisae. Paulum Megliettum, Venezia
292. Fabricius ab Aquapendente G (1641) Opera Chirurgica. Franciscum Balzettam, Padova
293. Fabricius ab Aquapendente G (1687) Opera omnia anatomica et phisiologica. Christianus Goezius per JF Gleditsch, Leipzig
294. Fabrizi P (1841) Sopra alcuni punti relativi alla rinoplastica. Tipografia Izzo, Malta
295. Falcon J (1649) Remarques sur la chirurgie de M. Guy de Chauliac. Jean Radisson, Lyons
296. Fallopius G (1567) Observationes anatomica. Marcum Antonium Ulmum, Venezia
297. Fallopius G (1569) De vulneribus Capitis Gabrielis Falloppii exposito. Petri Angeli Aghati Edita, Venezia
298. Fallopius G (1600) Tractatus de decoratione. Joann Petri Maphaei, Francofurti
299. Faltin R (1935) Bidrag till den Plastika Kirurgins historia i Finland. Finsk Läek Handl 78:188
300. Faltin R (1937) History of plastic surgery in Finland. Finsk Läk Sallsk Handl 80:97
301. Fantuzzi G (1790) Scrittori Bolognesi, vol III. Stamperi di San Tommas d'Aquino, Bologna

302. Faraday M (1818) Effects of inhaling the vapours of sulphuric ether. Quart J Sci Arts Miscellanae 4:158
303. Faye G de la (1743) Observations sur le bec-de-liévre. Memoires de l'Acad Royal de Chir 1:605
304. Fazio B (1745) De Viris Illustribus. Giovannetti, Firenze
305. Fergusson JD (1968) The urological records. Proc R Soc Med 61:417
306. Fergusson W (1844–1845) Observation on cleft palate and on staphyloraphy. Med Times Gaz 2:256
307. Fergusson W (1845) Cleft palate and staphyloraphy. Retrospect of Practical Med and Surg 9:118
308. Fergusson W (1850) Observations on harelip and cleft palate. Med Times Gaz 1:641 (*see also numerous refs pp 224–5 Patterson Index*)
309. Ferrari A (1885) Sugli innesti ossei. Arch d'Ortopedia 6:1
310. Feuvrier J (1865) Difformité congenital du pavillon de l'oreille droit. Strasbourg
311. Fienus T (Feyens) (1649) De Precipuis Artis Chirurgicae Controversii. Herm Conringi, Frankfurt
312. Filatov VP (1917) Plastic procedure using a round pedicle. Vestnik Oftalmol 34:149–158. Translated in: McDowell F (1977) Source Book of Plastic Surgery.Williams & Wilkins, Baltimore
313. Fioravanti L (1561) Il Capriccio Medicinale. Ludovico Avanzo, Venezia
314. Fioravanti L (1561) I Discorsi di Chirugia. Avanzo, Venezia
315. Fioravanti L (1565) Del Regimento della Peste. Andrea Ravenoldo, Venezia
316. Fioravanti L (1570) Il Tesoro della Vita Humana. Heredi di Melchior Sessa, Venezia
317. Fioravanti L (1570) Cirugia. Heredi di Melchior Sessa, Venezia
318. Fisher quoted by Neuhof H (1923) The transplantation of tissues. Appleton, New York
319. Fitch RH, Waters RM, Tatum AJ (1930) The intravenous use of barbituric acid hypnotics in surgery. Am J Surg 9:110
320. Flagg JFB (1851) Ether and chloroform: their employment in surgery, dentistry, midwifery and therapeutics. Lindsay & Blakiston, Philadelphia
321. Fleischmann A (1910) Die Kropfregion der Amnnioten. Morphology 41:615
322. Flourens MJP (1842) Recherches sur le development des os et des dents. Ann du Muséum d'Histoire Naturel
323. Flourens MJP (1847) Theorie experimentale de la formation des os. Masson et Fils, Paris
324. Flourens MJP (1847) Note touchant l'action de l'éther sur les centres nerveux. Acad Sci Paris 24:340
325. Foged J (1948) Operative treatment of abdominal obesity, especially pendulous abdomen. Br J Plast Surg 1:274
326. Fogh-Andersen FP (1961) Inheritance of cleft lip and palate: constant or increasing? Acta Chir Scand 122:106
327. Fomon S (1960) Cosmetic surgery: principles and practice. Lippincott, Philadelphia
328. Fomon S, Bell JW, Schattner A (1955) Ageing face: a surgical challenge. Arch Otolaryngol 61:554
329. Forbes D quoted by Maneksha RJ (1965) Plastic surgery in the tropics. Prakashan, Bombay
330. Forni GG (1948) La Chirurgia nello Studio di Bologna dalle Origini a tutto il XIX Secolo. Cappelli, Bologna
331. Fracastoro G (1536) Syphilis sive morbus gallicus. Johann Bebel, Basel
332. Franco P (1556) Petit traité contenent une des parties principalles de chirurgie. Vincent, Lyons
333. Franco P (1561) Traité des Hernies. Thibauld Payan, Lyons
334. Fred GB (1957) Jacques Joseph's last rhinoplasty. Eye Ears Nose and Throat Monthly 36:283–287
335. Freshwater F (1972) More about "BL", Mr Lucas and Mr Carpue, letter to the editor of Plast Reconstr Surg. Reprinted in: McDowell F (1977) The Source Book of Plastic Surgery. William & Wilkins, Baltimore, p 86
336. Freshwater F, Krizek M (1978) George David Pollock and the development of skin grafting. Ann Plast Surg 1:97
337. Freund A von (1882) Ueber trimethylene. Monatshefte f Chemie 3:625
338. Fricke JCG (1829) Die Bildung neuer Augenlieder (Blepharoplastik) nach dadurch hervorgebrachten Auswartswendungen derselben. Perthes und Basser, Hamburg
339. Friedberg SA (1917) Laryngology and otology in colonial times. Ann Med Hist 1:86
340. Fritze HE, Reich OFG (1845) Die Plastische Chirurgie. von Aug.Hirschuald, Berlin
341. Froelich H (1877) Baracken im trojanischen Kriege. Arch Path Anat Physiol 71:509
342. Frusci F (1861) Le scoperte e gli studi degli italiani sulla riproduzione della ossa. Tipografia del Filiatre-Sebezio, Napoli
343. Fukuda O (1968) Otoplasty and cryptotia. Jpn J Plast Surg 11:117
344. Fukuda O (1974) The microtic ear: survey of 180 cases in 10 years. Plast Reconstr Surg 53:458
345. Fulop-Miller R (1938) Triumph over pain. Translated by Eden and Cedar Paul, The Literary Guild of America, New York
346. Fulton FJ (1936) An introduction to a bibliography of the educational and scientific works of Joseph Priestley. Bibliographical Society of America 30:150
347. Furlan S, Mazzola R (1995) Alessandro Benedetti a fifteenth century anatomist and surgeon: his role in the history of nasal reconstruction. Plast Reconstr Surg 96:739
348. Galen C (1541–1545) Opera omnia sectio prima. Joannem de Farris et frateres Rivoltella, Venezia
349. Galen C (1544) Chirurgia ex Greco in Latinum conversa Vido Vidi Florentino Interprete. Pierre Gaultier, Paris
350. Galen C (1549) De ossibus. Galid Rouillium, Lyons
351. Galen C (1586–1625) Omnia quae extant opera in latinum conversa. Guinta, Venezia
352. Galen C (1605) De ossibus. Danielem van der Boxe, Leiden
353. Galen C (1822) Claudii Galena opera omnia. Kuhniana C Cnoblochii, Lipsiae
354. Galen C (1908) Corpus Medicorum Grecorum. Akademic, Lipsiae & Berlin

355. Gallie WE, Robertson DE (1918) The transplantation of bone. JAMA 70:1134
356. Ganzer H (1917) Die bildung von langgestielten Stranglappen bei Gesicgtplastik. Berl Klin Wochenschr 54:1095
357. Garanne R de la (1721) Sur la Réparation de quelques Parties du Corp Humain Mutilées. In: Historie de l'Académie Royal des Sciences Paris
358. Garmannus LCF (1687 and 1709) De miraculis mortuorum. Dresdae et Lipsiae
359. Garofalo I, Vegetti M (1978) Galeno. UTET, Torino
360. Garrison F (1917) History of Medicine. Saunders, Philadelphia
361. Garrison F (1924) An Introduction to the History of Medicine. Saunders, Philadelphia
362. Gattinari G (1894) Storia di Tagliacozzo. S Lapi, Città di Castello
363. Geib FW (1941) Vitallium skull. JAMA 117:306
364. Gerdsdorff H von (1517) Feldtbűch der Wundartznei. Johann Schott, Strasbourg
365. Gersuny R (1887) Plastischer ersatz der wangenschleimhaut. Zentralbl Chir 14:706
366. Gersuny R (1900) Ueber eine subcutane prothese. Z Heilk 21:199
367. Gersuny R (1903) Some cosmetic operations. Wien Med Wochenschr 53:2253
368. Gibson T (1961) Flagellation and free grafting. Br J Plast Surg 13:195
369. Gibson T, Medawar PB (1943) The fate of skin homografts in man. J Anat 11:299
370. Gibson T (1965) Early free grafting: The restitution of parts completely separated from the body. Br J Plast Surg 18:1
371. Gibson T, Davis WB (1960) A bank of living homograft cartilage: a preliminary report. In: Trans Int Soc of Plastic Surg 2nd Congress London. Livingstone, Edinburgh
372. Gilbert W (1540–1603) quoted by Bettman OL, Hench PS (1956) in A Pictorial History of Medicine, CC Thomas, Illinois. p 142 "Gilbert Explore Magnetism", p 214 "Healing Electrically"
373. Gillies HD (1920) The tubed pedicle in plastic surgery. N Y Med J 111:1
374. Gillies HD (1920) Plastic surgery of the face, based on selected cases of war injuries of the face including burns. Henry Frowde, Oxford Unversity Press, and Hodder and Stoughton, London
375. Gillies HD (1937) Reconstruction of the external ear with special reference to the use of maternal ear cartilage as the supporting structure. Rev Chir Structive 7:169
376. Gillies HD, McIndoe AH (1939) The technique of mammaplasty in conditions of hypertrophy of the breast. Surg Gynecol Obstet 68:658
377. Gilmer TL (1887) A case of fracture of the lower jaw with remarks on the treatment. Arch Dent 4:388
378. Giordano D (1920) Leonardo Fioravanti bolognese. Licinio Cappelli, Bologna
379. Gnudi MT, Webster JP (1935) Documenti inediti intorno alla vita di Gaspare Tagliacozzi. In: Studi e memorie per la Storia dell'università di Bologna, vol XIII. Instit per la Storia dell'Università Bologna
380. Gnudi MT, Webster JP (1950) The life and times of Gaspare Tagliacozzi. Hoepli, Milan
381. Gnudi MT, Webster JP (1950) The life and times of Gaspare Tagliacozzi, Surgeon of Bologna 1545–1599. With a documented study of the life of Bologna in the 16th century. Herbert Reichner, New York
382. Goebel R (1912) Freien autoplastischer Transplantation. Munchen Med Wochenschr 60:1577
383. Goebel R (1914) Mamma pendula und Mastodynie. Med Gef Kiel, June 1914
384. Goeliche AO (1738) Introductio in historiam litterariam anatomes. JG Corradi, Frankfurt
385. Goldman EE (1894) Ueber das Schksal der nach Verfhren von Thiersch verpflaften Hautstueckchen (Thiersch grafting). Beitr Klin Chir 11:229
386. Goldwyn RM (1985) An historical introduction to "Baronio G, On grafting on animals". Translated by Joan Bond Sax, The Boston Medical Library, Boston
387. Goleria KS (1966) Pedicle flaps: a historical review. Indian J Surg 28:4
388. Gould GM, Pylr WI (1898) Anomalies and Curiosities of Medicine. Saunders, Philadephia
389. Goumelenus S (1580) Chirurgiae Artis ex Hippocratis et aliorum veterum medicorum decretis et ratinis norman deductae. Lib III, Fol 73, Paris
390. Graefe CF von (1817) Kurze Nachrichten und Auszurge. Jour d pract Arznek u Wundarzk 44:116
391. Graefe CF von (1818) Rhinoplastik oder die kunst den verlust der Nase organisch zu ersetzen in ihren füheren Verhältissner forscht und durch neue verfahrrungs weissen zur höheren Volkmmenhelt gefördet. Realschulbuchhandlung, Berlin
392. Graefe CF von (1820) Die Gaumennath ein neuentdeckes Mittel gegen angeborene Fehler der sprache. Jour d Chir u Aufenh part I:1556
393. Graefe CF von (1825) Kurzer Auszug aus dem Berichte ueber das klinische chirurgisch-augenaerzlighe. Institut der Universitaet zu Berlin Journ d Chir u Augenh 7:371
394. Graefe CF von (1827) Die Gaumennath. Jour d Chir u Augenh 10:371 (*see also pp 130, 153 Zeis Index for von Graefe*)
395. Griffith HR, Johnson EG (1842) The use of curare in general anaesthesia. Anesthesiology 3:418
396. Griffith FL (1898) A Collection of Hieroglyphics: a contribution to the history of Egyptian writing. The Egyptian Fund, London
397. Grindlay JH, Clagett OT (1949) Plastic sponge prosthesis for use after pneumonectomy. Proc Staff Meeting, Mayo Clinic 24:538
398. Groddeck G (1733) De Judaeis praeputium attrehentibus ad illustrandum locum. Locum I Co VII Ahorae Hebraicae et Talmudicae, Dresdae et Lipsiae
399. Gross SD (1864) A system of surgery. Blanchard and Lea, Philidelphia
400. Guillemeau J (1598) Les oeuvres de Chirurgie. Chez Nicolas de Louvvain, Marchant, Paris
401. Guillemeau J (1598) Les oeuvres de Chirurgie. Viret, Rouen
402. Guinard A (1903) De l'ablation esthétique des tumeurs du sein. Bull Chir Paris 29:574

403. Gurunluoglu R, Gurunluoglu A (2002) Paulus Aegineta, a seventh century encyclopedist and surgeon: his role in the history of plastic surgery. Plast Reconstr Surg 110:1600
404. Haeseker B (1983) Dr JFS Esser and his influence on the development of plastic and reconstructive surgery. Doctoral Thesis, Erasmus University of Rotterdam
405. Hagerdon WHA (1884) Modification of the harelip operation. Zentralbl Chir 11:756
406. Hagerdon WHA (1892) Operation for harelip with zigzag suture. Zentralbl Chir 19:281
407. Haiken E (1997) Venus envy. The John Hopkins University Press, Baltimore and London
408. Hale RB, Coyle T (1988) Albinus on Anatomy. Dover, New York
409. Haller A von (1743–1756) Icones anatomicae quibus precipual partes corpori humani delineatae continentur (fasciculi I–IV). Abram Vandenhoech and widow, Goettingen (*see also von Haller in the Ziess Index p 31*)
410. Hamilton FH (1854) Elkoplasty or anaplasty applied to the treatment of old ulcers. Holman Gray, New York
411. Hanff W (1870) Ueber Wiederanheilung Vollstanding vom Körper getrennter. Hautstücke Thesis, Friedriech Wilhelms, Universitaet Berlin
412. Hardy J (1881) Observation concerning transplantation of bone, illustrated by a case of intra-human osseus transplantation. Proc R Soc Med 32:232
413. Harii K, Ohmori K, Ohmori S (1974) Hair transplantation and free scalp flaps. Plast Reconstr Surg 53:410
414. Hartley J (1976) Specific application of the double lumen prosthesis. Clin Plast Surg 3:247
415. Harvey W (1628) Excertitatio anatomica de motu cordis et sanguinis in animalibus. Guilelmi Fitzeri, Frankfurt
416. Harvey W (1651) Excertitationes de generatione animalium. Ludovicus Elzevirium, Amsterdam
417. Harvey W (1651) Excertitationes de generatione animalium. Pulleyn, London
418. Harvey W (1766) Opera omnia: a Collegio Medicorum Londinenis. edita Guilelmus Bowyer, London
419. Hauben DJ, Baruchin A, Mahler D (1982) On the history of the free skin graft. Ann Plast Surg 9:242
420. Hayward G (1847) Some account of the first use of sulphuric ether. In: Warren E (ed) Some Account on the Letheon: Who is the Discoverer? Dutton and Wentworth, Boston
421. Heekeren AJ Von (1835) Die operatione rhinoplastika. Dissertatio Kruger, Bonn
422. Heister L (1718) Chirurgie in welcher alles was zur Wund, Artzney gehoret nach der neuestern und besten. J Hoffman, Numberg
423. Heister L (1743) A general system in surgery in three parts. W Junys, London
424. Heister L (1770) Instituzioni chirugiche Francesco Pitteri, Venezia
425. Hellferich H (1899) Versuche ueber die der Transplantation des Intermediaeknorpel eachsenda Roehrenknochen. Dtsch Z Chir 51:564
426. Hellferich H (1911) Zur Frage der Transplantation des Intermediaeknorpel. Munchen Med Wochenschr 58:2796
427. Helmont JB von (1682) Opera omnia. Francofurti
428. Hermann L (1864) Ueber die physiologischen Wikungen des Stickoffoxydulgases. Arch Anat Physiol 1:521
429. Herodotus quoted by Rogers BO (1973) History of external genitalia surgery. In: Horton CE (ed) Plastic and Reconstructive Surgery of the Genital Area, chap 1. Little Brown, Boston
430. Hickman HH (1824) A letter on suspended animation containing experiments showing that it may be safely employed on animals with the view of ascertaining probable utility in surgical operations on the human subject. W Smith, Ironbridge
431. Highmore N (1651) Corporis humani disquisito anatomica. Comitis S Brown, Hagai
432. Highmore N (1673) De ovo incubatio observationes. J Martyn, London
433. Hilden WF von (Hildanus) (1614) Observationum et Curationum Chirurgicam Centuria Terti 1606–1641. Oppenhemio, Typis Hieronymi Galleri, aere Johan Theod de Bry, Basel, Frankfurt & Lyons
434. Hippocrates (1525) Octoginta Volumina. Francisci Minitii Calvi, Roma
435. Hippocrates (1544) Chirurgia e Greco in latinum Conversa. Vido Vidi Florentino Interprete. Pierre Gaultier, Paris
436. Hippocrates (1838–1861) Oeuvres Completes d'Hippocrate. Emile Littre, Paris
437. Hippocrates (1978) Hippocratic writings. GER Lloyd, Harmondsworth
438. His WE (1872) Ueber die Aufgaben und Zielpunkte der wissenschaftlichen Anatomie. Leipzig
439. His WE (1874) Unsere Koerperform und das physiologische Problem ihrer Entstehung. Leipzig
440. His WE (1901) Beobachtungen zur Gesichichte und Gamennbildung beim menschlichen Embryo. Kgl Akad Wiss 27
441. Holdsworth WG (1963) Cleft lip and palate. Heinemann, London
442. Hollander E von (1924) Surgical treatment of hypertrophy of breast. Dtsch Med Wochenschr 50:1400–1402
443. Hollander E von (1928) Die Operation der Mammahypertrophie und Haengerbrust. Dtsch Med Wchschr 7:603
444. Hollander E von (1932) Plastische (Kosmetische) Opertion: kritische Darstilung ihres gegenwaertigen Sandes. In: Klemperer G, Klemperer F (eds) Neue Deutsche Klinik, Urban & Schwarzenberg
445. Hollingsworth Smith H (1852) Operative surgery. Lippincott Grambo, Philadelphia
446. Holman E (1924) Protein sensitization in iso-skin grafting. Is the latter of practical value? Surg Gynecol Obstet 38:100
447. Holmes OW (1855) Puerperal fever as a private pestilence. Ticknor & Fields, Boston
448. Horner WE (1837) Clinical report on the surgical department of Philadelphia Hospital, Blockley for the months of May, June and July 1837. Am J Med Sci 21:99
449. Horton CE, Crawford HH, Adams JE (1961) John Peter Mettauer: American's first plastic surgeon. Plast Reconstr Surg 27:26

450. Houllier J (1623) Omnia opera practica. De Morbis Internis. Allobrogum excudebat Jacobus Stoer, Coloniae
451. Huard P, Grmek MD (1960) La premier manuscript Chirurgical Turc rédigé par Charaf ed- Din (1465) et illustré de 140 miniatures. Roge Dacosta, Paris
452. Hulke JB (1861) Medical Times & Gaz 2:213. Quoted by McDowell F in: The Source Book of Plastic Surgery. Williams & Wilkins, Baltimore
453. Humby G (1934) Apparatus for skin grafting. BMJ 1:1078
454. Humby G (1936) Modified skin grafting knife. BMJ 2:1086
455. Hunt HL (1926) Plastic surgery of the head face and neck. Lea & Febiger, Philadelphia
456. Hunter J (1803) The natural history of the human teeth. J Johnson, London
457. Hunter J (1840) Treatise on blood inflammation and gunshot wounds, with notes by James F Palmer. Haswell, Barrington and Haswell, Philadelphia (*first published in 1794*)
458. Hynes W (1950) Pharyngoplasty by muscle transplantation. Br J Plast Surg 3:128
459. Hynes W (1953) The results of pharyngoplasty by muscle transplantation in failed cleft palate cases. Ann R Coll Surg Engl 13:17
460. Ikuta U, Watari S, Kamwamura K, et al (1975) Free flap transfer by end to side arterial anastomosis. Br J Plast Surg 28:1
461. Israel J (1896) Zwei neue Methoden der Nasenplastik. Arch Klin Chir 53:255
462. Jakimowitsch (1881) Experiments on bone grafts. Dtsch Z Chir 15:201
463. Jensen CO (1903) Transplantation of mammary gland carcinoma in mice. Zentralbl Bakteriol 34:28
464. Jobert de Lamballe A (1849) Traité de Chirurgie Plastique. JB Bailliéres et fils, Paris
465. John of Arderne (1922) De arte phisicale et de chirurgia. Translated by D Power, John Bale, London (*originally published in 1378 in old English*)
466. Johnson T (1649) The workes of that famous chirurgion Ambrose Paré. Richard Cotes and William Dugard, London
467. Jones WHS, Withinton ET(1923–1931) Hippocrates, vol 1. Harvard University Press, Cambridge, Mass
468. Joseph J (1896) Eselohren. Verh Berl Ges 27:206
469. Joseph J (1898) Ueber die operative Verkleinerung einer Nase (Rhinomiosis). Berl Klin Wochenschr 40:882 (*see also translation by Aufricht G in The Source Book of Plastic Surgery (1977) McDowell F pp 164–169. Williams & Wilkins Balitmore*)
470. Joseph J (1902) Ueber einige weitere operative Nasenverkleinerungen. Berl Klin Wochenschr 39:851
471. Joseph J (1904) Intranasale Nasenhockerabtragung. Berl Klin Wochenschr 41:650
472. Joseph J (1905) More about nasal reduction. Munchen Med Wochenschr 52:1489
473. Joseph J (1907) Beitrage zur rhinoplastik. Berl Klin Wochenschr 44:470
474. Joseph J (1907) Die Korrektur der Schiefnase. Dtsch Med Schnschr 49:2035
475. Joseph J (1911) Nasekorrekturen. Verh Dtsch Ges Natursstorschor Aertzte 82 Versamlung (1910), Teil 2:340
476. Joseph J (1914) Beitraege zur totalen Rhinoplastik. Munchen Med Wochenschr 51:705
477. Joseph J (1921) Plastic operation on protruding cheek. Dtsch Med Wochenschr 47:287
478. Joseph J (1922) Beitrage zur totalen und partiellen Rhinoplastik nebst einem Vorschl age zur freien Hautueberpflanzung. Klin Wochenschr 1:678
479. Joseph J (1925) Zur operation der hypertophischen haengebrust. Dtsch Med Wochenschr 51:1103–1105
480. Joseph J (1925) Zur Operation de hypertrophischen Haengebrust (Diskussionsbeitraege). Berl Ges Chir 15 June
481. Joseph J (1931) Nasenplastik und sonstige Gesichsplastik nebst einem Anhang ueber Mammarplastik. C Kabitzsch, Leipzig
482. Joseph J (1987) Rhinoplasty and Facial Plastic Surgery with a Supplement on Mammoplasty and other Operations in the Field of Plastic Surgery of the Body. An Atlas and Textbook. Translation of 1931 edn by Milstein S, Jeremy Norman, Novato, CA
483. Jovanka, Morain WD (1983) Carl Manchot: the cutaneous arteries of the human body. Translated by Ristic WD, Springer, New York
484. Kampeleen W von (1791) Le Mèchanisme de la Parole, suivi de la description d'una machine parlante. Bauer, Wien
485. Kappis A (1915) Zur Deckung von Schaedeldefekten. Zentralbl Chir 42:897
486. Kausch W (1916) Die operation der Mammahypertrophie. Zentralbl Chir 43:713
487. Kazanjian VH (1946) The repair of nasal defects with the median forehead flap: primary closure of the forehead wound. Surg Gynecol Obstet 83:37
488. Kazanjian VH (1949, 1959 & 1974) (3 edns) The surgical treatment of facial injuries. Williams & Wilkins, Baltimore
489. Keating JM (1889) Cyclopaedia of the diseases of the children. Lippincott, Philadelphia
490. Keegan DF (1900) Rhinoplastic operations: with description of recent improvements in the Indian method. Balliere Tindall & Cox, London
491. Ketham J of (1491) Fasciculus Medicinae. Johannem et Gregorius, fratres de Forlivio, Venetiis
492. Keys TE (1978) The History of Surgical Anesthesia. Robert E Krieger, Huntington, New York
493. Kind H (1935) Curare. Nature 135:469
494. Kirkup J (2006) The Evolution of Surgical Instruments. An Illustrated History from Ancient Times to the Twentieth Century. Jeremy Norman, Novato, CA
495. Kircher A (1643) Magnes sive de Arte Magnetica opus Tripartitum. Coloniae Agrippinae, Roma
496. Kircher A (1667) Magneticum naturae regnum: sive disceptatio physiologica de triplici in natura rerum magnete. Typis Ignatii de Lazaris, Roma
497. Klap R (1912) Betraig zur Fet-transplantation. Dtsch Med Wochenschr 38:1569

498. Klasen HJ (1981) History of free skin grafting. Springer, Berlin New York
499. Kleiman M (1939) Histoire de l'anesthésie. Anesth Analg 5:122
500. Kleinert HE, Kasdan ML (1965) Anastomosis of digital vessels. J Ky Med Assoc 63:106
501. Kleinschmidt O (1941) Plexigas zur deckung von Schaedellucken. Chirurg 13:273
502. Koch SL (1941) The transplantation of skin. Surg Gynecol Obstet 72:1
503. Koch SL (1950) Some half forgotten chapters in the development of plastic surgery. Plast Reconstr Surg 6:97
504. Kolle FS (1911) Plastic and cosmetic surgery. Appleton, New York
505. Komatsu S, Tamai S (1968) Successful replantation of a completely cut off thumb. Plast Reconstr 42:374
506. König F (1890) Der knocherne Ersatz grosser Schaedeldefeckte. Zentralbl Chir 27:497
507. Kraske H (1923) Die Operation der atrophischen und hypertrophyschen Haengebrust. Munchen Med Wochenschr 70:672
508. Krause F (1893) Ueber die Transplantation grossen Ungestieelter Hautlappen. Arch Klin Chir 46:177
509. Krause F (1893) Transplantation of large non-pedicled skin flaps. Verh Dtsch Ges Chir 22:46 (*see classical reprint Plast Reconstr Surg 41:573 in 1968*)
510. Kriens O (1967) Anatomische Untersuchungen am gesplatenen wiche Gaumen Beitrag als Grundlage zur Veloplastik. Chir Plast Reconstr 4:14
511. Krogman WM (1940) The medical and surgical practice of pre and protohistoric man. Ciba Symp 2:444
512. Küster E (1926) Operation fur Haengebrust. Monatschr Gegurtsh Gynak 73:316
513. Labat L (1834) De la Rhinoplastie, art de restaurer ou de refaire le nez. Impriméri de Ducessois, Paris
514. Labat R (1951) Traitè akkadien de diagnostics et prognostics mèdicaux. Transcription et tradution. Collect de Trav de l'Acad Intern d'Hist des Scien. No 7. Brill, Leiden
515. Labat R (1954) A propos de la chirurgie babylonienne. J Asiatique 207
516. Laeke CD (1925) Valerius cordis and the discovery of ether. Isis 7:14
517. Lagarde M (1925) Nouvelle technique pour le traitment des rides de la face et du cou. Paris Chir 17:33
518. Lalardrie JP, Mouly R (1978) History of Mammoplasty. Aesthetic Plast Surg 2:167
519. Lallemand CF (1824) Plaie la Face avec Perte de Substance, Guéri par l'Application d'un Lambeau Détaché des Partes Voicines. Arch Gen 6:242
520. Lanfranchi da Milano (1481) Chirurgia Parva. in Chauliac G de, Chirurgia Magna Tract II, Cap II, Braemm, Louvain (also Collectio Veneta)
521. Lange GO (1856) Ad chirurgia plasticam simbolae. Cum tabula lithographica. Bonn
522. Langenbeck B von (1849) Fragmente zur Aufstellung von Grundregeln fur die operative Plastik. Gosch Deutsch Klin 2 pp 25 & 57
523. Langenbeck B von (1853) Zwei Falle zur Gaumenaht. Deutsche Klinic 5:3
524. Langenbeck B von (1859) Beitrage zur osteoplastik. Vorlaufighe Mitthellung Gosch Deutsch Klin 48:175
525. Langenbeck B von (1861) Professor Langenbeck on Uranoplasties: Med Times 2:69
526. Langenbeck B von (1861) Die Uranoplastik mittelst Ablösung des mucös-periostalen Gaumenüberzuges. Langenbeck's Arch f Klin Chir 2:205
527. Langenbeck B von (1862) Geheilter Fall von Gaumenspalte. Goesch deutsche Klin 14:1
528. Langenbeck B von (1861) Zur Geschichte der Uranoplastik. Gösch Deutsche Klin 19:436
529. Langenbeck B von (1877) Operation for cleft palate. Verhardl Deutsch Gesellsch Chir p73
530. Lanz O (1908) Dei Transplantation Betreffend. Zentralbl f Chir 35:3
531. Lascaratos J, Cohen M, Voros D (1998) Plastic surgery of the face in Byzantium in fourth century. Plast Reconstr Surg 102:1274
532. Lassus C (1970) A technique for breast reduction. Int Surg 53:69
533. Lassus C (1981) New refinements in vertical mammoplasty. Chir Plast 6:81
534. Lassus C (1987) Breast reduction: evolution of a technique. Aesthetic Plast Surg 11:107
535. La Trenta GS (1980) Otoplasty. In: Rees TD, La Trenta GS (eds) Aestetic plastic surgery. Saunders, Philadelphia
536. Lawson G (1871) On the transplantation of portions of skin for the closure of large granulating surfaces. Trans Clin Soc Lond 4:49 (*see also commentary by Peet E in The Source Book of Plastic surgery, McDowell F ed. (1977) Williams and Wilkins, Baltimore*)
537. Leca AP (1971) La Médicine Egyptienne au temps des Pharaohs. Roger Dacosta, Paris
538. Le Chat (1753–1783) Memoires sur le sujet proposè par l'Academie Royale de Chirurgie pour le prix de 1738. In: Recueil des pieces pour le prix l'Academie Royale de chirurgie, vol I. Delaguette Le Prieur, Lambert, Didot Paris
539. Leclerc MG (1701) The complete Surgeon: or the whole art of surgery explain'd in a most familiar method. Freeman W, Walthoe J, Goodwin T, Motton M, and Parker R, London
540. Leclerc L (1861) La chirurgie d'Albucasis. Bailliére, Paris
541. Le Dran HF (1749) The operation in surgery of Mons. Le Dran. Translated by T Gateker surgeon, with remarks of W Cheselden. Mem Acad R Chir Lond 1:440
542. Le Fort R (1901) Experimental studies on fractures of the upper jaw. Parts I and II Rev Chir Paris 23:208; Part III Rev Chir Paris 23:479
543. Lejour M (1994) Mammoplasty with liposuction of the breast. Plast Reconstr Surg 94:100
544. Lejour M (1999) Vertical mammoplasty: early complications after 250 person consecutive cases. Plast Reconstr Surg 104:764
545. Lejour M (1999) Vertical mammoplasty. Update and appraisal of late results. Plast Reconstr Surg 104:771
546. Lejour M, Abboud M (1990) Vertical mammoplasty without inframammary scar and with breast liposuction. Perspect Plast Surg 4:67

547. Lejour M, Abboud M, Declety A, et al (1990) Reduction des cicatrices de plastic mammaire. de ancre courte a al verticale. Ann Chir Plast Esthet 35:369
548. Le Manne F (1747) Dissertation au sujet d'un polype extraordinaire qui occupait la narine droite. Charles Giroud, Avignon
549. Le Mesurier AB (1949) A method of cutting and suturing the lip in the treatment of complete unilateral clefts. Plast Reconstr Surg 4:1
550. Leonardo da Vinci (1898–1901) Manoscritti di Leonardo da Vinci della reale biblioteca di Windsor. Dell'Anatomia. Edoardo Ronveyre and Roux & Viarengo, Paris and Torino
551. Leonardo da Vinci (1911) Quaderni di anatomia. Vangensten CI, Fonhaim A, Hopstock HJ (eds) Dyhwad, Christiania
552. Leonardo da Vinci (1977) Anatomical Drawings from the Royal Collection. Royal Academy of Arts, London
553. Leonicenus N (1497) Libellus de epidemia quam vulgo morbum Gallicum vocant. in domo Aldi Manutti, Venezia
554. Letterman G, Schurter M (1969) The surgical correction of gynaecomastia. Ann Surg 35:322
555. Letterman G, Schurter M (1974) Will Durston's "mammaplasty". Plast Reconstr Surg 53:48
556. Letterman G, Schurter M (1976) A history of mammaplasty with emphasis on correction of ptosis and macromastia. In: Goldwyn RM (ed) Plastic and Reconstructive Surgery of the Breast. Little Brown, Boston
557. Lewis CM (1985) Lipoplasty of the neck. Plast Reconstr Surg 76:268
558. Lewis JR (1978) Aesthetic blepharoplasty. In: Goulian D, Courtiss (ed) Symposium on Surgery of the Ageing face. Quality Medical Publish, St Louis
559. Lexer E (1925) Zur operation der Mammahypertrophie und der Haengebrust. Dtsch Med Wochenschr 51:26
560. Lexer E (1927) Die freien Transplantationen. Enke, Stuttgart
561. Lexer E (1931) Die Gesampte Wiederherstellungschirurgie. Barth, Leipzig
562. Lind Levi R (1975) Studies in pre-Vesalian anatomy. Biography, Translations, Documents American Philosophical Soc, Philadelphia
563. Linden JA von (1626) De formatio foetus. JB de Martinis & L Pascquatum, Padua
564. Linden JA van der quoted by Spieghel A van der (1645) Opera quae extenat omnia ex recensione. Joh. Antonides van der Linden Johannes Blaen, Amsterdam
565. Lisfranc J (1827) Rhinoplastie. Clin Hop de Paris 2:285 (*see also The Zeis Index pp 157–158*)
566. Lister J (1869) Observations on ligature of arteries on the antiseptic system. Lancet 1:451
567. Lister J (1870) A method of antiseptic treatment applicable to wounded soldiers in the present war. BMJ 2:243
568. Lister J (1881) An address on catgut ligature. Trans Clin Soc Lond 14:43 (*see also The collected papers of Joseph, Baron Lister (1909) Oxford University Press, Oxford*)
569. Liston R (1837) Practical Surgery. J & A Churchill, London
570. Liston R (1897) Practical Surgery; with one hunderd and thirty engravings. Lyon Med 85:198
571. Littlewood M (1967) Compound skin and sternomastoid flap for the repair of extensive carcinoma of the head and neck. Br J Plast Surg 20:403
572. Loeb J (1907) The chemical character of the process of fertilisation and its bearing upon the theory of life phenomena. Pub Physiol 3:61, University of California, Berkley
573. Loewe O (1929) Use of pieces of skin in deep plastic operations. Munchen Med Wochenschr 76:2125
574. Long CW (1849) An account of the first use of sulphuric ether by inhalation anesthetic in surgical operations. South M & SJ 5:705
575. Longacre JJ (1956) Surgical reconstruction of the flat discoid breast. Plast Reconstr Surg 17:358
576. Longacre JJ, Converse JM (1977) Deformities of the Forehead, Scalp and Calvariu. In: Converse JM (ed) Reconstructive Plastic Surgery. Saunders, Philadelphia
577. Lossen H (1898) Ueber Rhinoplastik mit Einfugen einer Prothesis. Munchen Med Wochenschr 45:1527
578. Lotsch F (1928) Ueber Haengenbrustplastik. Klin Wochenschr 7:603
579. Louis A (1768) Mémoires sur l'opération du bec de lièvre ou l'on établi le premier principe de l'art de reunir les plaies. Mém Acad R Chir 4:385
580. Lower R (1665) The method observed in transfusing blood out of one live animal to another. Philos Trans 1:353
581. Lower R (1669) Tractatus de corde. J Allestry, London
582. Luckett WH (1910) A new operation for prominent ears based on the anatomy of the deformity. Surg Gynecol Obstet 10:635
583. Lundy JS (1935) Intravenous anesthesia: preliminary report on the use of two new thiobarbiturates. Proc Staff Meeting, Mayo Clinic 10:536
584. Lupo G, Boggio-Robutti G (1970) Chirurgia plastica del seno e della regione mammaria. Edizione Minerva Medica, Torino
585. Lusitanus A (1556) Curationum medicinalium centuriae quatuor. H Frobenius, Basel
586. Lusitanus A (1672) Praxis historiaum accessit praxis medical admiranda, editio novissima. Sumpt Ioannis Antonii Huguetan, Ludguni
587. Lynch CD, MacGillycuddy CT, Sullivan VR (2005) Pierre Fauchard and his role in the development of obturators. Br Dent J 199:603
588. Maggius B (1552) De vulnerum scoletorum et bombardarum curatione Tractatus in Chirurgia. Bonardum, Bononiae
589. Magatus C (1733) De rara medicatione vulneum seu de vulneribus raro tractardi. Lib secondus. Franc, Lipsiae et Amstelad
590. Magill IW (1921) A portable apparatus for tracheal insufflation anaesthesis. Lancet 1:918
591. Magill I (1921) Warming ether vapour for inhalation anaesthesia. Lancet 1:1270
592. Magill I (1923) The provision of expiration in endotracheal insufflation. Lancet 2:68

593. Magill I (1923) An apparatus for the administration of nitrous oxide, oxygen and ether. Lancet 2:228
594. Magill IW (1928) Endotracheal anaesthesia. Proc R Soc Med 22:85
595. Magnus O (1535) (Archibiscopus Upsaliensis) Historia de gentibus septentrionalibus, De Leporum Varietate, Roma
596. Majno G (1982) The Healing Hand. Harvard University Press, Cambridge, Mass
597. Major J D (1667) Chirurgia Infusoria. Impremebat Joach Reumannus, Kiel
598. Malgaigne JF (1839) Traité d'Anatomie Chirurgicale et Chirurgie Expérmentale. G Ballière, Paris
599. Malgaigne JF (1843) Manuel dc Médecine Operatoire. G Bailliére, Paris
600. Malgaigne JF (1840) Oeuvres completes d'Ambroise Paré. JB Balliére, Paris
601. Malgaigne JF (1965) Surgery of Ambroise Paré, 1840 edn. Translated from French by Hamby WB, University of Oklahoma, Norman
602. Maliniak JW (1934) Prevention of necrosis in plastic repair of pendulous breasts. Am J Surg 26:292
603. Maliniak JW (1934) Sculpture in the living. Lancet Press, New York
604. Maliniak JW (1950) Breast deformities and their repair. Grune & Stratton, New York
605. Manchester WM (1965) The repair of bilateralcleft lip and palate. Br J Surg 52:878
606. Manchot C (1889) Die Hautarterien des menschlichen Körpers. FCW Vogel, Leipzig (*see also Jovanka and Morain (1983) and Morain WD (1985)*)
607. Mangold TF von (1900) Die einpflanzum von rippenknörpel in den kehlhopf zur heilung schewer stenoses und defekte und heilung der sattelnase durch knörpel ueber trangung. Verh Dtsche Ges Chir 29:460
608. Manna A (1950) I Vianeo e l'antica Autoplastica Italiana. Tip. Corpo Forest. dello Stato, Roma
609. Marc H (1952) La plastique mammaire par la méthode oblique. Rev Portug Obstet 5:363
610. Marinello G (1562) Ornamenti delle donne. De Franceschi, Venezia
611. Marini G (1931) Il Chirurgo dei Miracoli: Gaspare Trigambe da Tagliacozzo. Il Messaggero, 26 Feb. Roma
612. Marino H (1944) The work of J Joseph (1865–1934) Prensa Med Argen 31:449
613. Mascagni P (1784) Prodome d'un ovrage sur le systéme des vaisseaux lymphatiques. Vincenzo Pazzinni Carli e F, Siena
614. Mascagni P (1816) Anatomia per Uso degli studiosi di scultura e di pittura. Giovanni Merenigh a spese degli eredi, Firenze
615. Mascagni P (1823) Anatomiae Universae. Nichol Capurro, Pisa
616. Masiero F (1690) La chirurgia compendiata. Steffano Curti, Venezia
617. Mason F (1878) On the surgery of the face. J & A Churchill, London
618. Mauclaire P (1922) Les greffes chirurgicales. Librairie JB Balliére et Fils, Paris
619. Mauclaire P (1927) Surgical grafts. Rev Med Franc 8:9–30
620. Mauget JJ (1731) Bibliotheca scriptorum medicorum, vol IV. Perachon et Cramer, Geneva
621. May H (1944) Reconstruction of breast deformities. Surg Gynecol Obstet 77:532
622. May H (1947) Mammaplasty procedures: reconstructive and reparative surgery. FA Davies, Philadelphia
623. Mazzetti S (1840) Memorie Storiche sopra l'Università e l'Instituto delle Scienze di Bologna. Tip San Tommaso d'Aquino, Bologna
624. Mazzola R (2000) Albori e sviluppi della Illustrazione Anatomica. Collegio Ghisleri, Pavia
625. Mazzola R, Filippi A (1995) L'insufficenza velopalantina. Masson, Milano
626. Mazzola FR, Hueston JT (1990) A forgotten innovator in facial reconstruction: Pietro Sabattini. Plast Reconstr Surg 85:621
627. Mazzola FR, Lupo G (1984) Evolving concepts in lip reconstruction. Clin Plast Surg 2:583
628. McCarthy JG (1990) Introduction to plastic surgery. In: McCarthy JG (ed) Plastic Surgery, vol I, Saunders, Philadelphia
629. McCraw JB (1980) The recent history of myocutaneous flaps. Clin Plast Surg 1:3
630. McCraw JB, Arnold PG (1986) Atlas of muscle and musculatocutaneous flaps. Hampton Press, Norfolk Virginia
631. McCraw JB, Dibell DG, Carraway JH (1977) Clinical definition of independent myocutaneous vascular territories. Plast Reconstr Surg 60:341
632. McCraw JB, Massey FM, Shanklin KD (1976) Vaginal reconstruction with gracilis myocutaneous flap. Plast Reconstr Surg 58:176
633. McDowell F (1969) The "BL" bombshell. Plast Reconstr Surg 44:66
634. McDowell F (1976) History of Rhinoplasty. Aesthetic Plast Surg 1:321
635. McDowell F (1977) Carl Thiersch, microscopy and skin grafting. In: McDowell F (ed) The Source Book of Plastic Surgery. Williams & Wilkins, Baltimore
636. McDowell F (1977) The Source Book of Plastic Surgery. Williams and Wilkins, Baltimore
637. MacEwen W (1881) Inter human bone graft. Gaz Méd Paris 3:385
638. MacEwen W (1881) Observations concerning transplantation of bone. Proc R Soc Lond 32:232
639. MacEwen W (1887) The osteogenic factors in the development and repair of bone. Ann Surg 6:289 & 389
640. McGregor IA (1963) The temporal flap in intraoral cancer: its use in repairing the post-excisional defect. Br J Plast Surg 16:318
641. McGregor IA, Morgan G (1973) Axial and random pattern flaps. Br J Plast Surg 26:202
642. McIndoe AH (1938) Review of 80 cases of mammaplasty. Rev Chir Strt 8:39
643. McIndoe AH (1937) Surgical treatment of hypospadias. Am J Surg 38:176
644. McIndoe AH, Banister JB (1938) Operation for cure of congenital absence of vagina. J Obstet Gynaecol Br Emp 45:490

645. McIndoe AH, Rees TD (1958) Mammaplasty: indications, techniques and complications. Br J Plast Surg 10:307
646. McKissock PK (1972) Reduction mammaplasty with a vertical dermal flap. Plast Reconstr Surg 49:245
647. McKissock PK (1976) Reduction mammaplasty by a vertical bipedicle flap technique. Clin Plast Surg 3:309
648. Meckel JF (1808) Beitrage zur Gesichischte des menschlichen Foetus. Beitr Verlag Anat 1:72
649. Medawar PB (1944) The behaviour and fate of skin autografts and skin homografts in rabbits. J Anat 78:176
650. Medawar PB (1945) Second study on behaviour and fate of skin homografts in rabbits. J Anat 79:157
651. Medawar PB (1946) Immunity to homologous grafted skin: the suppression of cell division in grafts transplanted to immunised animals. Br J Exp Pathol 27:9
652. Medawar PB (1946) Immunity to homologous grafted skin: the relationship between the antigens of blood and skin. Br J Exp Pathol 27:15
653. Medawar PB (1948) Immunity to homologous grafted skin: the fate of skin homograft transplanted to the brain, to subcutaneous tissue and to the anterior chamber of the eye. Br J Exp Pathol 29:58
654. Medawar PB (1956) The storage of living skin. Proc R Soc Med 47:63
655. Medawar PB (1958) Immunology in transplantation. Harvey Lect 52:144. Academic Press, New York
656. Medawar PB (1973) Tolerance reconsidered: a critical survey. Transplant Proc 5:7
657. Medici M (1857) Compendio Storico della Scuola Anatomica di Bologna. Tip. Govern. della Volpe e del Sassi, Bologna
658. Meek'ren JAS van (1682) De fractures cranii, chap 1 In: Observationes medicochirurgicae. ex officina Henrici et Theodori Boom, Amstelodami
659. Mercklinus GA (1686) Lindenius renovatus sive Johannis Antonidae van der Linden de scripti medicis, libri duo. Norimbergae
660. Mercurialis H (1587) De Decoratione Liberere. Apud Joannem Wechelum, Frankfurt
661. Merrem DCT (1810) Anima diversiones quadeam chirurgicae experimentis in animalibus factis illustr. Tasche et Mueller, Giessiae
662. Mesmer FA (1779) Mémoires sur la découverte du magnétisme animal. PF Didot le jeune, Paris
663. Mettauer JP (1842) Practical observations on those malformations of the male urethra and penis, termed hypospadias and epispadias with an anomalous case. Am J Med Sci 4:43
664. Middeldorpf AT (1854) Plastische Operationen im Gesicht wegen Epithelialgeschwulst. Günsburg's Klin Ztschr Bd. 5, p 161
665. Middeldorph AT (1859) De fistulis ventricularis externis et chirurgia earum sanatione accedente historia fistulae arte chirurgicorum plastica prospere curatae. Commentatio, Vratislaviae
666. Mieli A (1925) Manuale di Storia della Scienza. Casa Ed Leonardo da Vinci, Roma
667. Millard RC (1976) Cleft Craft, vols I–III. Little Brown, Boston
668. Miller CC (1906) the excision of bag like folds of skin from the region about the eyes. The Medical Brief, St Louis 34:648
669. Miller CC (1907) Folds, bags and wrinkles of the skin about the eyes and their eradication by simple surgical methods. The Medical Brief St Louis 35:540
670. Miller CC (1907) Cosmetic Surgery: The Correction of Featural Imperfections. Oak Printing, Chicago
671. Miller CC (1907) Subcutaneous section of the facial muscles to eradicate expression lines. Am J Surg 21:235
672. Miller CC (1925) Facial bands as supports to relaxed facial tissue. Ann Surg 82:603–608
673. Milton SH (1969) The tubed pedicle flap. Br J Plast Surg 22:53
674. Milton SH (1969) The effects of "delay" on the survival of experimental pedicled skin flaps. Br J Plast Surg 22:244
675. Milton SH (1970) Pedicle skin flaps. The fallacy of the length-width ration. Br J Surg 57:502
676. Milton SH (1971) Experimental study on island flaps. I. Surviving length. Plast Reconstr Surg 48:574
677. Milton SH (1972) Experimental study on island flaps. II. Ischaemia and delay. Plast Reconstr Surg 49:444
678. Minodoi GT (1600) De Humani Corporis Turpitudinibus Cognoscendis Curandis. Libri Tres Francesco Balzetta, Padova
679. Mirault G (1844) Deux lettres sur l'opération du bec-de-lievre. J Chir 2:257
680. Mitz V, Peyronie M (1976) The superficial muscolaponeurotic system (SMAS) in the parotid and cheek area. Plast Reconstr Surg 58:80
681. Molinetti A (1669) Dissertationes Anatomicae et Pathologica Sensibus and eorum Organis. Matteo Bolzetto, Padova
682. Mondeville H de (1889) Die Anatomie. Translated by Papel J von, George Reimer, Berlin (*see also Nicaise F*)
683. Mondino dei Liucci (1493) Anatomia. Landsberg, Leipzig
684. Mondino dei Liucci (1513) De Omnibus Humani Corporis Interioribus Membris Anathomia. Impressit Argentien Martinus Flach, Strasbourg
685. Mondino dei Liucci (1540) Anatomia Mundini per Carpum caastigata. Melchiorre Sessa, Venezia
686. Monks GH (1898) Correction by operation of some nasal deformities and disfigurements. Boston Med Surg J 139:262
687. Montandon D, Millard GF, Morax S, et al (1988) Plasties et reconstruction orbito-palpebrales. Maloiner Ed. Médicine et Igiène, Geneve
688. Moodie R (1929) Surgery in pre-Colombian Peru. Ann Med History 1:689
689. Moodie R (1930) Prehistoric surgery in New Mexico. Am J Surg 7:689
690. Moore J (1784) A method of preventing or diminishing pain in several operations of surgery. T Cardell, London
691. Moore JC (1789) A dissertation on the process of filling up of cavities, healing of wounds and restoring parts which have been destroyed in the human body. John Richardson, London
692. Morain WD (1985) Carl Manchot, plastic surgery's missed opportunities. Med Herit 1:174

693. Morax V (1919) Plastic operation on the orbital region. Arch Orthop 48:625
694. Morax V (1919) Plastic operation on the orbital region including restoration of the eyebrows, eyelids and the orbital cavity. Trans Ophthalmol Soc UK 39:5
695. Morel-Fatio D (1971) Biographical sketch of Roux. Plast Reconstr Surg 47:181
696. Morestin H (1903) De l'autoplasty par déplacement du sein. Arch Gen Med 80:2686
697. Morestin H (1903) De la reposition et du plissement cosmetique du pavillon de l'oreille. Rev Orthop 14:289
698. Morestin H (1911) Difformité faciale consecutive à une ostéomyelite du maxillaire inferieur. Bull Soc Chir Paris p 236
699. Morestin H (1912) Cicatrice facial irréguliere deformé adhérente au malaire corrigée par l'insertion sous les teguments d'une greffe grasseuse. Bull Soc Chir Paris p 225
700. Morestin H (1914) De la correction des flexions permanents des doigts consecutive aux panaris et aux phlegmons de la paume de la main. Rev Chir Paris 50:1
701. Morestin H (1916) Les transplantations cartilagineuses dans la chirurgie réparatrice. Bull Mem Soc Chir Paris 42:1211
702. Morestin H (1916) Greffes de cartilage pour la difformité du nez. Bull Mem Soc Chir Paris 42:1375
703. Morestin H, Gossett A (1916) La cranioplasty: indications techniques suites operatoires et suites eloignées. Bull Mem Soc Chir Paris 42:1593 (*see also numerous references to Morestin H on pp 379–381 The Patterson Index*)
704. Morgagni GB (1705–1717) Adversaria Anatomica prima. Ferdinando Pisarri, Bologna
705. Morgagni GB (1761) De sedibus et causis morborum per anatomen indagatis libri quinque. Typographia Remondiniana, Venezia
706. Morgan J (1825–1826) Operation for new lip Lancet IX :394
707. Morgan J (1828–1829) Operation for a new under lip. Lancet II:537
708. Morgan J (1829–1830) Operation for a new upper lip. Lancet I:357
709. Morgan TH (1893) Experimental studies on teleost eggs. Anat Anz 8:803
710. Morley ME (1958) Cleft Palate and Speech. Livingstone, Edinburgh
711. Mornard P (1926) Mastopexie esthétique par transposition du mammelon pratique chirchurgical illustrée. C Doin et Cie, Paris
712. Morse WM (1934) Chinese Medicine. Hoeber, New York, p 129
713. Morton WT (1847) Letter to Am J Dent Sci 8:56
714. Morton WT (1850) On the physiological effects of sulphuric ether and its superiority to chloroform. D Clapp, Boston
715. Morton WT (1904) The first use of ether as an anaesthetic at the battle of the Wilderness in the Civil War. JAMA 42:1068
716. Morton LT, Norman JM (1991) Morton's medical biography: An annotated check list of texts illustrating the history of medicine (Garrison & Morton). Gower, Brookfield
717. Muhopadhyaya G (1913–1914) The surgical instruments of the Hindu with comparative study of the surgical instruments of the Greeks, Romans, Arabs and modern European surgeons. Calcutta University, Calcutta
718. Müller P (1915) Deckung von schaedeldefekten aus den Sternum. Zentralbl Chir 42:409
719. Mulliken JB, Glawochi J (1980) Induced osteogenesis for repair and construction in the craniofacial region. Plast Reconstr Surg 65:553
720. Mutter TD (1842) Cases of deformities from burns relieved by operation. Am J Med Sci 4:66
721. Myrrhen A (1721) Uvulae ab ortu, defectum resarciunt vicinae partes, sine incomodo. In: Magneti JJ (ed) Bibliotheca Chirurgica. Gabrielis de Tournes & Filiorum, Geneve
722. Nageotte J (1921) L'organisation de la matiére. Bull Mem Soc Chir Paris 47:33
723. Nannoni A (1797) Trattato chirurgico delle malattie delle mammelle. Adama Sappa, Venezia
724. Natvig P (1982) Jacques Joseph: Surgical Sculptor. Saunders, Philadelphia
725. Nélaton C (1902) Discussion au subjet de la Rhinoplasty. Bull Mem Soc Chir Paris 28:458
726. Nélaton C (1904) La rinoplasties. G Steinheil, Paris
727. Nélaton C, Ombrédanne L (1907) Les autoplasties: lévres joues oreilles tronc members. G Steinheil, Paris
728. Neuber G (1893) Fettransplantation. Chir Kong Verhandl 1:66
729. Neuhof H (1923) The transplantation of tissues. D Appleton & Co, New York
730. Neumann CG (1957) The expansion of an area of skin by progressive distention of a subcutaneous balloon. Plast Reconstr Surg 19:124
731. Nicaise E (1893) Chirurgie de maitre Henry de Mondeville composée de 1306 a 1320. G Bailliére e Cie, Felix Alcan, Paris
732. Nicolaus Salernitanum (1471) Antidotarium. Nicolaus Jenson, Venice
733. Niemann A (1860) Sur l'alcalode de Coca. J Pharm 37:474
734. Nöel A (1928) Aestetische chirurgie der weiblinchen Brust. Die Med Welt 2:51
735. Nöel A, Lopez Martinez H (1928) Nouveau procédés chirurgicaux de correction du prolapsus mammaire. Arch Franco-belge Chir 31:138
736. Nöel S (1926) La chirurgie esthetique: son role social. Masson, Paris
737. Nöel S (1928) La chirurgie esthetique: Thiron et Cie, Clermont Oise
738. Noordhoff MS (1977) Cleft lip and palate: the Asian connection. In: Transactions of 8th Int Congr on Cleft Palate and Related Craniofacial Anomalies, Singapore
739. Nové-Josserand G (1897) Traitement de l'hypospadias: nouvelle methode. Lyon Med 85:198

740. Nové-Josserand G (1919) Des hypospadias étendu par la tunnelization avec greffe dermo épidermique. J Urol 8:449
741. Nuttall GHF (1904) Blood immunity and blood relationship amongst animals by means of the preciptin test for blood. Cambridge University Press, Cambridge
742. Nylen CO (1954) The microscope in aural surgery: its first use and later development Acta Otolaryngol (Suppl) 116:226
743. Nylen CO (1972) The otomicroscope and microscopy 1921–1971. Acta Laryngol 73:453
744. O'Brien BM (1977) Microvascular Reconstructive Surgery. Churchill Livingstone, Edinburgh London New York
745. O'Brien BM, MacLeod WA, Hayhurst JW, et al (1973) Successful transfer of a large island flap from the groin to the foot by microvascular anastomosis. Plast Reconstr Surg 52:271
746. Olch PD, Harkins HN (1965) A history of surgery. In: Moyer CA, et al. (eds) Surgery, Principles and Practice. Lippincott, Philadelphia
747. Ollier LXEL (1860) Notes sur la transplantation d'os pris sur des animeaux morts depuis un certain laps de temp. C R Acad Sci Arch Med T 50:163
748. Ollier LXEL (1862) Des transplantations periostiques et osseuses sur l'homme. J Physiol de l'homme et animeauz 12:1
749. Ollier LXEL (1867) Traité experimental et clinique de la régeneration des os et de la production artificielle du tissu osseuz. V Masson et Fils, Paris
750. Ollier LXEL (1872) Sur les greffes cutanées ou autoplastiques. Bull Acad Med Paris 2:1:243 (*see also Zeis Index p 303*)
751. Ombrédanne L (1906) Hypospadias pèrinéoscrotal gueri par la procédé de la greffe autoplastique. Lyon Med 96:322
752. Ombrédanne L (1911) Hypospadias pénien chez l'enfant. Bull Med Soc Chir Paris 37:1076
753. Ombrédanne L (1939) Les Hermaphrodites et la Chirurgie. Masson et Cie, Paris
754. Oribasius (1544) Chirurgia ex Greco in Latinum Conversa. Vido Vidi Florentino, Interprete. Pierre Gaultier, Paris
755. Oribasius (1555) Oribasius Sardiani Collectorum Medicinalium. Apud B Turrisanum sub Offician Aldina, Paris
756. Oribasius, in Bussmaker & Daremberg (1851–1876) Oevres d'Oribase Texte Grec en grand partie inédit, vol 6. Imprimérie Nationale, Paris
757. Oribasius, in Raeder J (1931) Oribasii Collectionum Medicorum Reliquiae, part of Corpus Medicorum Graecorum 2:1 BG Teubner, Leipzig
758. Orlandi PA (1714) Notizie degli Scrittori Bolognesi. Constantino Pisani, Bologna
759. Orticochea M (1968) Construction of a dynamic muscle sphincter in cleft palates. Plast Reconstr Surg 41:323
760. Ortiz-Monasterio F, Serrano RA (1971) Cultural aspects of cleft lip and palate treatment. In: Grabb WC, RosensteinW, Bzoch KR (eds) Cleft Lip and Palate. Little Brown, Boston
761. Owens N (1955) Compound neck pedicle designed for repair of massive facial defects. Plast Reconstr Surg 15:369
762. Owens N (1946) A suggested pyrex form for support of skin grafts in the construction of an artificial vagina. Plast Reconstr Surg 1:350
763. Pancoast J (1844) A treatise on operative surgery. Carey and Hart, Philadelphia, p 317
764. Paracelsus (alias Hohenheim TB von) (1536) La grande chirurgie. Basel
765. Paracelsus (1658) Opera omnia medico-chemico chirugica. Sumtibus, Joan Antonii et Samuelis de Tournes
766. Paré A (1549) Briefe Collection de l'administration Anatomique. En la Boutique de Guillaume Cavellat, Paris
767. Paré A (1561) Anatomie Universelle du Corp humain. Iean le Royer, Paris
768. Paré A (1564) Dix Livres de la Chirurgie. Iean le Royer, Paris
769. Paré A (1575) Les oeuvres de M Ambroise Paré. Chez Gabriel Buon, Paris
770. Paré A (1840) Oevres completes etc Tome I–III. JF Malgaigne, Paris
771. Passavant G (1862) Ueber die Operation der angebornen Splaten des harten Gaumens und der damit complicirten Hasenscharten. Wagner's Arch f Heilk 3:196
772. Passot R (1919) La chirurgie esthétique des rides du visage. Presse Med 27:258
773. Passot R (1919) La correction chirurgicale des rides du visage. Bull Acad Méd Paris 82:112
774. Passot R (1925) La correction esthetique du prolaps mammaire par le procédé de la transposition du mamelon. Presse Med 33:757
775. Passot R (1931) Chirurgie Esthétique Pure. G Doin et Cie, Paris
776. Passot R (1933) Quelques généralitées sur l'operation correctrice des rides du visage. Rev Chir Plast 3:23
777. Pasteur L (1922–1929) Oeuvres. Pasteur Vallery Radat, Paris
778. Patten BM (1971) Embryology of the Palate and Maxillofacial region. In: Grabb WC, Rosenstein SW, Bzoch A (eds) Cleft Lip and Palate. Little Brown, Boston
779. Patterson TJS (1969) Experimental skin grafts in England 1663–1664. Br J Plast Surg 22:384
780. Patterson TJS (1971) "Mr Lucas" and the "BL" letter. A letter to the editor. Plast Reconstr Surg 48:68
781. Patterson TJS (1977) "Mr Lucas" and the "BL" letter. In: McDowell F (ed) The Source Book of Plastic Surgery. Williams & Wilkins, Baltimore
782. Patterson TJS (1977) The Zeis Index and History of Plastic Surgery 900BC to 1863AD. Williams & Wilkins, Baltimore
783. Peer LA (1955) Cell survival theory versus replacement theory. Plast Reconstr Surg 16:161
784. Peer LA (1959) Loss of weight and volume in human fat grafts. Plast Reconstr Surg 5:217
785. Peer LA (1959) Transplantation of tissues, vol 2. Williams & Wilkins, Baltimore

786. Peer LA (1964) Transplantation of Cartilage. In: Converse JM (ed) Plastic Reconstructive Surgery. Saunders, Philadelphia
787. Peer LA, Paddock R (1937) Histologic studies on the fate of deeply implanted dermal grafts: observations on sections of implants buried from one week to one year. Arch Surg 34:268
788. Peet EW (1971) Congenital absence of the ear. Livingstone, Edinburgh
789. Pennisi VR, Capozzi A (1972) The transposition of fat in cervicofacial rhytidectomy. Plast Reconstr Surg 49:423
790. Penso G (1984) La Medecine Romaine: l'art d'Esculape dans la Rome antique. Roger Dacosta, Paris
791. Percy PF (1815) Ente animale. In: Dictionaire des Sciences Médicales pour une Société de Medecins et de Chirurgiens Paris
792. Petersen NC (1973) Unknown lip-flap procedure by Stein. Scand J Plast Surg 7:82
793. Petersen NC (1977) Translation and commentary on "Lip repair (cheiloplasty) performed by a new method by Prof SAV Stein". In: McDowell F (ed) The Source Book of Plastic Surgery. Williams & Wilkins, Baltimore, p 328
794. Petrali N (1858) Due Parole sull'Arte di Rifare i Nasi. Gazz di Mantova 84:5 (*see also Petrali N (1845) Bericht uber den wissenschaltlichen. Congress zu Mailand. Lancet 1.29 reprinted 1972 by Aris and Phillips, Warminster*)
795. Petrie WMF (1914) Amulets. University College, London
796. Pfolsprundt H von (1868) Buch de Bűndth-Ertsnei von H von Pfolsprundt Brunder de deutschen ordens 1490. Herausgegeben von H. Haeser und A Middledorpf, Reimer, Berlin
797. Phemister DB (1914) The fate of transplanted bone and regeneration of its various constituents. Surg Gynecol Obstet 19:303
798. Piacentini M (1599) Oratio Bononiae habita in Funere Gasparis Taliacotii. Herdi Jonannes Rossii, Bolgona
799. Pierce GW (1930) Reconstruction of the external ear. Surg Gynecol Obstet 50:601
800. Pigott RW (1969) The nasoendoscopic appearance of the normal palatopharyngeal valve. Plast Reconstr Surg 43:19
801. Pigott RW (1993) The results of pharyngoplasty by muscle transplantation by Wilfred Hynes. Br J Plast Surg 46:440
802. Pigott RW (2000) Sir Harold Gillies Memorial Lecture: speak ye comfortably. Br J Plast Surg 53:641
803. Pitanguy I (1960) Breast hypertrophy. In: Trans of the 2*nd* Congr of the Int Soc of Plastic Surgery, London 1959. Livingstone, Edinburgh
804. Plinius the Elder quoted by Penso G (1895) La medicina Romana. Ciba Geigy, Milano (*Caius Plinius Secundus (23–79AD) author of Naturalis Historia*)
805. Pöhlmann GA (1930) Dissertation on the embryology of the face. Leipzig
806. Pousson M (1897) De la mastopexie. Bull Mem Soc Chir Paris 23:507
807. Pousson M (1897) Sur en cas de Mastopexie. J Med Bordeaux 27:495
808. Pollock GD (1870) Skin grafting and skin transplantation. BMJ 2:565
809. Pollock GD (1870) The operation of skin transplantation; clinical remarks. Lancet 2:669
810. Pollock GD (1871) On skin grafting and skin transplantation. Trans Clin Soc Lond 4:37
811. Pontén B (1960) Grafted skin: observations on reinnervation and other qualities. Thesis. Acta Chir Scand Suppl 257
812. Pontén B (1981) The fasciocutaneous flap: its use in soft tissue defects of the lower leg. Br J Plast Surg 34:215
813. Porzio C (1839) L'Istoria d'Italia nell'anno MDXLVII e la descrizione del Regno di Napoli. Tramier, Napoli
814. Porzio C (1846) Opere di Camillo Porzio per cura di C Monzani, Florence
815. Premuda L (1957) Storia dell'iconografia anatomica. Aldo Martello, Milano
816. Priestley WO, Stover TIR (1856) The obstetric memoires and contributions of James Y Simpson. Lippincott, Philadelephia
817. Prince D (1907) Plastics: a new classification and a brief exposition of plastic surgery. G Steinheil, Philadelphia
818. Pudenz RH, Odom GL (1942) Meningocerebral adhesions: experimental study on the effect of human amniotic membrane, amnioplastin, beef allantoic membrane, tantalium foil and polyvinyl alcohol film. Surgery 12:318
819. Purmann MG (1684) Grossen und gantz Neugewundener Lorbeerk-Krantz oder Wundartzney. Halberstadt
820. Putti V (1937) Beringario da Carpi. Cappelli, Bologna
821. Raeder J (1931) Oribasii Collectionum Medicarum reliquiae. BG Teubner Lipsiae et Berlino
822. Radovan C (1982) Breast reconstruction after mastectomy using the temporary expander. Plast Reconstr Surg 69:195
823. Radovan C (1984) Tissue expansion in soft tissue reconstruction. Plat Reconstr Surg 74:482
824. Radzimowski (1881) Ueber Replantation und Transplantation. Dissertation, Kiev
825. Ragnell A (1948) Breast reduction and lactation. Br J Plast Surg 1:99
826. Rambollà F (1998) La Chirurgia Plastica in Calabria ne XV e XVI secolo. Galassia Editrice, Cosenza
827. Randall P (1959) Triangular flap operation for unilateral clefts of the lip. Plast Reconstr Surg 23:331
828. Ranzano P (Bishop of Lucera) quoted by Auria V (1704) La Sicilia Inventrice. Con il divertimenti geniali di Dr Mongitore. Marino, Palermo
829. Ranzi A (1860–1863) Lezioni di Patologia Chirurgica date nella R Università di Pisa, vol III. Gazzini e Gianni-ni, Firenze, p 419
830. Rathke H (1832) Ueber die Bildung und Entwichlung des Oberkiefers und der Gerunchswerkzenge der Sangetiere. A Bild u Entw der Menschen und Tierre 1:95
831. Rees T, La Tenta G (1994) Aesthetic Plastic Surgery. Saunders, Philadelphia
832. Rehn E (1911) Fettransplantation. Ges Dtsch Naturf Aerzte 82:121
833. Rehn E (1912) Die Fettransplantation. Arch Klin Chir 98:1

834. Remensnyder JP, Bigelow ME, Goldwyn RM (1979) Justinian II and Camagnola: a Byzantine Rhinoplasty? Plast Reconstr Surg 63:19
835. Remondino PC (1891) History of Cirumcision from the earliest time to the present. FA Davies, Philadelphia
836. Rethi A (1934) Raccorcissement du nez trop long. Rev Chir Plast 2:85
837. Reverdin JL (1869) Greffe epidermiques. Experience faite dans le service de M le Docteur Guyon a l'Hopital Necker. Bull Soc Imp Chir Paris 10:493
838. Ricci JV (1945) One hundred years of gynecology: 1800–1900. Blakiston, Philadelphia
839. Richerand AB (1807) The elements of physiology: containing an explanation of the function of the human body. Translated by Robert Morrison, J & W Smith, London
840. Rickham PP (1958) The treatment of ectopia vescicae. Br J Plast Surg 10:300
841. Rigollot-Simonnot (1913) Fat grafts: a piece of a lipoma taken from another patient. Paris Chir 5:613
842. Rinieri V (1950) Diario delle Cose più Notabili, vol II quoted by Gnudi MT, Webster JP The Life and Times of Gaspare Tagliacozzi. Hoepli, Milan
843. Rintala A (1977) How a patient experienced a cleft lip operation in 1763. In: McDowell F (ed) The Source Book of Plastic Surgery. Williams & Wilkins, Baltimore, p 214
844. Rintala A (1998) Plastikka Kirurgian Historia Suomesa. Kirjapaino Grafia, Turku
845. Robbins T (1977) A reduction mammaplasty with the areola nipple based on an inferior dermal pedicle. Plast Reconstr Surg 59:64
846. Robert M (1764) Treatise on the principal aims of medicine. Lacombe, Paris
847. Roberts JB (1912) Surgery of deformities of the face including cleft palate. William Wood, New York
848. Roe JO (1887) The deformity termed "pug nose" and its correction by a simple operation. Med Rec N Y 31:621
849. Roe JO (1893) The correction of deformity of the nose resulting from abscess of the nasal septum. N Y Med J 57:319
850. Roe JO (1905) The correction of nasal deformities by subcutaneous operation: a further contribution. Med Rec N Y 68:1
851. Rogers BO (1971) A chronological history of cosmetic surgery. Bull N Y Acad Med 47:265
852. Rogers BO (1973) History of external genitalia surgery. In: Horton CE (ed) Plastic and Reconstructive Surgery of the Genital Area. Little Brown, Boston
853. Rogers BO (1976) The development of aesthetic surgery. Aesthetic Plast Surg 1:3
854. Rogers BO (1977) Harelip repair in colonial America. In: McDowell J (ed) The Source Book of Plastic Surgery. Williams & Wilkins, Baltimore
855. Rogge CWL (1976) Amboise Paré (1510–1590) and evolution of surgical instrumentarium. Plast Reconstr Surg 57:126
856. Romand MHL (1830) Dissertation sur les moyens réparateurs des pertes de substance de la face en general et des Lévres en Particulier. Thése. Collection de Paris, Didot
857. Romand MHL (1834) Chirurgie clinique de Montpellier, vol 2. Montpellier
858. Ronsil GA de (1768) Memoires de chirurgie devises en deux parties. J Nourse in the Strand, London
859. Roonhuysen H van (1674) Historischer heil-curen in zwei theil verfasste. Michael und Johann Freidrich Endtern, Nürnberg
860. Ropke W (1912) Zur frage der decking von schaedeldefekten. Zentralbl Chir 39:1192
861. Rose W (1891) On harelips and cleft palate. HK Lewis, London
862. Rosenstein NR von (1742) Dissertatio medico-chirurgia de Chirurgiae curtorum possibilitate. Uppsaliae Impressa, Uppsala
863. Rosenthal W (1924) Zur Frage der Gaumenplastik. Zentralbl Chir 51:1621
864. Rostinio P, Rostinio L (1564) Compendio di tutta la Chirurgia. Ava, Venezia
865. Roux JN (1828) Mémoires sur le cancer des lévres et sur une nouvelle méthode opératiore. Rev Med Etrang 1:30
866. Roux PJ (1819) Observation sur une division congénital du voile du palais et de la luette guérie au moyen d'ine operation analogue a celle du Bec-de-liévre, pratique par M. Roux. J Universel Sci Med 15:356
867. Roux PJ (1825) Staphyloraphie. Arch Gén Méd Paris 7:311, 465, 516
868. Roux PJ (1825) Mémoires sur la staphiloraphie ou la suture du voile du palais. JS Chaudé, Paris
869. Roux PJ (1827–1828) Division of the soft palate. Lancet 2:140
870. Roux PJ (1829–1830) Staphyloraphy. Lancet 2:350
871. Roux PJ (1845) Remarques cliniques sur les opérations autoplastiques en general et en particulier sur la staphiloraphie, à propos d'une operation pratiquée par ce professeur. Gaz Hop Paris 7:322
872. Roux PJ (1854) Congenital and accidental clefts of the soft and hard palate: their restoration. Quarante année de pratique chirurgicale 1:228
873. Rowbotham ES, Magill IW (1921) Anaesthesia in plastic surgery of the face and jaw. Proc R Soc Med 14:17
874. Ruding R (1964) Cleft palate. Anatomical and surgical considerations. Plast Reconstr Surg 33:132
875. Sabattini P (1838) Cenno storico dell'origine e progressi dell rinoplastica e cheiloplastica. Belle Arti, Bologna
876. Sabattini P (1847) Sull utilita del trafano nelle lesioni del capo. Tip. Galeati, Imola
877. Safian J (1935) Corrective Rhinoplastic Surgery. PB Hoeber, New York
878. Safian J (1970) Personal recollections of Dr Jacques Joseph. Plast Reconst Surg 46:175
879. Sahagun B de (1963) Codex Floreninus. General History of the things in New Spain, vol 13. University of Utah, Sante Fe
880. Saliceto G da (1476) Liber scientia medicinalis. Johannes Petrus de Ferrati, Placentia
881. Saliceto G da (1516) Vulgare in Chirurgia. Angelo Scinzenzeler, Milano
882. Salmon M (1936) Artéres de la peau. Masson et Cie, Paris

883. Salmon M (1936) Artéres des Muscles des Members e du Tronc. Masson et Cie, Paris
884. Salmon M (1988) Arteries of the skin.Translated from the French. Taylor GI, Tempest M (eds) Churchill Livingstone, London
885. Saltzman F (1886) Om cocainets anaesteserande verkan vid subcutan application. Finsk Läk Handl 28:154
886. Sancassiani DA (1731) Aforismi generali della cura delle ferite col modo di Magati. Delucidazioni fisico-mediche. Tom I–IV Venezia 1713 and Roma 1731
887. Sandison AT (1967) Sexual behaviour in ancient societies. In: Brothnell D, Sanison AT (eds) Diseases in Antiquity. Thomas, Springfield, Ill
888. Sandon RPG (1965) Plastic surgery of the breast. In: Battle RJV (ed) Clinical Surgery: Plastic Surgery. Butterworths, London
889. Santoni-Rugiu P (1961) Studi sulla conservazione della cute. Thesis. Omnia Medica XL: 113
890. Santoni-Rugiu P (1962) Comparative studies on the viability of skin stored by different methods. Plast Reconstr Surg 30:586
891. Santoni-Rugiu P (1969) Repair of skull defects by outer table osteoperiosteal free graft. Plast Reconstr Surg 43:157
892. Santoni-Rugiu P, Massei A (1982) The legend and the truth about the nose of Federico, Duke of Urbino. Br J Plast Surg 35:251
893. Santoni-Rugiu P, Mazzola R (1996) The Italian contribution to facial plastic surgery: an historical reappraisal. Facial Plast Surg 12:316
894. Santoni-Rugiu P, Mazzola R (1997) Leonard Fioravanti (1517–1588) A Barber Surgeon who influenced the development of reconstructive surgery. Plast Reconstr Surg 2:570
895. Santorini GD (1724) Observationes anatomicas. J Recurti, Venezia
896. Santorini GD (1775) Septem decim tabulae. Edited by Michele Girardi, ex Regia Typographia, Parma
897. Sanvenero-Rosselli G (1934) La divisione congenital de labbro e del palato. Luigi Pozzi, Roma
898. Sanvenero-Rosselli G (1931) Chirurgia Plastica del Naso. Luigi Pozzi, Roma
899. Sasaki GM (1985) Tissue expansion: guidelines and case analysis. Dow Corning, Wright, Arlington
900. Savariaud M (1912) Prothese du crane avec plaque d'argent extensibile. Bull Mem Soc Chir Paris 38:238
901. Scarpa A (1789) Anatomicae disquisitiones de auditu et olfactu. Petri Galeatii, Ticino
902. Scarpa A (1789) Anatomicarum Annotations. Giuseppe Galeati, Pavia & Milano
903. Schenck J von Graefemberg (1809) Observationum medicorum rerarum novarum admirabilium et monstrosarum volumen. Tomes septem. Joannes Georgiu Schenchius filius, Frankfurt
904. Schmidt GB (1916) Schaedelplastik: Besprechung. Beitr Klin Chir 98:604
905. Schoenborn K (1876) Ueber eine neue Methode der Staphyloraphie. Verh Dtsch Ges Chir 4:235
906. Schreiber F (1929) Operation der Haengebrust. Beitr Klin Chir 147:56
907. Schulten MW (1897) Eine Methode um Knockenhoelen in Femurund in Humerus durch plastische Operation auszufuellen. Arch Klin Chir 54:328
908. Schultes J (Scultetus) (1655) Armamentarium Chirurgicum. Balthasari Kuehnen, Ulm
909. Schultes J (Scultetus) (1674) The Chyrurgeon. John Starkey, London
910. Schwalbe E (1907) Die Morphologie der Missbildungen des Menschen un der Thiere. Jena
911. Schwarzmann E (1930) Die technique der mammplastik. Chirurg 2:932
912. Schwarzmann E (1936) Über eine neue methode der mammaplastik. Wien Med Wochenschr 86:100
913. Scott M, Wycis HT (1946) Experimental observations on the use of stainless steel for cranioplasty. J Neurosurg 3:310
914. Sedillot CE (1848) De l'application de la méthode autoplastique au treatment du cancer. Gaz Méd Strasbourg 9:20
915. Semmelweis IP (1847–1849) Hoechst wictige Erfahrunge ueber die Aetiologie der in Gebaeranstalten epidemischen Puerperalfieber. Z.K.K Wien Ges. Aertze, 4(2):242, 564
916. Semmelweis IP (1861) Die Aetilogie der Begriff und die Prophyslaxis des Kindbetfiebers, Pest., CA Harleben, Wien & Leipzig (*see also Childhood Fever: A scientific biography of Ignaz Semmelweis. Codell Carter K and Carter BR (2005) Transaction, New Brunswick NJ*)
917. Serre M (1842) Traité sur l'Art de Réstaurere les Difformités de la Face selon l Méthode par Displacement ou Methode Francais. L Castel, Montpellier
918. Serteurner FW (1806) Darstellung der reine Mohnsaeure (Opiumsaeure): nebst einer chemischen Untersuchung des Opiums, mit vorzueglicher Hinsicht auf einen darin neu entdeckten Stoff, J d Pharm Leipzig 14:47
919. Seydel H (1889) Eine neue Methode grosse knockendefekten des Schaedels zu Heckung. Zentralbl Chir 16:2209
920. Shah Tribowandas (1889) Rhinoplasty. A short description of one hundred cases. Junagahh Sakari Press, Junagadh
921. Shaw DT, Payne RL (1946) One stage tubed abdominal flaps. Surg Gynecol Obstet 83:205
922. Sheehan JE (1925) Plastic surgery of the nose. Paul Hoeber, New York
923. Sichel J (1844) Aphorismes pratiques sur divers points d'ophtalmologie. Ann Ocul 12:187
924. Siebold KK (1792) Ein in Zwey Theile bis an das Gaumenbein gespaltenes Zapfchen. In: Chirurgisches Tagenbuch obs XIII. Grattenauer, Nurnberg
925. Signoroni B (1833) Sulla rinoplastica. Memoria storico plastica. Ann Univ 67:225
926. Signoroni B (1836) Progetti Clinici della Scuola di Chirurgia Practica dell' Università di Padova. Tipografia Cartallier, Padova
927. Silex P (1896) Uber Lidbildung mit stiellosen Hautlappen. Klin Monatsbl Augenh 34:46
928. Simon G (1859) Ueber die Anwendung mehrfacher Nahtreien zur Vereininuus einer Wunde. Wunderl Arch 3:312

929. Simpson JY (1847) Discovery of a new anaesthetic agent more efficient that sulphuric ether. Lancet 2:519
930. Sims JM (1858) Silver Sutures in Surgery. S & SW Wood, New York
931. Sinclair SW, Davies DM, Bracha A (1982) The comparative reliability of nasal pharyngoscopy and videoflourography in the assessment of velopharyngeal incompetence. Br J Plast Surg 35:113
932. Singer CJ (1957) A short history of anatomy from the Greeks to Harvey. Dover, New York
933. Singer CJ Underwood EA (1962) A short history of medicine. Oxford University Press, New York
934. Skolnick ML (1970) Videofluoroscopic examination of the velopharyngeal portal during phonation in lateral and base projection. Cleft Palate J 7:803
935. Skoog T (1967) The use of periosteum and Surgicel for bone restoration in congenital clefts of the maxilla. Scand J Plast Reconstr Surg 1:113
936. Skoog T (1969) A head from ancient Corinth. Scand J Plast Reconstr Surg 3:49
937. Skoog T (1972) Principella sypunkter pa tekniken vid face lifting. Fifth Meeting of the Swedish Association for Plastic Surgery, Stockholm
938. Skoog T (1974) Plastic Surgery. New Methods and Refinements. Almqvist & Wiksel Intern, Stockholm
939. Smith GE, Dowson WR (1924) Egyptian Mummies. Unwin, London
940. Smith N (1826) Suture of the palate in infancy. Am Med Rev 3:396
941. Smith PJ (1973) Vascular base of axial pattern flaps. Br J Plast Surg 26:150
942. Smith PJ, Foley B, McGregor IA, et al (1972) The antatomical base of the groin flap. Plast Reconstr Surg 49:41
943. Smith T (1868) On the cure of the cleft palate in children with the description of an instrument facilitating the operation. Med Chir Tr 2:79
944. Snydacker EF (1906) Lid plasty with pedicle flap from the neck. Klin Monatsb Augenh 44:71 and 45:71 (1907)
945. Sömmering ST von (1778) De basi encephali et originbus nervorum cranio egredientium. Abram Vandenboech, Göttingen
946. Sömmering ST von (1791) Abbildungen und Beschreibungen einiger Misgeburten. Universitatsbehandlung, Mainz
947. Song R, GaoY, Song Y, et al (1982) The forearm flap. Clin Plast Surg 9:21
948. Spiegel A van de R (Spigelius) (1645) Opera quae extant omnia ex recensione. Joh. Antonides van der Linden, Johannes Blaen, Amsterdam
949. Stark RB (1975) The parable of the three doyens. Plast Reconstr Surg 56:487
950. Steffensen WH (1955) Comments on total reconstruction of the external ear. Plast Reconstr Surg 16:194
951. Steffensen WH (1965) Method of total ear reconstruction. Plast Reconstr Surg 36:97
952. Stein SAV (1848) Laebedannelse (Cheiloplastik) udfort på en ny methode. Hospitals Meddelelser 1:212
953. Stephenson KL (1972) The history of face, neck and eyelid surgery. In: Masters FW, Lewis JR Jr (ed) Symposium on Aesthetic Surgery of the Face, Eyelids and Breast. Mosby, St Louis
954. Stephenson KL (1977) The history of blepharoplasty for blepharocalasis. Aesthetic Plast Surg 1:177
955. Stephenson J (1820) De Velosyntesis: Thesis. University of Edinburgh. P Neil, Edinburgh
956. Sterpellone L (1990) La medicina Etrusca. Ciba Geigy, Milano
957. Sterpellone L, El-Sheikh MS (1995) La medicina Araba. Ciba Geigy, Milano
958. Sterzi G (1910) Il tessuto sottocutaneo (tela sottocutanea). Luigi Niccolai, Firenze
959. Stevens AH (1827) Staphyloraphy or palate suture successfully performed. North Am Med Surg J 3:233
960. Stieda A (1911) Betraig zur freien Fetrannspailantation. Veraien der Artze in Halle 58:108
961. Strömbeck JO (1960) Mammoplasty: report of a new technique based on a two pedicle procedure. Br J Plast Surg 13:79
962. Strömbeck JO (1964) Macromastia in women and its surgical treatment. Acta Chir Scand Suppl nr 341
963. Strömbeck JO (1971) Reduction mammoplasty. Surg Clin North Am 51:453
964. Strömbeck JO (1983) Late results after reduction mammaplasty. In: Georigiade NG (ed) Aesthetic Breast Surgery. Williams & Wilkins, Baltimore
965. Subczynsk JA (1977) One stage debridement and plastic repair of compound comminuted depressed skull fractures with methylmethacrylate. J Trauma 17:467
966. Syme J (1840) On the power of periosteum to form new bone. Trans R Soc Edinburgh 14:158
967. Syme J (1842) Principles of Surgery, London
968. Szymanowski J (1870) Handbuch der Operativen Chirurgie. F Viewug u Sohn, Braunschweig
969. Tagliacozzi G (1597) De Curtorum Chirurgia per Insitionem. Gaspare Bindoum, Venetia (*a pirated edition was also published in 1597 by R Meiettum of Venice*)
970. Tansini I (1906) Sopra il mio nuovo processo di amputatzione della mammella. Gaz Méd Ital 57:141
971. Tanzer RC (1959) Total reconstruction of the external ear. Plast Reconstr Surg 23:1
972. Taruffi C (1881–1895) Storia della teratologia. Bologna
973. Taylor GI, Daniel RK (1973) Free flap: composite tissue transfer by vascular anastomosis. Plast Reconstr Surg 55:642
974. Taylor GI, Miller GDH, Ham FJ (1975) The free vascularized bone graft, clinical extension of microvascular technique. Plast Reconstr Surg 55:533
975. Taylor GI, Palmer JM (1987) The vascular territories (angiosomes) of the body: experimental study and clinical observation. Br J Plast Surg 40:113
976. Teimourian B (1983) Face and neck suction assisted lipectomy associated with rhitydectomy. Plast Reconstr Surg 72:627
977. Tempest MN (1987) The British Journal of Plastic Surgery, chap 8. In: Wallace A (ed) The History of the British Association of Plastic Surgeons. Churchill Livingstone, Edinburgh, pp 57–73

978. Tennison CW (1952)The repair of unilateral cleft lip by the stencil method. Plast Reconstr Surg 9:115
979. Theodorico da Cervia (1498) Cyrurgia edita et compilata a Domino Fratre Theodorico episcop Cervionsi ordinis predicatorum Lib II, IV. In: Collectio Chirurgica Veneta, Venezia
980. Theodorico da Cervia Tractatus tres de Vulneribus in Universalis Tract III Doctr II. In: Chauliac G (1519) Cyrugia Magna. Novitea Impreressus, Venezia
981. Theodorico da Cervia. The Surgery of Theodoric. Translated from Latin by Campbell E & Colot J (1955) Appleton Century Crofts, New York
982. Thiersch K (1869) Ueber die Enstehungsweise und operative Behandlung der Epispadie. Arch Heilkunde 10:20
983. Thiersch K (1874) Ueber die feineren Anatomischen Veranderungen bei Aufheilung von Haut auf Granulationen. Verh Dtsch Ges Chir Berlin 3:6 (*this is translated by Dr and Mrs Hans May p 21 in McDowell F, A Source Book of Plastic Surgery (1977) Williams and Wilkins, Baltimore with an editorial comment*)
984. Thomas JH, Goldwyn RM (1996) Gaspare Tagliacozzi. Decourtorum chirurgia per insitionem (*with English translation*). Gryphons, New York
985. Thomas KB (1964) Curare its history and usage. Pitman, London
986. Thomas TG (1882) On the removal of benign tumours of the mamma without mutilation. N Y Med J Obstet Rev April, 337
987. Thompson CJS (1938) The evolution and development of surgical instruments. Br J Surg 25:726
988. Thompson H (1857) The history and practice of urethroplasty. Lancet 1:499
989. Thompson RC (1923) Assiryan Medical Texts from the originals in the British museum. Oxford University Press, Oxford
990. Thompson RC (1924 & 1925) Assiryan medical texts. Proc R Soc Med 17:1 and 19:29
991. Thomson J (1813) Lectures on inflammation. James Ballantyne, Edinburgh
992. Thorek M (1922) Possibilities in the reconstruction of the human form. N Y Med J 116:572
993. Thorek M (1930) Esthetic surgery of the pendulous breast, abdomen and arms in the female. Ill Med J 58:48
994. Törnroth LH (1849) Om behandling af bränsaar med kalla omslag af is. Notisbil 17
995. Trelat U (1846) De la valeur des operations plastiques sur le palais et de l'age auquel il convient de les ratiquer. J Acad Méd 12:1764
996. Trendelenburg F (1871) Beitrage zur den Operationene an den Luftwegen Tamponade de trachea. Arch Klin Chir 12:121 (*see Tribowandas [943]*)
997. Troja M (1775) De novorum ossium in integris aut maximus ob morbos deperditionibus regeneratione experimenta. FA Didot, Paris
998. Troja M (1779) Esperienze intorno alla rigenerazione delle ossa al callo delle fratture ed alla forza che la natura impiega in allungare le ossa mentre crescono. Stamperia Simoniana, Napoli
999. Ulmi MA (1601) Physiologia barbae humanae. Bologna
1000. Vagbat (Ayurvidie Therapies) translation and commentary by Shri Alri Der Gupta (1951) Astanga Sagrah, Nirnava Sagar Mundrainalaya, Bombay
1001. Vagbat (1980) Astranga Hirdya. Chaukhamba Sanskrit Sansthana, Varanasi
1002. Valsalva AM (1791) De aure humana tractus. Pisaro, Bologna
1003. Valverde Hamusco J de (1572) Vivae imagines partium corporis humani. Christophori Plantinie, Antwerp
1004. Valverde Hamusco J de (1586) La anatomia del corpo umano nuovamente stampata e con l'aggiunta di alcune tavole ampliata. d'Giunti, Venezia
1005. Veau V (1931) Division Palatine. Masson, Paris
1006. Veau V (1935) Bec de Liévre. Hypothése sur la malformation initiale. Ann Anat Pathol Paris 12:389
1007. Veau V, Recamiér J (1938) Bec de Liévre. Masson, Paris
1008. Verchère F (1898) Mastopexie latéerale contre le mastopatie hypertrophique. Méd Mod Paris 9:540
1009. Vellard J (1965) Histoire due curare. Les poisons de chasse en Amerique du Sud. Gallimard, Paris
1010. Velpeau AALM (1834) Manuéle de Médicine Opératoire. Germes-Bailliére, Paris
1011. Velpeau AALM (1839) Nouveaux Elements de Medicine Operatoire. Bailliére, Paris
1012. Verderame F (1909) Uber Fettransplantation bei adharenten knochnnarben om Orbitalrand. Arch Ottal Napoli 17:305
1013. Verneuil AAS (1877) Mémoires de chirurgie. Tomo I: Chirurgie Répartatrice. Masson, Paris
1014. Vesalius A (1543 & 1555) De humani corpori fabrica. Libri Septem. Joannis Oporini, Basel
1015. Vesalius A (1568) De humani corpori fabrica. Franscisсum Senensem & Johannes Criegher, Venezia
1016. Vesalius A (1604) De humani corpori fabrica. Apud Johannes Antonium et Jacobum de Franciscis, Venezia
1017. Vesalius A (1725) Opera omnia anatomica and chirurgica. Cura Hermanni Boerhaave et Bernardi Siegfried Albini. Apud Johannem du Vivie et Johannem et Hermannem Verbech, Leiden
1018. Vidi V (1544) Chirurgia e Greco in latinum Conversa. Vido Vidi Florentino Interprete Pierre Gaultier, Paris (*this reference occurs several times as it includes the latin version of the works of Hippocrates, Galen and Oribasius*)
1019. Vidi V (1839–1861) Oeuvres completes. Ed Emile Littre, Paris
1020. Viguerie C (1834) Cancer de la liévre inferieure, excision et reconstruction avec lambeau cervical. J Hebd 1:186
1021. Volkman R von (1872) Verhandlungen der deutschen Gesellschaft fur Chirurgie, quoted by Ferrari A (1885) Sugli innesti ossei. Arch Ortopedia 6:1
1022. Vrebos J (1982) Harelip surgery in Ancient China: further investigation. Plast Reconstr Surg 89:147
1023. Wadsworth OF (1876) A case of ectropion treated by transplantation of a large flap without pedicle. Boston Med Surg J 95:747
1024. Wallace AB (1966) Canadian-Franco-Scottish co-operation. Br J Plast Surg 19:1
1025. Wallace AF (1982) The Progress of Plastic Surgery. Willem E Meeus, Oxford

1026. Wallace AF(1985)The early history of clinical photography for burns, plastic and reconstructive surgery. Br J Plast Surg 38:451
1027. Wardill WEM (1926–1927) Discussion on the treatment of cleft palate by operation. Proc R Soc Med 5:178
1028. Wardill WEM (1928) Cleft palate. Br J Surg 16:127
1029. Warren JC (1828) On an operation for the cure of natural fissures of the soft palate. Am J Med Sci 3:1
1030. Warren JC (1833) Non existence of vagina remedied by an operation. Am J Med Sci 13:79
1031. Warren JC (1907) Plastic resection of the mammary gland. Ann Surg 45:801
1032. Warren JM (1843) Operation for fissure of soft and hard palate. N Engl Q J Med Sci 1:538
1033. Warren JM (1843) Taliacotian operation. Boston Med Sci J 28:69
1034. Warren JM (1848) Rhinoplastic operation with some remarks on the autoplastic methods usually adopted for the restoration of parts lost by accident or disease. Clapp, Boston
1035. Waters RM, Chen MY (1934) Cyclopropane anesthesia. JAMA 103:975
1036. Watson J (1959) Some observations of free fat grafts with reference to their use in mammaplasty. Br J Plast Surg 12:263
1037. Webster JP (1937) Thoracic-epigastric tubed pedicles. Clin North Am 17:145
1038. Webster JP (1945) Refrigerated skin grafts. Ann Surg 120:421
1039. Wecker L de, Landolt E (1880–1889) Traite complet l'opthalmologie in 4 vols. A Delabaye et Cie, Paris
1040. Weinold E (1926) Discussion zum Vortrag kuester: Operation bey haengebrust und haengebauch. Zentralbl Gynakol 40:2581
1041. Weir RF (1892) On restoring sunken noses without scarring the face. N Y Med J 56:449
1042. Wentscher J (1898) Wielange und untern welchen umstaenden bleibt die Labensfaehigkeit de menschlichen Epidermiszellen ausserhalb des organism erhalten. Zentralbl Chir 25:7
1043. Wheeler WM (1960) Ants: their structure and behaviour. Columbia University Press, New York
1044. Whipple AO (1963) The story of wound healing and wound repair. Thomas, Springfield, Ill
1045. White JC (1948) Late complication following cranioplasty with alloplastic plates. Ann Surg 128:743
1046. Witowski GJ (1903) Tetoniana: les seines dans l'histoire. A Maloine, Paris
1047. Wolfe JR (1875) A new method of performing plastic operations. Br J Med 2:360
1048. Wood A (1855) On a new method of treating neuroalgia by direct application of opiates to the painful points. Edinburgh Med Surg J 82:265
1049. Wood JB (1863) Autoplastic operation after a severe burn. Successful transplantation of integumentum from the abdomen to the arm. Lancet 1:92
1050. Woolfe JI, Walker AE (1945) Cranioplasty: a collective review. Int Abstr Surg 81:2
1051. Woolfe JI, Walker AE (1946) Cranioplasty: metallic inserts. Rev Oto-neuro-oftal 21:16
1052. Wrede L (1916) Ein Fettplastik der Mamma. Munchen Med Wochesch 6
1053. Wu LT Wong (1936) History of Chinese Medicine. Mercury Press, Shanghai
1054. Yang Guofan et al (1981) Forearm free skin flap transplantation. Nat Med J China 61:139 (*also abstract in Plast Reconstr Surg 69:1041*)
1055. Yperman J (1854) La chirurgie de maitre Yperman mise au jour et annotée par JMF Carolus. F & D Gyselynch, Gand
1056. Zahn FW (1855) Transplantation of fetal cartilage. Virchov's Arch Pathol Anat Vol 85
1057. Zahn FW (1884) The fate of transplanted tissues. Arch Pathol Anat 95:369
1058. Zeigler E (1890) Observations on wound healing after various injuries. Verh Schwiez Naturforsch Ges 79:179
1059. Zeis E (1838) Manual of plastic surgery with a foreword by Dieffenbach (with many woodcuts and two copper plates). Berlin
1060. Zeis E (1863) Die literature und Geschicthe der Plastiachen Chirurgie. Engelman, Leipzig

Recommended Reading

We have cited *The Source Book of Plastic Surgery* by McDowell F (1977), Williams and Wilkins, Baltimore, several times in the text and suggest that it warrants more than just passing reference. It contains many reprints of important articles from the past with commentaries by modern plastic surgeons with special knowledge of the authors. The following works may also be of value:

Aston SJ, Thorne TO (1980) History of Plastic Surgery. In: Rees TD (ed) Aesthetic Plastic Surgery. Saunders, New York
Berger A, Hiemer R (2005) Plastic Sugery: Kopf und Hals (Chapter I History of Plastic Surgery). Springer, Heidelberg
Davis JS (1941) The story of plastic surgery. Ann Surg 113:641
Gillies HD, Millard DR (1957) The Principles and Art of Plastic Surgery. Little Brown, Boston
Hayes H (1986) An Anthology of Plastic Surgery. Aspen, Rockville
Malley C, Sanders JB (1952) Leonardo da Vinci on the Human Body. Thomas, New York
McLeave H (1961) McIndoe, Plastic Surgeon. Muller, London
Paget A (1899) Amboise Paré and His Times (1510–1590). Putnams and Sons, New York
Pound R (1963) Gillies, Surgeon Extraordinary. Joseph, London
Rank B (1968) The story of plastic surgery 1868–1968. Practitioner 201
Rogers BO (1973) History of external genital surgery. In: Horton CE (ed) Plastic and Reconstructive Surgery of the Genital Area, chap 1. Little Brown, Boston (*this is also cited in the text and is a valuable historical chapter on genito-urinary plastic surgery*)

Thorek M (1943) A Surgeon's World: An Autobiography. Lippincott, Philadelphia

Wallace AF (1982) The Progress of Plastic Surgery. Meeuws, Oxford

Wallace AF (ed) (1987) The History of the British Association of Plastic Surgeons: The First Forty Years. Churchill Livingstone, Edinbugh (*a supplement to the British Journal of Plastic Surgery*)

Over the years several useful articles have appeared in the journal *Aesthetic Plastic Surgery* published by Springer, New York. We have refered to them where appropriate but again the reader may find them useful:

Vol I, pp 177–194 The history of blepheroplasty and blepharochalasis. Stephenson KL

pp 321–346 History of rhinoplasty. McDowell K

Vol II, pp 75–94 History of aesthetic surgery of the ear. Davis JE, Hernandez HH

pp 113–123 The history of abdomino dermolipectomy. Regnault P

pp 167–176 History of mammoplasty. Lalardrie JP, Mouly R

Vol XII, pp 129–152 History of occuloplastic surgery. Rogers BO

Vol XIV, pp 123–126 Early history of lipoplasty in the United States. Lewis CM

Other material which the authors found useful when compiling this book:

Adams RC (1940) Intravenous anesthesia: chemical, pharmacological and clinical considerations (Thesis). University of Minnesota, Graduate School

Ammon FA (1823) Parallele der franzosichen und deutschen Chirurgie. Hartmann, Leipzig, p 378

Angelicus B (1491) De proprietatibus rerum. Matgthias Huss, Lyon

Cecchini D (1714) La difesa dei diritta di Cesare Magati. A Ercole, Roma

Cecchini D (1715) La verita combattuta e sostenuta. A Ercole, Roma

De Takats G (1928) Local anesthesia. Saunders, Philadelphia

Dobson J (1962) Anatomical Eponyms. Livingstone, Edinburgh London

Ferrari F, Pitanguy I (1991) Chiruria Estetica, strategia operatoirie. Techniche chirurgiche. UTET, Milan

Halstead WS (1924) Surgical papers. John Hopkins Press, Baltimore

Hoffman P (1686) De labii leporinis. Bergman, Heidelberg

Jackson DE (1915) On the production of general anesthesia and analgesia with a description of the apparatus used. J Lab Clin Med 1:1

Kazi Rehan A, Rhys Evans P (2004) Sir Charles Bell: the artist who went to the roots. J Postgrad Med 50:158

Lindermann A (1916) in Die genenwärtigen Benhandlungswege de Kieferschussverletzungen. Haupmeyer F, Kühe M, and Lindeman A, Je Berbman, Wiesbaden

Lisfranc J (1859) Beitrage zur Osteplastik. Vorlaenfige Mittheilung Goesch deutsche Klin 48:475

Longacre JJ (1953) The use of local pedicle flaps for reconstruction of the breast after sub-total extirpation of the mammary gland and for correction of distortion and atrophy of the breast due to excessive scar. Plast Reconstr Surg 11:380

Mall FP (1908) A study and causes underlying the origin of human monsters. J Morphol 19:1

McGregor IA (1955) The vascularisation of homografts of human skin. Br J Plast Surg 7:331

Micheli-Pellegrini V (1991) Sintesi storica sullo sviluppo della chirurgia per l'imbellimento corpoeo. (*see Ferrari F and Pitanguy I*)

Péraire M, Bonamy (1914) Tumeur des deux seins chez une femme et transplantation lipomateuse. Bull Mem Soc Chir Paris 2:60

Pöhlman GA (1916) Die Embryonale Metamorphose der Physiognomic und Mundhole des Mutzenkopfer. Morphol Sh 41:617

Roux PJ (1830) Staphyloraphie. Rev Méd Franc et Étrangere Paris 1:17

Roux PJ (1834) Considérations sur la staphyloraphie, reunion par suture de voile du palais. Orthopédie clinicique sur les difformités dans l'espéce humaine 1:403

Roux PJ (1835) Congenital fissures of the soft palate. Lancet 1:694

Roux PJ (1843) Staphyloraphy in cases of soft palate. Am J Med Sci 6:229

Roux PJ (1850) Staphyloraphy. Med Times Gaz 1:71

Sacchi E (1894) Ulteriore contributo alle plastiche del cranio. Biol Acc Med Genova 9:71

Stark RB (1971) The development of the face. In: Hueston JT (ed) Transaction of the 5th International Congress of Plastic and Reconstructive Surgery. Butterworth, Sydney

Törnroth L-H (1844) Underraettelse från kliniska institutets i Helsingfors chirurgiska afdelning for aeren 1838–1844. Finsk Läk Handl

Wallace AB (1966) The 4th Kazanjian Lecture: burns past, present and future (a tribute to Lister and Kazanjian). Plast Reconstr Surg 37:385

Wallace AB (1967) An association of the holy family of special interest to plastic surgery. Plast Reconstr Surg 39:101

Wallace AB (1967) Thoughts on Lister's time. Br J Plast Surg 20:113

Wallace AB (1968) The first 21 years: the British Journal of Plastic Surgery comes of age. Br J Plast Surg 21:1

Wilks S, Bettany GT (1892) A biographical history of Guy's Hospital. Ward, Lock and Bowden, London

Subject Index

G

H

M

N

T

W

Z

MIX
Papier aus verantwortungsvollen Quellen
Paper from responsible sources
FSC® C105338

If you have any concerns about our products,
you can contact us on
ProductSafety@springernature.com

In case Publisher is established outside the EU,
the EU authorized representative is:
Springer Nature Customer Service Center GmbH
Europaplatz 3, 69115 Heidelberg, Germany

Printed by Libri Plureos GmbH
in Hamburg, Germany